Goodheart-Willcox presents a health science program focused on technical knowledge and skills

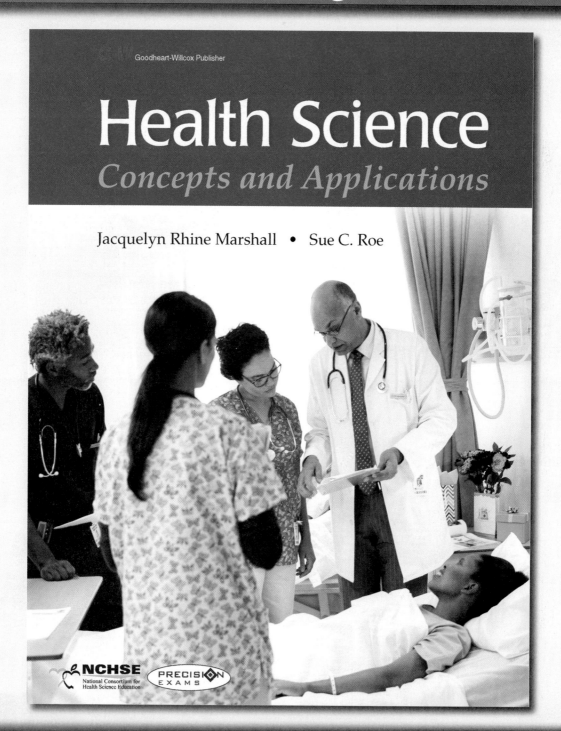

Goodheart-Willcox Publisher

Health Science
Concepts and Applications

Jacquelyn Rhine Marshall • Sue C. Roe

NCHSE
National Consortium for
Health Science Education

PRECISION EXAMS

includes extensive hands-on experiences for skill development

Inviting Layout Gets Students' Attention

Detailed anatomical illustrations offer visual explanations of key concepts.

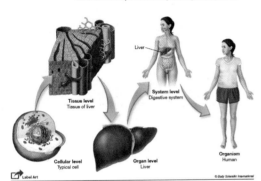

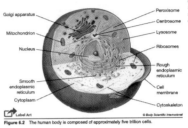

Engaging images get students interested in healthcare careers and procedures.

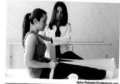

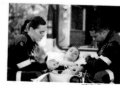

and Makes Content Accessible

It is not unusual for people to occasionally feel sad or get "the blues." Teenagers, especially, may have strong emotional reactions because they are experiencing a stage of life with many physical, emotional, psychological, and social changes. Occasional bouts of sadness, however, are different from **depression**, which is a medical condition characterized by feelings of hopelessness, worthlessness, or a general disinterest in daily life. For most people, feelings of sadness pass over time, but that is often not the case for people suffering from depression.

Adolescent depression is increasing at a fast rate. Recent surveys indicate that as many as one in five teens suffer from clinical depression. A family history of depression can increase the risk. This is a serious problem that calls for prompt, appro[...]. A related mental illness is called **bipolar disorder**, form[...] *manic-depression*. This form of depression alternates betw[...] **euphoria** and depression.

depression
mood disorder causing a persistent feeling of sadness and loss of interest

bipolar disorder
mental disorder characterized by alternating periods of euphoria, or an elevated mood, and depression

Did You Know? Beating Depression throug[...]

It's a scientific fact that exercise helps treat or prevent depr[...]. Many studies have shown that moderate exercise can have a significant effect on depression.

A study conducted at the Cooper Research Institute in Dalla[...] Texas, shows that as few as three hours of regular exercise a we[...] can reduce levels of depression. Participants who walked 35 min[...] a day for six days a week reduced their symptoms of mild to mo[...] depression by 47 percent. Exercise was as effective as the leadin[...] antidepressants in reducing depression.

Aerobic exercise, in particular, improves blood flow and oxy[...] to the brain. This type of vigorous exercise has the added benefi[...]

Marginal definitions highlight key terms so students can focus on important vocabulary.

Biotechnology

Technology that uses biological processes, organisms, or systems to manufacture products intended to improve the quality of human life is called **biotechnology**. Biotechnological advances in the world of medicine have restored, extended, and improved our lives, and will continue to do so in the future.

Biopharmaceuticals

New and exciting advances are being made today in the development of drugs and vaccines (Figure 10.11). Biotechnology and **biopharmaceuticals** may eventually help us eliminate certain diseases, alleviate pain, and extend our life span. In addition to studying new drugs in clinical trials, scientists are now identifying the previously unknown causes of many diseases. The Human Genome Project endeavored to find breakthroughs in treatment and possible cures. Biotechnology is making it possible for scientists to design new drugs that are products of **genetic engineering** (adding new DNA to an organism).

Approved biopharmaceuticals are now treating or helping prevent strokes. Other findings are making a difference in the treatment of multiple sclerosis, heart attacks, leukemia, hepatitis, lymphoma, kidney cancer, cystic fibrosis, and many other diseases. There are now over 900 biopharmaceuticals and vaccines in development to target more life-threatening diseases such as cancer and diabetes.

Gene Therapy

As you learned in chapter 7, gene therapy is a biotechnological [...]

biotechnology
technology that uses biological processes, organisms, or systems to develop products intended to improve the quality of human life

biopharmaceuticals
prescription drugs that are produced as a result of biotechnology

genetic engineering
the manipulation of genetic materials to eliminate undesirable traits or to ensure desirable traits

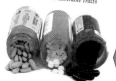

Figure 10.11 Biopharmaceuticals provide advanced treatment for many diseases and

Brian Chase/Shutterstock.com

Charts and graphs present information in an easy-to-understand manner.

Organizational Chart

- Board of Directors
- Medical Staff
- Administration
- Volunteers

Therapeutic Careers	Diagnostic Careers	Health Informatics/ Information Services Careers	Support Services Careers	Biotechnology Research and Development
Physician	Audiology	Health informatics	Central supply	Biological scientist
Dentistry	Cardiology	Admissions	Engineering	Bioengineer
Dietetics	Emergency	Clerical services	Food service	Forensic science
EMT	department	Finance	Grounds	technicians
Home health	Diagnostic imaging	Health education	maintenance	Biophysicist
Nursing	Laboratory	Human resources	Building	Microbiologist
Pharmacy	Neurology	Information	maintenance	Biochemist
Radiology	Optical	management		Biological
Rehabilitation	Pulmonary	Medical librarian		technicians
Dialysis	Radiology	Quality management		Physiologist
Respiratory therapy		Unit coordination		
Mental health		Utilization review		
		Health information		
		management		

Goodheart-Willcox Publisher

Figure 2.6 Organizational chart of a large healthcare facility.

Check Your Understanding boxes allow students to assess their progress throughout the text.

Understanding the differences among the learning sty[...] deal with an instructor whose teaching methods favor [...] you do not possess. You might benefit from a conferenc[...] to explain how your style differs from his or her teachin[...] allow the two of you an opportunity to brainstorm way[...] the instructor's classroom.

Check Your Understanding ✓

Which learning style might the following students favor?
1. Jeff does not like to sit still.
2. Maria finds charts to be helpful in class.
3. Joanna is really good at remembering names.
4. José enjoys loud music when studying.
5. Rachel likes to color code her notes.

Check Your Understanding ✓

1. Define "incident" as it relates to an incident report.
2. Name three types of people who could be involved in an "incident."
3. What information should you include when writing an incident report?
4. What is the purpose of the OSHA Hazard Communication Standard?
5. What is a material safety data sheet (MSDS)?

Electrical Safety

It is always possible to get an electrical shock when operating electrically powered equipment. Electrical shock injuries can result in moderate burns, severe skin dam[...] age, unconsciousness, or even death. Observance of safety guidelines concerning electricity can help reduce risk of such injuries.

Do not overload any electrical plugs or outlets, as an overloaded plug or outlet can become a fire hazard (Figure 4.6). All equipment must have a three-prong plug, which adds further safety benefits. Equipment must be in safe, working [...]

ajt/Shutterstock.com

Step-by-Step Procedures

Step-by-step procedures teach important skills students will need for healthcare careers.

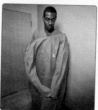

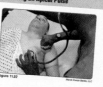

Procedure 4.3 — PPE: Putting on and Removing Gowns

Procedure 11.6 — Counting and Recording a Radial Pulse

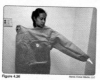
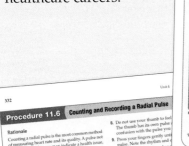
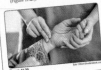

Procedure 11.7 — Counting and Recording an Apical Pulse

Procedure 11.9 — Taking a Patient's Blood Pressure—Manual and Electronic

High-Interest Features

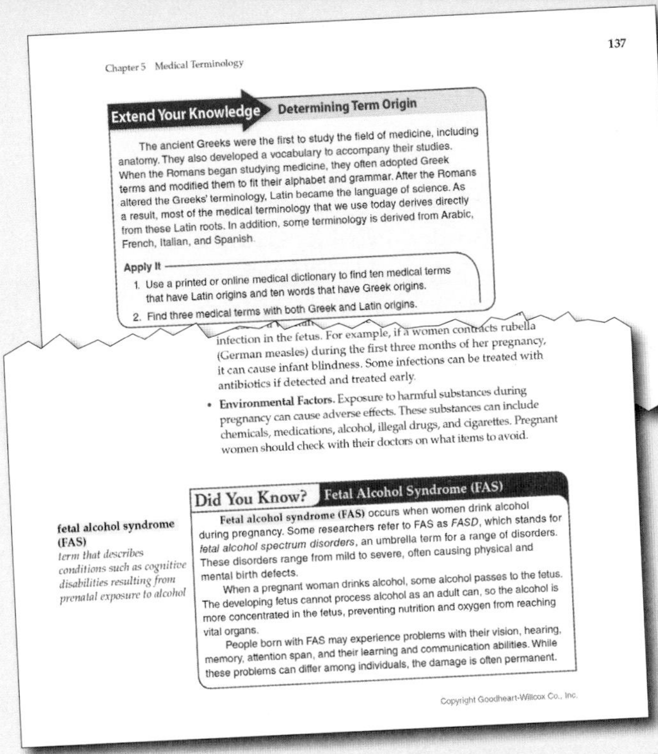
137

Chapter 5 Medical Terminology

Extend Your Knowledge Determining Term Origin

The ancient Greeks were the first to study the field of medicine, including anatomy. They also developed a vocabulary to accompany their studies. When the Romans began studying medicine, they often adopted Greek terms and modified them to fit their alphabet and grammar. After the Romans altered the Greeks' terminology, Latin became the language of science. As a result, most of the medical terminology that we use today derives directly from these Latin roots. In addition, some terminology is derived from Arabic, French, Italian, and Spanish.

Apply It

1. Use a printed or online medical dictionary to find ten medical terms that have Latin origins and ten words that have Greek origins.
2. Find three medical terms with both Greek and Latin origins.

infection in the fetus. For example, if a women contracts rubella (German measles) during the first three months of her pregnancy, it can cause infant blindness. Some infections can be treated with antibiotics if detected and treated early.

- **Environmental Factors.** Exposure to harmful substances during pregnancy can cause adverse effects. These substances can include chemicals, medications, alcohol, illegal drugs, and cigarettes. Pregnant women should check with their doctors on what items to avoid.

fetal alcohol syndrome (FAS)
term that describes conditions such as cognitive disabilities resulting from prenatal exposure to alcohol

Did You Know? Fetal Alcohol Syndrome (FAS)

Fetal alcohol syndrome (FAS) occurs when women drink alcohol during pregnancy. Some researchers refer to FAS as *FASD*, which stands for *fetal alcohol spectrum disorders*, an umbrella term for a range of disorders. These disorders range from mild to severe, often causing physical and mental birth defects.

When a pregnant woman drinks alcohol, some alcohol passes to the fetus. The developing fetus cannot process alcohol as an adult can, so the alcohol is more concentrated in the fetus, preventing nutrition and oxygen from reaching vital organs.

People born with FAS may experience problems with their vision, hearing, memory, attention span, and their learning and communication abilities. While these problems can differ among individuals, the damage is often permanent.

Copyright Goodheart-Willcox Co., Inc.

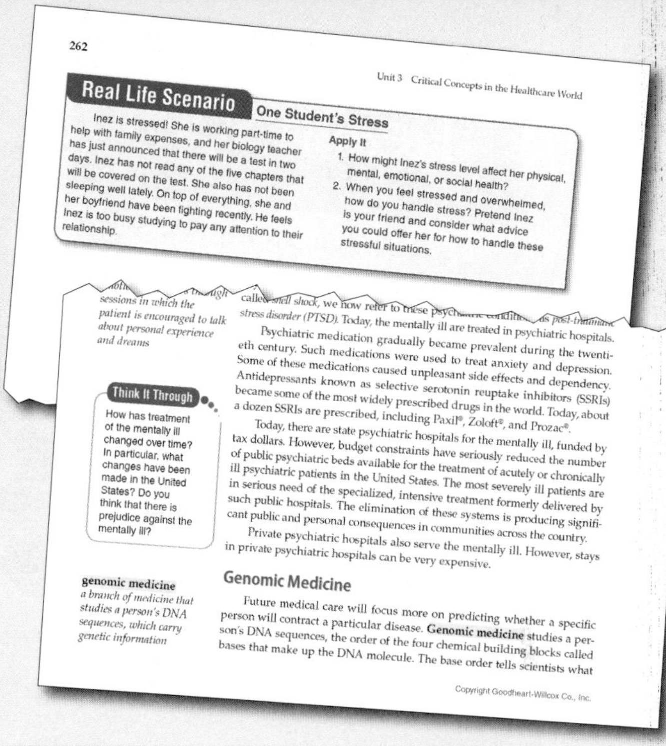
262

Unit 3 Critical Concepts in the Healthcare World

Real Life Scenario One Student's Stress

Inez is stressed! She is working part-time to help with family expenses, and her biology teacher has just announced that there will be a test in two days. Inez has not read any of the five chapters that will be covered on the test. She also has not been sleeping well lately. On top of everything, she and her boyfriend have been fighting recently. He feels Inez is too busy studying to pay any attention to their relationship.

Apply It

1. How might Inez's stress level affect her physical, mental, emotional, or social health?
2. When you feel stressed and overwhelmed, how do you handle stress? Pretend Inez is your friend and consider what advice you could offer her for how to handle these stressful situations.

sessions in which the patient is encouraged to talk about personal experience and dreams

called shell shock, we now refer to these psychiatric conditions as *post-traumatic stress disorder (PTSD)*. Today, the mentally ill are treated in psychiatric hospitals.

Psychiatric medication gradually became prevalent during the twentieth century. Such medications were used to treat anxiety and depression. Some of these medications caused unpleasant side effects and dependency. Antidepressants known as selective serotonin reuptake inhibitors (SSRIs) became some of the most widely prescribed drugs in the world. Today, about a dozen SSRIs are prescribed, including Paxil®, Zoloft®, and Prozac®.

Today, there are state psychiatric hospitals for the mentally ill, funded by tax dollars. However, budget constraints have seriously reduced the number of public psychiatric beds available for the treatment of acutely or chronically ill psychiatric patients in the United States. The most severely ill patients are in serious need of the specialized, intensive treatment formerly delivered by such public hospitals. The elimination of these systems is producing significant public and personal consequences in communities across the country.

Private psychiatric hospitals also serve the mentally ill. However, stays in private psychiatric hospitals can be very expensive.

Think It Through

How has treatment of the mentally ill changed over time? In particular, what changes have been made in the United States? Do you think that there is prejudice against the mentally ill?

genomic medicine
a branch of medicine that studies a person's DNA sequences, which carry genetic information

Genomic Medicine

Future medical care will focus more on predicting whether a specific person will contract a particular disease. **Genomic medicine** studies a person's DNA sequences, the order of the four chemical building blocks called bases that make up the DNA molecule. The base order tells scientists what

Copyright Goodheart-Willcox Co., Inc.

High-interest features such as *Did You Know?*, *Extend Your Knowledge*, *Real Life Scenario*, and *Think It Through* teach healthcare concepts in a unique way and offer self-assessment opportunities for students.

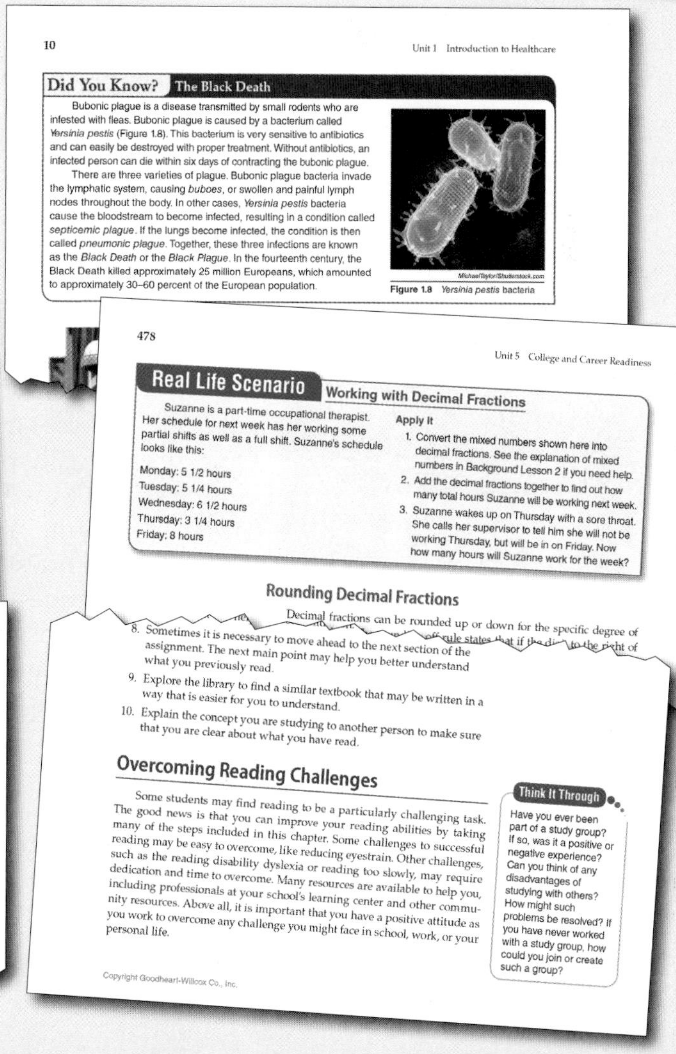
10

Unit 1 Introduction to Healthcare

Did You Know? The Black Death

Bubonic plague is a disease transmitted by small rodents who are infested with fleas. Bubonic plague is caused by a bacterium called *Yersinia pestis* (Figure 1.8). This bacterium is very sensitive to antibiotics and can easily be destroyed with proper treatment. Without antibiotics, an infected person can die within six days of contracting the bubonic plague.

There are three varieties of plague. Bubonic plague bacteria invade the lymphatic system, causing *buboes*, or swollen and painful lymph nodes throughout the body. In other cases, *Yersinia pestis* bacteria cause the bloodstream to become infected, resulting in a condition called *septicemic plague*. If the lungs become infected, the condition is then called *pneumonic plague*. Together, these three infections are known as the *Black Death* or the *Black Plague*. In the fourteenth century, the Black Death killed approximately 25 million Europeans, which amounted to approximately 30–60 percent of the European population.

MichaelTaylor/Shutterstock.com

Figure 1.8 *Yersinia pestis* bacteria

478

Unit 5 College and Career Readiness

Real Life Scenario Working with Decimal Fractions

Suzanne is a part-time occupational therapist. Her schedule for next week has her working some partial shifts as well as a full shift. Suzanne's schedule looks like this:

Monday: 5 1/2 hours
Tuesday: 5 1/4 hours
Wednesday: 6 1/2 hours
Thursday: 3 1/4 hours
Friday: 8 hours

Apply It

1. Convert the mixed numbers shown here into decimal fractions. See the explanation of mixed numbers in Background Lesson 2 if you need help.
2. Add the decimal fractions together to find out how many total hours Suzanne will be working next week.
3. Suzanne wakes up on Thursday with a sore throat. She calls her supervisor to tell him she will not be working Thursday, but will be in on Friday. Now how many hours will Suzanne work for the week?

Rounding Decimal Fractions

Decimal fractions can be rounded up or down for the specific degree of

8. Sometimes it is necessary to move ahead to the next section of the assignment. The next main point may help you better understand what you previously read.
9. Explore the library to find a similar textbook that may be written in a way that is easier for you to understand.
10. Explain the concept you are studying to another person to make sure that you are clear about what you have read.

Overcoming Reading Challenges

Some students may find reading to be a particularly challenging task. The good news is that you can improve your reading abilities by taking many of the steps included in this chapter. Some challenges to successful reading may be easy to overcome, like reducing eyestrain. Other challenges, such as the reading disability dyslexia or reading too slowly, may require dedication and time to overcome. Many resources are available to help you, including professionals at your school's learning center and other community resources. Above all, it is important that you have a positive attitude as you work to overcome any challenge you might face in school, work, or your personal life.

Think It Through

Have you ever been part of a study group? If so, was it a positive or negative experience? Can you think of any disadvantages of studying with others? How might such problems be resolved? If you have never worked with a study group, how could you join or create such a group?

Copyright Goodheart-Willcox Co., Inc.

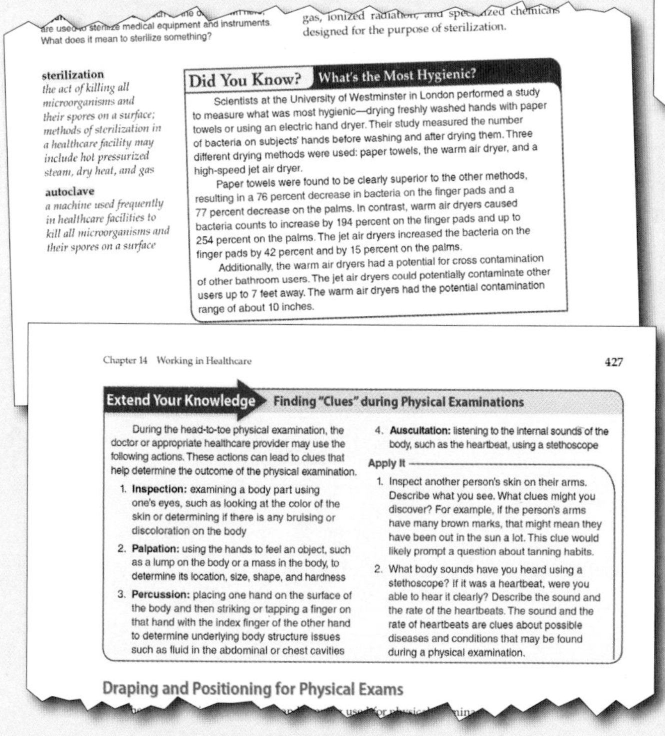
are used to sterilize medical equipment and instruments. What does it mean to sterilize something?

gas, ionized radiation, and specialized chemicals designed for the purpose of sterilization.

sterilization
the act of killing all microorganisms and their spores on a surface; methods of sterilization in a healthcare facility may include hot pressurized steam, dry heat, and gas

autoclave
a machine used frequently in healthcare facilities to kill all microorganisms and their spores on a surface

Did You Know? What's the Most Hygienic?

Scientists at the University of Westminster in London performed a study to measure what was most hygienic—drying freshly washed hands with paper towels or using an electric hand dryer. Their study measured the number of bacteria on subjects' hands before washing and after drying them. Three different drying methods were used: paper towels, the warm air dryer, and a high-speed jet air dryer.

Paper towels were found to be clearly superior to the other methods, resulting in a 76 percent decrease in bacteria on the finger pads and a 77 percent decrease on the palms. In contrast, warm air dryers caused bacteria counts to increase by 194 percent on the finger pads and up to 254 percent on the palms. The jet air dryers increased the bacteria on the finger pads by 42 percent and by 15 percent on the palms.

Additionally, the warm air dryers had a potential for cross contamination of other bathroom users. The jet air dryers could potentially contaminate other users up to 7 feet away. The warm air dryers had the potential contamination range of about 10 inches.

Chapter 14 Working in Healthcare

427

Extend Your Knowledge Finding "Clues" during Physical Examinations

During the head-to-toe physical examination, the doctor or appropriate healthcare provider may use the following actions. These actions can lead to clues that help determine the outcome of the physical examination.

1. **Inspection:** examining a body part using one's eyes, such as looking at the color of the skin or determining if there is any bruising or discoloration on the body
2. **Palpation:** using the hands to feel an object, such as a lump on the body or a mass in the body, to determine its location, size, shape, and hardness
3. **Percussion:** placing one hand on the surface of the body and then striking or tapping a finger on that hand with the index finger of the other hand to determine underlying body structure issues such as fluid in the abdominal or chest cavities
4. **Auscultation:** listening to the internal sounds of the body, such as the heartbeat, using a stethoscope

Apply It

1. Inspect another person's skin on their arms. Describe what you see. What clues might you discover? For example, if the person's arms have many brown marks, that might mean they have been out in the sun a lot. This clue would likely prompt a question about tanning habits.
2. What body sounds have you heard using a stethoscope? If it was a heartbeat, were you able to hear it clearly? Describe the sound and the rate of the heartbeats. The sound and the rate of heartbeats are clues about possible diseases and conditions that may be found during a physical examination.

Draping and Positioning for Physical Exams

The Complete Package for

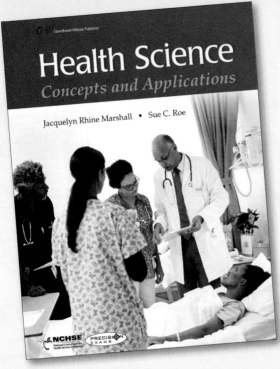

Student Textbook—Print or Online
The student edition of *Health Science: Concepts and Applications* is available as a printed textbook or as an interactive online text. Simply choose the format that works best for your students.

www.g-wonlinetextbooks.com

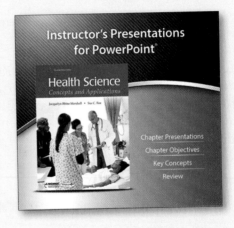

Instructor's Presentations for PowerPoint®
Visually reinforce key concepts with prepared lectures. Integrated review questions make the presentations interactive.

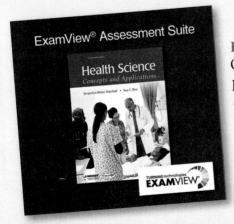

ExamView® Assessment Suite
Quickly and easily prepare and print tests with the ExamView® Assessment Suite. You can choose which questions to include in each test, create multiple versions of a single test, and automatically generate answer keys.

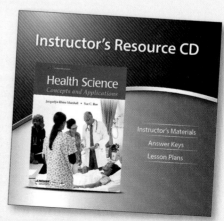

Instructor's Resource CD
Includes daily lesson plans, answer keys, and grading rubrics.

both students and teachers

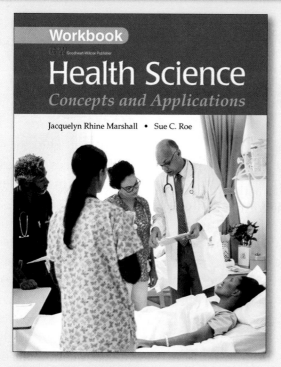

Student Workbook (available in print or online)
Workbook activities reinforce material presented in the textbook, offering students a hands-on learning experience.

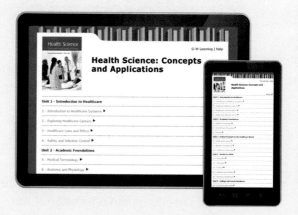

The G-W Learning Companion Website for *Health Science: Concepts and Applications* accompanies the **Student Textbook** and provides content to help students build skills and knowledge, extend textbook content, and reinforce learning. The website complements textbook chapters and is available to students at no charge.

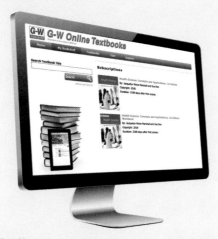

The Online Learning Suite for *Health Science: Concepts and Applications* is available as a classroom subscription. It includes the online student text, the companion website content, and the digital workbook.

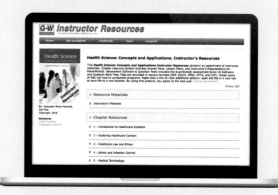

The Online Instructor Resources provide extensive support for instructors. Included in the online resources are Answer Keys, Lesson Plans, Instructor's Presentations for PowerPoint®, ExamView® Assessment Suite, and much more. These resources are available as a subscription and can be accessed at school or at home. They are also available on CDs.

Looking for a **Blended Solution**? G-W offers the Online Learning Suite bundled with the printed textbook in one easy-to-access package for school districts and instructors seeking a combination of print and digital tools. With this option, individual students and instructors have the flexibility of using solely print, solely digital, or a combination of print and digital versions of the *Health Science: Concepts and Applications* educational materials to best meet their particular learning and teaching styles.

Goodheart-Willcox Publisher Welcomes Your Comments

A leader in educational publishing since 1921, Goodheart-Willcox Publisher is now developing print and digital products for Health and Health Sciences courses. This brand-new *Health Science: Concepts and Applications* textbook program provides technical knowledge and skills for students interested in a healthcare career.

If you teach a health science class, or any course in the health and physical education area, and you have been unable to find a suitable text for your students, please let us know. We are eager to develop high-quality, innovative products that fill unmet needs in the educational market. Your suggestions may lead to the development of digital or print materials that benefit teachers and students across the country.

With each new product, our goal at Goodheart-Willcox Publisher is to deliver superior educational materials that effectively meet the ever-changing, increasingly diverse needs of students and teachers. To that end, we welcome your comments or suggestions regarding *Health Science: Concepts and Applications* and its supplemental components.

Please send any comments and suggestions to the managing editor of our Health and Health Sciences Editorial Department. You can send an e-mail to healthsciences@g-w.com, or write to:

Managing Editor—HHS
Goodheart-Willcox Publisher
18604 West Creek Drive
Tinley Park, IL 60477-6243

Health Science
Concepts and Applications

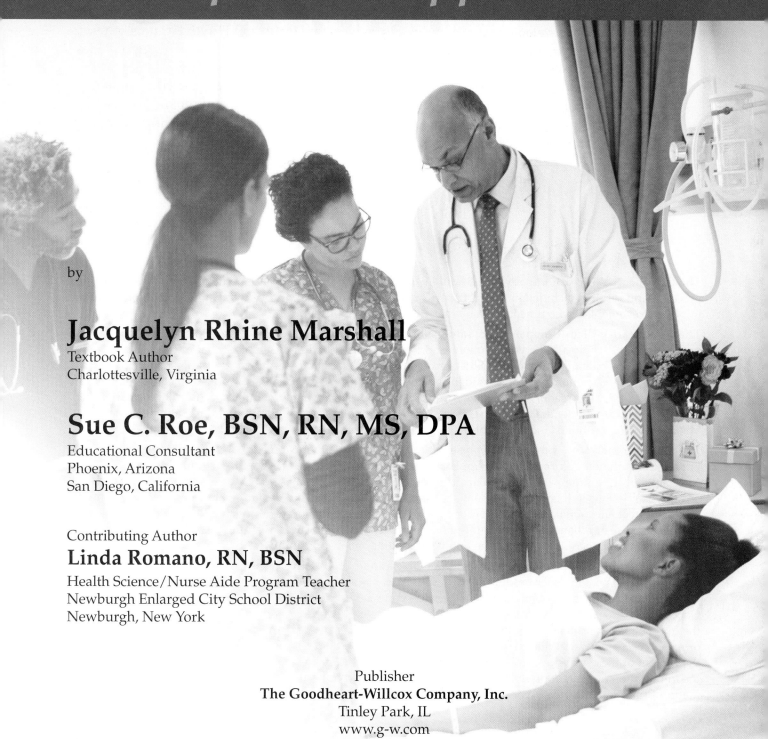

by

Jacquelyn Rhine Marshall
Textbook Author
Charlottesville, Virginia

Sue C. Roe, BSN, RN, MS, DPA
Educational Consultant
Phoenix, Arizona
San Diego, California

Contributing Author
Linda Romano, RN, BSN
Health Science/Nurse Aide Program Teacher
Newburgh Enlarged City School District
Newburgh, New York

Publisher
The Goodheart-Willcox Company, Inc.
Tinley Park, IL
www.g-w.com

About the Authors

For 35 years, **Jacquelyn Rhine Marshall** has been a medical professional; a medical careers instructor for Regional Occupational Programs, California; a medical writer; and a consultant/writer for the Center for Occupational Research and Development in Austin, Texas. Ms. Marshall's writing career includes authoring textbooks for Cengage Learning, Elsevier Publishing, Career Publishing, and Pearson Education, and writing medical course curriculum for the state of California. She has also developed several instructor guides and has edited or contributed to three medical series. Ms. Marshall holds degrees from the University of California, Berkeley; California State University, Hayward; and Notre Dame de Namur University.

Dr. **Sue C. Roe** has taught and designed academic courses for over 35 years at several public and private universities/colleges using a variety of delivery formats. She is co-editor of "Connections in Holistic Nursing Research," an online newsletter from the American Holistic Nurses Association, and was the Chapter Leader for the Phoenix Metro Holistic Nurses chapter of the American Holistic Nurses Association. She currently serves on a health system quality committee. Dr. Roe is Manager/Member of The Roe Group Enterprises, LLC and has a doctorate in public administration, with an emphasis in administration and policy. In addition, she has done graduate-level work in educational administration and instructional development. She has a Master of Science and Bachelor of Science degree in Nursing.

Contributing Author. Linda Romano currently teaches a Health Science/Nurse Aide program at Newburgh Free Academy-North Campus. She participated in the development of the 2006 New York State Nurse Aide Training Program Curriculum and several projects with the New York State Department of Health and Prometric. Linda is highly involved in her school community, serving as co-chairperson for the Building Leadership Team, serving on the Health and Safety Committee, mentoring new teachers, mentoring students, and volunteering for many other projects. In addition, she serves on the Executive Board for the New York State Health Science Educator Association. Linda has presented her project-based learning styles and creative strategies at both ACTE and NCHSE.

Reviewers

Goodheart-Willcox Publisher and the authors would also like to thank the following instructors who reviewed selected manuscript chapters and provided valuable input into the development of this textbook program.

Louise Braubach
Health Science Instructor
West Mesquite High School

Valerie Chin
Health Science Instructor
Spring High School

Nestelynn Friday
Master Health Science Teacher
Nimitz High School

Wendy Jackson
Registered Nurse Clinical Educator
Lakeview Centennial High School

Kelley Kirby
Health Science & Pharmacy
　Technician Instructor
Central High School

Maire Beth Mallard
Health Science Educator
Georgetown High School

Melissa Marek
Health Science Instructor
Cypress Springs High School

Oscar Martinez
Health Science Instructor
Socorro Independent School
　District

Sarah Moreno
Health Science Instructor
San Marcos High School

Joe Nolen
Health Science Technology Teacher
Texas High School

James Saunders
Health Science Teacher
Garland High School

Angela Vong
Health Science Technology
　Instructor
Clear Brook High School

Rebecca Ysaguirre, RN
Health Science Instructor
Health Careers High School

National Health Science Assessment (NHSA) Certification

Health Science: Concepts and Applications delivers thorough, comprehensive coverage of the technical knowledge and skills required for a career in healthcare. Goodheart-Willcox is pleased to correlate *Health Science: Concepts and Applications* to the National Consortium for Health Science Education's National Health Science Assessment (NHSA) exam, provided by Precision Exams. The NHSA standards and exam were created in concert with industry and subject matter experts to match real-world job skills and marketplace demands. Students who pass the National Health Science Assessment can earn a certificate validating their knowledge for colleges and employers. To see how *Health Science: Concepts and Applications* correlates to the NHSA exam provided by Precision Exams, please see the *Health Science: Concepts and Applications* correlations at www.g-w.com. For more information on the National Health Science Assessment, please consult the accompanying *Health Science: Concepts and Applications* Instructor Resources or go to www.healthscienceconsortium.org/assessment.

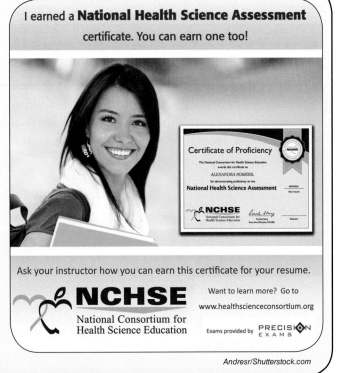

I earned a **National Health Science Assessment** certificate. You can earn one too!

Ask your instructor how you can earn this certificate for your resume.

NCHSE
National Consortium for
Health Science Education

Want to learn more? Go to
www.healthscienceconsortium.org

Exams provided by PRECISION EXAMS

Andresr/Shutterstock.com

Brief Contents

Contents

t-Willcox Co., Inc.

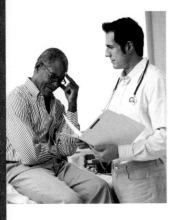

Unit 3
Critical Concepts in the Healthcare World 238

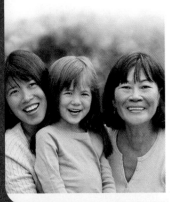

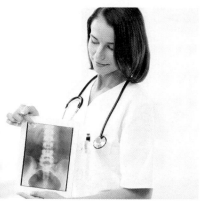

Unit 4
Healthcare Skills 314

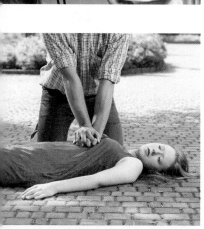

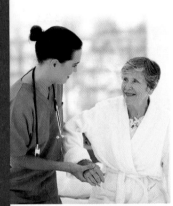

Chapter 13
Assisting with Mobility

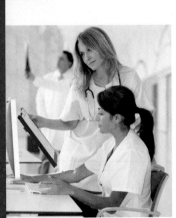

Chapter 14
Working in Healthcare

Unit 5
College and Career Readiness

446

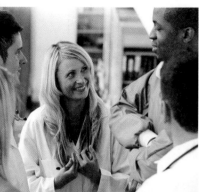

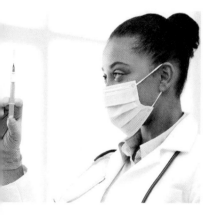

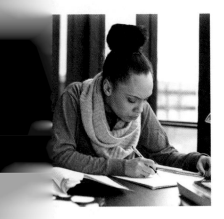

Chapter 17
Study Skills

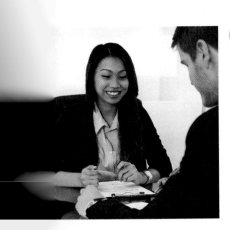

Chapter 18
Employability Skills

Background Lessons

Special Features

Career Exploration

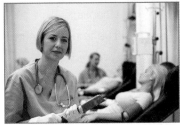
wavebreakmedia/Shutterstock.com

Did You Know?

Extend Your Knowledge

Real Life Scenario

Procedures

The thirty basic healthcare procedures listed below are explained and illustrated in a detailed, step-by-step manner in this text. All procedures should be practiced in a simulated laboratory setting under your instructor's supervision. The procedures should be performed with patients only after you have been observed performing the procedures by your instructor, and he or she has determined that your performance is competent.

Unit 1

Introduction to Healthcare

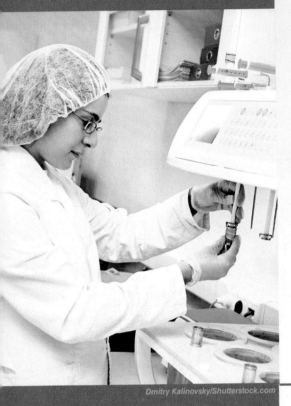

Dmitry Kalinovsky/Shutterstock.com

Chapter 1: Introduction to Healthcare Systems

Chapter 2: Exploring Healthcare Careers

Chapter 3: Healthcare Laws and Ethics

Chapter 4: Safety and Infection Control

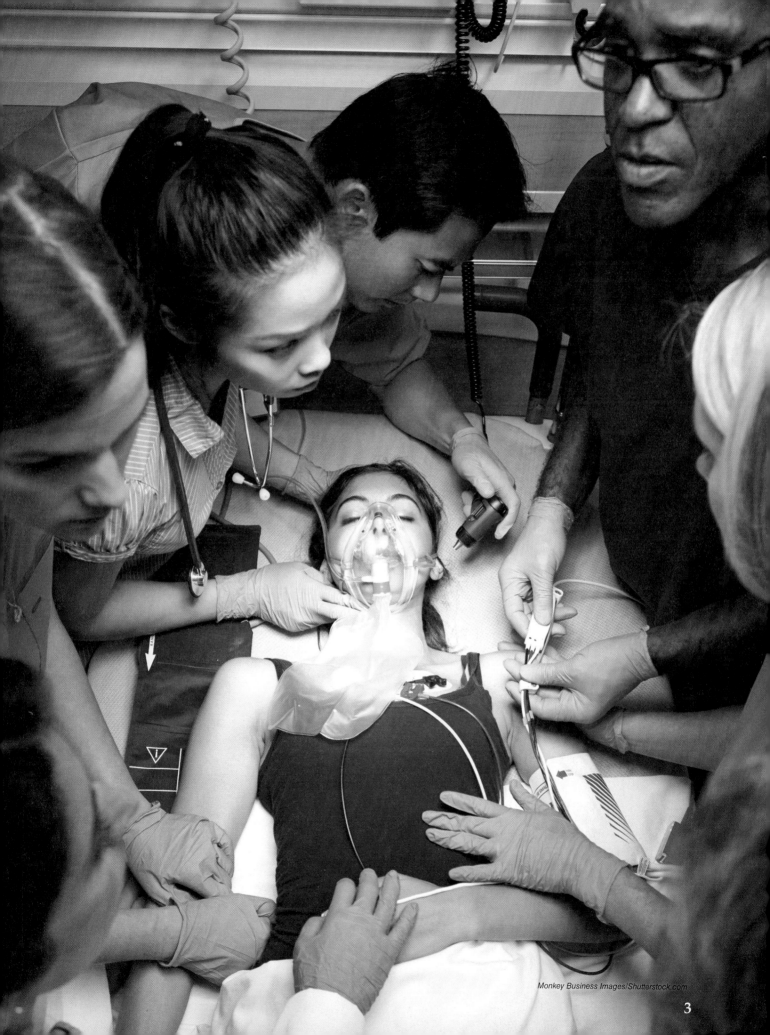

Chapter 1

Introduction to Healthcare Systems

Terms to Know Build Vocab

Affordable Care Act (ACA)

anesthesia

antibiotics

caduceus

Centers for Disease Control and Prevention (CDC)

copayment

deductible

epidemic

Food and Drug Administration (FDA)

genomic medicine

Hippocratic Oath

health maintenance organizations (HMO)

hospice

managed care

Medicaid

Medicare

microscope

National Institutes of Health (NIH)

Occupational Safety and Health Administration (OSHA)

pathogens

preferred provider organizations (PPO)

premium

psychoanalysis

quarantine

self-advocacy

United States Public Health Service

worker's compensation

World Health Organization (WHO)

vaccination

Chapter Objectives

- Discuss important contributions made in the advancement of medicine throughout history.
- Identify the importance of the Hippocratic Oath.
- Describe significant medical advancements made during the Renaissance and Industrial Revolution.
- Discuss the significance of vaccinations.
- Explain the importance of hand washing, hygiene, and sterilization in healthcare facilities.
- Identify the significance of Louis Pasteur's discovery of microbes.
- Compare and contrast Medicare and Medicaid.
- Discuss two common models of private, managed care insurance plans.
- Identify government and volunteer agencies that provide health services.
- List and describe various healthcare facilities found in the United States.

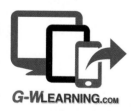

While studying, look for the activity icon to:

- **Build** vocabulary with e-flash cards and interactive games.
- **Assess** progress with chapter and unit review questions.
- **Expand** learning with animations and illustration labeling activities.
- **Simulate** EHR entry with healthcare documents.

G-WLEARNING.com

According to the United States Department of Labor, growth in two areas of employment—computer-related jobs and healthcare occupations—has soared above all others in the last decade. The future looks bright for those hoping to obtain excellent, challenging occupations in the healthcare industry. With the aging baby boomer generation (those born during the population increase following World War II) and the expansion of medical technology, health professions offer secure, well-paying employment.

The Patient Protection and Affordable Care Act (commonly called The **Affordable Care Act (ACA)** or *Obamacare*) was passed into law in 2010 by the US Congress. This act is the most significant government expansion and regulatory reform of US healthcare since the passage of Medicare and Medicaid in 1965.

Affordable Care Act
law passed in 2010 for a major regulatory reform of US healthcare

The National Consortium for Health Science Education publishes standards to provide a clear and consistent understanding of industry and post-secondary expectations for health science teachers and students. These standards reflect the knowledge that healthcare workers must possess in several academic areas to succeed in this industry, including reading, writing, math, life sciences, medical terminology, and the history of healthcare. Several states also publish standards that reflect the skills and knowledge needed to be successful as a healthcare student. This textbook focuses on several academic and healthcare areas, including

- oral and written communications;
- employability skills;
- legal and ethical responsibilities;
- safety practices;
- teamwork;
- health maintenance practices; and
- information technology skills.

Health career programs are competitive and demanding. This textbook will help the entry-level student review and improve the basic skills listed above. By mastering such skills, the student will be prepared to enter into a meaningful, challenging program leading to a rewarding career.

Some healthcare careers are stepping-stones to other careers. Because the healthcare field grows and changes so rapidly, careers that do not exist today may be needed tomorrow.

A Brief History of Healthcare

All societies have medical beliefs providing explanations for birth, death, and disease. Throughout history, illness has been attributed to witches, demons, astrological influences, or the gods making mischief. In many cases, the rise of scientific medicine over the past millennium has altered or replaced such mysticism.

Many people greatly influenced what we know as our healthcare industry today. Their contributions to modern medicine were often both significant and lasting. Reading about these pioneers may inspire you to conduct further research (either individually or with a group) to learn how these innovative and determined individuals made such discoveries.

The Chinese

Ancient Chinese doctors made many advancements in the practice of acupuncture, which is the strategic insertion of small needles into the body to treat disease and pain (Figure 1.1). Acupuncture is often used today as a treatment for chronic pain and infertility. The Chinese were also the first to study the pulse as a means of diagnosis. They believed that examining the characteristics of a patient's pulse—its strength, rate, and regularity, for example—could help determine the severity of an illness.

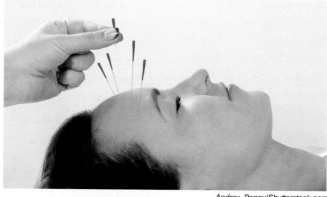

Figure 1.1 Chinese tradition explains that acupuncture is a way to balance the flow of energy in the body, which is known as qi. Modern western practitioners believe that acupuncture stimulates nerves, muscles, and connective tissue, and may work as a natural painkiller.

The Egyptians

Ancient Egyptians (and the Babylonians—people who lived in what is present-day Iraq and who made great advances in agriculture and science) developed a system of medicine that was quite advanced for the time period. The Egyptians began the practice of medical examinations and introduced the concepts of diagnosis (the process of determining the cause of the disease) and prognosis (forecasting the probable course and outcome of a disease). Figure 1.2 shows hieroglyphics, which the ancient Egyptians used to record their history and accounts of medical procedures.

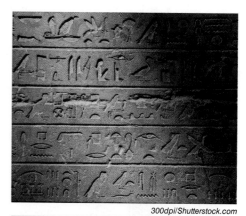

Figure 1.2 Ancient Egyptians recorded their history, including medical practices and developments, using hieroglyphics.

The Greeks

One of the biggest challenges to ancient medicine was sanitation. Ancient people did not understand germs and their role in transmitting disease. The Greeks, however, realized that some diseases were caused by poor sanitation, particularly contaminated water. They built aqueducts to bring clean water into cities and sewers to carry away waste (Figure 1.3).

Hippocrates was a Greek doctor who described many diseases and conditions in the fifth century BCE (before the Common Era). Hippocrates is credited with being the first person to believe that diseases were caused naturally and not as a result of superstition or the gods. He separated the discipline of medicine from religion, believing and arguing that disease was not a punishment inflicted by the gods, but rather the product of environmental factors, diet, and living habits.

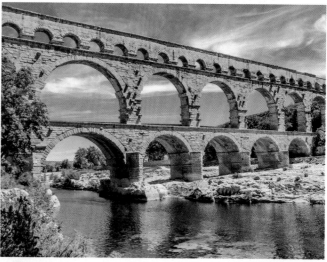

Figure 1.3 Aqueducts were built with a slight downward slope from the water source, allowing fresh water to flow into cities by the force of gravity.

Hippocratic Oath

a promise of professional behavior made by doctors beginning their careers; promises ethical and honest practice of the medical profession

caduceus

an emblem of medicine in the United States

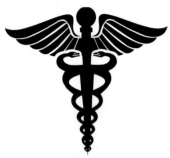

hkannn/Shutterstock.com

Figure 1.4 The caduceus has been used as a symbol for various medical groups, including the US Army Medical Corps and Nurse Corps.

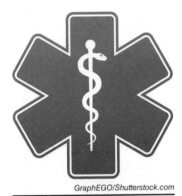

GraphEGO/Shutterstock.com

Figure 1.5 The staff of Aesculapius appears on the Star of Life, a common medical symbol.

Hippocrates has been credited with writing the **Hippocratic Oath**, a promise to practice medicine honestly, which doctors still make today. Although credited to Hippocrates, authorship of the oath has never been proved. A portion of the Hippocratic Oath states, "I will follow that method of treatment which according to my ability and judgment, I consider for the benefit of my patient and abstain from whatever is harmful or mischievous." Many people today consider Hippocrates to be the father of western medicine.

Another Greek doctor, Galen, was one of the greatest surgeons of the ancient world. Galen performed brain and eye surgeries that were not attempted again until 2,000 years after his death.

An emblem of the medical profession, the **caduceus**, has also been traced back to ancient times (Figure 1.4). The caduceus originally symbolized peace and was carried by Hermes, the messenger of the Greek gods. In the early 1900s, the caduceus was mistakenly adopted as the symbol of the US Army Medical Corps. Officials had confused it with the staff of Aesculapius, a Greek god of medicine. The staff of Aesculapius is a branch with a single snake wrapped around it, which resembles the caduceus (Figure 1.5). Today, both the caduceus and staff of Aesculapius are used to represent the medical profession, although the caduceus is used more commonly in the United States.

The Romans

The Romans were one of the first societies to use organized medical care. For example, Roman armies were accompanied by doctors, who carried medical equipment to care for wounded soldiers. Hospitals were created in Roman times, when doctors set aside a room in their houses to care for the ill. Eventually, separate buildings were built to accommodate the sick. The Romans also invented many surgical instruments such as forceps, scalpels, and surgical needles (Figure 1.6). Cataract surgery of the eye was first performed by Roman surgeons.

Native Americans

Native Americans were some of the earliest and most effective practitioners of the medical arts. Healers date back 40,000 years in North America.

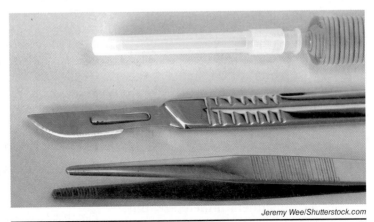

Jeremy Wee/Shutterstock.com

Figure 1.6 First developed by the Romans, forceps, scalpels, and surgical needles are basic tools used in healthcare today.

Because tribes did not have a written language, traditions were passed on orally from healer to healer. Healers believed that they should honor the patient's wishes and never force treatment on a patient.

Both the Navajo and Cherokee tribes used herbs and natural pain relievers (Figure 1.7). In many tribes, a person who recovered from a serious illness was thought to have supernatural powers after their recovery. Several tribes prayed to the spirits to intervene with a cure for the sick.

Dark and Middle Ages (400 CE to 1400 CE)

When the Roman Empire came under the rule of northern nomads called the Huns around 400 CE (Common Era), progress in the study of medical science slowed dramatically. For the next thousand years, medicine was practiced only in monasteries and convents. The Roman Catholic Church taught that life and death were in the hands of God, and there was little interest in learning how the body functioned or in curing disease by man's hands. Prayer was the preferred method of healing and curing disease. Doctors as we know them today did not exist.

Terrible **epidemics** (the plague, in particular) killed millions of people during this period. Other serious diseases without cures included smallpox, syphilis, tuberculosis, and diphtheria. Today, the plague, syphilis, and tuberculosis—which are all caused by different bacteria—can usually be cured by **antibiotics** and other antibacterial agents. According to the World Health Organization, smallpox has been officially eradicated, or done away with completely. This was done through a global effort involving **vaccination** and **quarantine**. Today, diphtheria is controlled by vaccinations.

The Islamic civilization rose to prominence in medical science during the Middle Ages. Arab doctors made significant contributions to medicine in disciplines such as anatomy, ophthalmology, pharmacology, physiology, surgery, and the pharmaceutical sciences. The Arabs were influenced by the Greeks, Romans, and the progress people in India had made. Like the Romans before them, Arab societies established hospitals dedicated to the care of the sick and injured.

Maimonides (1135–1204) was an extremely important Jewish philosopher and one of the most prolific and inventive biblical scholars and doctors of the Middle Ages. In his many writings, he described numerous medical conditions including asthma, diabetes, hepatitis, and pneumonia. Maimonides emphasized the importance of moderation and a healthy lifestyle. His writings influenced generations of doctors.

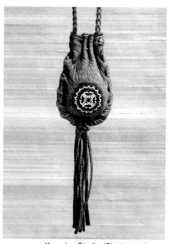

Knumina Studios/Shutterstock.com

Figure 1.7 Native American healers often carried medical bags containing items they believed held spiritual healing powers.

epidemic
an outbreak of a disease that affects many people and spreads rapidly

antibiotics
drugs that slow the growth of, or destroy bacteria; used to treat infections

vaccination
the use of medicines that contain weakened or dead bacteria or viruses to build immunity and prevent disease

quarantine
the process of isolating people who have been exposed to infectious or contagious disease

Check Your Understanding ✓

1. Name three incurable diseases that killed millions of people during the Dark and Middle Ages.
2. What is the Hippocratic Oath?
3. How did the Greeks use aqueducts to improve quality of life and prevent disease?
4. What medical concepts did the ancient Egyptians introduce to the world?
5. Which medical practice did the ancient Chinese invent that is still in use today?

Did You Know?   The Black Death

Bubonic plague is a disease transmitted by small rodents who are infested with fleas. Bubonic plague is caused by a bacterium called *Yersinia pestis* (Figure 1.8). This bacterium is very sensitive to antibiotics and can easily be destroyed with proper treatment. Without antibiotics, an infected person can die within six days of contracting the bubonic plague.

There are three varieties of plague. Bubonic plague bacteria invade the lymphatic system, causing *buboes*, or swollen and painful lymph nodes throughout the body. In other cases, *Yersinia pestis* bacteria cause the bloodstream to become infected, resulting in a condition called *septicemic plague*. If the lungs become infected, the condition is then called *pneumonic plague*. Together, these three infections are known as the *Black Death* or the *Black Plague*. In the fourteenth century, the Black Death killed approximately 25 million Europeans, which amounted to approximately 30–60 percent of the European population.

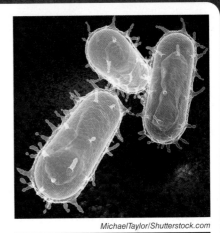

MichaelTaylor/Shutterstock.com

Figure 1.8   *Yersinia pestis* bacteria

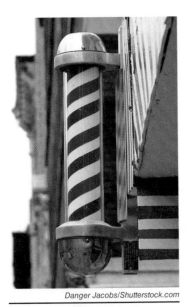

Danger Jacobs/Shutterstock.com

Figure 1.9   Placed on the outside of buildings, the barber pole has long signified the presence of a barber, or barber-surgeon, within.

The Barber-Surgeon

In the Middle Ages, a barber cut more than just hair. Barbers could also practice surgery, dentistry, and bloodletting (a procedure thought to rid the body of disease-causing substances circulating in the blood). The barber-surgeon also traveled with armies and often performed amputations.

Barber poles placed outside the home of a barber-surgeon were red, white, and blue. The red represented blood, the white bandages (or the tourniquet used to raise veins), and blue for the veins (Figure 1.9). The pole itself represented the stick squeezed by the patient to dilate, or enlarge, the veins.

During the Middle Ages, doctors first became licensed after completing formal training with an experienced doctor. Surgeons, like the barber-surgeons, had different training than doctors. Women were not allowed to practice medicine, but were allowed to be nurses and midwives.

Religion continued to play an important role in healthcare. In the Middle Ages, Christian and Muslim teachings encouraged members of their religions to care for those in need, including the sick. Prayer and rest continued to be prevalent treatments in many places.

Did You Know?   Bloodletting

The practice of bloodletting as a medical treatment came with the pilgrims to North America on the Mayflower. This medical practice was incredibly popular in the eighteenth and early nineteenth centuries. Doctors believed that removing blood from the body restored balance and eliminated the disease. In fact, President George Washington died in 1799 after being drained of 40 percent of his blood in an attempt to cure him of a sore throat and cold. By the end of the nineteenth century, the use of bloodletting as a medical treatment for illness was proved ineffective and considered quackery (an ignorant medical practice).

The Renaissance

There were many developments in healthcare during the Renaissance, a period that began in the fourteenth century and lasted until the seventeenth century. The invention of the printing press made it possible to mass produce books, allowing information about new medical discoveries to spread quickly. During the sixteenth century, scientists began to use the scientific method. Instead of guessing what made people sick, scientists could use the scientific method to make accurate conclusions based on observation and careful note-taking. You can learn more about the scientific method by reading *Background Lesson 4: Science Review*.

Another dramatic development during the Renaissance was the invention of the **microscope**. During the first century CE, some Romans experimented with making images larger by using crude lenses. It was not until 1,500 years later that a Dutch dry goods store owner, Antonie van Leeuwenhoek (1632–1723), used lenses to magnify and count threads in cloth. Van Leeuwenhoek became fascinated with making lenses and successfully produced magnifications up to 270 times. Van Leeuwenhoek later developed the device we know today as the microscope.

microscope
an instrument that uses a lens to magnify objects too small to be seen with the naked eye

Van Leeuwenhoek observed specimens no person had ever seen before—bacteria, yeast, red blood cells, sperm, and tiny microorganisms swimming in a drop of pond water. Van Leeuwenhoek has been called the father of microscopy. Robert Hooke (1635–1703), an Englishman who is sometimes called the English father of microscopy, also spent much of his life working with microscopes and improved their design and capabilities.

The Industrial Revolution

The Industrial Revolution of the mid- to late-eighteenth and nineteenth centuries brought great changes to industry, communication, and travel. Inventions such as the telegraph and railroad lines were developed to make communication and travel faster (Figure 1.10). Ideas could now be exchanged easily and more quickly.

Factories were developed using better technologies, allowing for the mass production of more sophisticated medical equipment such as finer syringe needles and microscope lenses. Considerable progress was made in the field of medicine with the invention of the stethoscope, which enabled medical professionals to listen to a patient's chest cavity, heart, and pulse points without an invasive procedure.

With the advent of industrialization, rural residents moved in great numbers to the cities to find work. The results of this mass exodus from the country to the city brought overcrowded conditions in which people lived close together, spreading infectious diseases in great numbers. During this period, public health laws designed to control the spread of disease were established.

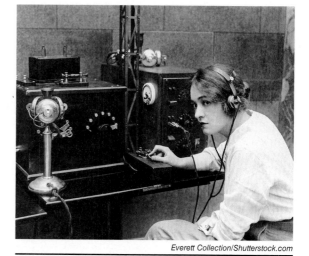

Everett Collection/Shutterstock.com

Figure 1.10   By 1861, telegraph lines spanned the United States, connecting the east and west coasts and vastly improving the speed at which messages could be sent across the country.

Vaccination

An English doctor named Edward Jenner (1749–1823) developed the practice of vaccination. Vaccination is the administration of dead or weakened microorganisms of a disease that increases a person's immunity, or resistance, to a particular disease.

Jenner observed that people who worked around cows and horses developed cowpox (a virus causing sores), but did not generally get a similar disease called *smallpox*. Smallpox was a highly infectious, and often fatal, disease caused by a poxvirus. The symptoms of smallpox included fever, headache, and inflamed skin sores. Jenner vaccinated people with the fluid from the cowpox blisters, which protected people from smallpox.

Throughout this period, vaccinations were developed for other diseases such as cholera, anthrax, rabies, tetanus, diphtheria, typhoid fever, and various plagues.

Pain Management

anesthesia
loss of feeling with or without the loss of consciousness

Before the nineteenth century, pain was a serious problem, especially during surgery. **Anesthesia** was not invented until the nineteenth century. Ether was first available as an inhalable anesthetic, followed by nitrous oxide and chloroform. Today, with the advent of more advanced methods of putting patients in deep sleep, anesthesia makes painless surgery possible.

Did You Know?   Early Pain Relief

In the early days of medicine, doctors used herbs, hashish (a product of cannabis), and alcohol to relieve pain during surgery. Some doctors choked patients into unconsciousness to stop pain. Unfortunately, many patients died from the terrible pain and shock caused by surgery.

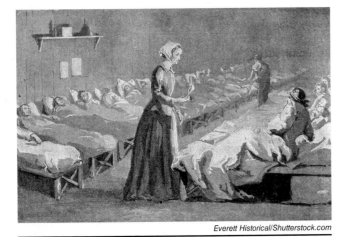

Everett Historical/Shutterstock.com

Figure 1.11 When a portrait of Florence Nightingale tending patients in Crimea by the light of a small lamp was published in the mid 1850s, she gained the nickname "Lady of the Lamp."

Women in Medicine

Before the Industrial Revolution, women played only a minor role in organized medical care, serving as cleaning women and midwives. However, the work of a few pioneering individuals opened up possibilities for women throughout the healthcare field.

Florence Nightingale. The work of Englishwoman Florence Nightingale (1820–1910) increased the participation of women in medical care (Figure 1.11). Nightingale demonstrated the critical role of nurses in the formerly male-dominated medical profession. Her goal was to reduce patient mortality that resulted from lack of hygiene and nutrition.

When the Crimean War broke out in the mid 1850s, Britain's Secretary of State at War, Sidney Herbert, sent Nightingale to the country's military hospital in Turkey. With her staff of nearly 40 nurses, she tended to wounded soldiers, saving many through the use of proper hygiene. Nightingale felt that disease was caused by an unclean environment. In hospital wards, she insisted that bed linens be changed frequently, rooms be well ventilated, chamber pots be emptied often, and the walls and floors scrubbed regularly.

Nightingale also laid the foundation for professional nursing with the establishment of her nursing school at St Thomas' Hospital in London in 1860. Nightingale's school was the first secular (nonreligious) nursing school in the world. The role of the nurse has expanded greatly since Nightingale's time, producing several levels of nurses' training. You will learn more about nurses' training in chapter 2. Today, the nurse's role has evolved into a professional and technological one, especially in acute care hospitals.

Elizabeth Blackwell. In 1849, Elizabeth Blackwell (1821–1910) graduated with her medical doctor (M.D.) degree, becoming the first woman to formally study and practice medicine in the United States. Blackwell's sister, Emily, followed in her footsteps as the third woman to earn a medical degree in the United States. The sisters worked together at the New York Infirmary for Indigent Women and Children for over 40 years. In 1868, the sisters founded the Women's Medical College in New York.

Clara Barton. In 1881, Clara Barton (1821–1912) formed the American Red Cross, which has become one of the largest humanitarian organizations in the world (Figure 1.12). During her life, Barton was first a teacher and then a clerk. However, during the Civil War, she dedicated herself to caring for soldiers on the front, gathering supplies from all over the country. After the war, Barton was recognized as a hero all over the world, receiving the Iron Cross, the Cross of Imperial Russia, and the International Red Cross medal.

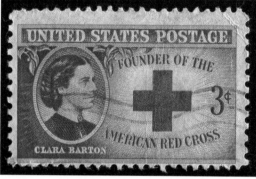

rook76/Shutterstock.com

Figure 1.12 Clara Barton was honored for her role as the founder of the American Red Cross with this stamp from the late 1940s.

Pathogens and Sterilization

In 1847, Hungarian doctor Ignaz Semmelweis (1818–1865) noticed a dramatic difference between the death rate of women who had babies at home and women who had babies in hospitals. In hospitals, mothers often came down with childbed fever, a severe vaginal or uterine infection. At the time, surgeons did not wash their hands before treating women in childbirth. Surgeons might deliver a baby after working with diseased patients, without first washing their hands. Semmelweis faced hostility from his fellow doctors for a time, until they began to realize the health benefits of hand washing.

Louis Pasteur (1822–1895), a French chemist, carried out experiments that helped develop the modern science of microbiology. Microbiology is the study of infectious microscopic organisms such as bacteria, viruses, fungi, and parasites. Pasteur developed the first vaccine for rabies and anthrax and developed the pasteurization (application of heat to destroy pathogens) of milk and wine.

Considered the father of antiseptic surgery, British surgeon Joseph Lister (1827–1912) insisted on using soap to disinfect instruments and clean hands before doctors moved from patient to patient. Today, sterilizing surgical equipment, disinfection, and hand washing are rigorously practiced as a way to prevent infection in patients.

Think It Through

Why do you think Dr. Semmelweis's colleagues doubted his research on the benefits of hand washing?

pathogens
disease-producing microorganisms

During the Industrial Revolution, German doctor Robert Koch (1843–1910) discovered that some diseases are caused by microorganisms called **pathogens**. The discovery of pathogens confirmed Lister's insistence upon maintaining medical asepsis (the practice of keeping things free of pathogens to prevent infection).

Check Your Understanding ✓

1. Which important concept did Ignaz Semmelweis introduce to the medical world?
2. Describe Florence Nightingale's contributions to healthcare.
3. Who is considered the father of antiseptic surgery?
4. What was Elizabeth Blackwell's important role in the medical history of the United States?
5. Which English doctor developed the practice of vaccination?

The Twentieth Century and Beyond

In 1928, Scottish doctor Alexander Fleming (1881–1955) discovered a mold that contained antibacterial secretions. Fleming's discovery, which he called *penicillin*, became the first antibiotic to treat bacterial infections. By 1943, mass production of penicillin had begun. The importance of penicillin was fully realized during World War II, when it prevented thousands of deaths by treating infected wounds. Along with other antibiotics, penicillin revolutionized healthcare, dramatically reducing death rates and giving birth to the modern pharmaceutical industry.

The development of X-ray technology by German physicist Wilhelm Röntgen (1845–1923) at the end of the nineteenth century opened up new and exciting possibilities in healthcare. X-ray technology has inspired the development of other noninvasive means of diagnosis using computers, such as magnetic resonance imaging (MRI) and computerized axial tomography (CT scans). An X-ray only produces a two-dimensional view of the body, but a computer can create a three-dimensional image, leading to more informed diagnoses. Another tool developed to monitor internal organs was the electrocardiogram (ECG or EKG). The electrocardiogram was developed by Willem Einthoven (1860–1927) in 1903 to monitor heart function.

Discovering Radium, Insulin, and DNA

Radium was discovered by French scientists Marie and Pierre Curie at the beginning of the twentieth century (Figure 1.13). After her husband died, Marie Curie dedicated herself entirely to the development of X-ray use in medicine, as well as therapeutic uses for radiation, including cancer treatment.

Insulin, an injectable hormone used to manage diabetes symptoms, was discovered in 1922 by Canadian doctor Frederick Banting and his student, Charles Best. These two men isolated the internal secretions of the pancreas, the organ that creates insulin, and were able to harvest insulin from these secretions.

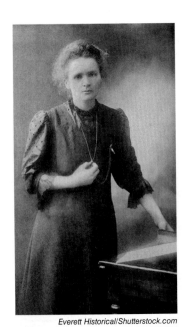

Everett Historical/Shutterstock.com

Figure 1.13 Working with her husband Pierre, Marie Curie discovered the elements radium and polonium. Polonium was named for Madam Curie's home country of Poland.

Insulin is used to regulate levels of glucose (a sugar) in the blood. Diabetics experience an inadequate production or utilization of insulin, resulting in excessive amounts of glucose in the blood and urine. Today, insulin is produced synthetically.

The discovery of deoxyribonucleic acid (DNA), the molecule that carries genetic information from one generation to the other, took place in April 1953. DNA's discovery has had an enormous effect on scientific and medical progress. Studying DNA involves the identification of genes that trigger major diseases and influences the creation and manufacture of drugs to treat these devastating diseases. The identification and analysis of these genes has greatly influenced therapeutic treatments.

The discovery of DNA has also resulted in many breakthroughs in criminal investigations because it can be used to trace the criminals by comparing the DNA samples found on the crime scene with those extracted from the suspects.

Although three men—James Watson (1928–), Francis Crick (1916–2004), and Maurice Wilkins (1916–2004)—were credited with the discovery of DNA, the research of Rosalind Franklin (1920–1958) helped them make their discovery. However, in 1962, Watson, Crick, and Wilkins were awarded the Nobel Prize in Physiology or Medicine for their discovery.

Check Your Understanding ✓

1. What did Alexander Fleming discover?
2. Why was the discovery of insulin so important?
3. Which German physicist developed X-ray technology?
4. What did Pierre and Marie Curie discover?

Medical Machines and Electronics

Machines can now serve as substitutes for certain organs, such as dialysis machines that replace the function of kidneys and heart-lung bypass machines that take over the heart's function during surgery. The first heart-lung bypass machine, which was invented by American doctor John Gibbon (1903–1973), was used on a human in May, 1953.

Organ transplantation continues to be increasingly successful. The first organ transplant was a kidney transplant performed in 1954 by Dr. John P. Merrill. Today, many organ transplants are possible, including combination heart-lung, bone marrow, stem cell, and liver transplants. Anti-rejection drugs have become increasingly successful in countering the body's reaction to foreign tissue introduced by an organ transplant.

Electronics and computer science have changed clinical medicine. One such change comes from the development of tiny robotic devices that assist in microsurgery. These devices view internal tissues during surgery. Fully mobile robots with computer screens for "heads" and video cameras for "eyes" and "ears" can be operated by a doctor using a joystick and wireless technology. Using this kind of robot, doctors can perform examinations on patients while being far away from them.

Robotics are also used in hospital pharmacies. Pharmacists enter prescriptions into a computer. A machine collects the dosages by scanning the barcode on a medication container and then packages a proper amount of the medication. The robots ensure that the correct medication reaches the correct patient. Pharmaceutical companies also use automated systems to package their medications (Figure 1.14).

Treating Mental Illness

Significant progress has been made in treating mental illness. At the beginning of the twentieth century, **psychoanalysis**—a method of treating mental and emotional disorders—became known to the medical community. Psychoanalysis is based on the concepts and theories of Sigmund Freud (1856–1939), an Austrian neurologist. Freud was known for his sessions during which the patient is encouraged to speak freely about personal experiences, particularly about his or her early childhood and dreams. Later in the twentieth century, psychoanalysis became a popular form of therapy for mental illness.

Before the twentieth century, mentally ill patients were placed in asylums. After World War II, soldiers received more consistent treatment thanks to the development of a new psychiatric manual for categorizing mental disorders. The contents of the manual were based on more knowledge of the mentally ill, instead of relying on outdated remedies that did not yield helpful results. After two world wars, the significant number of soldiers returning home with serious psychiatric conditions placed increased attention on such conditions. Originally called *shell shock*, we now refer to these psychiatric conditions as *post-traumatic stress disorder (PTSD)*. Today, the mentally ill are treated in psychiatric hospitals.

Psychiatric medication gradually became prevalent during the twentieth century. Such medications were used to treat anxiety and depression. Some of these medications caused unpleasant side effects and dependency. Antidepressants known as selective serotonin reuptake inhibitors (SSRIs) became some of the most widely prescribed drugs in the world. Today, about a dozen SSRIs are prescribed, including Paxil®, Zoloft®, and Prozac®.

Today, there are state psychiatric hospitals for the mentally ill, funded by tax dollars. However, budget constraints have seriously reduced the number of public psychiatric beds available for the treatment of acutely or chronically ill psychiatric patients in the United States. The most severely ill patients are in serious need of the specialized, intensive treatment formerly delivered by such public hospitals. The elimination of these systems is producing significant public and personal consequences in communities across the country.

Private psychiatric hospitals also serve the mentally ill. However, stays in private psychiatric hospitals can be very expensive.

Genomic Medicine

Future medical care will focus more on predicting whether a specific person will contract a particular disease. **Genomic medicine** studies a person's DNA sequences, the order of the four chemical building blocks called bases that make up the DNA molecule. The base order tells scientists what

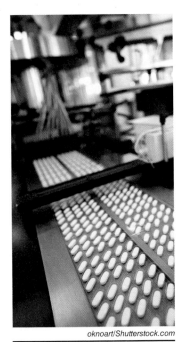

Figure 1.14 Mechanized tablet packaging at a pharmaceutical company.

psychoanalysis
a method of analyzing and treating mental and emotional disorders through sessions in which the patient is encouraged to talk about personal experience and dreams

Think It Through

How has treatment of the mentally ill changed over time? In particular, what changes have been made in the United States? Do you think that there is prejudice against the mentally ill?

genomic medicine
a branch of medicine that studies a person's DNA sequences, which carry genetic information

genetic information is carried in a particular DNA sequence. A genome is defined as the complete sequence of DNA for every chromosome in the human body. While 99 percent of genes are identical, a few will be different. These differences may explain why one person will develop a disease and respond to a certain drug and another will not.

For example, some women may carry BRCA genes (BRCA1 and BRCA2), resulting from mutations, or abnormalities, in normal genes. Women who have inherited mutations in these genes face a much higher risk of developing breast and ovarian cancers than the general population. If a doctor tests for such mutations and finds them, the patient can be monitored closely with frequent mammograms (a test that can often detect breast cancer). Some patients who have tested positive for this particular gene have elected to have a preventive double-mastectomy performed, removing all breast tissue before cancer begins to develop.

The United States' Healthcare Industry Today

Medical care in the United States receives a great deal of media attention today. The developments taking place in the healthcare industry are undoubtedly contributing to the larger history of healthcare. As a future healthcare employee, you should understand some of the components of our current healthcare system.

Government Health Insurance Programs and Laws

Two of the largest public health insurance programs run by the government are Medicare and Medicaid. Various factors determine whether a person is eligible for Medicare or Medicaid. In some cases, a person may qualify for both programs, which is known as *dual eligibility*. The US government also offers insurance coverage to active members of the military, veterans, and their families.

Medicare

Medicare is a government-funded insurance program for individuals over the age of 65 and people of any age who have a disability or illness that prevents them from working, such as permanent kidney failure. Medicare is funded by taxes, and eligibility is determined by the federal government. Many people who qualify for Medicare also have a supplemental insurance policy for costs not covered by Medicare, such as many prescription medications and portions of medical bills.

Medicare coverage is divided into four parts: A, B, C, and D. Part A of Medicare covers hospital and skilled nursing costs, while Part B provides medical insurance. Parts A and B are part of the original Medicare (signed into law in 1965), which is provided by the federal government when you reach 65 years of age. (Individuals are actually eligible to enroll for Medicare three months before turning 65, but coverage does not begin at that time.) Original Medicare does not pay for everything. You may pay a share of the cost in monthly **premiums** and **copayments**.

Medicare
a federal health insurance program for persons 65 or older and disabled individuals

premium
the amount an insured person pays to his or her insurance company to maintain coverage

copayment
a fixed amount (for example, $15) paid for a covered health care service, usually when service is provided; amount varies depending on type of health insurance a person has

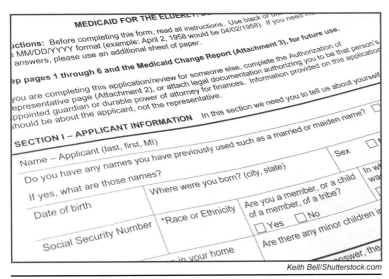

Figure 1.15 In order to receive Medicaid assistance, candidates must first apply and be found eligible for this insurance program.

Part C is Medicare coverage offered through private insurance companies. Called *Medicare Advantage*, this private insurance helps cover hospital stays and doctor visits. Some plans also include prescription drug coverage.

Part D covers prescription drugs. You can enroll in Part D to go with your original Medicare coverage.

Medicaid

Medicaid is an insurance program for people with low incomes and very few personal assets other than a home. It is a combined federal and state government insurance program, which means that it is paid for by state and federal taxes. States determine who is eligible for the program by following federal guidelines (Figure 1.15).

Medicaid
a program jointly funded by state and federal taxes that provides medical aid for low-income individuals of all ages; managed by the states

The Military Health System and TRICARE

The Military Health System offers TRICARE, the military's health insurance program. TRICARE offers basic options for care: TRICARE Prime, TRICARE Extra, and TRICARE Standard. Additional plans provide supplemental coverage to Medicare, covering active and retired National Guard Reserve members, as well as their families and dependent adult children. TRICARE offers coverage to everyone—active-duty members, retirees, and their families. However, retirees and their dependents have to chip in to cover the cost of their benefits.

Worker's Compensation

worker's compensation
a form of government insurance that provides wage replacement and medical benefits for employees injured at work

Worker's compensation is a form of government insurance that provides wage replacement and medical benefits for employees injured while at work. If an injured employee accepts worker's compensation, he gives up his right to sue the employer for negligence (failure to exercise care where their employees are concerned).

Worker's compensation plans differ among states. Most plans include payments instead of the employee's regular wages, compensation for past and future economic losses, payment for medical bills, and payments to dependents for workers killed on the job.

Most states require employers to have worker's compensation insurance. An injured employee must file for worker's compensation within a set time after the injury. This time frame varies depending on the state in which the employer resides. The insurance company decides on the merit of the case and determines if the injured employee wants a lump sum to treat the injury or if payment to compensate for wages is paid out over time. If an employer does not have such insurance, the employer must deal with the injury, which can end with an expensive lawsuit. Worker's compensation laws are designed to avoid lawsuits.

The Affordable Care Act (ACA)

The Affordable Care Act (ACA) was passed in 2010 with the intention of increasing the quality and affordability of health insurance. It is a long, complex piece of legislation that has significantly changed the US healthcare system. The law requires insurance companies cover all applicants within the new standards. People are to be offered the same rates regardless of pre-existing conditions. The ACA also allows dependents to be covered by their parents' insurance policies until age 26.

One goal of the ACA is to ensure that people can get treatment when they need it. Preventive care and immunizations are now offered at no cost to the insured individual. The ACA also creates state-based American Health Benefit Exchanges through which individuals can purchase coverage. Separate Exchanges exist through which small businesses can purchase coverage.

If you can afford health insurance but choose not to buy it, you must pay a fee called the *individual shared responsibility payment*. In some cases, you may qualify for an exemption from the requirement to have insurance. If you qualify for an exemption, you won't have to pay the fee. If your annual income is below approximately $11,000, you also do not have to pay the fee.

Since its inception, the ACA has faced challenges in Congress. The Supreme Court ruled in 2015 that the ACA's federal subsidies to help individuals pay for health insurance will be available in all states. Although most people agree that preexisting conditions should be covered and that children should be eligible to use their parents' insurance until age 26, there is much debate over healthcare mandates, or government-issued laws that require individuals to buy health insurance.

Private, Managed Care Insurance Plans

In the past, insurance payments were made based on the actual cost of a procedure. This caused providers of medical services to order additional procedures that were sometimes necessary. This situation resulted in increased costs for patients and insurance companies. To try to control costs, insurers have developed **managed care**. This is a general term for any healthcare plan that emphasizes wellness and provides healthcare through a network of doctors, hospitals, and other healthcare providers. Managed care plans are a form of private medical insurance. The most common models are the health maintenance organizations (HMOs) and the preferred provider organizations (PPOs).

Health Maintenance Organizations (HMO)

The Health Maintenance Organization Act of 1973 caused a rapid increase in the number of **health maintenance organizations (HMOs)**. HMOs are set up so that you receive most, or all, of your healthcare from a network provider. You select a primary care physician who is responsible for managing and coordinating your healthcare. Doctors are provided financial incentives to keep costs down. If you *choose* to have medical treatment outside of the HMO network, you will most likely pay the entire bill. If you cannot reach a network provider when outside the network area (for example, if you break your arm on vacation and need to visit the emergency room), you will probably be covered by your insurance for the out-of-network care you received.

managed care
a general term for any healthcare plan that emphasizes wellness and provides healthcare through a network of doctors, hospitals, and other healthcare providers

health maintenance organizations (HMO)
managed care organizations that provide prepaid, comprehensive healthcare at a flat rate and for a fixed period of time through a network of participating healthcare professionals and hospitals; policyholders select a primary care physician (PCP) and referrals from the PCP must be obtained to see a specialist

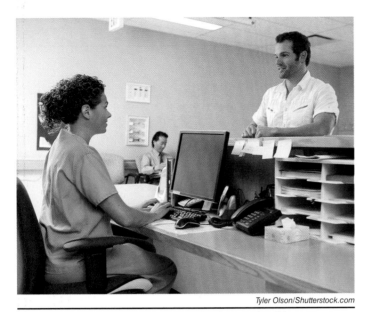

Tyler Olson/Shutterstock.com

Figure 1.16 If a copayment is required, many healthcare facilities will collect this fee when you arrive for your appointment.

preferred provider organizations (PPO)
health insurance organizations that contract with a network of preferred providers from which the policyholder can choose; often involves an annual deductible payment for service, but patients do not have a designated primary care physician and may self-refer to specialists

deductible
the amount you owe for covered healthcare services before your health insurance plan begins to pay

Most HMOs require a copayment at the time of a visit (Figure 1.16). Copayments may increase when you see a specialist and if you seek treatment from an emergency room. Some managed care plans require that you get a referral, or recommendation, from your primary doctor before seeing a specialist.

Preferred Provider Organizations (PPO)

Preferred provider organizations (PPOs) contract with a network of preferred providers from which you can choose. Under this plan, you do not have to select a primary care physician. Instead, you will have a choice of doctors, hospitals, and other providers within the PPO network. Although the PPO network is much wider than an HMO, you will still pay more for your care if you choose to visit an out-of-network healthcare provider.

Instead of a copayment, PPOs may require an annual **deductible** payment for services. Your annual deductible is the cost you must pay out of pocket before your insurance company begins covering your healthcare expenses.

Controlling Healthcare Costs

Healthcare costs in the United States have been rising rapidly for several years. The United States spends more on healthcare per person than any other country (Figure 1.17). To make health care coverage more affordable, our nation must address the high cost of medical care.

More than one-sixth of the US economy is spent on healthcare. For families and senior citizens, the cost of medical care means less money in their pockets and results in choices about balancing food, rent, and healthcare. These costs also affect businesses, making it harder to add new employees because health insurance has become expensive.

Real Life Scenario   Insurance Choices

Kevin is a twenty-seven-year-old student who has no medical insurance. His part-time job doesn't have any benefits and only pays him about $7,000 a year. Kevin's heavy academic load does not allow him time to get a full-time job with benefits. Kevin has been debating whether or not to buy medical insurance now that he is no longer covered by his parents' insurance. He decides that his tight budget won't stretch to cover the cost of health insurance, and he'll worry about health insurance when he is older.

Apply It

1. In your opinion, has Kevin made a wise choice for this time in his life?
2. Does he have any options for affordable health insurance?
3. How might Kevin go about obtaining health insurance utilizing the Affordable Care Act? What consequences will he face if he chooses not to purchase health insurance?

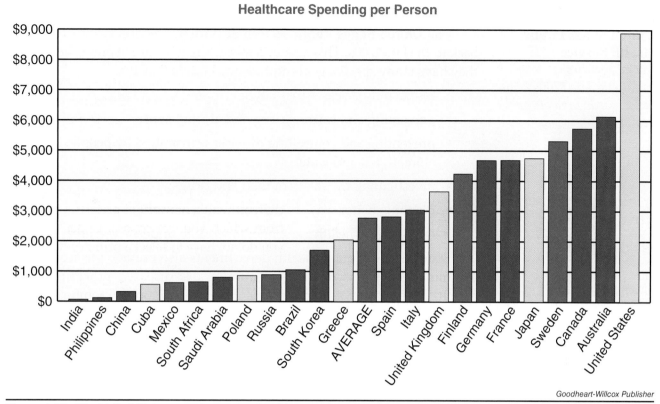

Figure 1.17   The United States spends more on healthcare per person than any other country.

Healthcare costs have risen for a variety of reasons, including the following:

- Americans are living longer as a result of better treatments for chronic illnesses.

- Poor diet and lack of exercise have increased obesity rates, most notably in children and teens, increasing the number of diagnosed diabetics who require many years of healthcare treatment.

As healthcare costs rise, so do healthcare insurance premiums. Expanding coverage to new populations, new taxes and fees, broader benefits, and the cost of healthcare services all affect health insurance premiums.

Many cost-reducing efforts have already been implemented. Limits have been placed on the amount paid to hospitals because, through research, Medicare and other health insurers have found many of the tests and procedures performed to be unnecessary. HMOs focus on providing preventive care for free or at little cost. If illnesses can be prevented, treatment costs can be eliminated. Some health plans reward doctors who provide consistently excellent care rather than rewarding them based on the number of patients seen in a short time. Healthcare reform such as the Affordable Care Act calls for major changes to provide affordable insurance for a larger number of Americans.

Government Agencies That Provide Healthcare Services

Federal, state, and local governments provide healthcare services that are funded by taxes. These programs give direct healthcare to citizens and promote health education. They also play a role in safeguarding our food and water supplies.

The United States Public Health Service

United States Public Health Service
federal agency that dates back to the late 1700s whose mission is to promote public health

The **United States Public Health Service** is a federal agency that dates back to the late 1700s. This agency's mission is to promote public health, but they have many specific goals and responsibilities, such as

- researching diseases that kill or cripple;
- preventing and treating drug and alcohol abuse;
- preventing and controlling diseases transmitted by people, insects, animals, air, and water;
- investigating the safety of food and drugs;
- planning better ways to deliver healthcare services; and
- encouraging health personnel to work in underserved areas.

State and local public health departments also provide services to local communities such as reporting communicable diseases, providing public health nursing, educating the public about health topics, monitoring environmental sanitation, providing maternal and child health services, and running public health clinics. Local public health departments report to their state's health agency.

Occupational Safety and Health Administration (OSHA)

Occupational Safety and Health Administration (OSHA)
a government agency that creates regulations to prevent work-related injuries, illnesses, and deaths

The acronym OSHA stands for the **Occupational Safety and Health Administration**. OSHA imposes safety and health legislation to prevent injury, illness, and death in the workplace. OSHA sets and enforces standards of safety and also provides training, outreach, education, and assistance to employers and employees to help ensure safe workplaces.

The Centers for Disease Control and Prevention (CDC)

Centers for Disease Control and Prevention (CDC)
a division of the United States Department of Health and Human Services that focuses on disease outbreaks and prevention in the United States

The **Centers for Disease Control and Prevention (CDC)** monitors and prevents disease outbreaks, responds to environmental emergencies and other health threats, and provides research-based health information to the public. The CDC also develops disease prevention strategies and keeps track of national health statistics.

The Food and Drug Administration (FDA)

Food and Drug Administration (FDA)
a government agency that regulates products in the food and drug industries and develops nutrition facts labels to help consumers make informed food choices

The **Food and Drug Administration (FDA)** is responsible for

- protecting the public health by ensuring that foods (except for meat from livestock, poultry and some egg products, which are regulated by the US Department of Agriculture) are safe and properly labeled;
- ensuring that human and veterinary drugs, vaccines, biological products, and medical devices intended for human use are safe and effective;
- regulating tobacco products; and
- advancing the public health by helping to speed product innovations.

The National Institutes of Health (NIH)

The **National Institutes of Health (NIH)** conducts and supports medical research. It is the world's leading agency for medical research. The National Institutes of Health's research programs include studies in the following areas:

- diagnosing, preventing, and curing disease;
- mental, addictive, and physical disorders;
- human growth and development; and
- effects of environmental contaminants.

The World Health Organization (WHO)

The **World Health Organization (WHO)** directs and coordinates health-related matters within the United Nations system. This organization provides leadership on global health issues, influencing health research, setting standards for good health outcomes, providing the required technical support to all the countries involved, and assessing and monitoring global health developments.

WHO's current priorities include reducing, and in some cases eradicating, communicable diseases such as HIV and AIDS, Ebola (Figure 1.18), malaria, and tuberculosis.

WHO is also involved in lessening the effects of noncommunicable diseases; promoting sexual and reproductive health, development, and aging; encouraging nutrition, food security, and healthy eating; ensuring occupational health; and providing education on and treatment for substance abuse.

Volunteer Health Agencies

Volunteer health agencies receive support from donations, gifts (including property or money), dues from members, and fundraisers. Examples of these agencies include

- the American Cancer Society;
- the Muscular Dystrophy Association;
- the National Association of Mental Health; and
- the American Red Cross (Figure 1.19).

Volunteer agencies play a very important role in advancing good health in our communities. Some also help with challenges such as disaster relief, educating people about diseases, and financially supporting critical research, to name a few. These volunteer health agencies often work closely with governmental health agencies.

National Institutes of Health (NIH)
a division of the Department of Health and Human Services that conducts research and provides information to promote and improve public health through 27 different agencies

World Health Organization (WHO)
an agency of the United Nations that is concerned with international public health

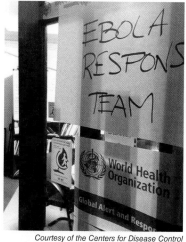

Courtesy of the Centers for Disease Control

Figure 1.18 The World Health Organization (WHO) offered aid to West Africa during the 2014 Ebola outbreak.

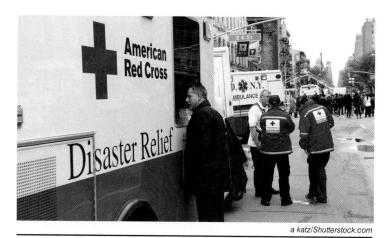

a katz/Shutterstock.com

Figure 1.19 The Red Cross responds to nearly 70,000 disasters, including home fires, hurricanes, flood relief, hazardous material spills, and tornadoes each year. Red Cross volunteers provide food, shelter, and support to the victims of these disasters.

Extend Your Knowledge ▶ Professional Healthcare Associations

Professional organizations in healthcare are formed to support specific careers in several ways. Many organizations offer certification to people who complete requirements for a certain profession. Organizations may also provide continuing education that is required of healthcare professionals to ensure they are up-to-date with advances in their field. Associations can provide important networking opportunities concerned with job openings, the latest and upcoming changes to the profession, and helpful information for new members of the profession. These organizations also publish journals and public relations materials about specific professions. They may advocate for members of the profession by working to improve benefits or promoting safety measures, for example.

Examples of professional organizations include the American Nurses Association, the American Medical Association, and the American Health Information Management Association.

Apply It

1. Choose two healthcare careers that interest you. Then research any professional associations that are relevant to those careers.

2. Research student healthcare associations such as the National Student Nurses Association, the Student National Medical Association, or the American Occupational Therapy Association. How can these organizations help you find more information related to your career interests?

Healthcare Facilities

When illness or injury occurs, patients have several types of healthcare facilities they can turn to in the United States. Remember that there are many options for employment in such institutions. The following are some of the most common healthcare facilities you might encounter in a city setting. Rural areas may only have a general hospital with few specialties.

Hospitals

There are over 6,500 hospitals in the United States today. They vary in size and types of service provided. Some hospitals operate as for-profit facilities, while others are nonprofit hospitals. Hospitals are further categorized as short-stay or long-term care facilities, depending on the length of time a patient stays before being discharged.

Nonprofit Hospitals

Nonprofit hospitals are a traditional means of delivering medical care in the United States. A nonprofit hospital does not pay state or local property taxes or federal income taxes. This type of hospital is considered a charity, and it operates in accord with state and federal guidelines for charities. Such hospitals are typically associated with a charity purpose or religious denomination. Nonprofit hospitals are distinct from government-owned, public hospitals and privately owned, for-profit hospitals.

Government-Owned Public Hospitals

In the United States, public hospitals receive significant funding from local, state, and federal governments. In addition, they may charge Medicaid, Medicare, and private insurers for the care of patients. Public hospitals, especially in urban areas, have a high concentration of free care as compared to other American hospitals. Many also provide graduate medical education. Public and nonprofit rural hospitals form a large part of the health care safety net for the uninsured and poor underinsured in the US.

For-Profit Hospitals

A for-profit hospital is investor-owned or publicly owned by shareholders. This type of hospital issues shares of stock to raise money to expand the hospital offerings. For-profit hospitals were traditionally located in the southern part of the United States, particularly in Texas and Florida. Recently, for-profit hospitals have expanded nationwide. Investors often buy financially distressed facilities that can no longer afford to operate on their own.

Short-Stay Hospitals

Short-stay hospitals are also referred to as *acute-care facilities*, where patients are admitted to treat acute, or severe, medical problems. However, these facilities are very expensive, and insurance companies only cover a certain number of days of the patient's stay before requiring their transfer to a long-term care facility. General hospitals treat a wide range of conditions and age groups, providing diagnostic, medical, surgical, and emergency departments. There are also specialty hospitals such as burn centers, cancer (oncology) hospitals, children's hospitals, and orthopedic hospitals (dealing with bone, joint, or muscle disease). In addition, university or college medical centers can be private or government-supported and often offer research and health education.

Emergency departments are most often found in short-stay hospitals. Patients are taken to the emergency department for treatment when they have life-threatening symptoms related to stroke, severe trauma, excessive bleeding, chest pains, and other serious situations (Figure 1.20). People without insurance or an established primary care physician often go to emergency departments for treatment of noncritical problems. The wait time for treatment may be lengthy, and the cost may be higher than what patients would normally pay. If the patient is not able to pay for this treatment, the hospital will set up a payment schedule. The hospital will also see if the patient qualifies for Medicare or Medicaid. If a patient's bill remains unpaid, the hospital may write it off as a bad debt.

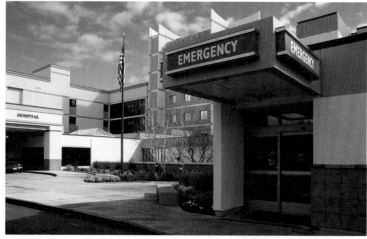

Galina Barskaya/Shutterstock.com

Figure 1.20 Emergency rooms often have separate entrances so that people recognize where to go to obtain rapid medical treatment.

Extend Your Knowledge ▶ Hospitals

If you live in the suburbs or in a city, you will most likely have a number of hospitals at your disposal. People living in rural areas may have to drive further for medical care. Your doctor may have privileges at only one hospital. Talk to your doctor to find out what hospital you are able to use. If your situation is serious, go to the closest hospital.

Apply It

1. Identify the hospital you would use if you needed a serious medical procedure. What do you know about this facility? Does your doctor have privileges at this facility? Is it a for-profit or nonprofit hospital?

2. How would you proceed if you wanted to gather information about what services your local hospital offers?

3. How can you find out if this hospital is the best one for your needs?

Long-Term Care Facilities

Long-term care facilities generally house elderly or disabled patients who have a medical problem or problems that keep them from being able to take care of themselves. While family members remain the primary caretakers of elderly, dependent, or disabled patients, the growing elderly population is increasing the demand for long-term care facilities. The number of long-term care facilities—often called *convalescent hospitals* or *nursing homes*—has gone up in recent years. Many patients have a short recovery stay at a nursing home after receiving treatment at an acute-care hospital. Others may live in long-term care for the rest of their lives.

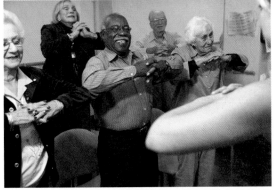

Monkey Business Images/Shutterstock.com

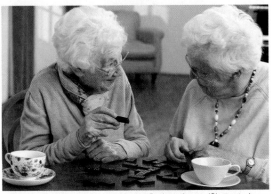

Monkey Business Images/Shutterstock.com

Figure 1.21   Many long-term care and independent-living facilities offer residents a variety of activities, including physical fitness classes and recreational games. Such activities are designed to strengthen the residents' physical, emotional, and mental health.

Independent-Living Facilities

Independent-living and assisted-living facilities are similar to long-term care facilities. Residents rent or purchase an apartment in the independent-living or assisted-living facility. Services such as meals, laundry, housekeeping, social events, transportation, and some basic medical care are provided (Figure 1.21).

These facilities are often associated with long-term care facilities. In some cases, an assisted-living resident may require additional medical care as he ages. When this happens, the person often moves from the assisted-living facility to the long-term care facility, where more around-the-clock medical care is offered.

Trauma Centers

Many hospitals are designated as trauma centers, which means that they are set up to handle the most serious of emergencies. Trauma surgeons and doctors trained in treating serious injuries are on staff at these centers. Highly sophisticated medical diagnostic equipment and treatment rooms designed for trauma injuries are available at these facilities. The leading causes of traumatic injuries are motor vehicle accidents, assaults, and falls.

Surgical Centers

Surgical centers are also called *ambulatory surgery centers*. These centers are designed to perform routine surgical procedures that do not require an overnight stay in the hospital. Minor surgeries such as biopsies, hernia repair, and cosmetic surgeries are performed in these centers.

Doctors' Offices

Doctors' offices can be found in almost every area of the country. Doctors often have family practices that focus on providing healthcare to people of all ages. These doctors provide continuing care such as annual checkups for all family members. Some doctors' offices focus on specialties such as orthopedics, pediatrics, cardiology, and obstetrics and gynecology. Doctors in these offices are often affiliated with a hospital where they will perform surgery or send their patients, if necessary.

Urgent-Care Centers

Urgent-care centers often serve as family practices as well. These facilities treat injuries or illnesses that are not life threatening, but require same-day intervention. Urgent-care centers usually do not take appointments, so the wait time may be significant, but not as long as an emergency room. Urgent-care facilities are often less expensive than an emergency room visit. Treatments at an urgent-care center might cover eye, ear, throat, and bladder infections; stomachaches; flu; asthma attacks; or broken bones and sprains. Both adults and children can be treated at urgent-care centers.

Walk-In Clinics

Walk-in clinics are found in some department stores, pharmacies, or shopping centers. There is much variation in the staff of these clinics—some are staffed by doctors, while others are staffed by nurse practitioners who have advanced degrees and training, and specialize in this line of work. These clinics are designed for the convenience of patients. Some are affiliated with hospitals. Most of these clinics treat colds, sinus infections, strep throat, muscle sprains, and other minor problems. Some walk-in clinics can also provide vaccinations, routine physicals, and pregnancy tests.

Dentists' Offices

Dentists' offices differ in size from office to office. Some dentists join together to form a dental clinic. There are also dental services in large retail stores. There are dentists that serve all ages and others who specialize in certain age groups, such as pediatric dentistry. Others may focus on certain dental conditions.

Optical Centers

Optical centers can be individually owned by an ophthalmologist or optometrist. There are also centers inside large chain stores.

Mental Health Facilities

These facilities provide mental health care for a variety of patients. Some of these patients are severely mentally ill, but may be able to function normally with treatment. Others are mentally disabled (such as accident victims and patients with developmental disabilities) or suffer from chronic mental disabilities and do not respond to treatment. Some facilities are clinics that treat patients at a same-day appointment. Others have patients stay for a certain period of time. Mental health facilities are often very expensive as funding for mental health services in the United States is declining.

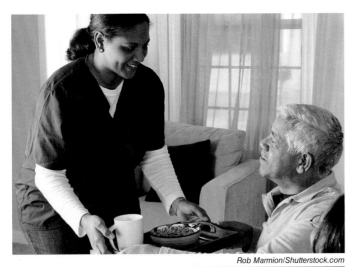
Rob Marmion/Shutterstock.com

Figure 1.22 The job outlook for home healthcare workers is expected to rise faster than average in the United States. Most home healthcare workers have graduated high school and receive on-the-job training.

Home Healthcare

Home healthcare is a popular alternative to long, costly hospital stays. Home healthcare agencies provide a wide variety of services for patients at home—from help with bathing, light housekeeping, and meal preparation, to skilled nursing care (Figure 1.22). Caregivers include registered nurses, practical nurses, and home health aides. Other caregivers may include physical therapists, social workers, and speech pathologists.

Hospice Care

hospice
a type of care designed to relieve pain and reduce suffering in terminally ill patients

Facilities that offer care for terminally ill (dying) patients are called **hospice** facilities, or *palliative care*. Hospice care focuses on relieving patients' pain and symptoms of their terminal illness without seeking to cure the illness. Hospitals can arrange for hospice services to be provided at the patient's home.

Kidney Dialysis Centers

Kidney dialysis is the process of removing waste products and excess fluid from the body (Figure 1.23). Dialysis centers provide comprehensive treatment for patients with chronic kidney disease. Patients visit the kidney dialysis center 3–4 times a week where machines serve as replacement kidneys.

Dialysis involves a machine that removes impurities and toxins from a patient's blood, which would normally be filtered and excreted from the body by the kidneys. People who undergo regular dialysis treatment usually have end-stage kidney disease and no more than 10–15 percent kidney function remaining. Dialysis patients are often waiting for a kidney transplant.

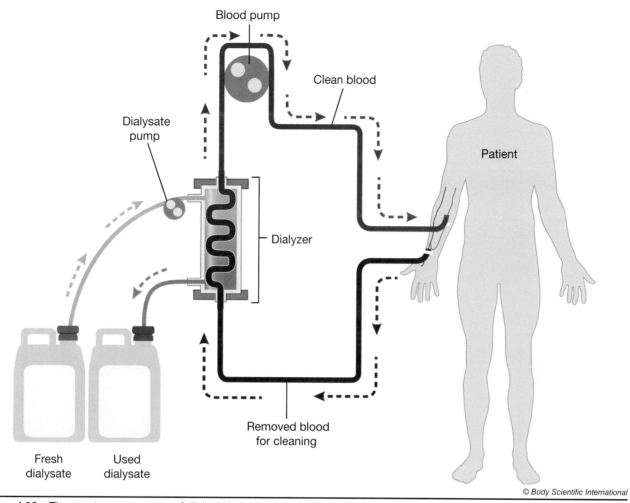

Figure 1.23   The most common type of dialysis is hemodialysis, a process by which blood is withdrawn from the body, filtered using a machine called a dialyzer, and then pumped back into the body. The filtering solution used by the dialyzer is called dialysate.

Rehabilitation Centers

Rehabilitation centers are facilities where patients work to reestablish or relearn abilities they lost because of a serious injury or illness, such as a stroke. Physical therapy helps with movement or previous loss of movement (Figure 1.24). Occupational therapy focuses on relearning activities of daily life or finding ways to perform them despite a disability.

Freestanding Laboratories and Radiology Facilities

For the convenience of patients, free-standing laboratory facilities are available for routine tests and blood drawing.

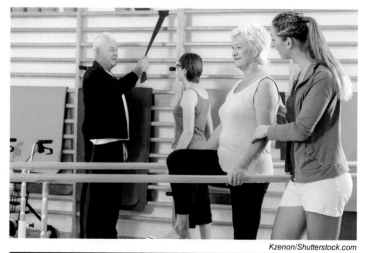

Kzenon/Shutterstock.com

Figure 1.24   Physical therapy exercises are designed to help a patient restore or improve their physical capabilities following an injury, surgery, or other medical condition.

Some of these facilities have the ability to produce rapid test results such as complete blood counts and throat cultures. Doctors often send their patients to freestanding laboratories when their own offices do not have the space or meet the staffing requirements for a lab. There are also radiology facilities separate from hospitals that perform routine radiology procedures.

Check Your Understanding ✓

1. What facility would a person go to after a serious car accident?
2. Where would you go if you needed a routine blood test?
3. What facility would be appropriate for a terminally ill person with no hope of recovery?
4. Where would you go if your kidneys failed?
5. What type of facility would be appropriate if you needed an appendectomy (surgery to remove the appendix)?

Consumer Responsibility

self-advocacy
refers to an individual's ability to effectively communicate, convey, negotiate, or assert his or her own interests, desires, needs, and rights

Within this complex healthcare system, you as a consumer must understand how the system can work for you. Although you are interested in a healthcare career, you will also utilize various healthcare facilities as a patient, or consumer, throughout your life. **Self-advocacy**, or protecting your own interests and making sure your needs are met, is an important element of being a healthcare consumer. It involves making informed decisions.

People often want to blame others when their needs are not met. You must be willing to advocate for yourself to receive the best care possible. You may need your doctor's help, support from your family, information about what treatment you need, and knowledge about the resources available to you.

Often, patients do not follow the directions given to them by their healthcare providers (possibly complaining that "I hate taking pills," or "I don't trust doctors"). Ultimately, it is the patient's responsibility to seek medical care, follow doctor's orders, and take advantage of available medical resources. Patients must comply with advice given by competent healthcare providers to get well. Healthcare is a two-way street—you must listen to medical advice just as your healthcare provider must listen carefully to you.

Rules and Regulations for the Healthcare Worker

It is important to understand the rules and regulations that apply to healthcare workers. Chapter 3, *Healthcare Laws and Ethics*, details the legal and ethical responsibilities of a professional healthcare employee. Depending on what state you live in and the type of facility in which you are employed, you will be given an employee handbook with all the rules and regulations you will be required to follow.

Generally, there are rules and regulations that cover

- treating patients with disabilities;
- patient rights;
- eligibility for Medicare and Medicaid;
- reporting facility accidents;
- reporting communicable diseases;
- how different facilities are run;
- treating patients with dignity; and
- maintaining confidentiality.

The Future of Healthcare

As healthcare in this country becomes more expensive, there will be continuing controversy over how to control costs. Should there be a different national health plan? Are healthcare mandates acceptable to the American public? Do we need more reform of our healthcare system?

The average life expectancy in the United States has dramatically increased since 1900, when the average life expectancy was 46.3 years for men, and 48.3 years for women. In the first decade of the 21st century, the average increased to 75.7 for men and 80.6 for women (Figure 1.25).

Hopefully, the future will bring cures for diseases like AIDS, and a decrease in cases of malaria, influenza, leprosy, and other diseases prevalent in developing countries. Much research is being done to cure genetically transferred diseases such as muscular dystrophy and cerebral palsy. Researchers are working aggressively on cures for heart disease, cancer, and Alzheimer's disease. In the future, new and exciting drugs will be developed that we cannot imagine at present.

There is still much to accomplish in the field of healthcare. Brilliant, innovative minds are continually at work in the spirit of such innovators as Hippocrates, Pasteur, Florence Nightingale, and the Curies. Medical technology continues to grow, with countries like the United States and Japan developing innovative medical devices to advance the healthcare industry. Hardworking healthcare workers will continue to provide outstanding care to those who are ill and suffering. Perhaps someday you, too, will contribute to this worthy cause.

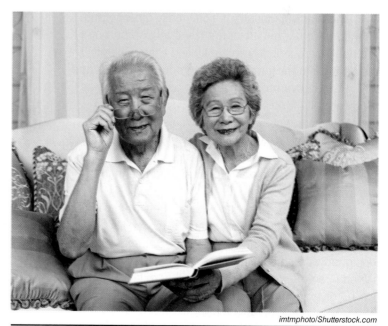

imtmphoto/Shutterstock.com

Figure 1.25   Thanks in part to medical advancements, the average life expectancy in the United States continues to rise.

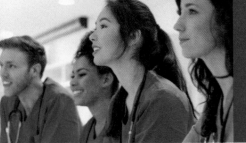

Summary

Healthcare has developed and changed dramatically throughout history. Healthcare discoveries that shaped the history of medicine and medical treatment have been made by cultures from around the world. The development of the printing press and the scientific method during the Renaissance allowed medical ideas and advances to spread quickly throughout the world.

The Industrial Revolution brought more effective communication tools and the development of sophisticated medical equipment. Vaccines were developed for smallpox, cholera, and tetanus. The introduction of anesthesia was an incredibly important contribution to the practice of surgery. Nursing became a respected profession and the importance of hand washing and sanitation was realized and promoted.

Scientists in the late nineteenth and twentieth centuries discovered the role of microorganisms in infection. Antibiotics and insulin were discovered. The discovery of DNA allowed researchers to begin unlocking the mysteries of heredity while advances in computers and electronics changed how clinical medicine is practiced.

The medical industry is continually growing and changing. Today, health insurance is a huge part of the healthcare industry. In the United States, health insurance is a mixture of private programs (HMOs and PPOs) and government insurance programs such as Medicare and Medicaid.

Government healthcare agencies such as the CDC, NIH, and OSHA play a critical role in our nation's health. Volunteer-based health service organizations also work to educate and promote good health in our communities.

Several types of healthcare facilities are available in communities across the country. Each facility has a unique set of rules and regulations, and many are designed with a specified purpose or patient in mind. When hired for a position at a healthcare facility, you will be given an employee handbook with all the rules and regulations you must follow.

As a healthcare consumer, you must advocate for yourself. Stay informed and keep an open mind about the advice you receive.

Review Questions

Answer the following questions using what you have learned in this chapter.

True or False Assess

1. *True or False?* The first vaccine developed was for polio.
2. *True or False?* Louis Pasteur developed a rabies vaccine.
3. *True or False?* Elizabeth Blackwell was the first woman to study and practice medicine in the US.
4. *True or False?* The American Red Cross is a government agency.
5. *True or False?* PPOs and HMOs are both examples of private insurance.
6. *True or False?* Psychoanalysis is a method of treating mental and physical disorders.
7. *True or False?* The caduceus and the staff of Aesculapius both feature two snakes wrapped around a staff.
8. *True or False?* The Hippocratic Oath is a promise of professional behavior made by doctors at the beginning of their careers.
9. *True or False?* Genomic medicine studies and identifies a person's DNA sequences.
10. *True or False?* FDA stands for the *Federal Drug Administration*.

Multiple Choice Assess

11. _____ are credited with the discovery of DNA.
    A. Marie and Pierre Curie
    B. James Watson, Francis Crick, and Maurice Wilkins
    C. Clara Barton and Alexander Fleming
    D. None of the above.

12. Which of the following is *not* a type of healthcare facility?
    A. Rehabilitation facility
    B. Emergency department
    C. Urgent care clinic
    D. Yoga studio

13. Which of the following health insurance plans is available in the United States?

    A. Medicare

    B. Medicaid

    C. Military Health System

    D. All of the above.

14. What are pathogens?

    A. harmless microorganisms

    B. vaccinations

    C. disease-producing organisms

    D. hand washing antiseptics

15. What is hospice care?

    A. a facility that rehabilitates addicts

    B. a physical therapy facility

    C. a facility that cares for the dying

    D. a long-term care facility

16. Many exciting inventions were made during the Renaissance, including the _____.

    A. forceps

    B. surgical needle

    C. microscope

    D. scalpel

17. Developments such as telegraph and railroad lines during the _____ enabled people to quickly and easily share ideas.

    A. Middle Ages

    B. Dark Ages

    C. Renaissance

    D. Industrial Revolution

18. Edward Jenner successfully vaccinated people for _____ using fluid from cowpox blisters, a symptom of a similar disease.

    A. cholera

    B. chicken pox

    C. smallpox

    D. rabies

19. _____ is the father of antiseptic surgery.

    A. Joseph Lister

    B. Louis Pasteur

    C. James Watson

    D. Alexander Fleming

20. _____ is a program jointly-funded by state and federal taxes that provides medical aid for low-income individuals of all ages.

    A. Medicare

    B. TRICARE

    C. Medicaid

    D. HMO

Short Answer

21. What roles do volunteer health agencies play in furthering health?

22. Name three government agencies tasked with improving our nation's health.

23. What causes bubonic plague?

24. What important invention did Antonie van Leeuwenhoek develop?

25. How did the development of aqueducts affect the people of ancient Greece?

26. What is an antibiotic?

27. Describe the practice of vaccination.

28. How has treatment of the mentally ill changed over time?

Critical Thinking Exercises

29. Research the effects of the bubonic plague in the Dark and Middle Ages. Why isn't the bubonic plague a huge problem for the world today?

30. Imagine your neighbor is a new mother confused by the conflicting information she hears through the media about vaccinations. She asks you for your opinions about vaccinating very young children. Research the pro and con arguments surrounding the vaccination of infants and children. How would you present your findings to your neighbor?

31. Imagine you are just starting a new job, and you're meeting with the human resources representative about your health insurance options. She tells you that you can choose either a PPO or HMO. Which plan do you think would best suit your needs? Why?

32. Are the hospitals in your area for-profit or nonprofit hospitals? What are the differences? If you had to choose to use one of the two, which would you pick and why?

33. What steps should you take to advocate for yourself when presented with a medical problem? Why is self-advocacy especially important when your health is concerned?

Chapter 2
Exploring Healthcare Careers

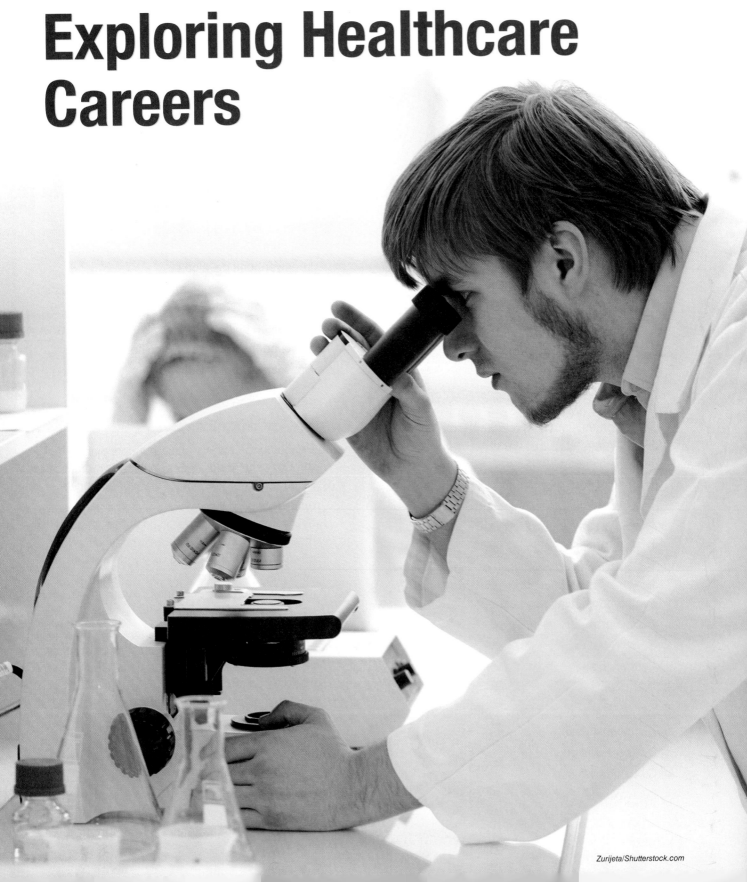

Terms to Know

 Build Vocab

associate's degree

bachelor's degree

biotechnology research and development

career ladder

certification

diagnostic-related groups (DRGs)

diagnostic services

doctorate

electronic health record (EHR)

health informatics services

job shadowing

licensure

master's degree

support services

therapeutic services

Chapter Objectives

- Understand the importance of self-assessment before embarking on a health career exploration.
- Identify the different levels of education required for various health careers.
- Compare and contrast licensure and certification for healthcare workers.
- Discuss the differences among the five pathways—therapeutic services, diagnostic services, health informatics, support services, and biotechnology research and development—as they relate to a healthcare setting.
- Identify careers in each of the five pathways, along with the educational requirements and responsibilities associated with each career.

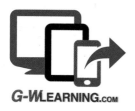

While studying, look for the activity icon to:

- **Build** vocabulary with e-flash cards and interactive games.
- **Assess** progress with chapter and unit review questions.
- **Expand** learning with animations and illustration labeling activities.
- **Simulate** EHR entry with healthcare documents.

G-WLEARNING.com

www.g-wlearning.com/healthsciences/

There are many career paths from which to choose, particularly in the healthcare field. Before selecting a future career, you might first ask yourself if you are suited for a career in healthcare. It is important to assess your goals and needs before you put time, energy, and money into pursuing a career. This chapter includes self-assessment questions as well as educational requirements and brief descriptions for many careers.

Planning for a Career in Healthcare

Many factors influence a person's choice of career. Some people pursue a career based on family expectations or suggestions of others. However, it's important not to take this decision lightly. You need to give serious thought to your talents, limitations, and goals for success before settling on a career. If you decide that your talents and goals are best suited for the healthcare field, you will need to choose a specific career path within the field. The following are tips for narrowing your desired career path in healthcare.

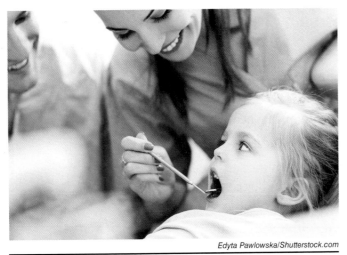

Edyta Pawlowska/Shutterstock.com

Figure 2.1 Some healthcare careers require working with patients of all ages.

Self-Assessment

Since the healthcare field offers a wide variety of career paths to choose from, it's important to consider what type of position would be best for you. Many factors will help you make this decision. As you begin researching careers in the medical field, ask yourself the following questions. Your answers to these questions will help guide you toward your ideal career:

- Do you like being with people of all ages (Figure 2.1)?

- Do you enjoy working as a team player, or do you prefer to work alone?

- Do you consider yourself a successful communicator?

- Do you enjoy working with computers more than interacting with others?

- Do you find helping others rewarding?

- Do you consider yourself an empathetic, compassionate person?

- Can you work with patients who may be scared, difficult, or uncomfortable?

- Are you comfortable making decisions?

- Is job security an important consideration for you?

- Do you want to work only a nine-to-five, weekday job?

- Are you comfortable supervising the work of other people?

- Do you like to be creative in your work, or are you more comfortable with having one way to do things?

- Are you open to continuing education or on-the-job training after you are hired?
- Do you enjoy solving problems?
- Do you imagine yourself advancing up the career ladder quickly?
- Do you aspire to become a leader?
- Do you see yourself as a high wage earner?
- Do you enjoy being in school?
- Do hospitals and sick people make you feel queasy?
- Would you rather work outside, or inside a healthcare facility?

> ## Did You Know? Working as a Team
>
> The ability to work as part of a team is considered one of the most important skills in today's job market. Employers value workers who can contribute their own ideas but also work collaboratively with others to create and develop projects and brainstorm ways to be efficient and productive.

It is critically important to find a career that matches your interests and abilities. Your school counselor should be able to help you identify a potential career path using career assessment testing (Figure 2.2). These tests are not perfect but may give you a starting point when looking for a career that will best suit you.

In addition to seeking the help of your guidance counselor, you can also access free career inventory tests online. Some helpful career assessments include the Holland Codes, the Myers-Briggs Type Indicator, and the Enneagram of Personality.

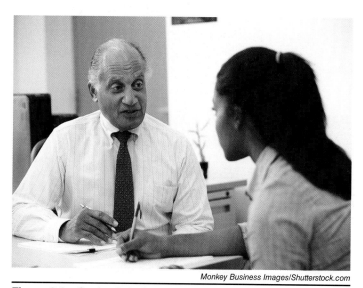

Monkey Business Images/Shutterstock.com

Figure 2.2 Getting help from your school counselor is an important way to assess your goals and needs for a career.

Job Shadowing

Another valuable resource that may be available to you is **job shadowing**. Before making a commitment to a particular career and its related courses, you may want to shadow a person who already has that job.

Job shadowing allows you to follow an employee completing the tasks of a job you find interesting. This allows you to see for yourself what the job entails. You might find that your concept of the career was not accurate, or that you are not suited for the day-to-day demands of the position. Another benefit of job shadowing is that it exposes you to the sights, sounds, and even smells you may encounter in the healthcare world.

job shadowing
a job exploration tool that involves following an employee while he or she completes the tasks of a job you find interesting

Your school counselor can help you set up job shadowing opportunities, or you can even contact a healthcare facility yourself and ask about job shadowing possibilities.

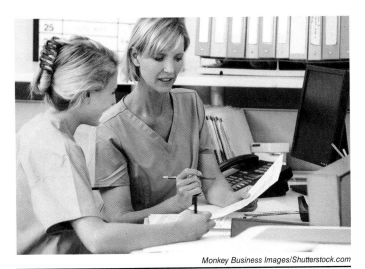

Monkey Business Images/Shutterstock.com

Figure 2.3 A clinical internship will allow you to use the knowledge and skills gained in class in a professional setting.

Clinical Internships

Many health science courses include a clinical internship. A course might consist of classroom instruction, laboratory exercises, skill practice, and the clinical application of knowledge and skills. Some classes start with classroom learning and contain hands-on experience in a healthcare facility before completing the course.

Clinical experience exposes you to healthcare professionals who will instruct and observe your practice of basic skills in the healthcare facility (Figure 2.3). You are also exposed to real, day-to-day experiences that allow you to observe several potential healthcare careers. Clinical internships can be as short as a few weeks or as long as a semester or a year. This experience also offers the unique opportunity to become known in a facility as a prospective employee.

Extend Your Knowledge ▶ The Importance of Forming Healthy Relationships

As you begin to decide on a career path and take courses to help you realize your goals, maintaining healthy relationships becomes very important. Maintaining strong relationships with friends and family and forming healthy relationships with classmates, teachers, and healthcare professionals you encounter will have a positive impact as you work toward your chosen career. The support and encouragement of these individuals will keep you focused and help ensure your success, both in school and your future career.

Forming strong relationships with your instructors is very important. These individuals are wonderful resources, with extensive knowledge to share. The grades you earn will also play a part in being hired or accepted into advanced programs. Your instructors may also write letters of recommendation when you begin your career, depending on whether or not they think you can contribute positively in that position.

When you are assigned to a clinical internship, the relationships you build with your fellow healthcare workers can enrich your experience. A positive clinical experience may increase your motivation to achieve the career goals you have set for yourself. Your fellow workers will also help you hone your skills and teach you how to provide patients with exceptional care. As you near graduation, these individuals can provide helpful career advice and possibly recommend you for a job.

Apply It

1. Do you feel that you have established good relationships with your healthcare instructors? Why or why not?

2. Think about the relationships you have with your family members, friends, classmates, and instructors. Then consider how each relationship might help you achieve your career goals. Do you think any of these relationships might hinder your career goals? Why or why not?

Choosing a Career Path

Once you have identified your personal strengths, talents, likes, and dislikes, you can begin to research the type of career you would like to pursue. In addition to evaluating your personality needs, you should consider how much education you are willing to complete, what kind of salary you want, and what type of workplace environment you would prefer. You will want to make sure there are plenty of opportunities available in the healthcare field you are researching.

The *Occupational Outlook Handbook* is a very useful starting point for researching a career. This resource can be found online. It provides career information, including working conditions, the training and education required, salary, and job outlook for hundreds of healthcare careers. A great deal of information about healthcare careers can be found elsewhere on the Internet, but you need to be aware of how current or accurate this information is. The United States government produces many publications related to jobs, such as guides for writing résumés, finding federal government jobs, and how to act while on a job interview. These publications can be found online. The National Institutes of Health (NIH), a government organization, also offers excellent Internet resources that discuss medical careers.

Many healthcare associations publish journals that include valuable career information. You can find these journals at your school or local library. Such journals include *The Journal of the American Medical Association (JAMA)*, *The Journal of Medical Ethics*, *The American Journal of Nursing*, *The Online Journal of Issues in Nursing*, and *The Journal of Physical Therapy*. Some communities also have a medical library, which is especially helpful when looking for specific periodicals and research materials that focus on medical issues and career possibilities. The career counselor at your school may be able to help you with your search. It is also helpful to cultivate relationships with professionals who are already working in a career in which you have some interest. They can give you invaluable, practical career advice.

Decision Making

People often say that making decisions is difficult. You probably know people who put off making decisions because they are afraid of making the wrong decision. People may endlessly search for more information or depend on others to make decisions for them. Are you one of these people?

The first important decision you will make in your career is choosing a career pathway to reach your goal. This decision will be the first of many you make throughout your career.

Making an informed decision is an important skill to master (Figure 2.4). Future employers will be impressed to know that you can make

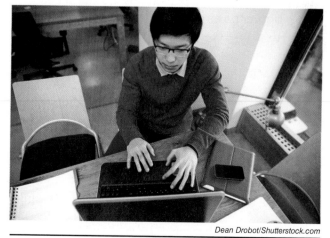

Dean Drobot/Shutterstock.com

Figure 2.4   Thorough research will help prepare you to make an informed decision about your future career path.

decisions after gathering facts and figures and use reasoning to come to conclusions. Of course, you do not want to go off on your own and make decisions without consulting your supervisor.

Do not let emotions affect your decisions. Try your best to be open and neutral about the issue. Poor decisions can be made when emotions drive the process instead of reason. Don't rush a decision. Get in touch with your intuition as well. Does the decision feel right to you?

When faced with decision making like choosing a career path, research the decision carefully, get advice if you are not sure how to proceed, and then follow through. Be confident in your decision and move on. Failure to make a decision can impede the progress of a task you are assigned. You may have to evaluate and modify a decision after making one. You may find that another career choice may work better for you. Be flexible if you need to modify your plan.

Real Life Scenario — Choosing a Career Path

Chase comes from a family of healthcare professionals. Chase has been encouraged to follow the family career path for most of his education. As a high school student, he has taken some health science courses and is being pressured by his family to choose a pathway. Several options are presented by family members, who are convinced they know what's best for Chase:

- Chase's dad wants Chase to become a doctor and join his medical practice.
- Chase's mom thinks he would make a great hospital administrator, so he should major in business.
- Chase's grandfather is a dentist and hopes Chase will take over his dental practice.

Chase feels he would not be comfortable working with his father, who can be very critical and controlling, in his practice. He also feels that he will never be as passionate about teeth as his grandfather, and does not feel he would enjoy a career in dentistry. Being a hospital administrator does not appeal to Chase either. He is not interested in business or being responsible for an entire hospital.

The one thing Chase does know is that he loves science, research, and working in a lab. He would love to develop a cure for a disease someday. Chase is shy and does not like the idea of interacting with patients.

Apply It

1. If you were Chase, how would you explain to the family that you do not want to follow in their footsteps?
2. What do you think would happen if Chase were to choose one of the options that his family wants?
3. Imagine you are Chase's school counselor. What steps would you suggest Chase take to learn more about a career in medical research?

Educational Requirements

As you begin to explore a career in healthcare, you should research how much education will be required for various careers. The amount of education you need varies from career to career and state to state. Ask yourself how much education you are prepared to pursue. You may not enjoy classroom work and find that on-the-job training would better suit you. Conversely, you might really enjoy classroom work and wish to take a variety of classes to satisfy your academic curiosity and explore different fields.

High School

A high school education will prepare a student for an entry-level position after graduation. Most occupations require at least a high school diploma. Specific classes that explore health careers or health occupations would be particularly helpful to take. Some high schools offer certification programs at the high school level. Graduates may start an entry-level career immediately following high school.

On-the-Job Training

During high school or after graduation, you can receive training to help advance your career. This training can be available for many careers such as home health aide, medical receptionist, food service worker, or central services worker. Though on-the-job training can be beneficial, further advancement will come through more formal education.

Technical Schools

Sometimes referred to as *vocational*, *trade*, or *proprietary schools*, technical schools provide training for specific careers beyond high school. Technical schools can be more expensive than training at a community college because technical schools are privately owned and operated. However, scholarships and loans are often available to cover these educational costs.

Two-year technical degrees and certifications are available, and some schools offer four-year degrees and higher degrees as well. Job placement guarantees are often part of a technical school's offerings. Many of these schools have agreements with local companies to place students in unpaid internships. Then companies are able to assess potential employees before making employment commitments. In turn, companies work with the schools to ensure their students are exposed to the skill sets they require of their employees.

Community College

A community college usually offers a two-year degree, called an **associate's degree**, in a specific course for a healthcare career. Students can use an associate's degree to transfer to a four-year college, where they can work toward a bachelor's degree. There are also many certificate programs at the community college level. Such programs might include emergency medical technician, medical assistant, health information technology, medical laboratory technician, and nursing.

Internships are often a part of community college programs. Internships (also called *the community classroom*, *externship*, or *clinical rotations*) involve placement and training in a healthcare facility. Internships are usually unpaid and require completion of a specified number of hours. These experiences give students the opportunity to observe and practice the skills learned in the program or course.

> **Think It Through**
>
> What attracted you to a career in healthcare? Did a family member who works in healthcare inspire you to explore the field? Do you have a mentor who encouraged you to follow this path? Are you motivated by a desire to help people?

associate's degree
a two-year college degree, often offered through a community college and awarded after completing 60 credit hours or more in a semester system

Four-Year College or University

bachelor's degree
a four-year college degree awarded after 120 credit hours or more in a semester system

Some healthcare careers require students to obtain a **bachelor's degree** and complete further training before starting a career. This training may include a clinical internship in which the student or recent graduate undergoes supervised training before becoming licensed or certified. Some clinical internships are unpaid, while others offer a small stipend (money given to offset costs such as transportation) during training. If you are taking classes full-time, a bachelor's degree typically takes about four years to complete.

Some professional-level careers may prefer candidates who have earned a further degree such as a **master's degree**. A master's degree can take one or more years of education to earn.

master's degree
academic degree awarded by a college or university to those who complete from one to two years (depending on the degree) of prescribed study beyond the bachelor's degree

High-level positions often require an advanced degree called a **doctorate** degree. Several professional schools offer such degrees. A student can earn a professional doctoral degree in medical fields such as medical doctor (MD) and veterinarian (DVM), or an academic doctorate such as a doctor of philosophy (PhD). Each of these doctoral degrees can take several years to attain.

Figure 2.5 shows the various levels of employment and the education they require, and provides examples of job titles found at each level.

doctorate
a degree awarded after two to six years of education beyond the bachelor's degree; available in many disciplines

Continuing Education

In many healthcare occupations, your education continues after you are hired. Some employers or government agencies require you to take additional courses to maintain professional status in your career. These requirements vary from state to state and among careers. In today's world, where changes and discoveries continually occur, continuing education is critical. Opportunities for continuing education may be offered at your place of employment; online; or through courses offered by schools, colleges, or private organizations or companies. If you are resistant to any change in your job, continuing education may be a challenge for you.

Healthcare Employment Levels		
Level	**Educational Requirements**	**Example**
Professional	four-year degree; advanced degree; clinical training; possible licensure	physician; registered nurse practitioner; registered nurse; pharmacist
Technologist	three to four years of college; clinical training; possible licensure	laboratory technologist; radiologic technologist
Technician	often associate's degree; clinical training; possible licensure	X-ray technician; health information technician; licensed vocational nurse
Assistant	up to one year of classroom and clinical training	physical therapy assistant; medical assistant; nursing assistant
Aide	high school diploma; on-the-job training	laboratory aide; central services aide

Goodheart-Willcox Publisher

Figure 2.5   Healthcare careers vary by level and educational requirements. Continuing your education is one way to advance in your healthcare career.

Licensure and Certification

In addition to educational requirements and training, some careers require **licensure** and **certification**. By obtaining licensure or certifications, employees ensure they have met all of the standards required for a particular healthcare career. In some cases, licensure or certification status must be maintained by meeting continuing education requirements, such as taking an additional course in your field.

Licensure

Licensure is awarded by a state agency when a person meets the qualifications for a particular occupation. People seeking licensure must pass a licensing exam. For instance, laboratory technologists must take a state examination and pass with a certain percentage before obtaining a license to work as a technologist. Registered nurses and licensed vocational nurses must pass a state board examination and receive a license to practice in a particular state.

Certification

Certification is given as recognition for completing a specific course of study and/or passing a certification exam. For instance, a phlebotomist (a person who draws blood) may earn a certificate after completing the clinical training hours required in the course of study. A health information technician must have an associate's degree and pass an examination given by a certifying agency to become a registered health information technician (RHIT).

In some occupations, certification is voluntary. An individual may choose to take a certification exam for professional advancement. In other cases, certification is required.

licensure
recognition given by a state agency when a person meets the qualifications for a particular occupation; given after the person passes a licensure examination; required to practice

certification
recognition given for completing a course of study and/or passing a certification exam

Check Your Understanding ✔

1. Explain the difference between licensure and certification.
2. What is the difference between a technical school and a community college?
3. What is the name of the handbook that can be helpful to you when researching careers?
4. What is job shadowing?
5. Explain why a clinical internship would be helpful as you prepare for your future career.

Healthcare Careers by Pathway

Do you follow the latest technology trends and enjoy working with computers? Are you interested in encouraging healthy lifestyles and helping promote wellness in patients of all ages? Does using your knowledge and training to diagnose and treat injuries and diseases appeal to you? Imagine being in a position to save someone's life—what an amazing feeling that would be!

If the job situations listed above appeal to you, then a career in healthcare is something to explore. To choose a specific path in the healthcare field, you should research and compare a variety of careers. In this section you will learn about several of these healthcare careers. These careers are divided into five pathways—therapeutic services, diagnostic services, health informatics, support services, and biotechnology research and development. Each of the five pathways contains a variety of careers that represent related areas of expertise, education, training, and skills. Figure 2.6 illustrates the five pathways presented in this chapter and how these careers are organized within a large healthcare facility.

It is important for you to be aware of your options before embarking on a path that may not be suitable for your long-term needs. This is when job shadowing and talking with a career counselor are very important steps to take.

Therapeutic Services

therapeutic services
career path that offers hands-on experience with patients and focuses on changing the health status of a patient over time

The **therapeutic services** pathway offers many career possibilities ranging from driving an ambulance to working with a child who has speech problems. Do hands-on experiences with patients seem like something you would enjoy? If so, you may find a career in the therapeutic services rewarding. Figure 2.7 presents some therapeutic services careers, along with their educational requirements. Use this figure to begin exploring careers that interest you.

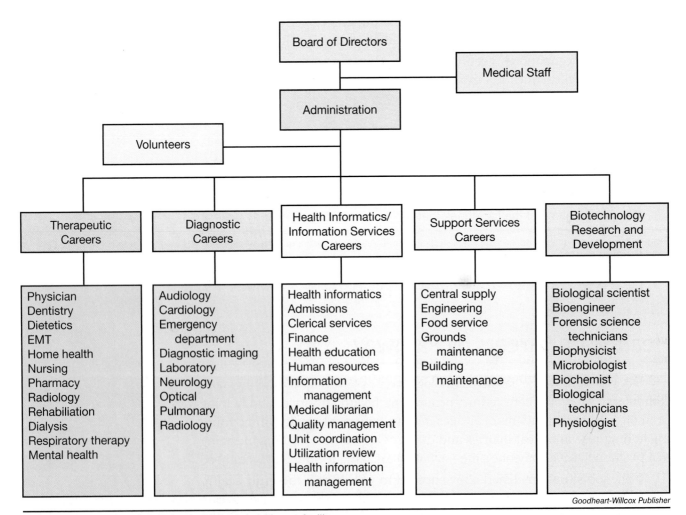

Goodheart-Willcox Publisher

Figure 2.6 Organizational chart of a large healthcare facility.

Educational Requirements for Common Therapeutic Careers			
High School Diploma/ Industry Certification/ On-the-Job Training	**Associate's Degree**	**Bachelor's Degree**	**Master's or Professional Degree**
home health aide; certified nursing assistant (CNA); patient care technician (PCT)	registered nurse (RN)	registered nurse (RN, BSN)	nurse practitioner (MSN, FNP); registered nurse (RN, BSN, MSN); doctorate of nursing practice (DNP)
respiratory therapist aide	respiratory therapy technician	respiratory therapist (RRT)	pulmonologist (MD)
emergency medicine tech (EMT)	paramedic	[required for admittance into advanced degree programs]	exercise physiologist
medical receptionist; file clerk; medical assistant (in some facilities)	administrative front office; clinical back office medical assistant; office manager	physician assistant (PA)	physician (MD); physician assistant (PA)
physical therapy assistant; sports medicine aide	physical therapy assistant; sports medicine assistant	athletic trainer; physical therapist	speech and language pathologist; physiatrist, MD; physical therapist (MPT); doctorate of physical therapy (DPT)
dental assistant	dental laboratory technician; dental hygienist	[required for admittance into advanced degree programs]	dentist (DDS)
pharmacy clerk	pharmacy technician	[required for admittance into advanced degree programs]	pharmacist (PharmD)
mental health aide	mental health technician; substance abuse counselor	counselor	counselor; psychologist; psychiatrist (MD)
veterinarian assistant	veterinarian technician	[required for admittance into advanced degree programs]	veterinarian (DVM)
occupational therapy aide	certified occupational therapy assistant (COTA)	occupational therapist (OT)	Masters of Science in Occupational Therapy (MOT)

Goodheart-Willcox Publisher

Figure 2.7   Many fulfilling career opportunities exist in therapeutic services. These careers vary greatly based on education.

Careers in the therapeutic services pathway are focused primarily on changing the health status of a patient over time. Health professionals in this pathway work directly with patients by providing care, treatment, counseling, and health education information (Figure 2.8). The amount of education required for therapeutic services careers varies.

There is much room for career advancement in this pathway. For instance, you can train on-the-job for an assistant or aide level career, and then go back to school to get an associate's degree in a related field. If you want to further advance your career to one with better pay and more responsibility, you can get a four-year degree or higher.

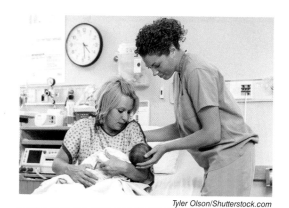

Tyler Olson/Shutterstock.com

Figure 2.8   Nurses, like many professionals in therapeutic services, must be comfortable working closely with patients.

career ladder

term for the progression from an entry-level position to higher levels of pay, skill, and responsibility

Nurses

Nursing is an exciting field that offers many opportunities for employment as well as advancement. For example, you may begin your career as a certified nursing assistant but eventually decide you would like more responsibility.

Licensed practical nurse (LPN) and licensed vocational nurse (LVN) are different titles for the same job. In Texas and California, this nurse is called a *licensed vocational nurse.* Throughout all other states, this nurse is called a *licensed practical nurse.* This nurse works under registered nurses. It can take as little as 13 months to earn this degree, which requires licensure after training.

To become a registered nurse (RN), you must obtain at least an associate's degree in nursing. Depending on the school, the name of the associate's degree may change; possibilities include an associate's degree in nursing (AN), an associate's degree of applied science in nursing (AAS), or an associate's degree in nursing (ADN).

Further professional development might lead you to pursue a bachelor's degree (BSN), a master's degree (MSN), or a doctorate degree (DNP, DNS, or PhD) in nursing. These advanced degrees will allow you to become a nurse administrator, manager, an instructor, or a nurse practitioner. RNs who hold a bachelor's degree rather than an associate's degree have opportunities for further career advancement, increased responsibility such as filling a supervisor role, and a higher salary.

There are many opportunities to climb the **career ladder** and receive a promotion in the medical field (Figure 2.9). If you originally earn an associate's degree in nursing, earning more degrees allows you to make a higher salary and opens up opportunities for specialization (for example, critical care nursing), and more responsibility.

Nurses are employed in many types of healthcare facilities. Many options are available if you would prefer to work in a small healthcare facility, including clinics, doctor's offices, and nursing homes. Figure 2.10 is a sample of the organization and hierarchy of the medical staff in a smaller facility. For current information about the careers mentioned in this organizational chart, see your school's job counselor or conduct further research online.

Doctors

Becoming a doctor (otherwise known as an *MD* or *physician*) requires many years of hard work that includes earning admission into colleges, universities, and medical school; studying; testing; writing; researching; and training.

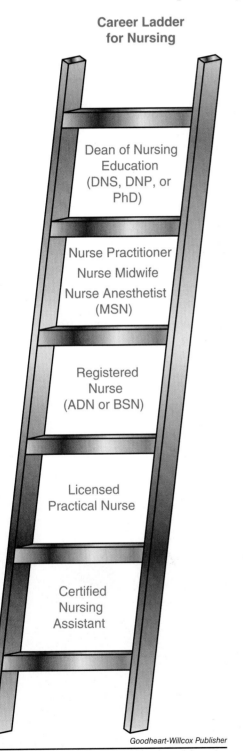

Career Ladder for Nursing

Dean of Nursing Education (DNS, DNP, or PhD)

Nurse Practitioner
Nurse Midwife
Nurse Anesthetist (MSN)

Registered Nurse (ADN or BSN)

Licensed Practical Nurse

Certified Nursing Assistant

Goodheart-Willcox Publisher

Figure 2.9   For members of the nursing staff, climbing the career ladder often requires additional education.

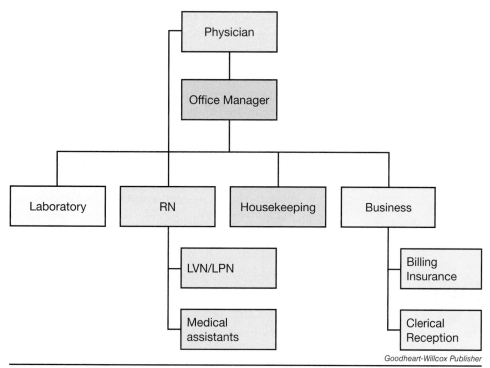

Goodheart-Willcox Publisher

Figure 2.10   Medical office organization chart

To achieve optimal success as a doctor of medicine, you should start preparing as early as possible, preferably in high school. The required education can take about 10 to 15 years after high school to complete, depending on what specialty (the specific area of medicine to be practiced) you choose. Although doctors are listed under the therapeutic careers, they are equally involved in diagnostic services.

As with many, if not most healthcare careers, successful doctors often exhibit strong leadership skills. A doctor, if in private practice, must be a capable leader of her staff. She must be able to work with hospital staff, building consensus among colleagues if necessary, and understanding group dynamics. Dealing with patients also requires that the doctor lead a patient through treatment. This means presenting each patient with options to consider and helping him make informed decisions about treatment.

Dentists

Dentistry is the branch of medicine that involves the study, diagnosis, prevention, and treatment of diseases, disorders, and conditions of the oral cavity and nearby structures (Figure 2.11). Individuals who have graduated from dental school are called *dentists*, or *doctors of dental surgery* (*DDS*).

After earning a bachelor's degree, candidates for dental school take the Dental Admissions Test (DAT) to ensure they are prepared for dental school training. The DAT is a multiple choice examination

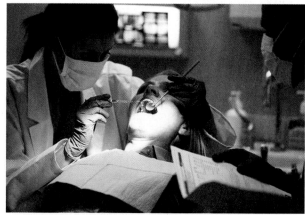

Monkey Business Images/Shutterstock.com

Figure 2.11   A dentist and dental hygienist work as a team to provide thorough, quality care for their patients.

that includes sections focused on the sciences (especially biology and chemistry), math, reading comprehension, and perceptual ability testing (the test taker's spatial visualization skills). To prepare for the DAT, future dentists should take courses in these areas during their undergraduate education.

Dental schools should be fully accredited, or *recognized*, by the American Dental Association's (ADA) Commission on Dental Accreditation. Dental school usually lasts four years, and graduates earn a doctor of dental surgery (DDS).

Veterinarians

Veterinarians care for animals by diagnosing, treating, or researching their medical conditions and diseases. In their practice, veterinarians treat pets, livestock, and animals found in zoos, racetracks, and laboratories (Figure 2.12).

Students who wish to enter a veterinary program typically obtain a bachelor's degree in a science-related area such as zoology, molecular biology, chemistry, animal science, or biochemistry. In some instances, veterinary programs do not require students to hold four-year degrees. However, students may experience difficulty gaining admittance into veterinary programs as these schools are extremely competitive, even with a degree.

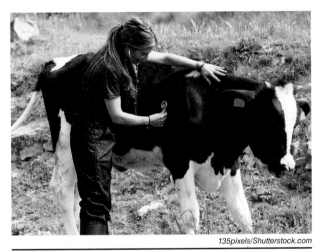
135pixels/Shutterstock.com
Figure 2.12 Veterinarians work in a variety of environments, depending on the type of animals in their care.

Veterinary students are required to complete a four-year doctor of veterinary medicine (DVM) program in addition to earning their bachelor's degree. These professionals are also required to obtain licensure to practice in the profession.

Respiratory Care Workers

Helping patients with their breathing is a critical part of healthcare. Without proper breathing, patients can suffer brain damage within a few minutes, with death following soon after.

Respiratory care workers perform many tasks to help patients who are having trouble with their breathing. Respiratory therapists test the patient's lung capacity and check oxygen and carbon dioxide levels in his or her blood. These workers give patients treatments and teach patients with chronic lung conditions to care for themselves. Respiratory therapists also provide emergency care to patients who have suffered strokes, electrical shock, heart failure, and other life-threatening conditions. As part of their responsibilities, respiratory therapists take care of their equipment and do a great deal of record keeping.

As Figure 2.7 shows, there is great potential for moving up the career ladder in this field. By continuing their education, respiratory care workers can advance from an aide to a technician-level position, or become a respiratory therapist after earning their bachelor's degree. Respiratory therapists might even advance to the level of pulmonologist, a doctor who specializes in the care and treatment of the lungs.

Physical Therapy and Occupational Therapy Workers

Physical and occupational therapists both provide rehabilitative care to patients who have been injured or have a disability. These careers share the goal of improving patient function and movement. Therapists require creativity and flexibility while working with patients to find the right equipment and tools to help the varying needs of each individual.

Physical therapists and physical therapy aides assist and direct patients in the process of rehabilitation after an injury or surgery. A physical therapist's goals are to reduce pain, restore physical function, and promote healing. Physical therapists use exercises, stretching, and equipment to prevent pain, improve wellness, and increase mobility (Figure 2.13).

Occupational therapy workers interact with people who are physically, mentally, developmentally, or emotionally disabled. These workers plan and develop programs that help restore, maintain, or develop the patient's ability to manage activities of daily living (ADL). An occupational therapist may also evaluate a patient's environment to determine assistive devices and equipment that may prove helpful.

Both physical and occupational therapists work in hospitals, schools, nursing homes, outpatient clinics, rehabilitation centers, and mental health facilities.

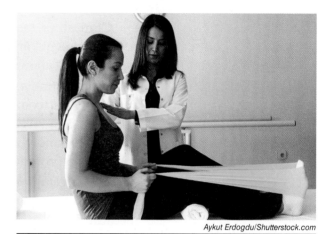

Aykut Erdogdu/Shutterstock.com

Figure 2.13 Physical therapists develop and implement treatment plans specific to each patient's needs and goals.

Emergency Medical Service Providers

Peoples' lives often depend on the quick reaction and competent care of emergency medical technicians (EMTs) and paramedics (Figure 2.14). Incidents as varied as automobile accidents, heart attacks, slips and falls, childbirth, and gunshot wounds require immediate medical attention. EMTs and paramedics provide this vital service as they care for and transport the sick or injured to a medical facility.

The primary difference between an EMT and a paramedic is the amount of education required and the tasks they are allowed to perform on the job. Both are highly skilled but are not equal in the level of care that they can provide.

In an emergency, EMTs and paramedics are typically dispatched to the scene by a 911 operator. When they arrive on the scene, EMTs and paramedics often work alongside police and firefighters. EMTs and paramedics immediately assess the nature of the patient's condition, while trying to determine whether the patient has any preexisting medical conditions. Following protocols and procedures, these workers provide emergency care

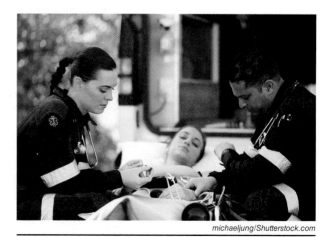

michaeljung/Shutterstock.com

Figure 2.14 Paramedics and EMTs must remain calm when dealing with life-and-death situations.

and transport the patient to a medical facility. EMTs and paramedics perform their duties in emergency medical services systems in which a doctor provides medical direction and oversight.

For more information about emergency medical service providers, refer to Chapter 14, *Working in Healthcare.*

Medical Assistants

Medical assistants work primarily in doctors' offices, clinics, and other outpatient medical facilities. They perform the administrative and clinical duties needed to assist doctors in providing patient care. Medical assistants may work with doctors who provide either general or specialized care.

Clinical, or *back office*, medical assistants help doctors with examinations, treatments, and diagnostic procedures. In many states, clinical medical assistants are allowed to give injections and draw blood.

Administrative, or *front office*, medical assistants manage the reception area. They also complete clerical duties, such as managing insurance claims, collections, and electronic medical records. Many medical assistants study to become comprehensive medical assistants, skilled in both administrative and clinical procedures.

Many community colleges, adult schools, and proprietary schools offer medical assistant programs. Although no license is required to practice as a medical assistant, many employers want medical assistants to be certified.

Additional careers that can be classified as therapeutic include certified athletic trainers (ATC), art therapists, massage therapists, radiation therapists, wellness coaches, and speech and language therapists.

Check Your Understanding ✓

1. What is the difference between an occupational therapist and a physical therapist?
2. What does a respiratory therapist do in the healthcare facility?
3. What are three nursing positions a person can hold after earning a master's or doctorate?
4. Name two types of medical assistants.

Diagnostic Services

diagnostic services
a healthcare pathway offering careers in implementing procedures to determine causes of diseases or disorders

When you choose the **diagnostic services** healthcare career path, you become an integral part of the diagnosing process. These careers involve procedures that determine the causes of diseases or disorders. Some workers in this pathway have direct contact with patients, but others do not.

Some careers are not only considered diagnostic, but fall into the therapeutic services category as well. An example of this is a cardiologist who diagnoses heart-related problems, but also works with patients and recommends therapies.

Diagnostic careers focus on planning services for patients as well as performing tests accurately. Those in this career path are responsible for quality control, which involves implementing a system for verifying and maintaining a desired level of quality in a product or process, use of proper equipment, continued inspection, and corrective action as required. If you are engaged in any testing procedures, you *must* produce accurate results and report them in a timely manner. Record keeping is also very important in this area.

Diagnostic services workers are often unseen by patients. They often work more with machines than with patients. If you enjoy working with technology, this might be the correct choice for you.

When you work in diagnostic services, attention to detail is critical. Sloppy handling of specimens to be tested, failure to correctly enter results into a computer, and an inability to meet deadlines can lead to termination. Remember, an incorrect test result could adversely affect the treatment of a patient. As with many healthcare fields, diagnostic services offer a variety of jobs depending on your level of education. As you read through the job titles in Figure 2.15, think about which diagnostic careers interest you the most.

The Clinical Laboratory

The clinical laboratory, often called the *medical laboratory*, is a separate section of a healthcare facility. The laboratory is the place where blood, urine, sputum (mucus coughed up from the lung), stool (feces), and tissues are analyzed in a precise, accurate, and timely manner. Analysis of these specimens provides valuable information about a patient's medical condition. A number of conditions can be rapidly diagnosed by the laboratory, including heart attack, diabetes, and strep throat.

Educational Requirements for Common Diagnostic Careers			
High School Diploma/Industry Certification/On-the-Job Training	**Associate's Degree**	**Bachelor's Degree**	**Master's Degree or Professional Degree**
clinical laboratory aide; phlebotomist; venipuncture technician; clinical laboratory clerical worker	clinical laboratory technician; cytologist; histologist	clinical laboratory technologist	clinical laboratory supervisor; laboratory administrator; chief technologist; pathologist
EKG technician	cardiovascular technologist	[required for admittance into advanced degree programs]	cardiologist
X-ray technician*; radiology aide	CT scan technologist*; radiologic technologist	diagnostic medical sonographer; radiologic technologist chief	radiologist; radiation oncologist
ophthalmology aide	optician	[required for admittance into advanced degree programs]	optometrist; ophthalmologist

*Note: An advanced degree may be required by some states.

Goodheart-Willcox Publisher

Figure 2.15 Advancement in diagnostic service careers can result from additional education.

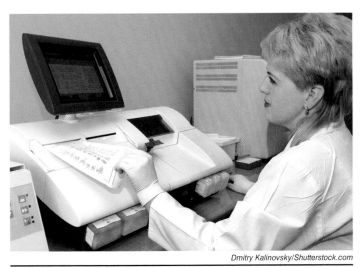

Figure 2.16   Clinical laboratory professionals work with sophisticated, often automated machinery.

Many tests in the clinical laboratory are very complicated and involve complex machines that require extensive training to operate (Figure 2.16). Clinical laboratory technologists train other staff members on the use of laboratory machines. Tests that are relatively simple and may not require the use of complex machines can be accomplished by the clinical laboratory technician or clinical laboratory aide. Each state has its own requirements for performing clinical laboratory tests.

There are many work environments available to clinical laboratory workers, such as acute care hospitals, private laboratories, doctor's office complexes, clinics, health maintenance organizations (HMOs), and research facilities. In a healthcare facility, the clinical laboratory continually interacts with almost every other department, providing critical services for all patients served by the facility.

Pathologists

Although pathologists are doctors, they do not treat patients of their own. Instead, pathologists conduct laboratory tests to diagnose diseases in the patients of other doctors. They perform or review tests on body tissues, secretions, and other specimens to see whether a disease is present and, if so, to determine its stage.

Clinical Laboratory Technologists

The clinical laboratory technologist (*clinical laboratory scientist* or *medical technologist*) typically has a bachelor's degree in a science discipline and has completed a yearlong internship in a healthcare facility. The clinical laboratory technologist often supervises one of the departments in the clinical laboratory, and is responsible for all test results produced in her department. With proper training, these workers are legally able to perform all tests in the clinical laboratory.

Clinical Laboratory Technicians

This position generally requires two years of community college or a vocational/technical program. In some states, these employees can perform many of the tests that clinical laboratory technologists can, but they are restricted from performing other tests. The laboratory technologist working with technicians is responsible for all tests produced in the specific department. Some states do not recognize this position, but it is becoming more acceptable.

Phlebotomists

Lab workers who are trained to draw blood from a live person or animal for tests, transfusions, donations, or research are called *phlebotomists*.

Phlebotomists collect blood primarily by performing venipuncture, a surgical puncture in which blood is extracted from a vein, or by taking small quantities of blood from the finger. Blood may be collected from infants by means of a heel stick, a procedure in which the infant's heel is pricked by a needle. Blood is then collected in a pipette (narrow tube) or on special paper. Some counties, districts, or states require phlebotomy personnel to be licensed or certified.

Clinical Laboratory Aides

Aides in the laboratory may clean laboratory equipment; prepare cleaning solutions; dry glassware; operate the autoclave (usually in small laboratories); and prepare stains, solutions, and culture media. Specific duties may vary from state to state and from laboratory to laboratory.

Real Life Scenario   Argumentative Patients

Daisy is a phlebotomist who works in the outpatient laboratory at Eastridge Hospital. A very nervous woman, Mrs. Rice, comes to her blood drawing station. Mrs. Rice's doctor wants her to have several blood tests, which requires Daisy to draw four vials of blood from Mrs. Rice.

Mrs. Rice is very upset that she has to have her blood drawn and immediately tells Daisy that she will not cooperate and gets up to leave.

Apply It

1. Imagine that you are Daisy; what would you do in this situation? Do you insist that Mrs. Rice sit down and give you her arm, not taking no for an answer? Do you try to talk Mrs. Rice into having her blood drawn?

2. What do you do if Mrs. Rice leaves without having her blood drawn?

Vision Care

Half of the people in the United States currently need some sort of vision care and 96 percent of people over the age of 65 have vision problems. As a result, there are many different types of vision care workers whose job it is to provide treatment for this high-demand area of healthcare. Due to our aging population, vision care will be a growing industry in the coming years.

There are three categories of eye care professionals—ophthalmologists, optometrists, and opticians. Vision care professionals need a great deal of scientific training, including anatomy and physiology, pharmacology (the study of drugs), mathematics, and other science disciplines. There is also considerable patient interaction in this field. Career opportunities include working in clinics, large medical facilities, private practice offices, and retail stores with an eye care section.

Ophthalmologists

Ophthalmologists are medical doctors who have received training beyond medical school with a specialty in vision care and eye diseases. They are licensed to diagnose, write prescriptions for, and treat all eye problems.

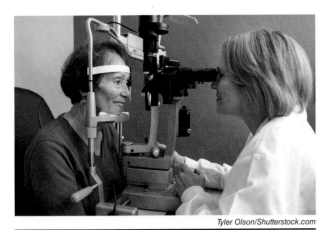

Tyler Olson/Shutterstock.com

Figure 2.17 According to the *Occupational Outlook Handbook*, job outlook for optometrists is expected to grow much faster than average in the coming years.

Optometrists

After obtaining their bachelor's degree, optometrists complete four years of graduate education at a college of optometry. They then receive a doctor of optometry (OD) degree and are able to examine patients for eye problems and fit eyeglasses and contact lenses. In some states, optometrists can diagnose eye diseases and prescribe and administer drugs to treat those diseases (Figure 2.17).

Opticians

Opticians fit and dispense glasses and contact lenses after receiving a prescription written by other professionals. Optician training varies from state to state. Becoming an optician requires a high school diploma or an approved GED equivalent, followed by formal education and training, or an apprenticeship.

Many opticians go to college to earn a two-year associate's degree in optometry, which involves coursework in basic anatomy, eye anatomy, algebra, trigonometry, optical physics, and administration.

Radiology Workers

Today, X-ray departments are also called *diagnostic imaging departments*. Radiology employees operate X-ray equipment to take pictures of internal parts of the body. X-rays can be used to diagnose lung diseases such as cancer or tuberculosis, as well as blood clots, ulcers, and fractures. As Figure 2.18 shows, sophisticated imaging technology is increasingly

Advanced Radiology Machines		
Diagnostic Imaging Technique	**Description**	**Operator**
Ultrasound	transmission of sound waves at high frequencies into a patient's body, resulting in an image called a sonogram; often used for prenatal care and for cardiology	ultrasound technologists; sonographers
Magnetic Resonance Imaging (MRI)	used to visualize detailed internal structures; provides good contrast between the different soft tissues of the body, making it especially useful in imaging the brain, muscles, the heart, and tumors	magnetic resonance technologist
Computer Axial Tomography (CT Scans)	an X-ray procedure that combines many X-ray images with the aid of a computer to generate cross-sectional views or three-dimensional images of the internal organs and structures of the body; used to define normal and abnormal structures in the body or assist in procedures by helping to accurately guide the placement of instruments or treatments	CT scan technologist
Mammography	a low-energy X-ray machine used to examine the breasts; helps to diagnose and screen for breast cancer, typically through detection of masses or calcium deposits in the breasts	mammographer

Goodheart-Willcox Publisher

Figure 2.18 Advanced radiology machines can be used for a variety of purposes.

being used to make more detailed diagnoses. Such technology includes ultrasound, computerized axial tomography (CT) scans, and magnetic resonance imaging, or *MRI* (Figure 2.19).

When working with radiation, workers must exercise caution and take the appropriate safety measures. Exposure to radiation can cause cell damage. A protective barrier should always be placed between the equipment operator and the source of radiation. Lead is the most common shielding material, and it is embedded in walls, gloves, aprons, partitions, and other protective items in diagnostic imaging rooms. Radiology workers must also maintain a safe distance of at least six feet from the radiation source.

Radiation badges called *dosimeters* monitor radiation exposure over a period of time. Employees working with radiation must wear dosimeters at all times to ensure that they are not being exposed to dangerous levels of radiation. Results of this monitoring are sent wirelessly to a computer.

Proper protection and adherence to safety guidelines ensure that radiation is not a problem for radiology employees. However, people under the age of 18 are not allowed to work around radiation because the tissues in their bodies are still growing and are more susceptible to injury from radiation. Because it is so important that people are aware of radiation, an internationally recognized symbol alerts people to its presence (Figure 2.20).

Excellent career opportunities exist in radiology. To qualify for most technician positions in this career path, you will need to learn to use sophisticated equipment. Much more education is required for positions such as radiologist or radiation oncologist.

Radiologists

Radiologists are medical doctors who specialize in the use of diagnostic imaging to diagnose and treat disease. Agents such as dyes are often administered to the body to help radiologists see imaging results more clearly. Radiologists also diagnose findings seen on X-rays.

Radiation Oncologists

Radiation oncologists are doctors who specialize in cancer treatment using radiation. A radiation oncologist determines a tumor treatment plan for each patient. Beams of radiation can be directed at cancerous cells or tumors to destroy or inhibit the cancerous cells' ability to grow.

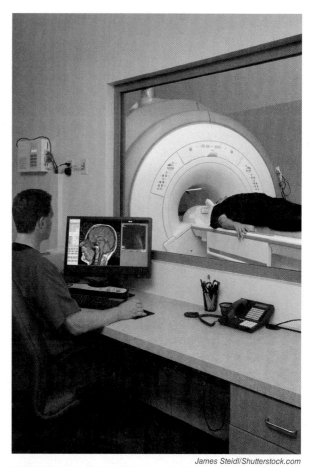
James Steidl/Shutterstock.com

Figure 2.19 An MRI machine can be used to create detailed images of internal structures such as the brain.

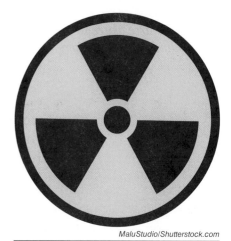
MaluStudio/Shutterstock.com

Figure 2.20 The radiation symbol is recognized internationally and alerts patients and healthcare workers that radiation is present.

Other Radiology Careers

There are several career opportunities in radiology that require an associate's degree:

- Radiation therapists deliver radiation to patients with cancer and other diseases.
- Nuclear medicine technologists prepare and administer radioactive drugs to patients undergoing scans; the radioactive drugs help identify abnormal areas of the body in the images.
- Diagnostic medical sonographers use sound waves to generate images used for assessing and diagnosing various medical conditions.
- Magnetic resonance imaging technologists operate MRI machines.
- Radiologic technologists perform diagnostic imaging procedures, such as X-ray examinations, magnetic resonance imaging (MRI) scans, and computed tomography (CT) scans.

Other diagnostic services careers include electrocardiogram (ECG) technician, cardiovascular technologist, and electroneurodiagnostic technologist.

Health Informatics Services

health informatics services
career field considered to be a bridge between medicine and technology, and which provides critical support to all other medical services; includes positions such as medical clerical worker, human resource workers, and medical records workers

Health informatics services involve the study of resources and methods for the management of health information. Health informatics technology includes the electronics and information technology used during the course of patient care. This service is an evolving specialization that links information technology, communications, and healthcare to improve the quality and safety of patient care.

Health informatics services careers serve as a bridge between the worlds of medicine and technology. Health informatics service workers such as hospital admitting department workers, various medical clerical positions, human resources workers, health unit coordinators, and medical records workers provide critical support to all other medical services in a healthcare setting.

There are many positions in this field that offer secure employment with excellent benefits. These positions vary greatly in a few key aspects—some require a high level of expertise with computers, some do not include contact with patients, and some deal directly with patients. All of these positions require people skills, whether or not you are working with patients or fellow employees. These careers also require exceptional attention to detail. Figure 2.21 lists some careers in health informatics and information services. Again, the requirements for these careers may vary among states.

Careers in Health Informatics

Health informatics is an exciting health career field. This area includes the knowledge, skills, and tools that enable information to be collected, managed, used, and shared to support the delivery of healthcare and to promote health.

Careers in health informatics involve incorporating advanced technology into patient care and facility operations. As technology continues to change, these professionals are needed to help implement these changes

Educational Requirements for Common Health Informatics Careers	
Career(s)	**Educational Requirements**
health unit coordinator, medical records clerk	one or more years in a career or technical education program; some on-the-job training opportunities
health information file clerk	high school diploma, industry certification, on-the-job training
health information management clerk	high school diploma or industry certification
registered health information technician (RHIT)	associate's degree
registered health information administrator (RHIA)	bachelor's degree
human resources assistant	high school diploma, industry certification, on-the-job training
human resources technician	associate's degree
human resources manager	bachelor's degree
human resources generalist	master's degree or professional degree
medical clerical worker	high school diploma, industry certification, on-the-job-training
medical office manager, medical records and health information technician	associate's degree
hospital admitting officer	bachelor's degree
medical librarian	master's degree in library science, certification or licensure required in most states
medical illustrator	bachelor's degree or master's degree, certification

Goodheart-Willcox Publisher

Figure 2.21   Various health informatics careers are available to you, depending upon your education level.

in healthcare settings. Jobs that fall under the health informatics category range from a health information assistant with an associate's degree to a member of health informatics management with a master's degree. Many career opportunities will exist for individuals with health information technology expertise to conduct or provide training for doctors and nurses as they adopt new electronic healthcare systems.

Job opportunities in health informatics are increasing at a rapid rate. According to the Bureau of Labor Statistics, employment in health information careers is expected to increase by 20 percent over the next few years—much faster than the average for all occupations. Job prospects are very good, especially for technicians with strong computer software skills. There are several occupations in this category that do not include any hands-on patient care.

Applicants for jobs in this area usually have at least an associate's degree. Career titles include the following:

- certified health information specialist
- chief information officer
- clinical informaticist
- informatics consultant
- medical and health services manager
- medical informatics specialist
- nursing information officer

Employment in the field of health informatics can be found in both rural and metropolitan areas in hospitals, clinics, universities, and biomedical research facilities.

Medical Clerical Workers

Medical clerical workers serve as support to all other medical services. These workers handle complaints, interpret and explain policies, prepare payrolls, resolve problems with billing, and collect overdue accounts. The following list includes some positions in the healthcare field of information services that may require on-the-job training or participation in a one- or two-year training program through a community college or vocational education program:

- appointment scheduler
- bill collector
- claim representative
- data processor
- insurance processor
- material or purchasing clerk
- payroll or timekeeping clerk
- personnel clerk
- medical receptionist
- administrative medical assistant

Medical clerical workers ensure that the everyday operations of healthcare organizations run smoothly and efficiently, while working to provide excellent customer service. Some of these workers deal directly with patients and their families, while others may not see patients.

Health Information Specialists

Detailed records are kept every time a patient receives care or interacts with a healthcare professional. Prescriptions, treatment plans, test results, diagnoses, the patient's medical history, and the description of symptoms are included in these records. These records are the primary responsibility of the health information technician, a position that was formerly called the *medical records technician* (Figure 2.22).

A traditional patient record was kept on paper and stored in medical facilities. However, electronic record keeping is quickly becoming the norm. Problems with paper medical records, such as illegible handwriting, can lead to serious errors in diagnosis, treatment, and billing. Also, there is only one copy of a paper record, making it difficult to share patient information and increasing the risk of misplacing a record.

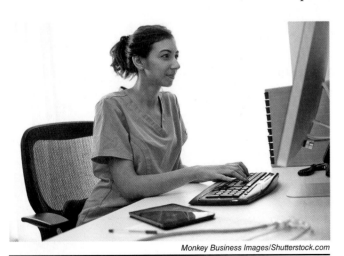

Monkey Business Images/Shutterstock.com

Figure 2.22   Keeping accurate medical records is critical for the correct diagnosis and treatment of patients.

There can also be a delay between the examination and completion of a doctor's notes. In some small doctor's offices, whose records may only be partially computerized, paper records are still used.

Electronic health records (EHRs) are now being used in many medical offices. The use of EHRs has been encouraged by the Health Insurance Portability and Accountability Act (HIPAA) and the federal government. Until all healthcare facilities have completely transitioned to electronic records, health information department employees must be able to work with both paper and electronic health records, making sure that the information recorded is correct and complete.

electronic health records (EHR)
a digital record that contains information about a patient and spans his or her entire medical history and experiences

The health information specialist's career ladder includes

- health information clerks, who have completed a vocational education program;

- registered health information technicians (RHIT), who have graduated from a program accredited by the Commission on Accreditation for Health Informatics and Information Management of Education (CAHIIM) and have passed a national certification exam; and

- registered health information administrators (RHIA), who have attained a bachelor's degree, received a passing grade on a certification examination given by the American Health Information Management Association (AHIMA), and usually act in a supervisory or consulting capacity.

The responsibilities of a health information technician depend largely on the size of the institution in which he is working. Smaller facilities may employ an experienced health information technician to supervise the entire records department, while facilities with medium-sized and larger departments usually have technicians specializing in various areas of healthcare. For example, a large records department might employ a medical coder who specializes in coding patient information for reimbursement purposes.

Did You Know?   HIPAA

The Health Insurance Portability and Accountability Act (HIPAA) was passed by the US Congress in 1996. The act resulted in the creation of a law that included a privacy provision for patient health records, to be fully enforced in 2006. Under this law, patients must be aware of this privacy policy and be notified when their information is shared. Staff must be trained to respect the privacy of patients. Chapter 3, *Healthcare Laws and Ethics*, discusses patient confidentiality in greater detail.

Diagnostic Coding Specialists

Diagnostic coding specialists use several hundred **diagnostic-related groups**, or *DRGs*, to maintain electronic health records. DRGs group patients by diagnosis. A code is assigned for each diagnosis and medical procedure and is used for insurance purposes and maintaining patient health records.

diagnostic-related groups (DRGs)
a system that categorizes patients according to their diagnoses

Coding specialists are known as *health information coders*, *medical record coders*, or *coders/abstractors*. These are occupations that are related to medical records and require completion of a community college program or a course offered in a technical school. Employment settings for these occupations may include acute-care hospitals, long-term care hospitals, doctor's offices, public health departments, health information systems manufacturers, and insurance companies.

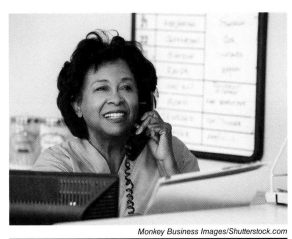

Monkey Business Images/Shutterstock.com

Figure 2.23   Health unit coordinators interact directly with staff, patients, family, and visitors.

Health Unit Coordinators

The health unit coordinator (HUC), also referred to as the *unit secretary* or *unit clerk*, is often the first person you encounter when you enter a hospital nursing unit. The health unit coordinator, stationed at the desk on a nursing unit, coordinates activities on the unit and handles telephone calls. The health unit coordinator reports to the nurse manager or unit manager (Figure 2.23).

A HUC helps to keep the facility organized and coordinates communication between patients and medical staff. The health unit coordinator may greet and check in patients, and schedule appointments or procedures. Receiving new patients, ordering supplies, preparing forms for admission and discharge, transcribing doctors' orders, and preparing birth or death certificates are additional duties.

Today's health unit coordinator often completes a vocational education program for a unit secretary or health unit coordinator. There is also a national certification examination for health unit coordinators. The National Association of Health Unit Coordinators, or NAHUC, provides continuing education and other membership benefits for people in this field. National certification is available through an examination given by NAHUC.

Additional job titles in the health informatics field include epidemiologist, medical illustrator, medical librarian, health educator, community services specialist, and certified compliance technician.

Check Your Understanding ✓

1. Describe what a pathologist does in a healthcare facility.
2. What is the difference between an ophthalmologist and an optometrist?
3. What is another name for the X-ray department?
4. Name three careers in health informatics.
5. What are four duties a health unit coordinator might perform?

support services
a sector of a healthcare facility that plays a critical role in providing a clean, safe environment for all who enter a healthcare facility

Support Services

Support services in a healthcare facility focus on such functions as safety, sanitation, equipment maintenance, counseling services, marketing, and food preparation (Figure 2.24). Workers in the support services occupy a variety of jobs throughout a healthcare facility.

Employees in the support services include housekeepers, central services workers, food service workers, grounds and building maintenance workers, and biomedical technicians. Some support services jobs, and their educational requirements, are listed in Figure 2.25. These are only a few of the jobs available in this field.

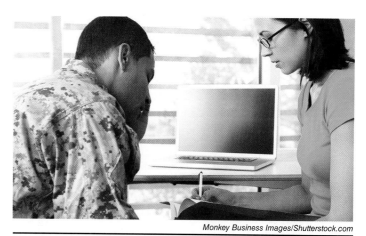

Monkey Business Images/Shutterstock.com

Figure 2.24   The support services staff includes counselors who help patients improve their mental health, recover from addiction, or overcome behavioral problems.

Educational Requirements for Support Services Careers	
Career(s)	**Educational Requirements**
support services aide, support services attendant, support services crew leader	high school diploma; industry certification; or on-the-job training
support services technician	associate's degree
director of support services	bachelor's degree
director of support services and central services	master's degree or professional degree
central services worker	high school diploma; industry certification; or on-the-job training
central services technician	associate's degree
central services supervisor or coordinator	bachelor's degree
food service worker	high school diploma; industry certification; or on-the-job training
dietetic technician	associate's degree
dietetic intern, registered dietitian	bachelor's degree
administrative dietitian	master's degree or professional degree
biomedical technician aide	high school diploma; industry certification; or on-the-job training
biomedical equipment technician (BMET)	associate's degree
health technology manager (HTM), biomedical technologist	bachelor's degree
rehabilitation counselor, mental health counselor, substance abuse counselor, or behavioral disorders counselor	master's degree or professional degree
central or sterile supply technician	one or more years in a career or technical education program; some on-the-job training opportunities; certification for a sterile processing technician

Goodheart-Willcox Publisher

Figure 2.25   Many rewarding careers are available in support services.

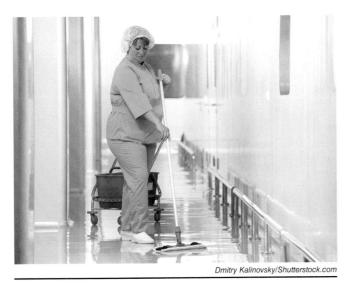

Dmitry Kalinovsky/Shutterstock.com

Figure 2.26 The housekeeping staff plays a critical role, ensuring the safety of patients, visitors, and staff.

Housekeeping Services

A health facility's housekeeping services workers are responsible for the cleanliness of the healthcare environment (Figure 2.26). Their labors help prevent the spread of infection, creating a more pleasant, safe environment for everyone who enters the hospital, including patients and staff. Hospital housekeepers have many job opportunities in acute-care hospitals, long-term care facilities, and clinics.

Healthcare facility cleaning requires specialized training and compliance with various local laws and regulations, some of which dictate how to clean up potentially infectious materials. Hospital-acquired infections (also known as *nosocomial infections*) are a reality in any healthcare facility. Housekeeping employees work continually to see that patients' rooms and the general environment of the facility are free from infectious agents. You will learn more about safety and infection control in chapter 4.

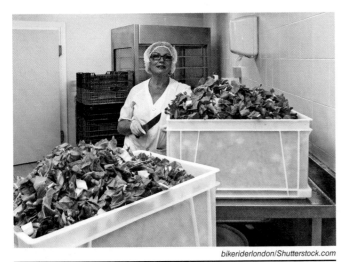

bikeriderlondon/Shutterstock.com

Figure 2.27 Food service workers prepare and serve meals to the patients, visitors, and staff in a healthcare facility.

Food Services

Employees in food services are responsible for providing patients with safe, nutritional meals. Food service workers plan special diets such as low-sodium, low-fat, and restricted-carbohydrate meals (Figure 2.27). Food service employees also bring menus to patients, prepare food trays, and deliver food to the patients. Hospitals typically have cafeterias where staff and visitors may eat their meals.

There are many career options in food services, including food service workers, dietetic technicians, dietetic interns, and registered dietitians. All of these employees provide a critical service, making sure patients are given balanced meals to help the recovery process.

Dietitians

Dietitians have degrees in nutrition, dietetics, public health, or a related field from accredited colleges and universities. Registered dietitians have successfully completed internships and passed an examination for their credentials. Dietitians work with patients newly diagnosed with a disorder that requires a special diet, such as heart disease, diabetes, kidney failure, and many other conditions.

Extend Your Knowledge ▸ **Dietary Needs**

Americans are flooded with articles, books, TV commercials, magazines, and newspapers about the latest diets. One diet wants you to avoid carbohydrates, and another tells you that carbs are fine. Other diets want you to eat nothing but meat and vegetables.

Apply It

1. Research what constitutes a healthful diet. Use the United States Department of Agriculture's (USDA) website as a resource.

2. People with particular health problems may require a special diet. Research dietary recommendations for people with diabetes, kidney failure, or heart disease. Compare these diets to the recommended diet for a healthy individual. Discuss your findings in class.

Central Services

Another support services occupation is the central processing services worker. These workers keep an inventory of supplies and equipment for the facility in which they work. Supplies and equipment must be properly packaged, cleaned, and sterilized. Central services workers play a key role in making sure patients are not exposed to infectious diseases and ensuring that doctors and nurses have proper, sterile equipment with which they can perform various procedures. Jobs in central services can be found in acute-care hospitals and large outpatient clinics.

Biomedical Equipment Technicians

A biomedical equipment technician (BMET) is responsible for medical equipment maintenance. This job is also referred to as a *biomedical electronics technician* or *biomedical engineering technician*. A BMET maintains, installs, and repairs a wide variety of healthcare technology and equipment (Figure 2.28). They may work on ventilators, X-ray or ultrasound machines, or medical laboratory equipment. A BMET also trains health facility staff to ensure they understand how to properly operate biomedical equipment.

Technology is a critical component of patient care that improves medical outcomes and safety. Highly skilled and trained biomedical equipment technicians are increasingly sought by hospitals, the medical equipment industry, and many other healthcare employers to ensure medical equipment is up-to-date and functioning efficiently and safely for optimal patient care.

A biomedical equipment technician is required to earn an associate's degree or a bachelor's degree in a related field, such as electronic technology.

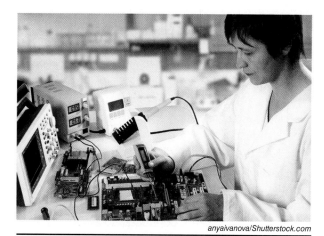

anyaivanova/Shutterstock.com

Figure 2.28 The biomedical equipment technician is a highly skilled and trained person.

Some employers may only require a high school diploma and provide on-the-job training.

Other careers in support services include dietary manager, environmental services facilities manager, materials manager, transport technician, maintenance engineer, and central services manager.

Biotechnology Research and Development

biotechnology research and development
highly science-oriented career pathway that uses living systems and organisms to create and develop products used in healthcare

The **biotechnology research and development** careers pathway includes jobs that are highly scientific. Biotechnology is the use of living systems and organisms to create and develop products. Some of the ways biotechnology has been used in healthcare include producing new drugs, manufacturing medical devices, and developing diagnostic tests. The science of biotechnology also works on discoveries in other fields such as helping to clean up the environment, creating biofuels, and helping to make our foods safer by developing crops that do not need pesticides. Healthcare continues to be the most active focus of biotechnology.

In general, employees in the biotechnology research and development pathway work in laboratories rather than healthcare facilities. Many of these employees have a strong research background in biology and chemistry.

To enter this field, a person needs a strong background in and love of science. This field also requires excellent communication skills. Many of the tasks involved in this job consist of sharing research results through speeches, articles, and reports. These careers also require exceptional attention to detail, accuracy when performing tasks in the lab, and strong problem-solving skills.

Positions in biotechnology research include assistants, technicians, educators, researchers, and scientists (Figure 2.29). Individuals may work in the food industry, agriculture, pollution control, pharmaceuticals, government agencies, water treatment plants, or education. Educational requirements range from a two-year technical degree from a community college to 8–12 years of study to earn a doctoral degree or PhD.

Think It Through

Jason is not comfortable around sick people and prefers working with computers instead of interacting with others. He is very interested in the medical field but isn't interested in the traditional medical professions. What might be some other healthcare career options for Jason to explore?

Extend Your Knowledge ▶ Deep Brain Stimulation for Parkinson's Disease

Parkinson's disease (PD) is a degenerative disorder that affects the nervous system. People with Parkinson's disease experience tremors that often affect their coordination and speech, among other bodily functions.

An exciting biomedical therapy that continues to develop is successfully treating the symptoms of Parkinson's. Deep brain stimulation is performed by electrodes that are surgically inserted into the brain. These electrodes are connected to a pacemaker placed under the skin of the chest, near the collarbone.

The pacemaker sends continual electrical impulses to the areas of the body responsible for producing the tremors. These electrical impulses work to prevent the debilitating tremors associated with Parkinson's.

Apply It

1. Research other ways biotechnology is being used to treat or cure diseases. Draft a one-page report and share your findings with the class.

2. Does a career in biotechnology interest you? Why or why not?

| Educational Requirements for Common Biotechnology Careers ||
Career(s)	Educational Requirements
biological scientist	bachelor's, master's, or doctoral degree in a science discipline with licensure required in some states
chemical technician	associate's and bachelor's degree in a science discipline, depending on the state
microbiologist	bachelor's degree in microbiology or closely related field; graduate degree to carry out independent research
biological technician	associate's degree, but often requires bachelor's degree
laboratory assistant	on-the-job training; associate's degree in biological science
laboratory technician	associate's degree in biological science
biotechnological engineer	bachelor's degree in bioengineering; master's degree and advanced degree also available

Goodheart-Willcox Publisher

Figure 2.29   Careers available in the Biotechnology Research and Development pathway vary by education and experience.

Biological Scientists

A biological scientist studies living organisms such as bacteria, viruses, protozoa, fungi, and other organisms that can cause infection. These scientists may assist in the development of vaccines, medicines, and treatments for disease. Some biological scientists work on researching genes associated with specific diseases. This is a technical career, requiring a strong background in science and love of scientific inquiry. Laboratory experience in undergraduate work is highly recommended (Figure 2.30). Biological scientists typically do not work closely with patients.

Microbiologists

A degree in microbiology or a related field such as biochemistry or cell biology is required for this career. Laboratory experience is important for becoming a microbiologist.

As in other biotechnology careers, microbiologists should be able to effectively communicate their research progress and findings. Excellent organizational and writing skills are particularly important in this career. Also, attention to detail is very important in any career that is involved with experimentation and analyzing results with accuracy and precision.

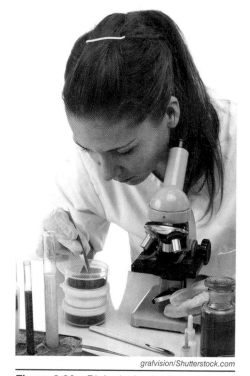

grafvision/Shutterstock.com

Figure 2.30   Biological scientists work with microorganisms in laboratories.

Bioengineers

Bioengineers (or *biotechnological engineers*) have an engineering background, typically having earned a bachelor's degree in biotechnology or a related field. These engineers strive to improve existing medical devices such as pacemakers (small device placed in the chest or abdomen to help control abnormal heart rhythms) or defibrillators (device that gives an electric shock to a person's heart to make it beat normally again).

Bioengineers also develop brand new medical devices. Bioengineers may design or construct artificial organs, research metals that can be used as implants without fear of the body rejecting the metal, and discover other exciting solutions to medical challenges (Figure 2.31).

Biological and Chemical Technicians

A biological technician assists biological scientists or bioengineers in the study of living organisms, helping to perform experiments. They can also help in the development, testing, and manufacturing of medications. Biological technicians must be able to work as a team member and take direction well. They must have strong communication and writing skills, work with accuracy, and be skilled in the use of laboratory equipment and computers.

A chemical technician, also known as a *process technician*, takes direction from the biological scientist or a research doctor to monitor and operate machinery used to produce biotechnology products. These professionals are responsible for following quality improvement programs for laboratory equipment and the products they create. They are also assigned to make sure that anyone who uses the equipment follows the necessary safety regulations. A biological technician must pay careful attention to detail and must possess the mechanical ability to work with all kinds of machines.

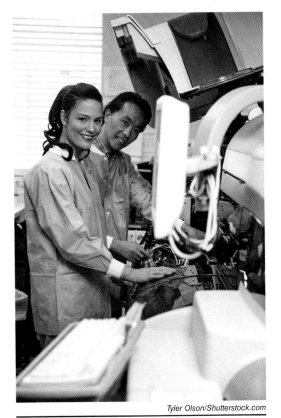

Tyler Olson/Shutterstock.com

Figure 2.31 Bioengineers often work as members of a team to improve or develop medical equipment and processes.

Extend Your Knowledge ▶ Career Research

Research a specific health science career that appeals to you by following these steps:

1. Make a list of the five things you think you want most from a career (for example, a flexible schedule, good salary, patient contact, or making a difference may be on your list).

2. Then list five of your strongest abilities, such as math skills, excellent organizational talents, and strong people skills.

3. Next, answer the questions from the self-assessment section of this chapter.

4. Research a career you are interested in online in the *Occupational Outlook Handbook*.

5. Talk with your school counselor about opportunities for employment in your area and what further education would be required, if any. Does this career require an associate's or bachelor's degree? What about graduate work?

6. Set up an informational meeting or job shadowing experience with someone who works in the field to find out what they like or dislike about their job. Your counselor or instructor may be able to help you identify a professional in the field.

7. Talk with your health science instructors about related clinical experience or coursework available to you.

Apply It

1. What career did you research and why?

2. Based on your answers to the questions above, do you think this career would be a good fit for you? Why or why not?

3. What did you learn about yourself after completing this exercise?

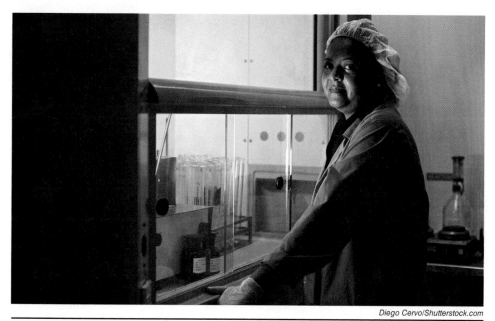
Diego Cervo/Shutterstock.com

Figure 2.32   A laboratory assistant cleans test tubes in the lab.

Laboratory Assistants and Technicians

Laboratory assistants maintain the equipment used in a laboratory. This position typically requires a high school diploma. Further education and laboratory experience is required to climb the career ladder in this field. Lab assistants clean and store glassware, maintain inventory, reorder supplies, and may test glassware to verify that it is free from contamination (Figure 2.32).

Laboratory technicians commonly have an associate's degree. The biological and chemical technician positions are specialties of the laboratory technician. Lab technicians must follow directions with a great deal of accuracy. They analyze and graph data from experiments. A lab technician must possess excellent math skills and maintain accuracy while completing repetitive tasks. Lab technicians with a bachelor's degree may become research associates, who supervise lab technicians and assistants. The research associates may create new processes for developing new products.

Check Your Understanding ✔

Determine which of the five pathways each of the following healthcare careers belongs to.

1. dentist
2. research scientist
3. housekeeping supervisor
4. physical therapist
5. massage therapist
6. clerical worker
7. biomedical technician
8. nurse
9. laboratory aide
10. veterinarian
11. dietetic technician
12. human resources manager
13. mammographer
14. cardiologist
15. respiratory therapist
16. occupational therapy aide

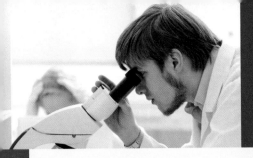

Summary

It is important to assess your goals and needs before you put time, energy, and money into pursuing a career. In exploring a career in healthcare, you will find that there are many career pathways from which to choose. Therapeutic services, diagnostic services, support services, health informatics, and biomedical research and development all contain wonderful positions with impressive career ladders.

Only a fraction of the careers in healthcare are discussed in this chapter. Making the correct choice means matching your needs and interests with a career. Your career decision will include how much education you are willing to complete, how much time you can dedicate to your education, your budget, and the availability of your chosen career where you live. Be sure to see the school counselors at your school, take career inventory tests, volunteer in a healthcare facility where you can observe career professionals at work, and interview someone who has a career about which you are curious. Remember also that your state may have different educational requirements for each healthcare career.

Review Questions

Answer the following questions using what you have learned in this chapter.

True or False Assess

1. *True or False?* Becoming an optometrist only requires a bachelor's degree.
2. *True or False?* You must take a licensing exam in order to receive a license for certain healthcare professions.
3. *True or False?* Respiratory therapists help patients walk after surgery.
4. *True or False?* Phlebotomists draw blood from patients' veins.
5. *True or False?* Dosimeters are what patients use to call the nursing station.
6. *True or False?* Biotechnology research and development careers all require a master's degree or higher.

7. *True or False?* The primary responsibility of a bioengineer is to maintain lab inventory and clean and store glassware.
8. *True or False?* Being a nurse is a diagnostic services position.
9. *True or False?* Continuing education opportunities after being hired as a healthcare worker are restricted to doctors.
10. *True or False?* HIPAA is an organization for physical therapists.

Multiple Choice Assess

11. Which of the following statements can be used to describe the responsibilities or qualifications of a hospital dietitian?
    A. plans balanced meals for patients
    B. earns a degree in nutrition, dietetics, public health, or a related field from an accredited college or university
    C. becomes licensed as a dietitian
    D. All of the above.

12. Which of the following careers is *not* considered a therapeutic career?
    A. physical therapist
    B. dental assistant
    C. nurse
    D. medical laboratory technician

13. Which of these machines is used in the radiology department?
    A. MRI
    B. CT scan
    C. mammography
    D. All of the above.

14. Which of the following healthcare professions does *not* require at least a bachelor's degree?
    A. medical doctor
    B. dentist
    C. paramedic
    D. nurse practitioner

15. What career is categorized under diagnostic services?

    A. physical therapist

    B. dental laboratory technician

    C. pharmacist

    D. medical doctor

16. Which of the following occupations does *not* work in the clinical laboratory of a healthcare facility?

    A. phlebotomist

    B. laboratory aide

    C. radiologist

    D. pathologist

17. Which of the following occupations is *not* categorized as part of the health informatics pathway?

    A. medical clerical worker

    B. data processor

    C. EMT

    D. health unit coordinator

18. Support services in a healthcare facility include _____.

    A. food service workers

    B. central services workers

    C. biomedical equipment technicians

    D. All of the above.

19. Which of the following certifications is granted in the area of health information?

    A. PA

    B. DPT

    C. RHIT

    D. DDS

Short Answer

20. Make a list of three occupations that appeal to you in the healthcare world.

21. Name five healthcare careers in therapeutic services.

22. Name five healthcare careers in diagnostic services.

23. Name five careers in health informatics and information services.

24. Name three careers in healthcare facility support services.

25. What kind of student would be attracted to jobs in the biomedical technology field?

26. List six strengths you have that will serve you well for a career in healthcare.

27. What does health informatics mean?

28. Name five careers in biotechnology research and development.

29. Name three types of degrees that might be required of a healthcare professional.

30. Why is a clinical experience an important step in your education and when deciding on a future career?

Critical Thinking Exercises

31. Take career aptitude tests through your school counselor or online. Remember, these tests are simply a tool to help you assess what careers might best suit your personality and abilities. Analyze your results. Do your results seem to accurately reflect your interests?

32. Consider the time, money, and effort you would like to invest in your education. How much education do you wish to complete in order to realize your career goals? on-the-job training? one to two years of training? associate's degree? bachelor's degree? advanced degree and training beyond a four-year degree? Why does a particular level of education appeal to you?

33. Choose an occupation in the medical field in which you are particularly interested. Answer the following questions in as much detail as possible:

    A. What are the educational requirements for this occupation?

    B. Are these jobs currently available in your community? Research projected job availability online. Using government resources like the Bureau of Labor Statistics might be a good place to start.

    C. What is the salary range for this job?

    D. If possible, interview one or two people who currently work in this position. Ask them what personality traits and skills are needed to do this job well.

    E. Do you think this is a job you might be interested in pursuing? Why or why not?

34. Based on the information in this chapter and your personal strengths, which careers do you think would be the best fit for you? Why?

Chapter 3
Healthcare Laws and Ethics

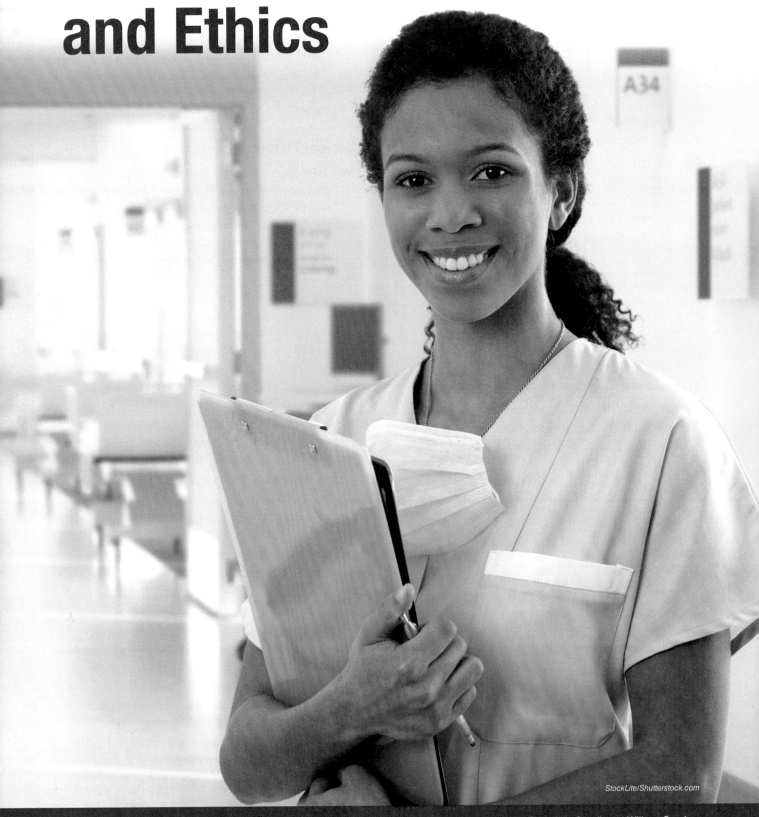

StockLite/Shutterstock.com

Terms to Know

 Build Vocab

advance directive (AD)

arbitration

assault

battery

civil law

confidentiality

criminal law

defamation

discrimination

do not resuscitate (DNR)
    document

durable power of attorney

duty of care

emancipated minor

ethics committee

Good Samaritan laws

guardian

Health Insurance Portability and
    Accountability Act (HIPAA)

informed consent

invasion of privacy

libel

malpractice

medical ethics

medical law

negligence

ombudsman

Patients' Bill of Rights

Patient Self-Determination Act

reasonable care

scope of practice

sexual harassment

slander

standard of care

statute of limitations

values

Chapter Objectives

- Discuss the difference between ethical and legal issues in healthcare.
- Explain the role of ethics committees in a healthcare facility.
- Understand the concept of values.
- Explain the importance of an ombudsman in a hospital setting.
- Understand important legal terms, including *advance directive*, *assault*, *battery*, *durable power of attorney*, *duty of care*, *emancipated minor*, *Good Samaritan laws*, *guardian*, *libel*, *malpractice*, *negligence*, *reasonable care*, *scope of practice*, *slander*, and *statute of limitations*.
- Explain why maintaining patient confidentiality and privacy in healthcare is critical.
- Identify the importance of patient consent forms.
- Explain how to recognize sexual harassment and other reportable behaviors in the workplace.
- Discuss the concept of discrimination in the workplace.

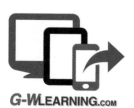 **While studying, look for the activity icon** **to:**

- **Build** vocabulary with e-flash cards and interactive games.
- **Assess** progress with chapter and unit review questions.
- **Expand** learning with animations and illustration labeling activities.
- **Simulate** EHR entry with healthcare documents.

G-WLEARNING.com

www.g-wlearning.com/healthsciences/

When you are sick or injured, or when a family member or a friend needs healthcare, you want to be certain that care is given in a safe, ethical, and legal manner. Many of us can think back on a time when a healthcare professional treated us with special care. Most healthcare workers perform their duties in an ethical manner, but you may have encountered a few who did not. Healthcare workers must be educated as to their ethical and legal responsibilities for the protection of patients, coworkers, employers, and themselves.

Medical Ethics and Legal Responsibilities

medical ethics
standards concerned with whether a healthcare worker's actions are right or wrong

medical law
standards concerned with whether a healthcare worker's actions are legal or illegal

It is important for healthcare workers to make legal and ethical decisions. **Medical ethics** are concerned with whether a healthcare worker's actions are right or wrong. **Medical law** focuses on whether a healthcare worker's actions are legal or illegal. These concepts can be related to one another as well. Illegal acts are always unethical; however, unethical behavior may or may not be illegal.

It is important to know that the application and impact of ethics and laws can vary widely depending on the facts involved in an incident, the institution's policies, and specific laws in each jurisdiction. Also, keep in mind that law is dynamic—it is constantly changing. This is especially true in health law. Courts and legislatures continually respond to issues and technologies that require a new interpretation of existing law or the creation of new laws.

Medical Ethics in the Workplace

Medical ethics have a long history, dating back to our earliest practicing doctors. You learned about Hippocrates in chapter 1. The oath written for doctors and attributed to Hippocrates implies that doctors should do no harm to their patients. Similar to the Hippocratic Oath, many healthcare organizations today have a code of ethics for doctors and other healthcare providers to follow.

Ethical Behavior

Ethical behavior represents ideal conduct for a certain group. Medical ethics in the healthcare setting are established as a framework for describing ideal behavior for employees. Licensed healthcare professionals adopt a specific code of ethics when they become licensed. All healthcare workers at a facility are expected to know, understand, and comply with codes of ethics. Descriptions of workplace ethics are usually found in an employee handbook or a policy and procedure manual.

Ethics Committees in Healthcare Facilities

ethics committee
a committee made up of individuals who consider ethical problems in the healthcare facility and recommend solutions for resolving the issues

Ethics committees in healthcare facilities consider ethical problems that affect the care and treatment of the facility's patients. Members of an ethics committee might include healthcare providers, consumers, and members of the clergy. The committee forms a recommendation for how to resolve the ethical problem and presents it to those responsible for resolving the problem.

Responsible parties may include the facility's governing board, healthcare workers, attending doctor, or other persons. The decision makers are not obligated to follow the committee's recommendations, but the recommendations should be seriously considered as a possible solution. An ethics committee may refer to The Code of Medical Ethics of the American Medical Association for guidance when making their own recommendations.

In the case of denominational healthcare institutions (for example, a Catholic hospital), the recommendations of the ethics committee will be consistent with published religious beliefs and principles.

Examples of ethical behavior include treating all patients and coworkers with mutual respect and providing excellent service to everyone. As a healthcare professional, you are expected to

- be well groomed;
- respect the privacy of others;
- be aware of your limitations;
- avoid taking on tasks for which you are not trained; and
- be honest and trustworthy as you perform your job.

Extend Your Knowledge ▶ Ethical Issues in Healthcare Today

For some people, the following issues might not be considered unethical, while others find some or all of these issues unethical and believe they should be illegal, if they are not already. *Warning: Some, if not all, of these issues invoke strong emotional reactions. Calm, respectful discussions of the issue are always best, but remember that you may not always reach an agreement.*

Euthanasia is the practice of intentionally ending a patient's life to relieve pain and suffering. Euthanasia is illegal in most states, regardless of the circumstances. States such as Oregon, Washington, Montana, and Vermont have enacted legislation allowing a patient to request life-ending drugs from a doctor. In these states, the patient must be a resident and have a terminal illness. Several countries have made euthanasia legal, including Ireland, Mexico, the Netherlands, India, Belgium, and Colombia. Whether euthanasia is murder or an act of compassion is a common debate.

In vitro fertilization, the fertilization of a human egg or eggs in a laboratory, is another ethical issue in healthcare. In vitro fertilization is accomplished by mixing sperm with eggs that have been surgically removed from an ovary. The fertilized egg, or eggs, is implanted in the uterus in the hopes that it will develop into an embryo. Often, several eggs may be successfully fertilized but only two or three are implanted.

In vitro fertilization is legal in the United States. Ethical considerations arise when one considers what to do with any unused, fertilized eggs that are no longer needed. Some feel these eggs are human lives and therefore, should not be destroyed or used for research. Others believe that the eggs should be used to research possible cures for disease.

Apply It

1. Many other ethical issues are debated in healthcare every day, including organ donation, vaccination, abortion, and stem cell research. Using one of these topics, or a topic of your choosing, research the arguments presented by those on both sides of the issue. Write a brief report summarizing the ethical debate.

2. Take a moment to reflect on the ethical debate you researched above. Now that you have learned the arguments from either side, what is your opinion?

Unethical practices in the workplace include displaying rude behavior toward any patient; being impatient with a patient who moves or talks slowly; arriving at work with dirty clothes and hair; gossiping about patients and coworkers; and lying about a mistake you made. It is also unethical for an employee to discuss salaries with coworkers. To do so can be cause for termination.

Values

values
the concepts, ideas, and beliefs that are important and meaningful to a person

Values are the concepts, ideas, and beliefs that are important and meaningful to a person. Your values can be influenced by the people around you, and they help you make decisions by defining what you think is good or bad. Values greatly influence your behavior and serve as broad guidelines in all situations. Your employer may describe what values are important to perform your job and how to put them into practice. As you perform your job in a healthcare facility, your values and behaviors are a reflection of your ethics.

Medical Law

civil law
directives that pertain to disputes between individuals, organizations, or a combination of the two in which monetary compensation is awarded; also known as tort law

Medical law governs the legal conduct of members of the medical professions. Medical law includes laws to be followed at the federal, state, and local levels. Breaking such laws subjects the offender to civil or criminal prosecution (Figure 3.1). **Civil law** (also known as *tort law*) refers to any laws that enforce private rights, not criminal behavior. **Criminal law** deals with criminal behavior that could have consequences such as imprisonment.

Breaking a medical law can lead to loss of a professional license, a fine, and even a prison sentence.

criminal law
directives that pertain to a crime in which the guilty party is punished by incarceration and possible fines

Think It Through

Make a list of the values you believe should be most important to a healthcare worker. Then, make a list of the personal values that are important in your life. How do these two lists compare? Are the values you associate with a healthcare worker different than those you feel are important in your life?

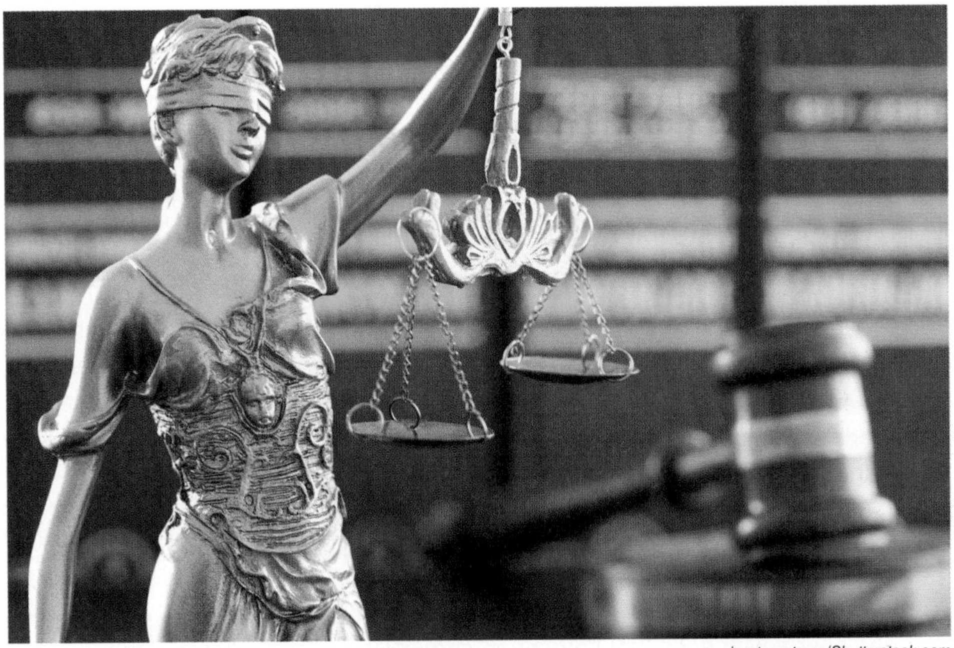

izzet ugutmen/Shutterstock.com

Figure 3.1   In this statue, a blindfolded Lady Justice holds the scales of justice. The blindfold she wears symbolizes the importance of impartiality.

Check Your Understanding ✓

1. Explain the difference between criminal and civil law.
2. Name three ethical issues in healthcare today.
3. What is the purpose of an ethics committee in a healthcare facility?
4. What is the difference between medical ethics and medical law?
5. What are values?

Legal Protection for Patients and Healthcare Workers

When a patient and a doctor form a relationship, their relationship is considered a contract (Figure 3.2). The practice of medicine is carried out within a framework of laws that includes protections for patients, healthcare workers, and healthcare facilities. Knowledge of medical laws will help you avoid legal trouble while carrying out your duties as a healthcare professional. There are various legal protections in the healthcare world—some relate to the patient and some to healthcare workers.

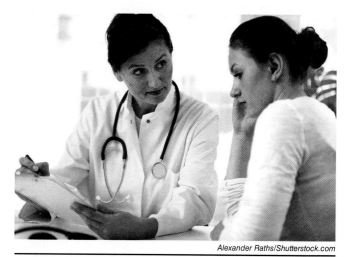

Alexander Raths/Shutterstock.com

Figure 3.2 The patient and doctor's relationship exists within a framework of laws.

Extend Your Knowledge ▶ Civil Law and Criminal Law

Civil law, also known as *tort law*, deals with disputes between individuals, organizations, or a combination of the two, in which monetary compensation is awarded. An example of a civil law case is a healthcare worker telling a patient's employer that the patient has a disease that would keep him from being an effective employee. The patient then loses his job, resulting in a loss of wages. This case would be filed by a private party, and that party must present believable evidence that this patient had been injured by the healthcare worker.

Criminal law deals with a crime in which the guilty party is punished by incarceration (jail or prison), fines, or both. The state (prosecution) files the case and has the responsibility of proving the case "beyond a reasonable doubt." An example of breaking a criminal law in a healthcare setting is a pharmacy technician stealing drugs and selling them.

Apply It

1. Some crimes are subject to both civil and criminal law, allowing a person to be charged twice for the same crime. One famous instance of this occurred in the 1990s, when former football star O.J. Simpson faced both criminal and civil charges for the murder of his ex-wife, Nicole Brown Simpson, and Ronald Goldman. Research these cases. How did the civil and criminal trials and verdicts differ?

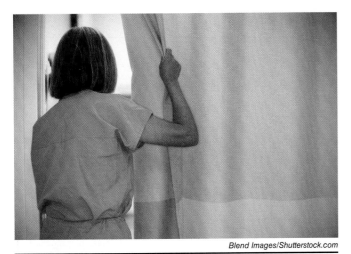

Blend Images/Shutterstock.com

Figure 3.3 Every patient has a right to physical privacy while receiving care. Properly draping a patient and screening the bed or room is one way to protect a patient's modesty.

Invasion of Privacy

There are two types of **invasion of privacy**. The first is physical. An example of a physical invasion of privacy is a healthcare worker who does not protect the modesty of a patient by draping him during a procedure or properly screening his hospital bed (Figure 3.3). The second type is informational invasion of privacy. This occurs when a healthcare worker reveals a patient's personal information without the patient's consent. For example, a healthcare worker who gives information to an insurance company without the patient's written permission has invaded her privacy. Invasion of privacy could lead to legal action.

Patients' Bill of Rights

A **Patients' Bill of Rights** is a list of guarantees for those receiving medical care. It may take the form of a law or a nonbinding declaration. A Patients' Bill of Rights guarantees patients access to health services, information to help them make informed medical decisions, and fair treatment, among other rights. There have been a number of attempts in the past to create a universal Patients' Bill of Rights in the United States and make it law. The Affordable Care Act of 2010 includes a list of patient rights that are now law.

The American Hospital Association has developed a pamphlet highlighting the Patients' Bill of Rights, with the belief that it promotes more effective patient care. The pamphlet, which outlines how patients should be treated by healthcare workers, should be given to patients when they arrive at the healthcare facility. Hospitals are urged to adhere to rules about providing information regarding patient rights, as they apply to its healthcare workers, employees, and patients.

Ombudsman

The role of an **ombudsman** is to ensure that patients are not abused and that their legal rights are protected. An ombudsman may be a nurse, a trained volunteer, or a social worker. In most facilities, there will be a person acting as an ombudsman and a phone number posted for employees to use when reporting violations of patients' rights. Employees can also discuss the issue with the ombudsman in person.

The Patient Self-Determination Act

The **Patient Self-Determination Act** was passed by Congress in 1990. This law requires that most healthcare institutions inform patients about their rights, under state law, at the time of admission. These include the right of patients to

- participate in and direct their healthcare decisions;
- accept or refuse medical or surgical treatment;

invasion of privacy
intrusion on another's personal life; applies to personal information as well as a person's body

Patients' Bill of Rights
summary of a patient's rights regarding fair treatment and appropriate information

ombudsman
a member of the healthcare team who ensures that patients are not abused and that their legal rights are protected; investigates complaints and advocates for patient rights

Patient Self-Determination Act
a law passed by the US Congress in 1990 that requires most healthcare institutions to inform a patient about his or her rights at the time of admission

- prepare an advance directive;
- view information on the facility's policies about recognizing advance directives; and
- know how the facility educates its staff regarding advance directives.

Advance Directives (AD)

An **advance directive (AD)** is a legal document in which a patient gives written instructions about healthcare decisions to be used in the event that he becomes incapable of making such decisions in the future. An example of an advance directive is a request by the patient to instruct his doctor that "heroic measures," such as using feeding tubes and respirators, must not be taken if there is no expectation of recovery.

A **do not resuscitate (DNR) document** is made by a patient as part of an advance directive (Figure 3.4). This document states that cardiopulmonary resuscitation (CPR) or advanced cardiac life support (ACLS) should *not* be performed if the patient stops breathing or the patient's heart stops. The DNR document should be kept with the patient's medical record. Some people also have a DNR document posted in their homes.

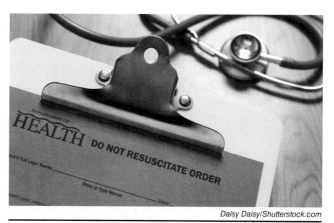

Daisy Daisy/Shutterstock.com

Figure 3.4 Healthcare providers in all states accept DNR orders.

advance directive (AD)
a legal document in which a patient gives written instructions about healthcare issues in the event the patient becomes unable to make such decisions in the future

do not resuscitate (DNR) document
a legal document made by a patient, which states that CPR or other advanced cardiac life support should not be performed if a patient stops breathing or a patient's heart stops

Durable Power of Attorney

The **durable power of attorney** is a legal document that grants another person, or *agent*, the authority to make legal decisions for you. The Durable Power of Attorney for Health Care (DPAHC) allows the patient to express her healthcare decisions and outline how much authority the agent should be given. This power is often granted to a family member of an elderly relative.

durable power of attorney
a legal document that grants another person the authority to make legal decisions for you

Guardianship

If a patient is not able to make his or her own decisions due to mental or physical incapacity, a court-appointed **guardian** may make decisions to protect the interests of the patient.

guardian
a court-appointed person who may make decisions for a patient who is mentally or physically incapable of making such decisions

Emancipated Minors

In most states, parents are required to sign medical consent forms for any child under 18 years of age. However, this is not the case for an **emancipated minor**. An emancipated minor is a person under 18 years of age who has legally established that he does not live with his parents. The emancipated minor is financially and legally responsible for himself and can consent to treatment.

emancipated minor
a person under 18 years of age who has legally established that he or she does not live with parents

duty of care
a legal obligation for healthcare personnel to take reasonable care to avoid causing harm to a patient

negligence
performing an act that a reasonable person would not have done, or not doing something that a reasonable person would have done in the same or a similar circumstance, resulting in harm to a patient

Good Samaritan laws
laws that protect people from legal action after voluntarily giving emergency medical aid while using reasonable care

reasonable care
legal protection for the healthcare worker if proven that the worker acted reasonably as compared to other members of the profession in the same or a similar circumstance

arbitration
a cost-effective alternative to litigation

Duty of Care

Every patient is entitled to safe care. **Duty of care** is a legal obligation for healthcare personnel to take reasonable care of a patient to avoid causing harm. If this duty is not met, a charge of negligence may be made against the healthcare provider.

Negligence

In the healthcare world, **negligence** refers to performing an act that a reasonable person would not have done. Negligence can also mean failing to do something that a reasonable person would have done, resulting in injury or harm to a patient. An example of negligence is a nurse ignoring a resident's bedsore and leaving it untreated while in a long-term care facility.

Good Samaritan Laws

Good Samaritan laws are designed to protect people from legal action after they have given free, emergency medical aid while using reasonable care. These laws are designed to encourage healthcare professionals to give first aid in an emergency situation without fear of being sued for negligence (Figure 3.5). Unfortunately, these laws are not always clearly written, sometimes creating confusion for healthcare professionals. Additionally, these laws differ from state to state. In some states, these laws apply to the general public as well as trained healthcare professionals.

Reasonable Care

Reasonable care is a legal protection for healthcare workers. This protection applies if it can be proven that the worker acted reasonably as compared to actions that other members of the profession would take in similar circumstances. If the healthcare worker does not meet such a standard and the patient is harmed, negligence may be proven.

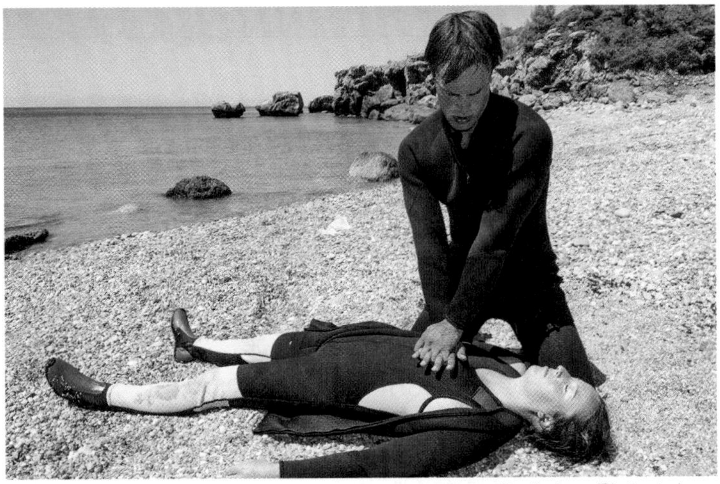

Arbitration

Arbitration is a method of resolving disputes outside the courtroom. Rather than let the case go into litigation (to be settled by a court of law), healthcare professionals may choose arbitration, which does not involve a trial. Hospitals, doctors, and other healthcare professionals often ask patients to sign arbitration agreements before care is provided. This protects the healthcare facility from involvement in a costly trial, should something go wrong.

Roy Pedersen/Shutterstock.com

Figure 3.5 Good Samaritan laws are designed to protect from legal action those who perform cardiopulmonary resuscitation (CPR) and other first aid measures. Only those who are properly trained should perform conventional CPR in case of an emergency.

Medical Malpractice

Malpractice, also known as *professional liability*, is defined as any misconduct or lack of skill that results in patient injury. When filing a malpractice claim, you must present information stating that a professional does not meet the standard of care. Most claims of this nature are filed against doctors or hospitals, but any healthcare worker can be named in a malpractice suit. Insurance policies may be purchased to protect healthcare workers against potential malpractice suits. Insurance policies often allow doctors to cover their employees, but healthcare workers may also purchase their own policies. In some cases, a healthcare facility may provide malpractice insurance for their healthcare providers. Some medical malpractice lawsuits must be settled in a court of law (Figure 3.6).

malpractice
any misconduct or lack of skill that results in patient injury; also known as professional liability

Assault and Battery

When a person's words or actions make another person fear that he or she may be harmed, that is deemed an **assault**. **Battery** refers to touching a person without permission. Often, assault and battery are charged together. Both actions are considered crimes.

If a patient who is capable of making medical decisions refuses a procedure, you should not insist she cooperate and perform the procedure anyway. If a healthcare worker argues with a patient who does not want a procedure, it may be considered an assault. If the healthcare worker performs a procedure without the patient's consent, it can be considered battery. Sometimes family members can talk the patient into the procedure. If not, the doctor who ordered the procedure must be informed about the refusal. A child who is fearful of needles or other tests may consent if a parent helps to calm him.

assault
any words or actions that lead an individual to fear that he or she will be harmed by another person

battery
touching a person without consent

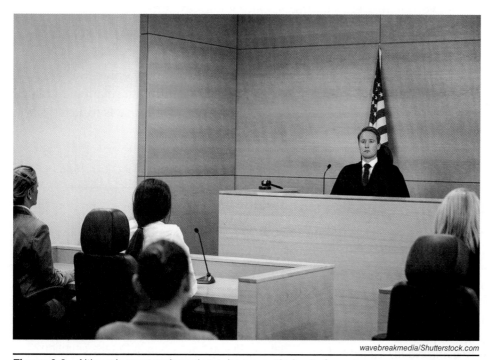

wavebreakmedia/Shutterstock.com

Figure 3.6   Although most malpractice suits are settled out of court, some go to trial.

Check Your Understanding ✓

1. What is the difference between assault and battery?
2. What is meant by *arbitration* in a hospital setting?
3. Who is an emancipated minor?
4. Define *duty of care*.
5. What is an ombudsman?

Defamation

defamation
damaging someone's good name or reputation

slander
saying something that damages someone's good name or reputation

libel
damaging someone's good name or reputation in writing

Defamation is the act of damaging someone's good name or reputation. Verbal defamation is **slander**. Gossip could be categorized as slander. **Libel** is defined as damaging someone's good name or reputation in writing. For instance, if you post something damaging about another person online, it could be considered libel.

Abuse

Abuse is any action that results in physical or mental harm. Unfortunately, abuse may occur in the healthcare facility, or victims of abuse may seek medical care in your facility. There are several types of abuse:

- **Physical abuse:** hitting, depriving someone of food and water, restraining a patient when it is not necessary (some states forbid the use of restraints altogether), or refusing to administer physical care
- **Psychological abuse:** threats, intimidation, or making fun of someone in a cruel manner
- **Verbal abuse:** swearing, speaking harshly, and name calling
- **Sexual abuse:** sexual touching and acts, using sexual gestures, or suggesting sexual behavior

Other forms of abuse can take place before a patient enters the hospital. Domestic abuse occurs when one partner in an intimate relationship such as a marriage abuses the other. Child abuse or elder abuse is inflicted upon individuals of a particular age.

Real Life Scenario — Assault or Proper Patient Care?

Ada is an 89-year-old patient who is being admitted to the hospital after breaking her hip. Ada is in pain and is very confused. Shortly after Ada is admitted, Peter, a phlebotomist, appears at her bedside to take a blood sample.

Ada is having trouble understanding where she is and thinks Peter is going to harm her. Peter knows that the doctor wants the results of the blood test as soon as possible. Ada yells as Peter secures her arm and tells Peter to go away. Peter restrains Ada and gets the sample.

Apply It

1. Could Peter's actions be considered assault and battery? Why or why not?
2. What would you have done in Peter's situation?

Physical signs of abuse include fractures, burns, serious bruising, or other injuries. An abuse victim may have irrational fears, display aggressive or withdrawn behavior, or be hesitant to explain what happened.

If you witness abuse or suspect abuse is taking place, you must report it to the proper authorities as outlined in your facility's handbook. Abuse can be charged as a crime, depending on its seriousness. Any mistreatment of a patient by a healthcare worker can mean being permanently barred from caregiver jobs.

Standard of Care

Standard of care refers to the skill and care that healthcare providers such as doctors, nurses, medical assistants, and phlebotomists must use as determined by their state license or certification. Such practitioners must perform a procedure in the way that someone with similar qualifications would have performed in the same or similar situation.

Suppose a patient comes to the emergency room complaining of rapidly worsening pain in the lower-right side of her abdomen. The doctor fails to explore her complaint thoroughly and sends her home without checking for appendicitis. (The symptoms described are classic signs of appendicitis and the possibility of appendicitis should have been explored.) Consequently, the patient's appendix ruptures. The doctor did not provide the standard of care expected in this case and could be sued for malpractice.

standard of care
reasonable and prudent care that a practitioner of similar qualifications would have performed in the same or similar situation

Statute of Limitations

When a patient decides that something has been done to him that could lead to a lawsuit, there is a **statute of limitations**. The statute of limitations concerns the amount of time that can pass before any legal action is taken. After that time period, a lawsuit may not be filed.

statute of limitations
the amount of time during which any legal action may be taken; after such time a lawsuit may not be filed

Scope of Practice

A healthcare worker's **scope of practice** includes all the skills she is trained for and allowed to use. The more responsibility a worker is given, the more skills are required of her. Scope of practice is a legal concept. A healthcare worker can be held legally responsible (liable) for not performing tasks within her scope of practice. For example, a registered nurse (RN) is not working in her scope of practice if she delegates a task she is licensed to perform to a coworker who is not licensed to perform the task, such as a certified nursing assistant (CNA). Conversely, scope of practice places limits on what healthcare workers are allowed to do (Figure 3.7). Working outside your scope of practice is illegal. An example of this is a laboratory technician performing a blood test on a machine that his scope of practice does not permit him to use.

scope of practice
tasks that an employee is legally allowed to perform based on his or her training and certification

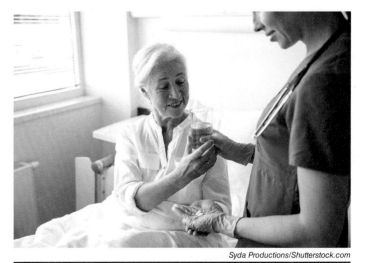

Syda Productions/Shutterstock.com

Figure 3.7 In some states, administering medication is outside of the scope of practice for CNAs.

Real Life Scenario — Scope of Practice

Maria is an ultrasound technician. She is performing an ultrasound on Mona, a very anxious patient. While scanning Mona's gallbladder, Maria sees that the gallbladder contains many gallstones. "Well, do I need to have my gallbladder removed?" asks Mona. Maria's proper response to her patient is "your doctor will see the results of the ultrasound and will let you know as soon as possible." If Maria comments on what she sees, she is acting beyond her scope of practice.

Jamil is a phlebotomist who has been sent to draw blood twice today on a patient who is suspected of having a serious blood disorder. The doctor is anxious to make a diagnosis and needs more blood. The patient wants to know why Jamil is back again for more blood so soon. Jamil would be acting beyond his scope of practice to explain that the doctor suspects a serious blood problem and needs more blood for confirmation. Instead, Jamil tells the patient that more tests are ordered and apologizes for the inconvenience of two blood draws.

Apply It

1. Why would Maria be acting beyond her scope of practice if she tells Mona that her gallbladder will need to be removed?
2. Why would Jamil be acting beyond his scope of practice if he tells his patient the reason for the second blood draw?
3. What should you do if you see a fellow healthcare worker act beyond his scope of practice? What if his actions result in a mistake that causes harm to a patient? Can you think of a situation in which that might occur?

Check Your Understanding ✔

When you pursue a career in healthcare, it is very important that you understand the laws that protect both patients and healthcare professionals. Which legal concept applies to each of the following situations?

1. A nurse performs CPR on a man who experiences cardiac arrest in a restaurant.
2. A patient is injured by a worker who incorrectly performed a procedure that met the standard of care for other members of the worker's profession.
3. Rosie was disappointed that she couldn't sue her doctor because too much time had passed since the incident.
4. A healthcare professional performed a procedure she is not qualified to perform and a patient was injured.
5. A nurse performs a procedure on a patient who refused to give permission for the procedure.

Confidentiality

confidentiality
the practice of allowing only certain individuals the right to access information; ensures that others do not obtain the personal information of patients

Confidentiality allows only certain individuals the right to access personal information. Confidentiality protects a patient's personal information, ensuring that others do not have access. As a future healthcare worker, you are responsible for upholding the confidentiality of your patients' information. In a digital age in which privacy is increasingly threatened, the issue of confidentiality has never been more important.

Healthcare agencies and providers *must* provide confidentiality and privacy of any health-related information that is collected, maintained, used, or transmitted (Figure 3.8).

Confidentiality has been, and always should be, a critical aspect of the relationship between a patient and healthcare worker. Common knowledge of some diagnoses or treatments could destroy a patient's reputation. Mental illness, drug or alcohol addiction, sexually transmitted infections, and other types of problems can be misunderstood and unfairly judged by others. An example of this occurred when people first reacted to AIDS in the early 1980s. When word spread that someone had AIDS, ignorance caused employers to fire employees, insurance carriers to deny insurance to people with AIDS, and landlords to refuse to rent to someone with AIDS. Although laws are now in place to protect patients' confidentiality, problems still occur because of ignorance about many diseases and disorders.

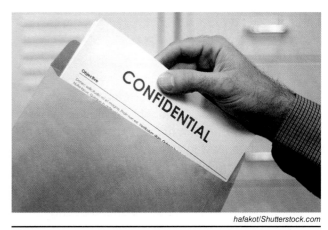

hafakot/Shutterstock.com

Figure 3.8   Healthcare workers must protect patients by keeping their personal information confidential.

HIPAA Privacy Protections

As you learned in chapter 2, Congress passed the **Health Insurance Portability and Accountability Act (HIPAA)** in 1996. One main purpose of the act was to guarantee continuation of health insurance coverage if a person changes jobs. It also provided standards for health information transactions, as well as confidentiality and security of patient data.

The HIPAA Privacy Rule has been enforced by the US government's Office of Civil Rights since April of 2003. This rule establishes national standards to protect individuals' medical records and other personal health information. It also gives patients rights regarding their health information, including the right to examine and obtain a copy of their health records, and to request corrections.

Violating the HIPAA Privacy Rule can result in civil penalties ranging from $100 per violation up to $25,000. These penalties can apply to healthcare facilities as well as individuals. Criminal penalties are also possible and may include a fine of $50,000 with the possibility of one year in prison if information is illegally disclosed. If there is intent to sell confidential information, penalties can include a maximum fine of $250,000 with the possibility of ten years in prison. Maintaining confidentiality is a serious matter. Something as seemingly harmless as gossiping about a patient's condition can result in such penalties (Figure 3.9).

Health Insurance Portability and Accountability Act (HIPAA)
an act approved by the US Congress in 1996 and fully enforced in 2006; includes a privacy provision for patient health records

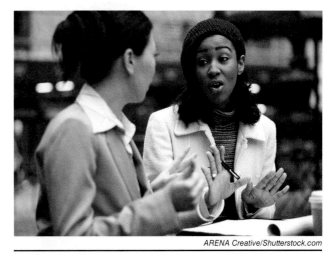

ARENA Creative/Shutterstock.com

Figure 3.9   Gossip can lead to breaches of patient confidentiality.

Real Life Scenario — Confidentiality

Jane is a phlebotomist at Eastridge Hospital. One morning she is assigned to draw blood on the alcohol rehabilitation floor. One of Jane's patients is her sister's neighbor. Jane knows that the patient is part of a car pool that takes Jane's niece and nephew to school. The possibility of an alcoholic driving the children to school makes Jane very nervous. Jane adores her niece and nephew and is very concerned that they might be in danger.

Apply It

1. Should Jane tell her sister about the situation? Why or why not?
2. Jane is working with Jessie, a fellow phlebotomist. Jane goes to lunch with Jessie and wants to let her know that a patient Jane has just drawn blood from is really abusive toward the staff. She and Jessie have a long discussion about how to deal with the patient. The discussion takes place in the hospital cafeteria. Is this a violaton of confidentiality? Why or why not?

Exceptions for Releasing Patient Information

Healthcare workers are both *ethically* and *legally* bound to protect the privacy and confidentiality of patient-doctor interactions. Doctors may share information about patient confidences *only* if required by law. Breaches, or breaks, in confidentiality can result in lawsuits against the doctor and her employees, or against a healthcare facility.

A patient's medical record is a confidential, legal document that should not be discussed with anyone who does not have a need to know this information. Before information can be released for insurance billing purposes, a release-of-information form must be signed by the patient (Figure 3.10).

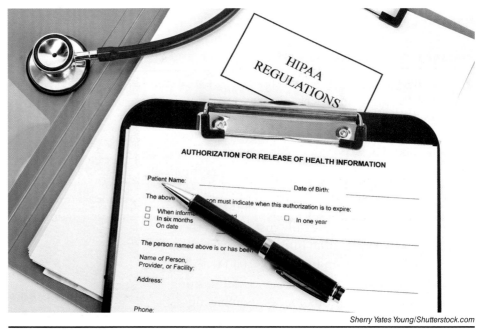

Sherry Yates Young/Shutterstock.com

Figure 3.10   Personal information cannot be released without the patient's signed consent or a court order.

As a healthcare worker, you will be exposed to a wide range of confidential information about many patients. Acting in a professional manner is absolutely mandatory.

There are some exceptions for releasing patient medical information. Doctors are sometimes required by law to release medical information to authorities without the patient's consent. This situation may arise when authorities, including doctors, have concerns that a patient may be at risk for immediate harm. Doctors must release medical information when ordered to by the court. Even so, privacy rules require a doctor to make reasonable efforts to disclose only the minimal amount of information necessary for the purpose requested. Rules about confidentiality are different in some healthcare facilities, schools, and social service agencies. You must be aware of specific policies of the facility in which you work.

Patient Consent Forms

When a doctor makes a diagnosis and recommends a specific treatment, the patient has the responsibility to decide whether or not to accept the diagnosis and method of treatment. The doctor must inform the patient, or the patient's guardian, of the risk of the procedure, using easily understandable words. The benefits and risks of a procedure or treatment plan must be explained to a patient or guardian before permission is given. If the patient is willing to accept the risks involved, a consent form—called an **informed consent**—is signed. You may be asked to prepare such a form. All signatures must be in ink. Patients *cannot* be forced to sign a consent form.

informed consent
a form, given to a patient by a doctor, explaining the benefit and risks of a procedure; the patient accepts the risk by signing the informed consent form

Sexual Harassment

Sexual harassment can occur in any workplace. According to the United States Equal Employment Opportunity Commission (EEOC), sexual harassment is a form of sex discrimination. Employers must have a process in place to take immediate steps when they receive a sexual harassment complaint. Unwanted sexual advances or other forms of offensive sexual behavior should be reported immediately to a supervisor.

sexual harassment
unwanted sexual advances and other forms of offensive sexual behavior; both men and women can be sexually harassed

Both men and women can be sexually harassed. Your training manual or employee handbook should include definitions of sexual harassment, along with measures to stop the harassment. You may not realize that something you say in an offhanded way might be considered sexual harassment. An example of sexual harassment is a man commenting to a woman that he really appreciated the tight blouse she wore to work yesterday.

Sexual harassment is unethical and illegal. You can be disciplined for such behavior and lose your job. For example, if an employer is found to have denied a promotion to an employee because the employee did not return the employer's sexual advances, that is illegal behavior.

> **Think It Through**
>
> Johanna and Emily are both working with a 1-year-old patient who was born with fetal alcohol syndrome. Both women want to discuss how they feel about the case, so they wait until they are in the hospital cafeteria to discuss their reactions. They didn't want to talk about it near their supervisor or the patient and her family. Are they right in waiting to talk in the cafeteria?

Real Life Scenario   The New Employee

Mallory and Sadie are young, single women who work in the Financial Services Office of Eastridge Hospital. When a new employee, Mark, is hired to work with them, both women agree he is "hot." When Mark walks by Sadie and Mallory's desks, both women comment under their breath about Mark's physique so that Mark can hear. They also compliment him on his trousers, giggling as they say that they could be tighter.

Apply It

1. Is Mallory and Sadie's behavior considered sexual harassment? Why or why not?
2. What should Mark do if he feels uncomfortable in this situation?

Recognizing Reportable Behavior

Healthcare workers are responsible for helping to protect everyone in the workplace. If you suspect that there is unethical or illegal behavior occurring in the workplace, or you have observed such behavior (not just relying on gossip), the incident must be reported. A reportable incident is an event that can affect the health, safety, or welfare of those around you. A few examples of reportable behavior include

- an employee harassing another employee;
- an employee stealing medication (Figure 3.11);
- an employee making fun of a patient;
- evidence of misuse of hospital funds;
- a breach of confidentiality;
- a worker striking or otherwise harming a patient;
- an employee stealing property from the employer; and
- an employee stealing property from a patient or a coworker.

Incident reports are discussed in further detail in Chapter 4, *Safety and Infection Control*.

There should be instructions for reporting illegal and unethical conduct in your employee handbook. Your supervisor or human resources representative can help you report such behavior. If you suspect your supervisor is acting illegally or unethically, contact your human resources representative. Acting ethically and obeying laws that relate to the healthcare environment is essential to maintaining a high degree of professional behavior.

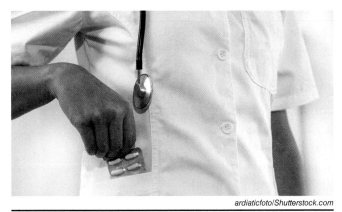

ardiaticfoto/Shutterstock.com

Figure 3.11   Stealing medication is both unethical and illegal. It must be reported.

Real Life Scenario Acceptable Speech

Brad is a receptionist for Dr. Winston's dental practice. One day a new patient arrives in the reception area. This patient is an obese woman wearing unwashed clothes. After the patient is brought into an examination room, Jane—Dr. Winston's dental assistant—overhears Brad saying, "Wow! That patient is as big as a house and smells terrible! Someone should tell her how gross she is."

Apply It

1. What should Jane do? Is this a reportable offense? Should Jane report Brad to Dr. Winston?
2. Is Brad acting unethically or illegally?
3. What would you do if you were Jane?

Discrimination in the Workplace

Healthcare workers must be sensitive to the diversity of their patients. Recognizing and understanding cultural, social, ethnic, and racial differences will help you treat patients with respect and empathy (Figure 3.12). **Discrimination** based on illness, age, weight, or a disability can also occur in the healthcare setting. For example, patients with HIV and AIDS have experienced discrimination in the past, even from their healthcare providers. Chapter 15, *Communication Skills*, provides additional guidance for communicating with diverse populations.

discrimination
the act of unfairly treating a person or a group of people differently from others

Discrimination toward your fellow employees is also unacceptable. Most healthcare facilities present a code of ethics for their employees, clearly stating that discrimination of any sort will not be tolerated. The American Health Information Management Association Code of Ethics states: "Respect the inherent dignity and worth of every person."

Not only is discrimination unethical, it is also illegal in most states. Healthcare workers can lose their job, be fined, and face more drastic penalties if they violate a patient's right to ethical and fair treatment. Healthcare workers must ensure patient safety and privacy while treating each and every patient and fellow worker with respect and dignity.

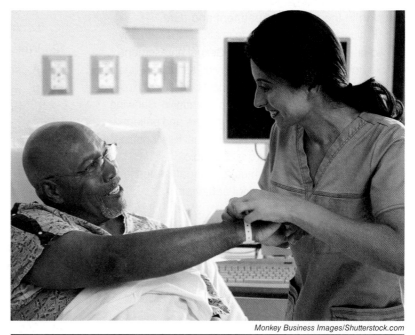

Monkey Business Images/Shutterstock.com

Figure 3.12 To establish positive relationships with coworkers and patients, healthcare workers must always respect others. Discrimination of any kind is unacceptable.

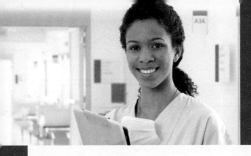

Summary

It is important for healthcare workers to understand the concepts of medical ethics and medical law. A healthcare employee must make decisions that are both ethical and legal. Unethical or illegal behavior may lead to termination of employment and even legal actions.

An employee must understand the various legal protections that exist for both patients and healthcare workers. Healthcare workers should understand the definitions of the following terms: *advance directive*, *assault*, *battery*, *durable power of attorney*, *duty of care*, *emancipated minor*, *Good Samaritan laws*, *guardian*, *libel*, *malpractice*, *negligence*, *reasonable care*, *scope of practice*, *slander*, and *statute of limitations*.

The issue of confidentiality has never been more important than in this digital age, in which privacy is increasingly threatened. A healthcare worker must never discuss a patient's personal or medical information with anyone except fellow employees involved in the patient's treatment and care.

Ethical behavior extends to relationships with any individual in the healthcare facility. Sexual harassment should not be tolerated. Such behavior, as well as stealing, misuse of facility funds, or abuse must be reported to a supervisor or human resources representative. Showing respect for the diversity of your coworkers and patients is part of establishing healthy professional relationships. Discrimination of any sort is unacceptable.

Continual focus on ethical and legal issues is a necessity for truly professional behavior.

Review Questions

Answer the following questions using what you have learned in this chapter.

True/False 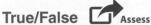Assess

1. *True or False?* Only a doctor can be sued for malpractice.

2. *True or False?* Telling your friends that your patient, Jane Maxwell, has a sexually transmitted disease is both unethical and illegal.

3. *True or False?* Breaking a medical law can lead to losing your professional license.

4. *True or False?* The standard of reasonable care protects the healthcare worker.

5. *True or False?* Confidentiality is a relatively recent concern for the medical world.

6. *True or False?* A civil law enforces private rights rather than punishing criminal behavior.

7. *True or False?* If something is illegal, it is always unethical.

8. *True or False?* Good Samaritan laws are the same in every US state.

9. *True or False?* If you hear "through the grapevine" that someone is being unethical, you should report the person immediately.

10. *True or False?* Libel and slander are the same.

Multiple Choice Assess

11. Which of the following would be seen as unethical?
    A. being rude to a patient
    B. gossiping about a fellow team member
    C. ignoring supervisor requests
    D. All of the above.

12. Which scenario would be considered illegal?
    A. striking a patient
    B. revealing a patient's condition to someone outside the workplace
    C. coming to work with an illness
    D. Both A and B.

13. Which of the following could be considered sexual harassment?
    A. any unwanted touching by someone in the workplace
    B. a male employee telling a female team member that she has really "hot" legs
    C. telling a dirty joke
    D. All of the above.

14. Assault and battery in the healthcare setting includes _____.
    A. gossiping and being rude to a patient
    B. stealing from a patient and performing a task that isn't in your job description
    C. threatening and hitting a patient
    D. ignoring your supervisor and hitting a patient

15. Which of the following statements is *false*?

    A. Every patient is entitled to safe care.

    B. An emancipated minor is a person over 18 years of age.

    C. Insurance policies can be purchased to protect employees from malpractice suits.

    D. Reasonable care is a legal protection for healthcare workers.

16. Professional liability is also known as _____.

    A. negligence

    B. malpractice

    C. reasonable care

    D. duty of care

17. _____ created a law including a privacy provision for patient health records.

    A. Civil law

    B. Durable power of attorney

    C. Good Samaritan laws

    D. HIPAA

18. Ethical behavior includes _____.

    A. treating all patients with respect if they show respect to you

    B. respecting the privacy of others

    C. understanding the limitations of your training

    D. B and C only.

19. The Patient Self-Determination Act of 1990 states that _____.

    A. healthcare institutions must inform the patient of rights under state law at the time of admission

    B. a patient can refuse medical or surgical treatment

    C. patients have the right to participate in healthcare decisions

    D. All of the above.

20. Which exception can be made for release of patient medical information?

    A. A woman's fiancé wants information about her surgery.

    B. A concerned citizen wants to know the diagnosis of her next door neighbor.

    C. A doctor is ordered by the court to reveal patient medical information.

    D. A reporter wants to know the status of a hospitalized celebrity.

Short Answer

21. According to Hippocrates, what should doctors never do?

22. Is ethics about legal/illegal or right and wrong?

23. Name two types of invasion of privacy.

24. Failure to perform duty of care results in what crime?

25. What is an advance directive?

26. Define each of the following terms.

    A. malpractice

    B. duty of care

    C. Good Samaritan laws

    D. guardian

    E. negligence

    F. standard of care

    G. scope of practice

27. What does DNR mean?

28. What is another name for civil law?

29. What is the role of the ombudsman in a healthcare setting?

Critical Thinking Exercises

30. At your past jobs, did you ever see unethical or illegal behaviors? If so, did you report such behavior to a supervisor? If you did not report this information, what was your reason for doing so?

31. Is it unethical to play games, send your friends personal e-mails, or shop online when using a work computer? What could you do on a work computer that would be considered illegal?

32. Research on the Internet to find three cases in which healthcare workers were accused of unethical or illegal behavior. You may also find cases in newspapers as well. In your experience, have you found this type of behavior to be common or uncommon?

33. Research and describe the roles of professional associations and regulatory agencies involved in medical law and ethics.

34. When can gossip become unethical or even illegal? Give two examples of cases where gossip can become damaging.

35. Investigate the legal and ethical ramifications of unacceptable behavior.

36. Search online for the Affordable Care Act's Patient Bill of Rights. Choose three protections from the document and explain the legal and ethical ramifications of each.

Chapter 4
Safety and Infection Control

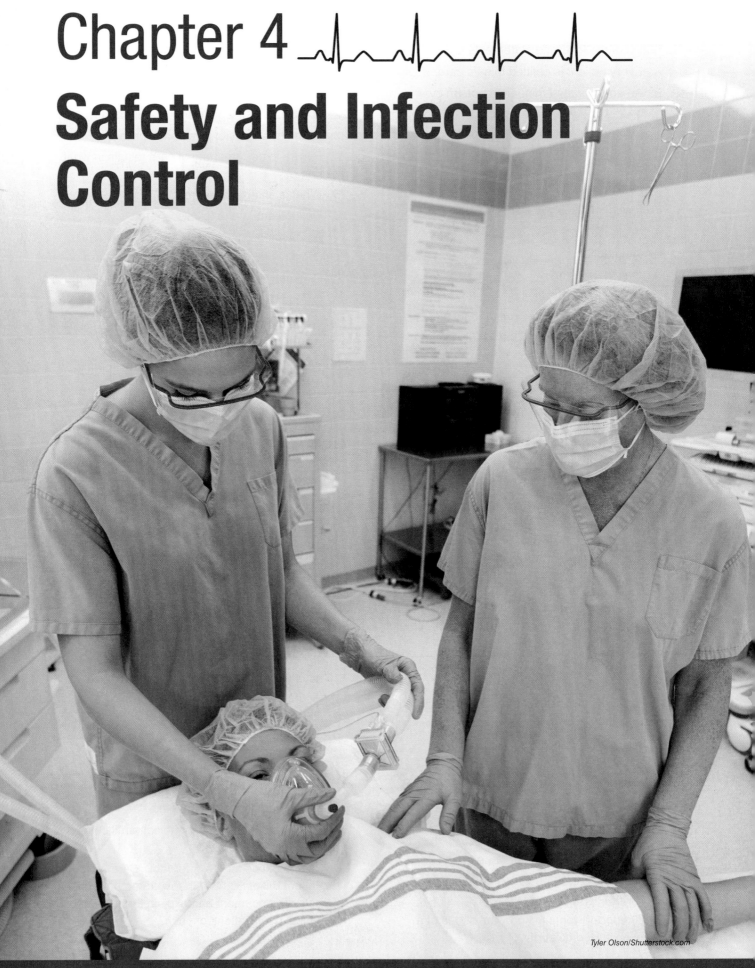

Tyler Olson/Shutterstock.com

Terms to Know

 Build Vocab

- aerobe
- anaerobe
- antisepsis
- asepsis
- autoclave
- bacteria
- biohazard sharps container
- biopsy
- bloodborne pathogens
- body mechanics
- carpal tunnel syndrome
- chain of infection
- direct contact
- disinfection
- ergonomics
- fire triangle

- fungi
- hand hygiene
- hospital emergency codes
- incident reports
- indirect contact
- infection con~~trol~~
- i~~solation~~
- m~~aterial safet~~y data sheet (~~M~~SDS)
- Methicillin-resistant *Staphylococcus aureus* (MRSA)
- morphology
- needlesticks
- Needlestick Safety and Prevention Act
- nosocomial infections

Study These

- OSHA Bloodborne Pathogens Standard
- OSHA Hazard Communication Standard
- parasites
- personal protective equipment (PPE)
- potentially infectious materials (PIM)
- protozoa
- quality improvement (QI)
- rickettsiae
- sanitization
- sharps
- standard precautions
- sterilization
- vectors
- viruses

Chapter Objectives

- Explain the role of several organizations, including OSHA, that work to improve healthcare delivery.
- Understand the basic safety rules of a healthcare facility.
- Describe how to avoid chemical, electrical, radiation, and fire dangers in a healthcare facility.
- Discuss the proper responses to fires and other emergencies.
- List some ways to practice proper body mechanics when lifting objects and patients.
- Discuss the importance of proper hand washing.
- Explain the importance of infection control.
- List the parts of the chain of infection and explain how to break it.
- Discuss the need for isolation procedures and how the procedures differ.

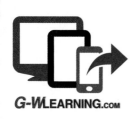

While studying, look for the activity icon to:

- **Build** vocabulary with e-flash cards and interactive games.
- **Assess** progress with chapter and unit review questions.
- **Expand** learning with animations and illustration labeling activities.
- **Simulate** EHR entry with healthcare documents.

G-WLEARNING.com

www.g-wlearning.com/healthsciences/

infection control
term for all efforts made to prevent the spread of infection

In this chapter, you will learn about two extremely important healthcare topics: safety and infection control. Safety must be a primary concern of anyone choosing a career in healthcare. Maintaining safe conditions means avoiding danger, risks, injury, and infection for patients, healthcare workers, and visitors. **Infection control** includes all the activities involved with preventing the spread of infection. Every possible effort must be made to maintain infection control to protect patients from further health problems and keep employees and their families safe and healthy. After completing this chapter, you will be more aware of and better prepared to follow safety and infection control procedures.

Safety

As a future healthcare worker, when you think of safety, you probably think of making sure that patients are safe. Keeping patients safe is indeed a critical part of healthcare safety, but there is much more to healthcare safety. If you work in healthcare, you must be aware at all times of conditions that could negatively impact not only the safety of patients, but also the safety of your coworkers, visitors to your facility, and of course, yourself. Let's take a closer look at these different aspects of safety.

Safety in Healthcare Facilities

Some healthcare facilities have special safety regulations that apply to their specific environment, equipment, or patients. You will need to learn and practice these regulations at each healthcare facility at which you work. In addition, there are some general safety rules that all healthcare workers at all healthcare facilities should remember.

Safety Manuals

Every healthcare facility has policies regarding safety and should have written safety instructions readily available to all employees. These policies are usually spelled out in the facility's safety manual. Instructions for following the facility's safety guidelines will most likely be part of the in-service training given to all new employees. You will also be required to attend all staff training regarding patient safety issues. It is important that you follow all safety procedures in the safety manual of your facility.

Individual departments within the facility may have additional written safety rules specific to their operations. For example, a department using hazardous chemicals will have rules for the safe handling of chemicals. The diagnostic imaging department will have manuals dealing with radiation safety. It is also important that you follow all of your department's safety rules.

General Safety Rules

The following are some of the most important standard safety rules for all healthcare facilities. These are the types of rules you will find in the safety manuals of the different healthcare facilities at which you work.

- **Whenever possible, walk on the right-hand side of hallways and stairways.** Avoid walking alongside more than two people. Leave hallways open so that there are no "traffic" problems (Figure 4.1).

- **Always hold on to handrails when using stairs.** If you are in a hurry and are not holding on to the railing, you may fall and injure yourself.

- **Never run in a hallway.** If you run, you can fall and injure yourself, or you may collide with another person or object. Running can also cause a panic. Walk, don't run!

- **Report any lights that do not work in your facility.** No one should be injured due to faulty lighting. Additionally, report any faulty electrical sources, such as electrical cords, machinery, and power outlets.

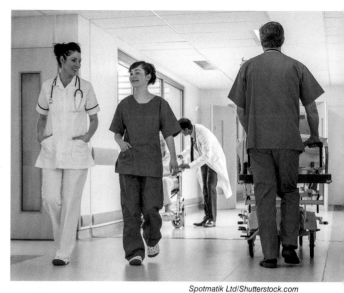

Spotmatik Ltd/Shutterstock.com

Figure 4.1 Walk on the right side of a hallway whenever possible. Doing so will greatly reduce the chances of blocked pathways and collisions.

- **Cautiously open swinging doors.** Take care to check that someone is not on the other side of a swinging door. Otherwise, you can injure yourself or someone else.

- **Remove obstructions from floors and hallways.** Obstructions on floors and in hallways are possible tripping hazards. They might include out-of-place equipment or patients' personal items.

- **Do not prop open fire safety doors.** Keep all equipment away from these doors.

- **Wear sensible shoes.** Open-heel and open-toe shoes expose the foot to potential injury. A biohazard spill could damage your skin if you were wearing open-heel or open-toe shoes.

- **Make sure your uniform is neat and clean in appearance.** This includes clean shoes, clean scrubs, long hair tied back, and name badge securely in place.

- **Store items in a safe, yet easily accessible manner.** Avoid placing items on the top of cabinets, as they might fall off when you open the cabinet doors. Do not overfill shelves, as you do not want items falling off the shelves and posing a safety hazard. Heavier items should be stored close to the floor to allow everyone to reach and remove them safely.

- **Recognize and obey evacuation routes posted throughout the facility.** It is important to be familiar with evacuation routes and plans in the event of an emergency. Floor plans should be posted with clearly marked exit routes.

- **Be aware of everyone around you.** If you see something that concerns you, or could be dangerous, say something to the appropriate supervisor.

- **Practice safety in your daily life.** It is easier to prevent accidents than to treat them. Be aware of potential hazards in your home and school environments.

Hospital Emergency Codes

Hospital emergency codes are used in hospitals to alert healthcare workers to various emergencies. These codes quickly convey essential information while preventing stress and panic among patients and visitors to the hospital. Some hospitals are phasing out codes because they can lead to confusion due to the variation of codes among different facilities. Efforts have been made to establish uniform codes throughout the United States.

All healthcare facility employees must know the meanings of their facility's various codes. Some facilities print the codes on the back of workers' ID badges to avoid confusion and serve as quick reference. Some frequently used hospital emergency codes are

- Code Red—fire in the facility;
- Code Blue—cardiac arrest;
- Code Pink—infant or child abduction;
- Code Orange—hazardous materials spill;
- Code Silver—dangerous person with a weapon; and
- Code Black—bomb threat.

When codes are announced, the location of the emergency is identified as well. An example of this is, "Code Blue, Cardiac Care Unit." When the danger is over, there will be an "all clear" announcement.

Disaster Preparedness in the Healthcare Facility

A disaster is any sudden event that brings great damage, loss, or destruction. Individuals in the healthcare profession must be prepared for unexpected events due to terrorism, catastrophic accidents, earthquakes, explosions, fires, tornadoes, hurricanes, and gun violence. In the event of a disaster, you will most likely find yourself working alongside police, firefighters, and emergency medical personnel.

Healthcare facilities are required to develop and implement plans for dealing with disasters. The facility in which you work will also have disaster drills. When you are hired, you will be given instructions for how to handle a disaster and what your specific role will be in those situations. These instructions may include procedures for evacuating patients, recognizing evacuation routes, and working as part of a team in emergency situations.

Many communities offer CERT programs (Community Emergency Response Training). CERT educates individuals about disaster preparedness for hazards that may impact their area. CERT also trains workers in basic disaster response skills, such as fire safety, light search and rescue, team organization, and disaster medical operations.

During a disaster, you must act in a professional manner, remain calm, and carry out your assigned task without complaint. Always obey directions given by your supervisor.

Safety in the Science Laboratory

As part of your education to become a healthcare worker, you will probably take several science courses. Science courses often include labs.

There are several safety issues to keep in mind while working in the science laboratory. These considerations can also apply to any career that involves working in scientific research laboratories, hospital labs, or independent laboratories.

There are significant safety risks in the science laboratory. When working in a laboratory, you must adhere to the following guidelines:

- Obey all of the rules your instructor or supervisor has posted in the laboratory. These rules are often also printed and given to students. A zero tolerance policy for disobeying safety rules will probably be in effect.

- Be aware of all safety symbols in the laboratory. For instance, the label on a bottle of a particular chemical may have a warning symbol indicating that the chemical within the container is flammable. Figure 4.2 illustrates some safety symbols that you should be familiar with when working in a laboratory.

Laboratory Safety Symbols			
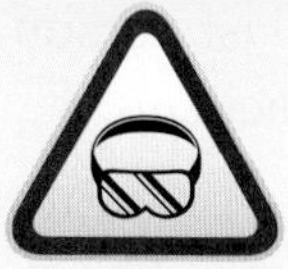 **Safety goggles**	Safety goggles must be worn to protect the eyes while performing any task that involves chemicals, flames, heating, or glassware.	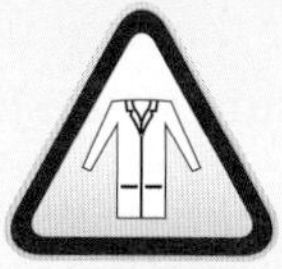 **Lab coat**	A lab coat or apron must be worn to protect the skin and clothing from harm.
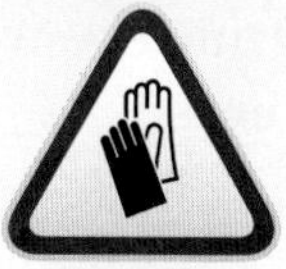 **Gloves**	When working with harmful chemicals or microorganisms, disposable gloves must be worn at all times. Dispose of used gloves properly.	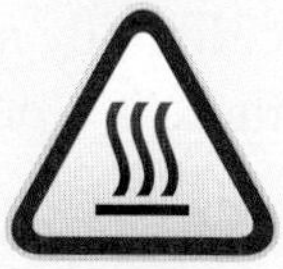 **Heat**	Do not touch hot objects with your bare hands; instead use a clamp or tongs.
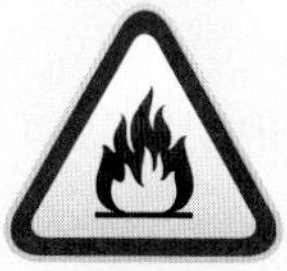 **Flames**	Follow your instructor's or supervisor's directions when working with flames. Tie back loose hair and clothing before working with flames.	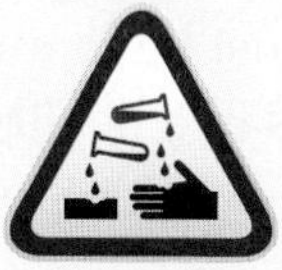 **Corrosive chemical**	When working with a corrosive chemical, avoid contact with the skin, eyes, or clothing and do not inhale the vapors. Wash your hands thoroughly after working with corrosive chemicals.
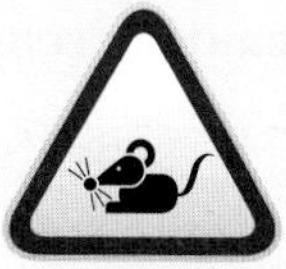 **Animal safety**	Avoid harming any animals or yourself when working in the lab. Wash hands thoroughly after handling any animal.	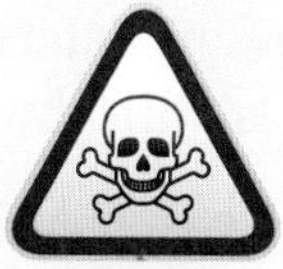 **Poison**	Avoid contact with poisonous substances and do not inhale vapors. Wash hands thoroughly after working with poisonous substances.
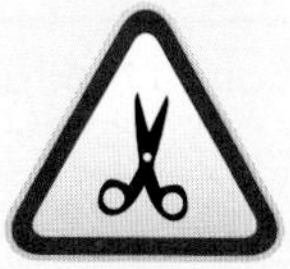 **Scissors**	Sharps, including scissors, knives, scalpels, or needles must be handled with care to avoid puncturing or cutting the skin. Always direct the sharp point of the object away from yourself and others.	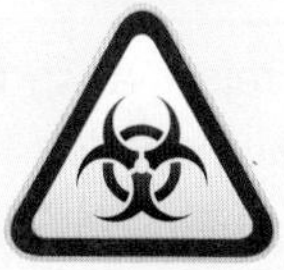 **Biohazard**	Materials that are harmful and pose a threat to your health must be handled with care. Avoid contact with biohazards including used needles, toxins, infectious substances, and other medical waste.

Ecelop/Shutterstock.com; Max Griboedov/Shutterstock.com; andromina/Shutterstock.com; Miguel Angel Salinas Salinas/Shutterstock.com; Barry Barnes/Shutterstock.com

Figure 4.2   Test yourself on these laboratory safety symbols. Can you identify each symbol if the label is covered?

- Clothing is an important consideration when working in a laboratory. Exposed heels and toes are vulnerable to injury so it is best to avoid shoes that expose your feet. Do not wear loose-sleeved blouses or shirts if fire sources are in use.

- Protective safety equipment must be worn when working with chemicals, blood, and other items that pose a safety risk. If you are not sure when to use such equipment, ask your instructor or supervisor. You will learn more about the use of protective safety equipment later in this chapter.

- When doing a laboratory exercise, you may be tempted to read through the directions quickly in an effort to complete the exercise on time. For the sake of safety, read all directions carefully. Instructions for safely working with equipment and handling substances are most likely included in the laboratory exercise directions. If you are confused, ask your instructor or supervisor to explain.

- When working in a laboratory setting, make sure that your workspace is neat and clean during and after the procedure. You will be given instructions on how to leave your laboratory station for the next user. Imagine how you would react if the last person using your station left behind a puddle of dangerous acid.

- In the event of an accident, refer to the instructions and procedures for avoiding and treating injuries. Eyewash stations should be available if you are working with any liquid chemicals that might accidentally splash into your eyes. Protective eyewear must be worn if there is a possibility of chemicals splashing into the eyes.

- Burns, fires, and equipment failures that result in injuries are considered emergencies. Read through all emergency policies before starting any laboratory exercise. All accidents, no matter how minor, must be reported to your instructor or supervisor immediately. As in a healthcare facility, you may have to fill out an incident or accident report.

- Familiarize yourself with the location and operation of safety equipment such as a safety shower and eyewash station(s).

Following safety guidelines in all areas of healthcare, including science training, is critical whether you are a student or an employee.

Check Your Understanding ✔️

1. Why might an individual department have safety rules in addition to the rules contained in the facility's safety manual?
2. On which side of a hallway in a healthcare facility should you walk?
3. Give two examples of the importance of wearing proper clothing in a laboratory.
4. What are hospital emergency codes? Give three examples of commonly used codes and their meanings.

Patient Safety

Caring for patients requires serious attention to detail to provide competent care and prevent accidents. As a conscientious healthcare worker acting in a professional manner, you are responsible for the safety of your patients. Even if you do not work directly with patients, you must still be observant. It is important that you act quickly if you see safety hazards, such as liquid spills, loose rugs, or confused and disoriented patients.

Universal Patient Safety Guidelines

useful

If you do work directly with patients, follow the guidelines of your facility. The following are some universal guidelines for patient safety:

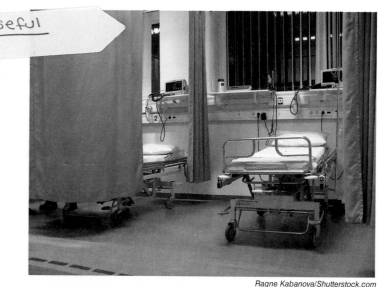

Figure 4.3 Curtains surround these hospital beds for a reason. Always close them when working with patients to respect their privacy.

Ragne Kabanova/Shutterstock.com

1 • Always identify the patient before you interact with him or her. Check the patient's identification bracelet and your paperwork to make sure that you have the correct patient. Ask the patient to tell you her name.

2 • Make sure your patient has privacy during all procedures (Figure 4.3). It is your responsibility to ensure the safety and comfort of a patient at all times.

3 • When leaving a patient, make sure the bed is in a low position. The call button must be within reach of the patient.

4 • Be sure that the patient knows the location of the bathroom, call buttons, emergency call lights, handrails, and safety rails.

5 • Before performing a procedure, explain the entire procedure and make sure you have the patient's consent. For example, if a patient does not want you to take his or her blood and refuses permission, you must tell the nurse in charge that the patient has refused. Make sure that the patient understands you. If language is a barrier, your facility may have designated translators available to help. If the patient cannot understand you because of a medical challenge, make sure someone who can speak for the patient is there, such as a guardian or a close relative. *Always remember that the patient has the right to refuse treatment!* If an employee performs a procedure that the patient has refused, the employee may be sued for battery, or unlawful touching.

6 • Never start or perform a procedure that you are not trained to perform. Never take shortcuts such as skipping a time-consuming step because you are in a hurry. If a particular step is part of the approved procedure, it is important. Operating within your scope of practice is not only ethical but legal.

7 • Immediately report safety hazards to a nearby supervisor. What is a safety hazard? Tangled or frayed wires, any kind of liquid spill in the patient's room or hallway, hot beverages served to a patient who cannot manage them, the smell of smoke, and a patient who will not stay in bed when bed rest is required are just a few examples. Additionally, a patient's room crowded with equipment can become a hazard if the patient gets out of bed.

8 • Observe the patient carefully so that you can identify any changes in status. If you see increased coughing, changes in skin color, difficulty breathing, increased restlessness, change in the level of consciousness, unexpected bleeding, or increased pain, report these events to a supervisor as soon as possible. Do not leave a patient alone when you observe that he or she may be disoriented and confused. Again, report the situation to a supervisor to make sure the patient is safe.

9 • Patients can develop allergies to medications and food, as well as environmental conditions. Watch for signs of allergic reactions. Such signs include rash, difficulty breathing, coughing, sneezing, tightness in the throat, nausea, skin itching, tingling, redness, or swelling. Allergic reactions can be life threatening if not treated quickly.

10 • Wash your hands upon entering and leaving a patient's room. Never wear gloves out of a patient's room. Discard them and wash your hands prior to leaving the room and in between procedures. Frequent hand washing is the best way to prevent the spread of disease.

Check Your Understanding

1. Name three safety hazards that could occur in a patient's room.
2. Before you leave a patient's room, what precautions should you take with the patient's bed?
3. Before interacting with a hospitalized patient, what must you do?
4. Does a patient have the right to refuse a treatment prescribed by the doctor?

Expand

Incident Reports

An incident is any event that is not a part of the routine operation of the healthcare facility. An incident could be a patient or visitor falling, a healthcare worker hurting his or her back while lifting a patient, or a patient receiving an incorrect medication. There are also incidents that are not safety-related, such as theft or abusive language from a patient or employee. **Incident reports** should be used to document both safety- and non-safety-related occurrences.

If you see unsafe practices or situations, you must immediately report these incidents to a supervisor in the area. You may be asked to fill out an incident report documenting the problem (Figure 4.4). An incident report is an internal document and should not be included in a patient's medical record. Some facilities use separate reports for employee accidents versus other types of incidents. The reports should be readily available at all times.

incident reports

forms used in a healthcare facility to document both safety- and non-safety-related events that are not part of a routine operation in the facility

I. OCCURRENCE:				STATUS	
DATE	TIME	LOCATION	NAME	❑ INPT ❑ VISITOR ❑ OUTPT ❑ OTHER	

AGE	SEX ❑ M ❑ F	Diagnosis or Procedure	Witness Yes ❑ No ❑ Name _____ Dept. _____

Condition Prior to Occurrence ❑ Alert ❑ Disoriented ❑ Asleep ❑ Anesthetized	Meds in last 12 hrs (falls only)

II. MEDICATION (All that apply)	INTRAVENOUS (Note all that apply)	FALL (Complete both sides)	
❑ Wrong medication ❑ Wrong amount ❑ Wrong date/time ❑ Wrong pt ❑ Wrong route ❑ Transcription error ❑ Allergic reaction ❑ Omission ❑ Incorrect narcotic count ❑ Other _____ ❑ Name of Med	❑ Wrong solution ❑ Wrong medication ❑ Wrong rate ❑ Wrong time ❑ Infiltration ❑ Transcription error ❑ PCA error ❑ Blood transfusion ❑ Hyperalimentation ❑ Other _____	❑ Ambulating ❑ In BR ❑ Out of bed ❑ To FRM B/R ❑ Other	❑ PT has fallen prev ❑ Restrained ❑ Side rails up ❑ Side rails down

		Surgical — Please Comment	
Consent	**Equipment**	❑ Delay ❑ Consent mismatch ❑ Unplanned return ❑ Incorrect count ❑ Unplanned repair/removal ❑ Arrest ❑ Death ❑ Anestheia related ❑ Other _____	
❑ Name written ❑ Mismatch ❑ Refused to sign ❑ Incomplete ❑ Other _____	❑ Not available ❑ Disconnected ❑ Procedure not followed ❑ Nonsterile ❑ Malfunction ❑ Other _____ ❑ Descript. of item _____		

AMA	**Pressure Sore (Complete both sides)**		**Other**	
❑ AMA signed ❑ Not signed ❑ AWOL ❑ Other _____	❑ On admission ❑ Hospital acquired ❑ Picture taken	❑ Stage I ❑ Stage II ❑ Stage III ❑ Stage IV	❑ Security ❑ Engineering ❑ Combative pt ❑ Suicide attempt ❑ Fire ❑ Respiratory ❑ Pharmacy ❑ Code blue expired ❑ Code blue survived ❑ Complaint	❑ Self abuse ❑ Lost/damaged article ❑ Hazardous exposure ❑ Burn ❑ Lab ❑ X-ray ❑ Food services ❑ Housekeeping ❑ Other (comment) _____

III.   **Severity of Outcome**
❑ No Injury   ❑ Inconsequential   ❑ Consequential

IV. **Comments & Action**	V. **Follow-up** (Director to complete)

Name of MD notified	Date	Time	Seen by MD? Yes ❑ No ❑

❑ Communicated with
_____
❑ Employee counseled
❑ In-service
❑ Policy change/new
❑ Trend
❑ Other _____

X-ray / Lab / Tests ordered	Equipment
Yes ❑ No ❑ State _____	❑ Sent for repair ❑ Removed from service

Reported by — Date — Dept.	Persons Involved Dept.	Department Director Sign — Date

Goodheart-Willcox Publisher

Figure 4.4 Most healthcare facilities will have an incident report similar to the one above. What are the major categories of incidents included in this report?

An incident report must be filled out accurately, completely, and immediately after the incident. You must use a black pen to fill in an incident report, as it is a legal document. Do not use whiteout on the report. Avoid being wordy in your report—simply state the facts. Healthcare facilities use a variety of incident report forms. The following information is included on most report forms:

- date of incident
- names of persons involved
- location and time of incident
- person to whom the incident is reported
- date and time of the reporting
- brief description of what happened
- names of any witnesses
- name of any machine or piece of equipment involved
- action taken to prevent recurrence
- signature of person filling out the report

Patients' Bill of Rights

As you learned in chapter 3, patients have detailed rights, which are stated in the Patients' Bill of Rights. These rights have been written to ensure that patients receive high-quality healthcare services, particularly regarding their safety. You may want to review the Patients' Bill of Rights.

Employee Safety

For a healthcare facility to operate successfully, it must maintain employee safety as well as patient safety. Employee illness and injury can affect patient care. An injury can also have serious professional consequences and may result in loss of a job. For example, a nurse who suffers a serious back injury might not be able to perform his or her nursing duties.

The **OSHA Hazard Communication Standard** directly affects healthcare workers. This standard ensures that employees are educated about chemical hazards in the workplace. Chemical injuries can result from inhaling toxic fumes or from splashing acid into the eyes. Members of the housekeeping, custodial, laboratory, and food service teams, as well as pharmacy assistants, medical assistants, nursing staff, radiology employees, and dental assistants are just a few of the employees who may be at risk of a chemical injury.

OSHA Hazard Communication Standard
rules established by the Occupational Safety and Health Administration (OSHA) that require employers to educate employees about chemical hazards in the workplace

Real Life Scenario   Reporting Accidents

James does clerical work in a pediatrician's front office. One day James notices a 5-year-old boy running in the reception area. Suddenly, the boy trips over his untied shoelaces and bumps his head on a chair. His mother assures James that it is no big deal, as the boy is clumsy. James doesn't notice a cut or any bleeding on the boy's head.

Apply It

1. Should James tell his employer about the boy's fall?
2. Should James write up the incident even though the mother says not to bother?
3. Have you ever had to report an incident while on the job? If so, what procedure did you follow?

The most common chemical injury is a burn. The site of the chemical contact should be flushed with water immediately. The skin might simply turn red at the site, but proper first aid must still be applied right away. Various chemicals may also produce harmful gases, which can cause burns to the respiratory tract, shortness of breath, a certain type of pneumonia, or other respiratory distress. To reduce the risk of chemical injury

- wear gloves when using chemicals (goggles and protective safety clothing may also be required);
- do not use chemicals in unlabeled containers;
- read chemical labels carefully, double-checking before use;
- never mix unknown chemicals;
- use chemicals in a well-ventilated area;
- clean up all spills immediately using a special spill kit (only if you know what the spill contains and are trained to clean it up); and
- immediately flush the skin or eyes if they come in contact with a chemical, and continue to do so for up to 10 minutes. Your facility may have a safety shower or an eyewash station for you to use (Figure 4.5).

Contact lenses are not protective safety gear. Contact lenses must be protected by safety goggles to prevent serious injury to the eye. Some healthcare facilities prohibit contact lens wearers from handling certain chemicals. Check with your facility for guidelines.

Every chemical used in your healthcare facility should be accompanied by a **material safety data sheet (MSDS)**. Read this sheet carefully—it contains important information about the chemical's makeup, dilution and mixture concentration, and instructions for use. It also explains the possible hazards of using the chemical and the appropriate first aid treatment needed in case of an accident or spill. These sheets should be placed in easily accessed and known locations for everyone using the chemicals and near where the chemicals are used.

material safety data sheet (MSDS)
a document containing comprehensive information about a particular chemical used in a healthcare facility; each chemical used has a corresponding MSDS

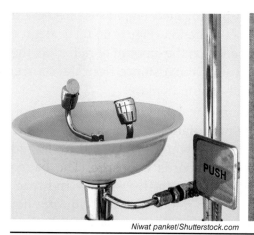
Niwat panket/Shutterstock.com

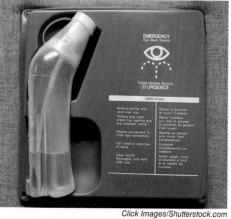
Click Images/Shutterstock.com

Figure 4.5 You will encounter different types of emergency eyewash stations if you pursue a career in healthcare. Know where these stations are located in your facility.

Check Your Understanding ✓

1. Define "incident" as it relates to an incident report.
2. Name three types of people who could be involved in an "incident."
3. What information should you include when writing an incident report?
4. What is the purpose of the OSHA Hazard Communication Standard?
5. What is a material safety data sheet (MSDS)?

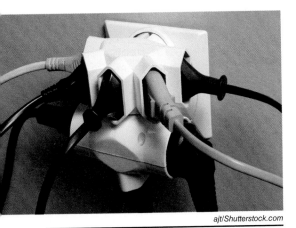

ajt/Shutterstock.com

Figure 4.6 Overloading electrical outlets increases the likelihood of a fire.

Electrical Safety

It is always possible to get an electrical shock when operating electrically powered equipment. Electrical shock injuries can result in moderate burns, severe skin damage, unconsciousness, or even death. Observance of safety guidelines concerning electricity can help reduce risk of such injuries.

Do not overload any electrical plugs or outlets, as an overloaded plug or outlet can become a fire hazard (Figure 4.6). All equipment must have a three-prong plug, which adds further safety benefits. Equipment must be in safe, working condition with no frayed cords or loose wires. Minimize the use of extension cords.

Follow all electrical safety regulations found in the safety manual when working with electricity in a healthcare setting. It is also important to receive proper training before operating a piece of equipment. When operating electrical equipment, make sure your hands, the patient's hands, and the floor are dry. Do not perform any routine maintenance on a piece of equipment until you make sure the equipment is unplugged. Be sure to inspect equipment before use to ensure that it is safe, looking for frayed wires or other maintenance issues.

Radiation Safety

As a healthcare worker, you must be aware of radiation safety procedures. Radiation exposure can occur when unprotected employees are near a machine that uses radiation (Figure 4.7). The degree of exposure depends on the amount of radiation, the duration of exposure, the distance from the source, and the type of shielding in place.

The radiation hazard symbol will alert you to the presence of radiation. If you are frequently exposed to radiation, you are required by law to wear a badge that records exposure. The badge should be checked periodically (sent in and read, typically monthly) to make sure that you are not being exposed to damaging levels of radiation. Failure to wear a badge may result in the loss of your job.

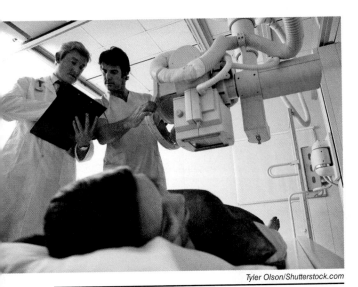

Tyler Olson/Shutterstock.com

Figure 4.7 These radiographers have been trained to protect their patients and themselves from excessive and unnecessary radiation exposure.

The radiation safety principle is represented by the acronym *ALARA*, which stands for <u>A</u>s <u>L</u>ow <u>A</u>s <u>R</u>easonably <u>A</u>chievable. This principle takes into account three factors:

1. time, or duration of exposure

2. distance from the source of radiation

3. shielding devices used

Fire Safety

Fire is one of the most feared disasters in healthcare facilities. A fire, or a threat of fire, is extremely frightening to patients, especially those who are unable to leave the facility on their own. Healthcare workers must be trained to recognize fire risks and respond in a professional manner.

The most common causes of fire include matches, heating and cooking equipment, electrical equipment, flammable liquids, and smoking (which is prohibited in all healthcare facilities). Fire can occur in any situation where three elements—fuel, heat, and oxygen—are present. These three elements form what is called the **fire triangle**. If one of these elements is missing, a fire will not take place. A fire extinguisher stops the actions of a fire triangle and puts out the fire.

There are five types of fire extinguishers (Figure 4.8 on the next page). Fire extinguishers must be placed at various locations in the healthcare facility and kept in working order at all times by regular, careful inspections.

Think It Through

Does your family have a fire evacuation plan? Do you have fire extinguishers in the home? If so, do you know where they are located or how to use them? If your family has a fire evacuation plan, explain it. If you do not have a plan, discuss creating one with the members of your household.

fire triangle
term for the three elements—fuel, heat, and oxygen—needed to start and maintain a fire

Extend Your Knowledge ▶ Burn Degrees

Burns are classified in degrees. The three degrees of burns that are most relevant to the healthcare worker include first-, second-, and third-degree burns.

- First-degree: the skin is usually red and very painful, and it heals in 3–5 days.

- Second-degree: blisters can be present, and the wound will be pink or red in color, painful, and appear to be wet. These burns will take several weeks to heal.

- Third-degree: all layers of the skin are destroyed, extending into tissue. Affected areas can be black or white, and are typically dry. Third-degree burns may take months to heal, and could require skin grafts—the surgical transfer of healthy skin to the burned area.

You will learn more about burns in chapter 12.

Apply It

1. Have you ever had a burn that was more serious than a first-degree burn?

2. Name situations in your home or workplace that could possibly result in burns.

Types of Fire Extinguishers				
Pressurized Water	**Carbon Dioxide (CO_2)**	**Dry Chemical**	**Class D Dry Chemical**	**Multi-Purpose Dry Chemical**
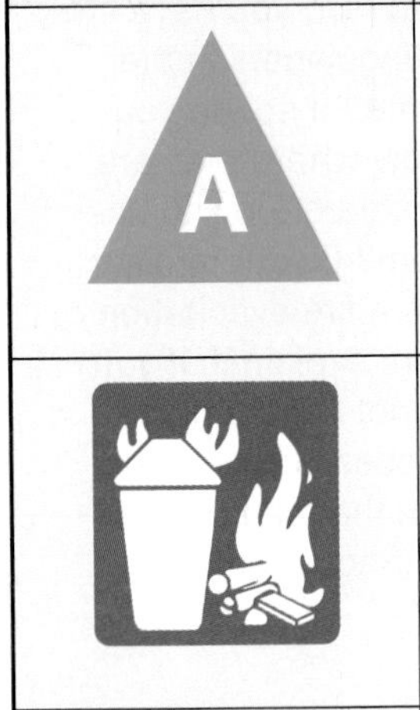 A	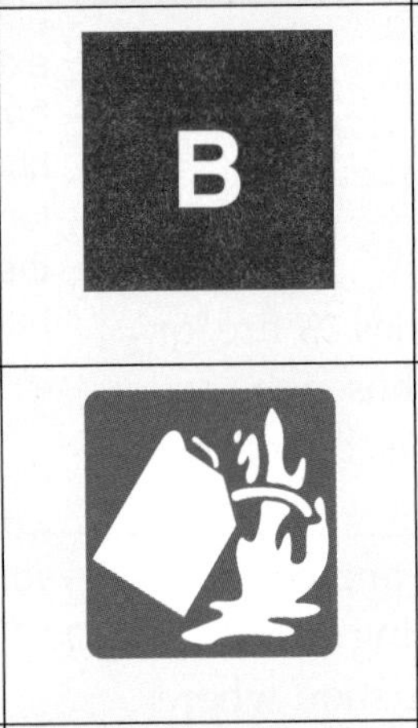 B	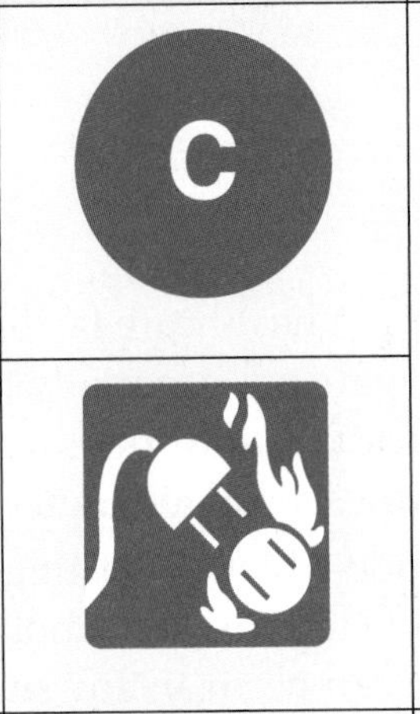 C	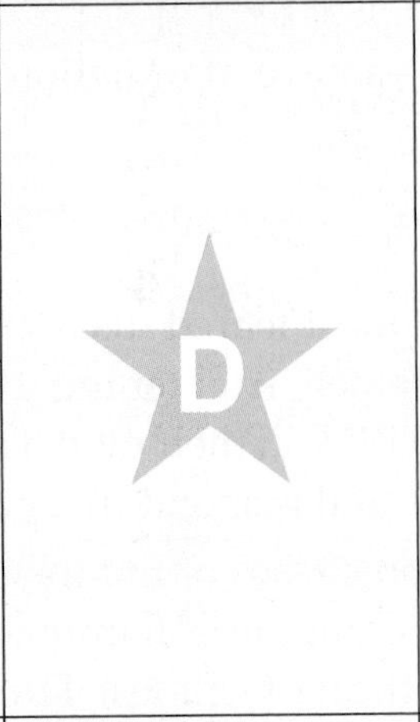 D	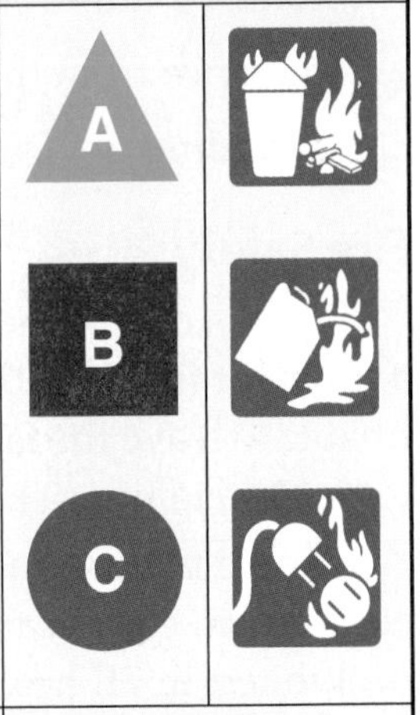 A B C
Ordinary combustibles (wood, paper, or textiles)	**Flammable liquids** (grease, gasoline, oils, and paints)	**Electrical equipment** (wiring, computers, and any other energized electrical devices)	**Combustible metals** (magnesium, potassium, titanium, and sodium)	Labeled for use on ordinary combustibles, flammable liquids, and electrical equipment fires

Figure 4.8 Study this chart to familiarize yourself with the different types of fire extinguishers. Which types are located in your school? in the facilities where you work?

If a fire occurs, you should stay calm. Knowing how to react will prepare you to ensure the safety of patients and yourself. It is important to familiarize yourself with your facility's evacuation routes and plans in case of a fire. In addition to familiarizing yourself with your facility's fire emergency plan, remember the following rules to keep yourself and your patients safe during a fire:

1. Know where the fire extinguishers and the fire alarms are located (they should be in plain view) and how to use them. Make sure fire extinguishers are inspected on a routine basis.
2. Keep areas uncluttered and free of debris.
3. Evacuate ambulatory patients (those able to walk) first, then the patients who need wheelchairs, and finally any bedridden patients.
4. Do not prop open any fire doors.
5. Never use an elevator during a fire.
6. Don't evacuate unless instructed to do so by an authority.
7. Participate professionally during drills to ensure proper participation during a real emergency.
8. If there is no way out, close all doors between you and the fire. *Do not* open the doors without first checking to make sure they are cool to the touch. Place towels at the bottom of the door, if possible.

Another way to remember how to deal with a fire is the acronym **RACE**:

1. **Rescue**: immediately stop what you are doing and remove anyone in immediate danger from the fire to a safe area.

2. **Alarm**: activate the nearest fire alarm pull stations (if applicable).

3. **Contain**: close all doors and windows that you can safely reach to contain the fire. During evacuation, close the doors behind you.

4. **Extinguish**: only attempt to extinguish the fire if it is safe to do so.

When attempting to extinguish the fire, retrieve the nearest fire extinguisher and follow the **PASS** procedure:

1. **Pull**: pull the pin to break the tamper seal.

2. **Aim**: aim low, pointing the extinguisher nozzle (also called the *horn* or *hose*) at the base of the fire. Warning: *do not* touch the plastic discharge horn on CO_2 extinguishers. It gets very cold and may damage your skin.

3. **Squeeze**: squeeze the handle to release the extinguishing agent.

4. **Sweep**: sweep from side to side at the base of the fire until it appears to be out. Watch the area; if the fire reignites, repeat steps 2 through 4. Keep in mind that fire extinguishers only last about 30 seconds.

Body Mechanics

Healthcare workers move, lift, and carry all types of supplies and equipment. They also help move or position patients. Healthcare workers can injure themselves if they move patients improperly. Patients may struggle or twist during movement, making them more difficult to handle. Healthcare workers should educate themselves on **body mechanics** to ensure they do not hurt themselves.

Without the use of proper body mechanics, healthcare workers risk injury, particularly to their backs. Back injuries can result in long periods of lost wages and even permanent disability. You can greatly reduce the possibility of a workplace injury by following simple **ergonomic** practices, which are designed to minimize physical effort and discomfort and maximize efficiency. Following are some basic ergonomic practices.

Sitting. Many healthcare workers spend several hours a day working on a computer. It is important for these workers to have ergonomic chairs and to maintain proper body mechanics.

When sitting in a chair, make sure your buttocks are at the back of the chair. Your back should be straight, which means your shoulders should not be hunched (Figure 4.9 on the next page). Bend your knees at right angles and place them at the same height as, or higher than, your hips. Your feet should be flat on the floor.

The height and back of the chair should be adjustable. The use of a footrest might help you avoid posture problems. Larger fonts help reduce eyestrain, and performing deep breathing exercises helps to reduce stress. Following these guidelines will help you avoid repetitive strain injuries (RSI).

When sitting for extended periods of time, you should relax periodically by standing and moving your body. If there is a glare on your computer screen, change the lighting or your position to eliminate it. A vertical document holder, either attached to a flexible equipment arm or freestanding, eases eyestrain and improves posture.

body mechanics
the proper use of body movements to prevent injury during the performance of physical tasks, such as lifting and sitting

ergonomics
the practice or science of maximizing efficiency and preventing discomfort or injury during the time a person is performing work tasks

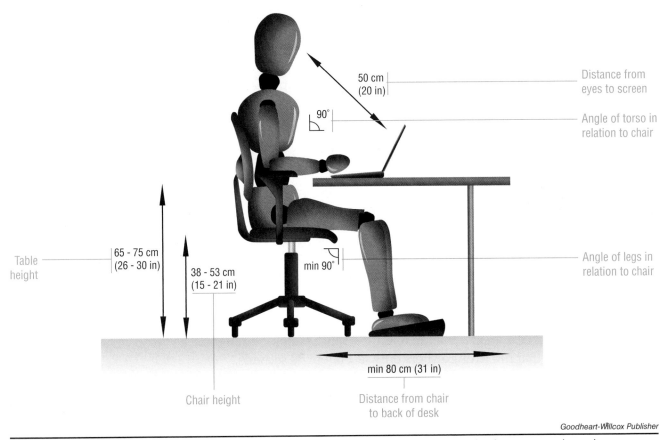

Table height
65 - 75 cm (26 - 30 in)
38 - 53 cm (15 - 21 in)
Chair height
90°
50 cm (20 in)
Distance from eyes to screen
Angle of torso in relation to chair
min 90°
Angle of legs in relation to chair
min 80 cm (31 in)
Distance from chair to back of desk

Goodheart-Willcox Publisher

Figure 4.9   If you must spend many hours at a computer station, make sure your work station is set up as shown here. Observing proper ergonomic principles can help you avoid painful conditions such as carpal tunnel syndrome.

carpal tunnel syndrome
a painful, progressive hand and arm condition caused by compression of a key nerve in the wrist; can be caused when wrists are not supported during keyboard use

A good wrist support should be available to keep your wrists as straight as possible. The support should have rounded edges and padding, and should be about two inches high. **Carpal tunnel syndrome** is a progressively painful hand and arm condition caused by a pinched nerve in the wrist. This condition can be prevented, or lessened, by maintaining a proper wrist position while operating a computer keyboard. The fingers should be lower than the wrist.

Real Life Scenario   Repetitive Strain Injury (RSI)

Laura has been an administrative assistant in the radiology department at Eastridge Hospital for four years. Laura spends a significant amount of time working on the computer, and was recently diagnosed with repetitive strain injury (RSI). Her condition is caused by the repetitive motion of keyboarding and sitting in one position for long periods of time in front of a computer. Laura's back and neck ache on the job, and she feels more and more fatigued as her condition worsens. Recently she has been experiencing shooting pains up and down her back.

Laura's doctor suggested that she take a short walk every hour or whenever possible at work, stretching her neck, back, and fingers.

Apply It

1. Do you spend significant time sitting at a computer or a desk?

2. What activities in addition to the ones mentioned above could you do to avoid RSI?

3. What actions are recommended to travelers who are on a plane for several hours to avoid discomfort?

Standing. When standing, your shoulder blades should be back, chest forward, knees straight, and the top of your head should align with the ceiling. Your pelvis should not tilt, and the arches of your feet should be supported by your shoes.

Reaching. When reaching for an object, stand directly in front of it, making sure you are close to it. Avoid twisting or stretching. Use a stool or ladder for high objects but check the stool or ladder first to make sure it is stable and will support you. Do not try to move the object if it is too large or heavy.

Lifting. Practicing good body mechanics when lifting a heavy object requires you to keep your body in an upright position, with your back straight at all times. Your leg muscles should do most of the lifting work. Good body mechanics can be achieved by obeying the following principles when lifting objects:

- **Think before you lift.** First, think how you will lift the object. Plan your path and make sure it is clear of any equipment or hazards.

- **Test the weight.** Before you lift, assess the weight and make sure you can lift the item safely. If not, get help or use an assistive device such as a hand truck.

- **Bend at the hips and knees.** With the lower back upright, the forces are distributed safely.

- **Maintain a wide base of support.** A solid and wide base will help reduce the possibility of slipping while lifting.

- **Hold objects as close to you as possible.** This technique reduces stress on your back.

- **Do not twist when carrying.** Always move or change directions with your feet. This decreases the stress and load on your back. Twisting often occurs when moving a patient.

- **Tighten abdominal muscles when lifting.** Your abdominal muscles help you lift while reducing strain on your lower back.

- **Lift with your legs.** Using the large muscle groups in the legs helps reduce the forces exerted on the lower back.

- **When lifting a patient, communicate with her to let her know what you are doing.** If possible, have the patient help you by moving her body as much as she can.

- **Lower your body down to meet the object you are trying to pick up.** Never bend at the waist with your legs straight; this is called *stooping*.

- **Lift straight up in one smooth motion.** Use your leg muscles to return to an upright position.

Did You Know? Back Injuries

More musculoskeletal injuries are suffered by healthcare workers, such as orderlies, attendants, nurses, and nursing aides, than workers in any other industry. Back injuries in the healthcare industry are estimated to cost over $7 billion every year. You do not want to injure your back, so be sure to practice good body mechanics at all times.

- **Maintain good communication if two or more people are lifting.** Communicating with any helpers will ensure good timing when lifting, thereby reducing the likelihood of jerky or unexpected movements.

- **Push rather than pull.** It is easier to use your weight advantage when pushing.

- **Eliminate repetitive lifting duties if possible.** Store supplies that you frequently use at a reachable height to decrease lifting challenges.

- **When in doubt, get help.** Remember, some back injuries can last a lifetime.

Check Your Understanding ✓

1. When moving a heavy object, you should _____ rather than _____.
2. What is ergonomics?
3. How can you reduce your chance of getting carpal tunnel syndrome?
4. What elements form the fire triangle?
5. The radiation safety principle is represented by the acronym **ALARA**, which stands for _____.

Quality Improvement and Safety

quality improvement (QI)
term for policies that motivate or require healthcare facilities to monitor and evaluate their services based on predetermined criteria for the purpose of improving those services

Since the 1960s, serious efforts have been made to initiate **quality improvement (QI)** policies, which are also called *quality assurance policies*. QI policies are put in place to ensure that healthcare organizations monitor and evaluate services based on predetermined criteria. These policies are aimed at improvement, measuring the facility against specific criteria and then figuring out ways to improve performance. These policies attempt to avoid blame and to create systems to prevent errors.

Examples of quality improvement in a healthcare facility include keeping records of incidents that occur in the facility; ensuring that all machinery is monitored on a regular basis, with strict records of maintenance; and completing patient care documentation in a clear, consistent, accurate, complete, and timely manner. Because so many tasks are involved in maintaining quality improvement, most medium-sized and large facilities have a separate department dedicated to providing the best possible quality of care.

Of course safety criteria are a major part of quality improvement. Quality healthcare begins with strictly observing *all* safety procedures. Today, healthcare facilities report their quality measures, many of which include safety, to several national organizations that publish safety definitions and standards. Three governmental agencies (in addition to OSHA) involved in protecting the health and safety of patients and the public are the FDA, NIH, and the CDC.

The following list includes these three and other important organizations:

- **The Food and Drug Administration (FDA)** is responsible for protecting and promoting public health through the regulation and supervision of food safety, prescription and over-the-counter pharmaceutical drugs (medications), vaccines, biopharmaceuticals, blood transfusions, and medical devices, to name several responsibilities.

- **The National Institutes of Health (NIH)** is an agency of the United States Department of Health and Human Services. It is the primary agency of the United States government responsible for biomedical and health-related research.

- **The Centers for Medicare and Medicaid** is also part of the US Department of Health and Human Services. Its mission is to strengthen and modernize America's healthcare system.

- **The Centers for Disease Control and Prevention (CDC)** conducts and supports health promotion, disease prevention, and preparedness activities in the United States with the goal of improving overall public health. The CDC tracks disease throughout the United States and sponsors a great deal of research on disease control and prevention (Figure 4.10).

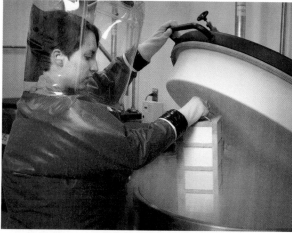

The Centers for Disease Control and Prevention

Figure 4.10 The CDC conducts research to help prevent and control the spread of diseases. This CDC scientist is placing biological specimens in liquid nitrogen for storage.

- **The Joint Commission (TJC)** is a healthcare accrediting agency. A nonprofit agency, the TJC accredits more than 20,000 healthcare organizations and programs in the United States. The TJC publishes national patient safety goals for hospitals, home care, laboratory services, long-term care, office-based surgery, and others. TJC focuses on workers correctly using medicines; carefully identifying patients; and preventing infections, falls, and bedsores. The TJC also presents safety goals for improving staff communication, identifying patient safety risks, and preventing surgical errors. TJC does not share all of its findings with the public. However, it does share the accreditation decision, the date that accreditation was awarded, and any standards that were cited for improvement. An organization must be in compliance with all, or most, of the standards to become accredited.

- **The Institute of Medicine (IOM)**, an independent organization, focuses on the following guidelines for healthcare delivery: safety, timeliness, effectiveness, efficiency, equitable care, and patient-centered care. The IOM believes that people should not be harmed by healthcare intended to help them. Care should be scientifically sound, and it should be designed around individual preferences, needs, and values. The number of necessary waits and delays should be reduced, and care should not be wasteful or vary in quality because of patient diversity. The IOM stresses transparency in reporting safety issues.

- **The Agency for Healthcare Research and Quality (AHRQ)** is the lead federal agency charged with improving the safety and quality of America's healthcare system. AHRQ develops the knowledge, tools, and data needed to improve the healthcare system and help American citizens, healthcare professionals, and policymakers make informed health decisions. AHRQ works with Department of Health and Human Services (HHS) agencies and other partners to achieve the goals of better care, smarter spending of healthcare dollars, and healthier people.

- **The World Health Organization (WHO)**, created in 1948 as part of the United Nations, is tasked with "directing and coordinating" international health policy. WHO defines patient safety as the prevention of errors and harmful effects to patients. These effects are defined as a process of not performing the right procedure or implementing the wrong procedure, resulting in hazardous healthcare conditions or unintended harm.

- **The National Quality Forum (NQF)** is a nonprofit organization dedicated to improving the quality of healthcare in the United States. The NQF has a three-part mission—to set goals for performance improvement, to endorse standards for measuring and reporting on performance, and to promote educational and outreach programs.

Private and governmental organizations continually monitor healthcare organizations with the goal of eliminating errors in medical care that are damaging as well as preventable. The important points to remember from these efforts, both nationally and privately, are to

- be aware and mindful of safety at all times;

- always work toward preventing errors or harm;

- learn from the errors that do occur; and

- work to ensure a culture of safety involving healthcare staff, organizations, and patients.

Infection Control

Healthcare facilities battle continuously to prevent the spread of microorganisms that can cause infectious disease. These microorganisms, known as *pathogens,* can present major problems both for patients and employees. Today, most healthcare facilities have a separate department devoted exclusively to infection control. Many facilities call this the *Department of Hospital Epidemiology and Infection Control (HEIC).* In this section, you will learn some basic information about pathogens and the standard procedures for preventing them from spreading.

Introduction to Microorganisms

Microorganisms such as **bacteria**, **viruses**, and **fungi** are everywhere in our environment—in the air, on our skin, in food, and on everything that we touch. You cannot see bacteria without a microscope. Viruses, which are much smaller than bacteria or fungi, cannot even be seen using a standard microscope.

Not all microorganisms cause illness. The ones that do not cause illness are called *nonpathogenic* microorganisms. Nonpathogenic microorganisms, such as the bacteria in our intestines, maintain a balance in the environment and in our bodies. When in balance, these bacteria do not cause health problems; instead, they contribute to good health by helping to break down waste and nutrients.

Under normal circumstances, nonpathogenic microorganisms do not cause disease, but there are exceptions to this rule. For example, in some circumstances, such as surgery that perforates (punctures) the bowel, the bacteria in the colon can spill into the body cavity and cause serious infection.

bacteria
small, one-celled microorganisms that cannot be seen by the naked eye; can be pathogenic (cause disease)

viruses
pathogenic microorganisms, much smaller than bacteria, that depend on a living cell to survive; cause many serious diseases and illnesses

fungi
parasitic organisms that live in the soil or on plants; include disease-causing microorganisms such as yeasts and molds

In addition, people who have compromised immune systems are susceptible to infections and may become ill from microorganisms that do not usually affect individuals with healthy immune systems. Nonpathogenic organisms can become pathogens to such patients.

For microorganisms to live and thrive, they must have certain elements in their environment. For example, some microorganisms require oxygen to live. They are called **aerobes**. Others live in an environment with little or no oxygen. They are called **anaerobes**.

Bacteria

Bacteria are initially classified by their **morphology** (form and structure) as seen under a microscope. After observing bacteria under the microscope, a clinical microbiologist identifies the actual family of the bacteria through testing.

The basic forms of bacteria are spherical (*coccus*) and rod-like shapes (*bacilli*). Figure 4.11 illustrates several shapes of bacteria, including those that appear as twisted cylinders (*spirochetes*), spherically-shaped cocci arranged in clusters (*Staphylococcus*), cocci forming chains (*Streptococcus*), and cocci in pairs (*Diplococcus*).

aerobe
an organism that requires oxygen to live

anaerobe
an organism that requires little or no oxygen to live

morphology
the science or study of the form and structure of organisms

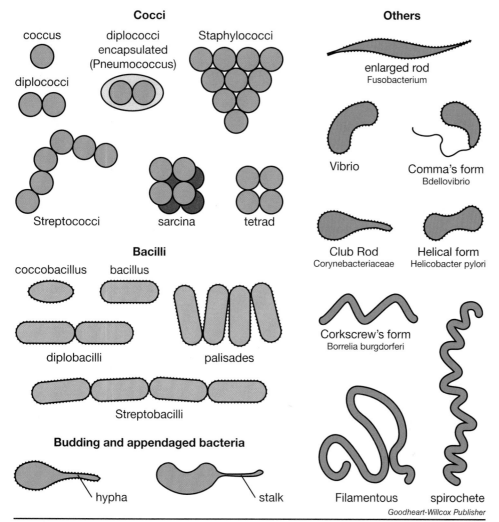

Goodheart-Willcox Publisher

Figure 4.11 These illustrations show a few simple representations of the many different shapes and sizes of bacteria. Which bacteria names do you recognize?

Bacteria can cause major illness in our bodies. Here are some examples:

- Hospital stays can be prolonged by the bacterium called *Staphylococcus aureus* (*S. aureus*). The infections caused by these bacteria are commonly called *staph infections*.

- The Black Death that killed approximately 25 million people in fourteenth-century Europe was a plague caused by the rod-shaped bacterium, *Yersinia pestis*. Today, *Yersinia pestis* is easily treated with antibiotics.

- Syphilis is a bacterial infection caused by a spiral bacterium called a *spirochete*.

Bacterial infections are treated with antibiotics—drugs that kill the disease-inducing microorganism.

Viruses

Much smaller than bacteria, viruses depend on a living cell to survive because they cannot reproduce on their own. Viruses are the cause of the common cold, smallpox, chicken pox, measles, influenza, human papillomavirus (HPV), herpes simplex, and AIDS. Many more illnesses are caused by viruses.

Antibiotics do not kill viruses. Usually, time and rest are necessary to let most of these illnesses run their course. Doctors will advise patients to stay home, take non-aspirin pain relievers, and get plenty of rest. However, vaccines have been developed against many viral diseases. A vaccine introduces small amounts of the microorganism into the system in an effort to boost the immune system against the microorganism. An increasing number of antiviral remedies are being developed. These remedies prevent the virus from replicating, or reproducing itself.

Fungi

Microscopic fungi include yeasts and molds. Some fungi can cause disease, especially if the immune system has already been compromised by a different disease or disorder.

Examples of fungal infections include athlete's foot, thrush (an infection of the mouth or throat), vaginitis, and certain lung diseases. Fungal infections are treated with topical, oral, or injectable medications.

protozoa
microorganisms that depend on a host cell to survive and replicate; can cause serious illness

Protozoa

Although they are larger than viruses, protozoa also depend on a host cell to survive and replicate. **Protozoa** are found in water and soil and cause amoebic dysentery, an inflammation of the colon that results in fever, abdominal pain, and severe diarrhea. They also cause amoebiasis, trichomoniasis, and malaria (a disease contracted via a mosquito bite). In a malaria patient, the protozoan lives in red blood cells. Protozoal infections are treated with oral and injectable anti-protozoal medications.

Rickettsiae

Rickettsiae are **parasites**, or organisms that live in or on another organism. Parasites such as **rickettsiae** normally choose fleas, lice, ticks, or mites as their host organism. If one of these creatures bites a human, that human's body becomes the parasite's host. Rickettsiae cause Rocky Mountain spotted fever and types of typhus, both of which are severe infections that have been known to cause serious epidemics. Rickettsiae are treated with appropriate antibiotics.

parasites
organisms that live in or on another organism

rickettsiae
parasites that normally choose fleas, lice, ticks, or mites as their host organisms; can cause severe infections

Extend Your Knowledge ▶ Super Bugs

In the news today, you hear a great deal about antibiotic-resistant bacteria, or *super bugs*. Over the years, certain bacteria have developed a resistance to antibiotics. This resistance makes some infections difficult to treat.

Some bacteria are resistant to most antibiotics. This resistance can develop when antibiotics are used improperly, such as when

- patients do not take all of their prescribed antibiotics (the bacteria may not be completely killed, which will cause further illness or even drug resistance);

- antibiotics are prescribed when not needed or indicated (antibiotics will not be effective against the flu, which is caused by a virus);

- antibacterial substances are contained in cleaning products;

- antibiotics are found in animals consumed as food; or

- genetic mutation of bacteria has occurred.

Some bacteria that have become resistant to antibiotics include *Mycobacterium tuberculosis*, *Streptococcus*, *Klebsiella*, *Acinetobacter*, *Pseudomonas*, *Clostridium difficile*, vancomycin-resistant *Enterococcus*, and *Enterobacter*. One of the most highly publicized bacterium in this category is **Methicillin-resistant *Staphylococcus aureus* (MRSA)**. MRSA is responsible for a difficult-to-treat infection. MRSA is prevalent in hospitals, prisons, schools, and nursing homes, where residents with open wounds and weakened immune systems are confined in close quarters. These patients are at greater risk of infection than the general public.

Careful monitoring of antibiotic use is necessary to prevent the development of antibiotic resistance and to reduce the spread of antibiotic-resistant bacteria.

Apply It

1. Have there been incidences of antibiotic-resistant bacteria at one of your local healthcare facilities?

2. After completing this chapter, identify the infection control procedures that you believe should be followed when antibiotic-resistant bacteria are involved.

Methicillin-resistant *Staphylococcus aureus* (MRSA)
an antibiotic-resistant bacterium responsible for a difficult-to-treat infection; sometimes prevalent in hospitals, prisons, schools, and nursing homes

The Chain of Infection

During a hospital stay, a patient does not expect to acquire an infection. Unfortunately, patients often do acquire new infections while in the hospital. Hospital-acquired infections are called **nosocomial infections**, also known as *healthcare-acquired infections* or *healthcare-associated infections*. Nosocomial infections can cause pneumonia and infections of the bloodstream, the urinary tract, and other parts of the body. The reduced infection resistance of hospitalized patients contributes to the rate of nosocomial infections. Learning the various aspects of infection can help you prevent nosocomial infections.

There are many modes of transmission of infection. As a healthcare worker, you should be familiar with all of them. One mode is **direct contact**, such as person-to-person contact or contact with infectious body secretions (contamination on hands). Another is **indirect contact**, in which a pathogen comes from food, air, soil, feces, instruments, equipment, clothing, and so on. **Vectors**, such as insects, rodents, or other small animals, can spread pathogens by biting a host.

As part of a team working continually to prevent the spread of infection, you need to understand the various ways that infection can be transmitted from person to person. The **chain of infection** is used to visualize the sequence of events that allows infection to invade the human body. This sequence consists of an infectious agent, reservoir or host, portal of exit, mode of transmission, portal of entry, and susceptible host (Figure 4.12).

The infection control department of a healthcare facility focuses on interrupting the chain of infection before the infection spreads throughout the hospital. Once it becomes clear that an infection has developed, the clinical laboratory must identify the infectious agent as soon as possible. Appropriate treatment must be started immediately.

Several methods are used to break the chain of infection to control the spread of infection. The remaining sections of the chapter examine the most common and important methods.

Hand Hygiene

Employees must maintain excellent hygiene, which includes **hand hygiene**. Hand hygiene is considered the single most important way to prevent the spread of infection. It can be accomplished through hand washing with a detergent or antimicrobial soap and water, or by applying an alcohol-based hand rub. Hand sanitizers do not kill the microorganisms that cause severe gastrointestinal infections such as *Clostridium difficile* (or *C. difficile*) or the Norovirus. Alcohol-based hand wipes have been found to be useless against any viruses not coated in lipid envelopes.

In an effort to prevent the spread of infection, the CDC has issued hand hygiene guidelines for healthcare workers. These guidelines state that hands should be washed

1. before and after eating;

2. after the restroom has been used; and

3. when dirt or body fluids such as blood, mucus, urine, and feces are visible on the hands.

nosocomial infections
infections acquired in hospitals and other healthcare facilities; also known as healthcare-acquired infections

direct contact
a type of infection transmission in which the pathogen travels directly from one host to another, such as in person-to-person transmission

indirect contact
a type of infection transmission in which the pathogen takes an indirect path—such as through food, air, or clothing—to its next host

vectors
carriers—such as insects, rodents, or other small animals—that spread pathogens from host to host

chain of infection
the sequence of events that allows infection to move from one source or host to another

hand hygiene
hand washing with a detergent or antimicrobial soap and water, or by applying an alcohol-based hand rub; considered the single most important way to prevent the spread of infection

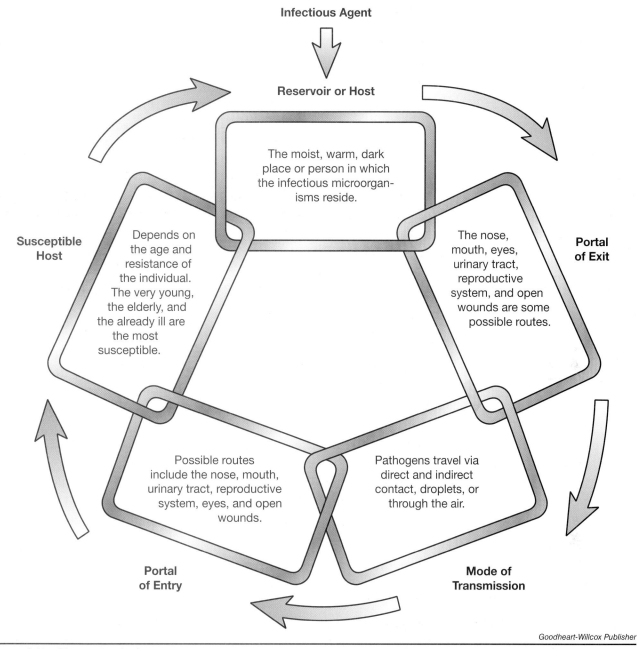

Infectious Agent

Reservoir or Host

The moist, warm, dark place or person in which the infectious microorganisms reside.

Susceptible Host

Depends on the age and resistance of the individual. The very young, the elderly, and the already ill are the most susceptible.

Portal of Exit

The nose, mouth, eyes, urinary tract, reproductive system, and open wounds are some possible routes.

Portal of Entry

Possible routes include the nose, mouth, urinary tract, reproductive system, eyes, and open wounds.

Mode of Transmission

Pathogens travel via direct and indirect contact, droplets, or through the air.

Goodheart-Willcox Publisher

Figure 4.12   The chain of infection is a sequence of events allowing infection to invade the human body. Including the infectious agent, how many steps are there in a chain of infection? How many of these steps must be eliminated to stop the spread of the infection?

It takes at least twenty seconds to wash your hands properly. Twenty seconds is about how long it takes to sing "Happy Birthday to You" twice.

The use of alcohol-based hand products is acceptable throughout the day, except under the previously stated circumstances. Alcohol-based hand rubs have become popular today because they do not dry out the skin as much as hand washing. As a result, alcohol-based hand rubs are widely used in healthcare facilities.

In addition to practicing good hand hygiene, hospital employees and healthcare workers must not come to work when sick with a contagious disease.

Procedure 4.1   Hand Washing

Rationale

Standard precautions require routine and proper hand washing to remove and prevent the spread of microorganisms.

Preparation

1. Locate a sink near where care will be given. The sink must have
   - a sufficient supply of antimicrobial soap or an antimicrobial soap dispenser;
   - warm running water;
   - a dispenser by the sink with clean paper towel(s); and
   - a proper waste container by the sink.

2. If your uniform sleeves are long, push them up your arms so they are close to your elbows.

3. Remove your watch and rings, if possible. If you cannot remove your watch, push it up your arm so it is away from your hands. If you cannot remove your rings, you must lather soap underneath them.

4. Stand far enough away from the sink so that your clothes do not touch it (Figure 4.13). Do not touch the inside of the sink at any time. Rewash your hands if they touch the sink at any time.

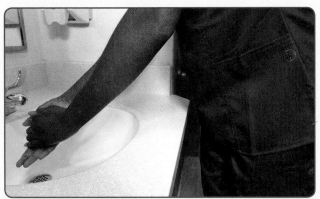

Figure 4.13   Wards Forest Media, LLC

The Procedure

5. Turn on the faucet and adjust the water temperature until it is warm.

6. Thoroughly wet your hands, wrists, and your arms a few inches above your wrists.

7. Apply soap and work into a thick lather over your hands, wrists, and at least 1 to 2 inches above your wrists (Figure 4.14).

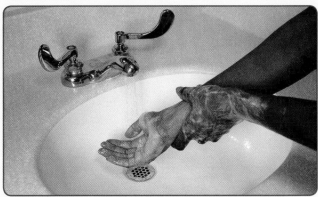

Figure 4.14   Wards Forest Media, LLC

8. Keep your hands and forearms below your elbows. Water must always flow down off your fingertips and never go up your arms.

9. Rub your palms together (to create friction) and rub between your fingers and thumbs. Work up a good foam as you wash every part of your hands and wrists.

10. Clean under your fingernails by rubbing them against the palm of the other hand to force soap to go underneath them (Figure 4.15). Clean around the tops of your nails.

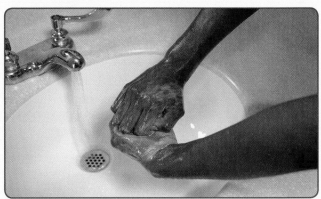

Figure 4.15   Wards Forest Media, LLC

11. Wash your hands for at least 20 seconds.

12. Under the running water, rinse your wrists and hands thoroughly, holding your hands so that your fingertips point downward (Figure 4.16). Do not shake water from your hands.

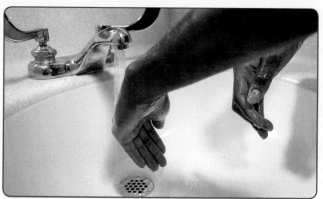

Figure 4.16   *Wards Forest Media, LLC*

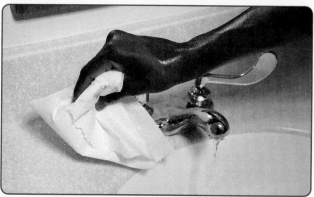

Figure 4.17   *Wards Forest Media, LLC*

13. Dry your wrists and then your hands thoroughly with a clean, dry paper towel.

14. Drop the used towel into the proper waste container. Do not touch the waste container.

Follow-up

15. Use a clean, dry paper towel to turn off the sink faucet. The paper towel, not your hand, should always touch the sink faucet (Figure 4.17). The faucet is considered contaminated.

16. Discard the towel into the proper waste container. Do not touch the waste container.

17. Use lotion or hand cream after washing to avoid dry, chapped skin.

Reporting and Documentation

18. Hand washing is an accepted and established standard procedure. It does not need to be reported or documented.

Check Your Understanding ✓

1. What is meant by the *chain of infection*?

2. What is considered the single most important way to prevent the spread of infection in a healthcare facility?

3. What are healthcare-acquired infections called?

4. Healthcare workers conform to guidelines and regulations from which nine agencies described in this chapter?

> **Think It Through**
>
> How seriously do you take hand hygiene in your everyday life? How many times a day do you wash your hands? How do you clean your hands? Under what daily circumstances do you practice hand hygiene?

Cleaning the Healthcare Facility

The absence of bacteria, viruses, and other microorganisms is called **asepsis**. In some facilities, the terms *medical asepsis* and *surgical asepsis* are used. Medical asepsis, or *clean technique*, includes procedures used to reduce the number of organisms present and prevent the transfer of organisms. Surgical asepsis, or *sterile technique*, prevents contamination of an open wound, serves to isolate the operative area from the unsterile environment, and maintains a sterile field for surgery.

The term **antisepsis** refers to using an antiseptic to prevent or inhibit growth of pathogenic organisms. Antiseptics (alcohols and iodine, for example) are not effective against spores and viruses.

asepsis
term that describes the absence of bacteria, viruses, and other microorganisms

antisepsis
the process of using an antiseptic to prevent or inhibit the growth of pathogenic organisms

sanitization

the use of antimicrobial agents on objects, surfaces, or living tissue to reduce the number of disease-causing microorganisms

disinfection

the use of antimicrobial agents on nonliving objects or surfaces to destroy or deactivate microorganisms

At least three levels of cleaning take place in healthcare facilities to prevent the spread of pathogens. These levels include sanitization, disinfection, and sterilization.

Sanitization is defined as the use of antimicrobial agents on objects, surfaces, or living tissue to reduce the number of disease-causing microorganisms to nonthreatening levels. An example of sanitization is cleaning tables in a hospital cafeteria before disinfection.

Disinfection involves the use of antimicrobial agents on nonliving objects or surfaces to destroy or deactivate microorganisms. Disinfectants are applied and allowed to dry according to the directions of the chemical manufacturer. The floors and walls of a hospital room, for example, are disinfected.

Disinfecting an object does not mean that all of the bacteria, viruses, and fungi have been removed. Some microorganisms form thick walls around themselves to protect themselves from harsh environments. This makes it difficult for disinfectants to completely remove the microorganisms.

To kill all microorganisms on a surface, the surface must be sterilized. The most common method of **sterilization** in many healthcare facilities is the use of the **autoclave**. An autoclave is a machine that employs hot, pressurized steam for cleaning purposes. The steam's high temperature kills all microorganisms and their spores (Figure 4.18). Other methods of sterilization include dry heat, gas, ionized radiation, and specialized chemicals designed for the purpose of sterilization.

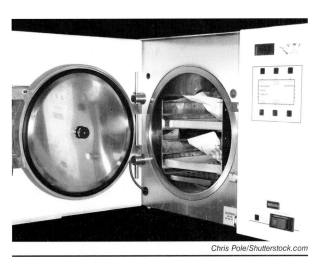

Chris Pole/Shutterstock.com

Figure 4.18 Autoclaves, such as the one shown here, are used to sterilize medical equipment and instruments. What does it mean to sterilize something?

sterilization

the act of killing all microorganisms and their spores on a surface; methods of sterilization in a healthcare facility may include hot pressurized steam, dry heat, and gas

autoclave

a machine used frequently in healthcare facilities to kill all microorganisms and their spores on a surface

Did You Know? What's the Most Hygienic?

Scientists at the University of Westminster in London performed a study to measure what was most hygienic—drying freshly washed hands with paper towels or using an electric hand dryer. Their study measured the number of bacteria on subjects' hands before washing and after drying them. Three different drying methods were used: paper towels, the warm air dryer, and a high-speed jet air dryer.

Paper towels were found to be clearly superior to the other methods, resulting in a 76 percent decrease in bacteria on the finger pads and a 77 percent decrease on the palms. In contrast, warm air dryers caused bacteria counts to increase by 194 percent on the finger pads and up to 254 percent on the palms. The jet air dryers increased the bacteria on the finger pads by 42 percent and by 15 percent on the palms.

Additionally, the warm air dryers had a potential for cross contamination of other bathroom users. The jet air dryers could potentially contaminate other users up to 7 feet away. The warm air dryers had the potential contamination range of about 10 inches.

In a hospital, the Central Services Department handles sterilization procedures. Autoclaves are widely used in doctors' offices, but many supplies used in patient care are prepackaged and sterilized by the manufacturer and are disposable. As a result, the use of an autoclave has declined somewhat in the healthcare facility.

Preventing the Spread of Bloodborne Pathogens

To avoid exposure to potentially harmful substances, employees must strictly follow instructions stated by the **OSHA Bloodborne Pathogens Standard**. This standard went into effect in the United States in 1992. It was designed to reduce the risk of transmitting **bloodborne pathogens** within the healthcare facility.

Bloodborne pathogens are infectious microorganisms found in human blood that can cause disease in humans. Examples of these pathogens include, but are not limited to, hepatitis B (HBV), hepatitis C (HCV), and human immunodeficiency virus (HIV).

The rules set forth by the OSHA Bloodborne Pathogens Standard apply to all patients receiving care in any healthcare facility, regardless of their diagnosis or infection status. The standard lists **potentially infectious materials (PIM),** which include a range of body fluids. To protect themselves and their patients, healthcare workers should always proceed as if these body fluids are infectious. Several body fluids have the potential to transmit harmful pathogens:

- human blood and its components (plasma, serum, platelets, and immunoglobulin)

- semen and vaginal secretions

- body fluids such as cerebrospinal, synovial (joint), pleural (lung), pericardial (heart), peritoneal (abdominal cavity), and amniotic (surrounding unborn baby) fluids

- body fluids visibly contaminated with blood or other unidentified substances (such as saliva in dental procedures)

- human tissue such as tissue removed during a **biopsy** (procedure to obtain tissue for examination and diagnosis)

- any bodily substance from a patient known to be infected with HIV

In addition to practicing good hand hygiene and cleaning contaminated surfaces, employees *must* dispose of all potentially infected materials in a biohazard receptacle.

Gloves are not always worn when giving patient care, but they *must* be worn when there is the possibility of an employee being exposed to blood and body fluids. Healthcare workers must always wash their hands before putting on gloves and again after removing their gloves between patients. Used gloves that are visibly contaminated with blood or other body fluids must be disposed of in a biohazard receptacle.

OSHA Bloodborne Pathogens Standard *guidelines developed by the Occupational Safety and Health Administration (OSHA) that list potentially infectious materials and mandate all healthcare workers to proceed at all times as if the materials are infectious*

bloodborne pathogens *infectious microorganisms in human blood that can cause disease*

potentially infectious materials (PIM) *substances designated by OSHA that require healthcare workers to proceed as if they are infectious*

biopsy *a piece of tissue removed from the body for examination; the process of removing tissue for examination*

Patient Isolation

The purpose of isolation is to separate patients with certain infections from other patients to prevent the transmission of pathogenic microorganisms in hospitals. Reverse isolation, also called *protective isolation*, protects susceptible patients from contagious diseases by isolating them from others. Guidelines for patient isolation have been identified by The Centers for Disease Control and Prevention (CDC) and the Hospital Infection Control Practice Advisory Committee (HICPAC).

isolation rooms
rooms in a healthcare facility used to prevent the spread of infections, either by containing patients who have contagious diseases or by protecting immune-compromised patients from infectious diseases

Healthcare facilities often have special **isolation rooms**. Signs are placed on the doors of these rooms to signal the type of isolation in place. Standard precautions are always used, with great attention paid to hand hygiene.

Protective gloves, masks, and face shields serve as barriers against infection. Various types of gowns are worn to prevent contamination of clothing and to protect the skin from blood and other body fluids. Impermeable gown, leg, and shoe covers are available when greater protection is required. Special handling of patient supplies and equipment is important. Disposable dishes and other items are often used. Thorough cleaning and disinfection of the room and equipment is done regularly and upon patient discharge.

Patients in isolation should be moved outside of the room as little as possible. When it is necessary for an isolated patient to be transported in the hospital and airborne or droplet precautions are in place, the patient should wear a mask. Caregivers must never forget that the patient in isolation is especially in need of compassionate care and understanding so that the patient does not feel unnecessarily shut off from the world.

Healthcare facilities use a variety of isolation practices. Many facilities divide these practices into two levels of isolation precautions: standard precautions and transmission-based precautions.

Standard Precautions

standard precautions
a set of basic practices intended to prevent transmission of infectious diseases from one person to another

Standard precautions apply to all patients, regardless of their diagnosis. **Standard precautions** are a set of basic infection prevention practices intended to prevent transmission of infectious diseases from one person to another. These precautions include guidelines for hand hygiene, personal protective equipment, respiratory hygiene, needlestick and sharps injury prevention, cleaning and disinfection, waste disposal, and safe injection practices.

Because we do not always know if a patient has an infectious disease, standard precautions are applied to *every person, every time* to ensure that transmission of disease does not occur. These precautions were formerly known as *universal precautions*. These precautions apply to all body fluids and any secretions or excretions (except perspiration), whether they contain visible blood or not. These also apply to non-intact skin and mucous membranes.

Transmission-Based Precautions

Transmission-based precautions are designed for patients with highly transmissible infections. Transmission-based precautions are used in addition to standard precautions. Transmission-based precautions are divided into three categories—airborne precautions, droplet precautions, and contact precautions—based on how the infections are transmitted.

Airborne Precautions. Airborne precautions are used to prevent the spread of diseases, such as tuberculosis, that are transmitted by tiny, airborne droplet residue or dust particles containing microorganisms. Airborne precautions require that the patient be placed in a private room or with another patient who has the same disease. The door to the room must be kept closed and the room must have special ventilation.

Respiratory protection in the form of an N95 respirator should be worn when giving patient care. An N95 respirator is a respiratory protective device designed to achieve a very close facial fit and very efficient filtration of airborne particles. N95 respirators are not designed for children or people with facial hair. Because a proper fit cannot be achieved on children and people with facial hair, the N95 respirator may not provide full protection for these individuals.

Droplet Precautions. Droplet precautions are used to prevent infection spread through large droplet transmission. In these cases, disease transmission occurs through coughing, talking, and sneezing. People within a three-foot radius are susceptible. Patients should be placed in a private room or with a patient who has the same diagnosis. Masks should be worn within three feet of the patient (Figure 4.19). Because the droplets do not remain suspended in air, no special air handling or ventilation is required. Influenza and *Bordetella pertussis* (whooping cough) are examples of infectious diseases requiring droplet precautions.

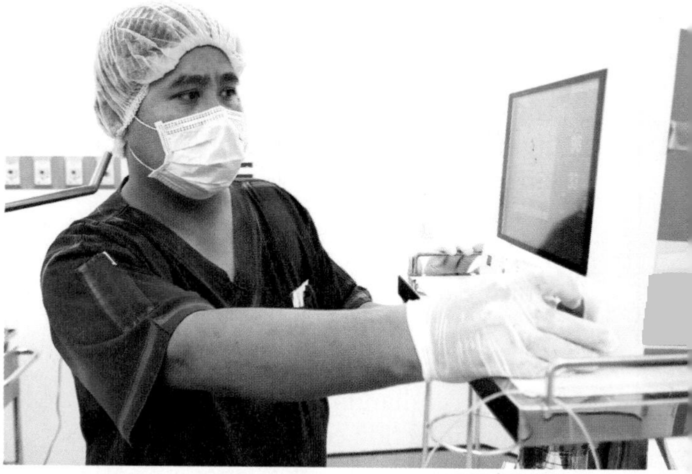

nimon/Shutterstock.com

Figure 4.19 This healthcare worker is wearing a mask to prevent the spread of an infection through droplets, which can occur during coughing or sneezing.

Contact Precautions. Contact precautions are designed to reduce the risk of transmission of certain infectious microorganisms through direct or indirect contact. Direct contact transmission occurs when a patient is touched by a healthcare worker providing care. Indirect contact transmission occurs when pathogens are transferred from a contaminated object or surface to a susceptible host. Whenever possible, patients should be placed in a private room or with another patient with the same condition. Hepatitis A and impetigo are examples of infectious diseases requiring contact precautions.

Personal Protective Equipment

OSHA requires that all workers be provided with the appropriate **personal protective equipment (PPE)** for their position. PPE protects workers from serious workplace injuries or illnesses resulting from contact with hazards of a microbial, chemical, radiological, physical, electrical, or mechanical nature. The protective equipment can include face shields, safety glasses, goggles, gowns, gloves, and face masks.

You should wear a face mask if your patient has a respiratory infection and is coughing and sneezing. In a doctor's office, wear a face mask if you have a cold or if you are going to be exposed to a patient with a cold.

personal protective equipment (PPE)
equipment worn by workers to protect them from serious workplace injuries or illnesses

Procedure 4.2 PPE: Putting on and Removing Disposable Gloves

Rationale

Standard and transmission-based precautions require the use of disposable gloves when performing different procedures. Properly putting on and removing gloves helps ensure infection control.

Preparation

1. Locate a pair of new disposable gloves in the correct size. Find, at minimum, one extra pair of gloves in case they are needed.

2. Before putting on the gloves, inspect them for cracks, holes, tears, or any discoloration. (Be aware that gloves may become punctured by rings and nails that extend beyond your fingertips.) If any gloves are damaged, discard them.

3. If a gown is required, put the gloves on after putting on a gown.

The Procedure: Putting on Disposable Gloves

4. Wash your hands according to procedure to ensure infection control.

5. Dry your hands well. Gloves are easier to put on with dry hands.

6. Pick up one glove by its cuff (Figure 4.20). The outside of a glove is always considered contaminated, so keep gloved hands away from your clothing or other areas that can be contaminated.

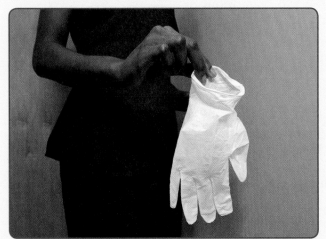

Figure 4.20 Wards Forest Media, LLC

7. Pull the glove onto your hand (Figure 4.21).

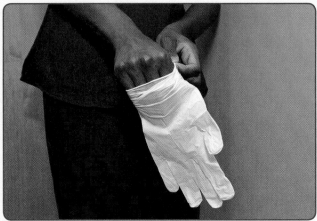

Figure 4.21 Wards Forest Media, LLC

8. Repeat the same procedure with the glove for your other hand.

9. Interlace your fingers to adjust the gloves on your hands.

10. If wearing a gown, pull the cuffs of the gloves up over the sleeves of the gown (Figure 4.22).

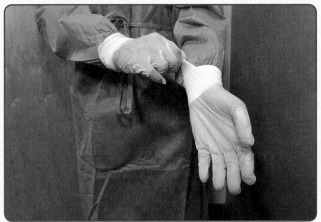

Figure 4.22 Wards Forest Media, LLC

The Procedure: Removing Disposable Gloves

11. Always remove gloves if they become torn or soiled during a procedure. Wash your hands to ensure infection control and then put on another pair of gloves using the procedure described previously.

12. To remove a glove, grasp the gloved hand just below the cuff of the glove with the gloved fingers of the other hand.

13. Pull the cuff of the glove down, drawing it over your hand while turning it inside out (Figure 4.23).

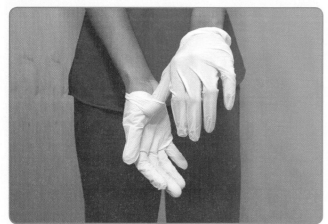

Figure 4.23   *Wards Forest Media, LLC*

14. Pull the glove off your hand and hold the removed glove with the other gloved hand (Figure 4.24).

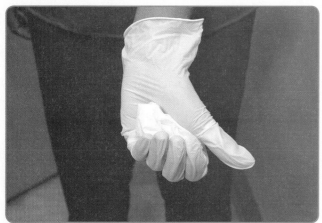

Figure 4.24   *Wards Forest Media, LLC*

15. Insert the fingers of the ungloved hand inside under the cuff of the glove on the other hand.

16. Pull the glove off inside out, drawing it over the first glove (Figure 4.25).

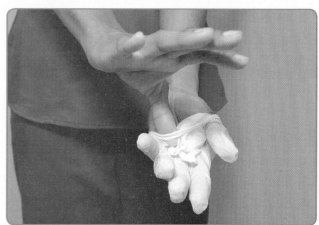

Figure 4.25   *Wards Forest Media, LLC*

17. Drop both gloves into the proper waste container. Never wash or reuse the gloves.

Follow-up

18. Wash your hands according to procedure to ensure infection control.

19. Dry your hands with a clean, dry paper towel. Discard the paper towel into the proper waste container.

20. Use a clean, dry paper towel to turn off the sink faucet. Discard the paper towel into the proper waste container.

Reporting and Documentation

21. Putting on and removing disposable gloves are accepted and established standard procedures. They do not need to be reported or documented.

Procedure 4.3   PPE: Putting on and Removing Gowns

Rationale

Standard and transmission-based precautions require that healthcare workers wear a gown when they might be exposed to or transmit microorganisms. The gown creates a barrier that protects the healthcare worker.

Preparation

1. Select a clean or isolation gown, as appropriate.
2. Remove your wristwatch and jewelry.
3. If wearing long sleeves, roll them up above your elbows.
4. As much as possible, carry out procedures at one time to avoid re-gowning and unnecessary waste of supplies.

The Procedure: Putting on a Gown

5. Wash your hands according to procedure to ensure infection control.
6. Hold the clean or isolation gown by the shoulders and out in front of you. The back of the gown should face you.
7. Unfold the gown carefully. Do not shake it open.
8. Slide your hands and arms into the sleeves of the gown (Figure 4.26).

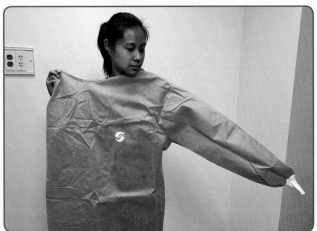

Figure 4.26   Wards Forest Media, LLC

9. Place the gown around your neck so your scrubs are covered.
10. Reach behind and tie the neck ties using a simple shoelace bow.

11. Reach behind the gown again. Grab the open edges of the gown and pull them together so they overlap. Your uniform should be covered completely.
12. Tie the waist ties in the back using a simple shoelace bow (Figure 4.27).

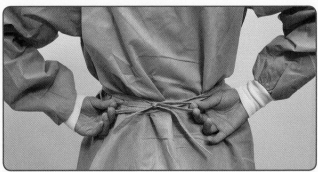

Figure 4.27   Wards Forest Media, LLC

13. Put on gloves according to Procedure 4.2. This is always done after putting on a gown.

The Procedure: Removing a Gown

14. If you are wearing gloves, remove and discard the gloves first, being careful not to contaminate yourself.
15. Wash your hands according to procedure to ensure infection control before removing the gown.
16. Untie both the waist and the neck ties of the gown.
17. Slide your hands back into the sleeves of the gown. Hold the cuff of one sleeve with your opposite hand (still inside the other sleeve) and begin pulling your arm out of that sleeve (Figure 4.28).

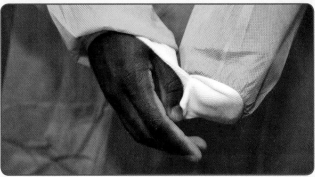

Figure 4.28   Wards Forest Media, LLC

18. Repeat the procedure to begin pulling the other arm out of its sleeve. Do not to touch the outside of the gown with your bare hands as you pull the gown down off your shoulders and arms (Figure 4.29).

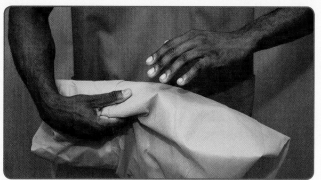

Figure 4.30 *Wards Forest Media, LLC*

22. Dispose of the contaminated gown in the appropriate waste container. Do not wear the gown again. It must be discarded as infectious waste. A reusable cloth gown is worn only once. Then it is handled as contaminated linen.

Follow-up

23. Wash your hands according to procedure to ensure infection control.
24. Dry your hands with a clean, dry paper towel. Discard the paper towel in the proper waste container.
25. Use another clean, dry paper towel to turn off the faucet.
26. Discard the paper towel in the proper waste container.

Reporting and Documentation

27. Putting on and removing gowns are accepted and established standard procedures. They do not need to be reported or documented.

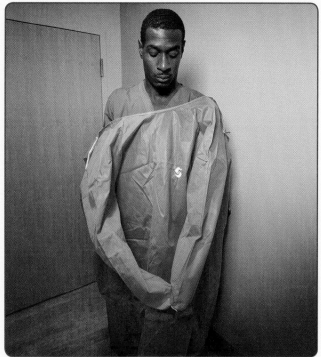

Figure 4.29 *Wards Forest Media, LLC*

19. Turn the gown inside out as it is being removed.
20. Hold the gown away from your scrubs with it turned inside out.
21. Roll the gown with the contaminated side facing in (Figure 4.30).

Needlesticks and Other Sharps-Related Injuries

sharps
needles or any other objects that could puncture or cut the skin

Needles and other **sharps** (any objects that could puncture or cut the skin) are a hazard in the healthcare environment. Injuries related to **needlesticks** (any accidental punctures of the skin) or other sharp-related injuries can be both painful and dangerous.

In the healthcare environment, all needles are considered sharps, including needles with syringes and attached tubing, or needles from vacutainers (devices that enable phlebotomists to draw several blood tubes at one time). Sharps also include blades such as razors, scalpels, and lancets.

needlesticks
any accidental punctures of the skin by needles; can be dangerous in a healthcare setting because the puncture can cause a potentially serious infection

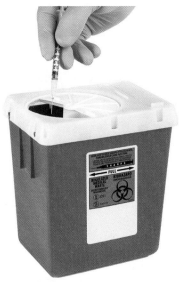

Figure 4.31 As a healthcare worker, you will need to develop the habit of putting used sharps into the proper disposable containers. Any object that is contaminated with biohazard waste and can puncture through a garbage bag must be placed in a biohazard sharps container.

biohazard sharps container
a puncture-resistant container used for disposing of waste-contaminated sharps, including needles, scalpels, glass slides, and broken glassware

Needlestick Safety and Prevention Act
a law enacted in 2000 requiring employers to identify, evaluate, and introduce safer medical devices to avoid needlesticks

These items must be placed in a **biohazard sharps container**, whether or not they are contaminated with biohazardous waste (Figure 4.31).

Any object that has been contaminated with biohazardous waste and has the potential to puncture a garbage bag must be placed in the biohazard sharps container. Such items might include broken glassware, glassware with sharp edges or points, pipettes, or glass slides. If these items are *not* contaminated with biohazardous waste, they may be placed in a rigid container and marked with the words "broken glassware."

Preventing Infections

A needlestick or other sharp-related injury immediately opens the skin to the potential of infection with bloodborne disease and other pathogens. Any skin abrasion, including acne, presents an opening for pathogens to enter your body. Be sure to bandage any cuts or breaks in the skin, and keep your hands away from your eyes and face to avoid infection.

Nurses, EMTs, paramedics, phlebotomists, clinical medical assistants, housekeeping personnel, and other healthcare workers may be at risk of exposure to bloodborne pathogens. A highly effective hepatitis B vaccine is available. Employers must offer this injection if their employees are at risk of being exposed to bloodborne pathogens. There is no vaccine for HIV or hepatitis C, but much research is being conducted in an attempt to find vaccines for these viral illnesses.

Needlestick Safety and Prevention Act

The **Needlestick Safety and Prevention Act** was signed into law on November 6, 2000. Under this act, OSHA requires employers to identify, evaluate, and introduce safe medical devices. Devices are available to shield a needle as soon as it is withdrawn from the patient. A needle should never be recapped. OSHA requires that safety-engineered needles—such as ones that have needle shields—must be used. After use, needles should be immediately placed in a puncture-resistant biohazard sharps container to prevent accidental exposure to a needlestick.

If you are stuck by a needle or another sharp object, or get blood or potentially infectious materials in your eyes, nose, mouth, or on broken skin, immediately flood the exposed area with water. Clean all wounds with soap and water or a skin antiseptic, if available. Immediately report the incident to your employer and seek medical attention. Your facility safety manual should clearly explain how to proceed after such an exposure.

The OSHA Standard requires the following:

- Sanitize your hands after direct contact with each of your patients.
- Use protective barriers such as gloves when working with blood and other potentially infectious body fluids. In addition, gowns, aprons, masks, and goggles must be used when there is a danger of being splashed or sprayed with body fluids. Remember, gloves that are worn when giving patient care are not puncture-proof.
- Collect and properly dispose of needles and other sharps in a biohazard sharps container.

- Do not recap needles.

- Cover all of your cuts and broken skin with a waterproof dressing before putting on gloves and handling blood or other potentially infectious body fluids.

- Promptly and carefully clean up spills of blood and other body fluids as directed by your facility safety manual.

- Facilities should use a safe system for healthcare waste management and disposal.

Real Life Scenario — Needlestick Incidents

Isabella just started her job as a phlebotomist at Eastridge Hospital. It is her first week drawing blood, and her supervisor is very strict about procedures. Isabella already feels that her supervisor does not have much faith in her abilities.

Isabella's next patient is a male adult who admits to being afraid of needles, increasing Isabella's anxiety. Isabella's hands are shaking, and she worries that her supervisor will come into the room to watch, so she hurries through the blood draw. She is able to draw the blood quickly, but in her haste to put away the needle she sticks herself with it. Isabella immediately decides that she won't tell anyone about the needlestick for fear of getting in trouble, or possibly fired.

Apply It

1. What could be the possible consequences of Isabella's failure to report this incident?
2. Do you think her supervisor should fire her?
3. What could happen if her patient has a bloodborne disease?
4. What would you do in Isabella's position?

Protocol for Disposal of Hazardous Materials

The Joint Commission requires hospitals to have hazardous-materials and waste-management plans or protocols describing how the facility will safely control hazardous materials and waste. Infectious materials are considered hazardous.

Written orientation and education programs must be created to train all personnel who come into contact with hazardous materials and waste. These programs must address the following:

- proper precautions in selection, handling, storage, and disposal of hazardous materials and waste

- proper emergency procedures for spills and exposures

- orientation and education about incident reporting

Recycling and Waste Reduction

Most of the waste generated in a healthcare facility is nonhazardous. This means that you need not follow the protocols for disposal of hazardous materials for most waste materials. You should, however, use recycling procedures when disposing of nonhazardous materials. Recycling practices save money for the facility and help protect the environment.

Paper usually makes up the largest amount of waste in a healthcare facility. Paper waste includes cardboard, high-grade office paper, newspaper, and mixed paper. Other recyclable materials include plastics, food waste, and disposable linens. Efforts should be made whenever possible to purchase products made from recycled materials.

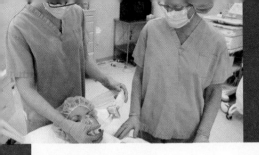

Summary

Safety definitions and standards for healthcare facilities and providers are published by several national organizations and government agencies. All healthcare workers are responsible for the safety of the patients, visitors, and their coworkers. General safety rules must be obeyed in the healthcare facility, and you must be aware of potential safety hazards in the facility, such as liquid spills, loose rugs, and disoriented patients. Healthcare workers should also practice proper body mechanics to avoid injuring themselves.

Your department's safety manual contains specific safety concerns in your area. Incident reports must be filled out whenever the safety and health of a patient, visitor, or employee is compromised. This could include any event that is not a part of the routine operation in the healthcare facility, such as a patient falling, abuse from a patient or an employee, or an accidental needlestick. OSHA oversees employee safety in the workplace.

As a healthcare worker, you must know and practice safety regulations regarding chemical, electrical, radiation, and fire hazards. Follow instructions for disaster preparedness and participate in disaster drills.

Infection control is a constant battle in healthcare facilities. The chain of infection may be interrupted using strategies such as observing proper hand hygiene, wearing appropriate personal protective equipment, and properly disposing of all potentially infectious materials. Employees should also follow proper procedures regarding patients in isolation areas.

Needles and other sharps are prevalent in the healthcare environment. Accidental needlesticks are dangerous and must be avoided. Used needles and other sharps should be placed in a puncture-resistant biohazard sharps container.

Safety must be a serious concern for students and healthcare professionals working in a healthcare facility or the science laboratory. Following safety guidelines in school, the workplace, at play, and at home is critical for the healthcare student and worker.

Review Questions

Answer the following questions using what you have learned in this chapter.

True or False Assess

1. *True or False?* Isolation rooms can be used to contain contagious diseases such as tuberculosis.

2. *True or False?* Hands do not need to be washed after you have removed your gloves.

3. *True or False?* A carpal tunnel injury is often a result of incorrect lifting.

4. *True or False? Streptococcus* and *Staphylococcus* are parasites that cause disease.

5. *True or False?* Viruses are the cause of the common cold.

6. *True or False?* The friction caused by rubbing hands and fingers together is a desirable part of proper hand washing.

7. *True or False?* Always check the patient's identification wristband and ask the patient's name before carrying out any procedures.

8. *True or False?* Personal protective equipment is only worn by employees of the fire department.

9. *True or False?* Antibiotic-resistant bacteria are also known as *super bugs*.

10. *True or False?* Gloves do *not* need to be worn when attending to a cut on a patient's arm.

Multiple Choice Assess

11. Which of the following situation(s) could merit filling out an incident report at a hospital?

    A. an employee yelling at a patient

    B. a patient falling while walking to the restroom

    C. a patient experiencing a serious allergic reaction to an ingredient in his dinner

    D. All of the above.

12. To avoid back injury, which of the following should be avoided?

    A. holding objects as far away from you as possible

    B. lifting with your legs

    C. tightening stomach muscles when lifting

    D. pushing rather than pulling objects

13. Which of the following is a correct procedure for infection control?

    A. use a puncture-proof biohazard container to dispose of needles and other sharps

    B. follow proper hand hygiene procedures between contact with each patient

    C. use protective barriers when in direct contact with blood

    D. All of the above.

14. In a fire emergency, which step should *not* be followed?

    A. Follow facility evacuation plans.

    B. Keep areas uncluttered and free of debris.

    C. Run through the halls shouting "Code Blue!"

    D. Know how to operate fire extinguishers.

15. Antibiotic resistance can be caused by _____.

    A. not taking the full prescription of antibiotics

    B. prescribing antibiotics when not needed

    C. antibacterials contained in cleaning products

    D. All of the above.

16. The acronym PASS stands for _____.

    A. pinch, aim, spray, stop

    B. pull, aim, sweep, spray

    C. pin, aim, shake, squeeze

    D. pull, aim, squeeze, sweep

17. Which of the following is true of anaerobic organisms?

    A. They are not pathogenic.

    B. They need little or no oxygen.

    C. They do not require gloves when handling.

    D. They are people who are exercising.

18. Which of the following is true of the Joint Commission?

    A. It is a non-profit organization.

    B. It is a healthcare agency.

    C. It is an organization that publishes national patient safety goals.

    D. All of the above.

19. Which of the following do you know to be true of OSHA?

    A. It is a waste management organization.

    B. It is an administration established by the Occupational Safety and Health Act of 1880.

    C. It is a state-funded agency.

    D. It requires that all workers be provided with PPE.

20. It takes at least _____ seconds to wash your hands properly.

    A. 25

    B. 30

    C. 20

    D. 15

Short Answer

21. What is an incident report?

22. What is a nosocomial infection?

23. Name the five types of fire extinguishers.

24. List three basic principles of body mechanics involved in safely lifting an object.

25. What is meant by the chain of infection? Name six parts of the chain.

26. Name at least three types of microorganisms.

27. What is meant by hand hygiene?

28. What is a biohazard sharps container and why is it used?

29. Describe two OSHA standards that apply to the healthcare facility.

30. Define quality improvement.

Critical Thinking Exercises

31. Do you and your family have disaster preparedness plans? Establish response plans for any natural disasters that might occur in your city or town.

32. Develop a plan to support recycling and waste management in a facility such as your school or a local hospital. Explain how your plan would contribute to both cost containment and environmental protection.

33. What are the differences between bacterial and viral infections? What treatments are available for both infections?

34. Sanitization, disinfection, and sterilization are three levels of cleaning that take place in the healthcare environment. Explain the significance and use of each level.

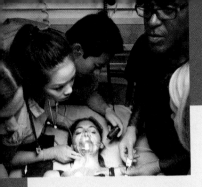

Unit 1
Cumulative Review Assess

Review Questions

Answer the following questions using what you have learned in this unit.

True or False

1. *True or False?* Criminal law is also known as tort law.

2. *True or False?* A paramedic has more training and responsibilities than an EMT.

3. *True or False?* OSHA is a government agency that imposes safety regulations to prevent injury and death in the workplace.

4. *True or False?* AHRQ focuses on helping healthcare professionals, not consumers, make informed decisions.

5. *True or False?* PPOs and HMOs are set up the same way.

6. *True or False?* Used needles, razors, scalpels, and lancets must be placed in a biohazard sharps container.

7. *True or False?* An ombudsman must be a doctor.

8. *True or False?* Job shadowing allows you to follow an employee completing job tasks.

9. *True or False?* A DNR is a document instructing a doctor to use cardiopulmonary resuscitation if the patient's heart stops.

Multiple Choice

10. The bubonic plague is caused by the bacterium _____, which is transmitted by small rodents infested with _____.
    A. *Staphylococcus aureus* and mites
    B. *E. Coli* and mosquitoes
    C. *Yersinia pestis* and fleas
    D. None of the above.

11. The chain of infection includes each of the following events *except* _____.
    A. a portal of exit
    B. the mode of transmission
    C. the final stage
    D. a susceptible host

12. What is considered reportable behavior in the healthcare workplace?
    A. applying lipstick while working
    B. bad breath
    C. a breach of confidentiality
    D. smoking outside the facility

13. What is *not* true about health maintenance organizations (HMOs)?
    A. You can pick any doctor you want, inside or outside the HMO.
    B. HMOs are set up so the patient receives most, or all, of her healthcare from a network provider.
    C. Most HMOs require a copayment at the time of a visit.
    D. Bonuses may be paid to doctors for keeping costs down.

14. Which of the following is the best body mechanics practice?
    A. holding the item you are lifting away from your body
    B. pull rather than push
    C. lift with your back
    D. tightening abdominal muscles when lifting

15. All of the following careers are classified as support services *except* _____.
    A. food service worker
    B. biomedical equipment technician
    C. health unit coordinator
    D. administrative dietitian

16. Which agency of the US government regulates and supervises food and drug safety?
    A. FDA
    B. CDC
    C. NIH
    D. TJC

17. The career pathways in healthcare include all the following *except* _____.
    A. support services
    B. therapeutic services
    C. recreational services
    D. diagnostic services

18. Which of the following developments did *not* occur during the Industrial Revolution?

    A. the invention of the stethoscope

    B. factories developed more sophisticated medical equipment

    C. the development of the personal computer

    D. public health laws began to control disease spread

19. Which statement describes genomic medicine?

    A. medicine focused on the elderly

    B. the study related to psychiatric medicine

    C. the study of a person's DNA sequences

    D. the military health system

Short Answer

20. What is a health insurance copayment?

21. Describe the procedure that must be followed after sticking yourself with a contaminated needle or other sharp object.

22. What is an advance directive?

23. Which elements constitute the fire triangle?

Critical Thinking Exercises

24. Review the US regulatory agencies that impact the healthcare industry, such as OSHA, the FDA, and the Joint Commission. Then, explain which regulations you feel will be most important for your future healthcare career and why.

25. Identify a situation in which a healthcare worker's actions might be considered unethical. Then, research the ethical ramifications of that behavior. Do you feel the consequences are appropriate? Why or why not?

26. Antibiotic resistance has become a worldwide problem. Using the Internet or your school's library, research the current bacteria that have become antibiotic resistant and those that have the potential to become antibiotic resistant. Then brainstorm possible solutions to this problem.

Career Exploration

Public Health Nurse

Public health nurses educate people about health issues unique to their location. They create and implement health education and disease prevention campaigns, such as health screenings and immunization clinics. Public health nurses may also work with both government officials and members of the community to improve access to healthcare. They also monitor health trends and research health risk factors for individual communities.

Public health nurses work for government agencies, nonprofit organizations, community health clinics, and other groups that work to improve health in communities.

Public health nurses are registered nurses (RNs) with a bachelor's degree in nursing. Job outlook looks promising in the coming years. Public health nurses may earn between $50,000 and $55,000 each year.

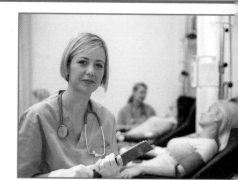
wavebreakmedia/Shutterstock.com

Further Research

1. Research one of the related careers using the *Occupational Outlook Handbook* and other reliable Internet resources. What is the outlook for this career?

2. Review the educational requirements for this career. What level of education is necessary? What classes would you need to take to pursue a related degree?

3. What is the salary range for this job?

4. What do you think you would like about this career? What might you dislike? Compare the job you have researched to the description of a public health nurse. Which job appeals to you more? Why?

Related Careers

Environmental health manager

Epidemiologist

Medical investigator

Public health information officer

Public health supervisor

Unit 2

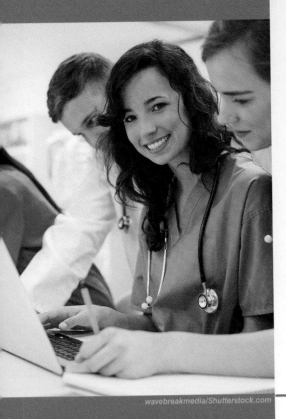

wavebreakmedia/Shutterstock.com

Academic Foundations

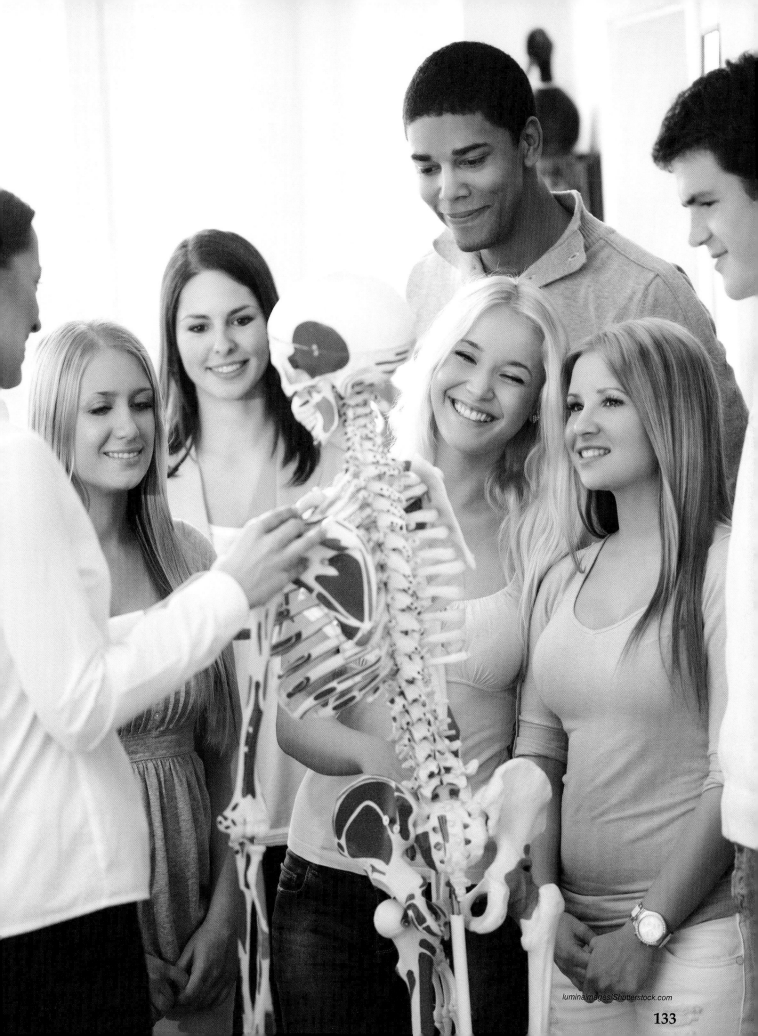

Chapter 5
Medical Terminology

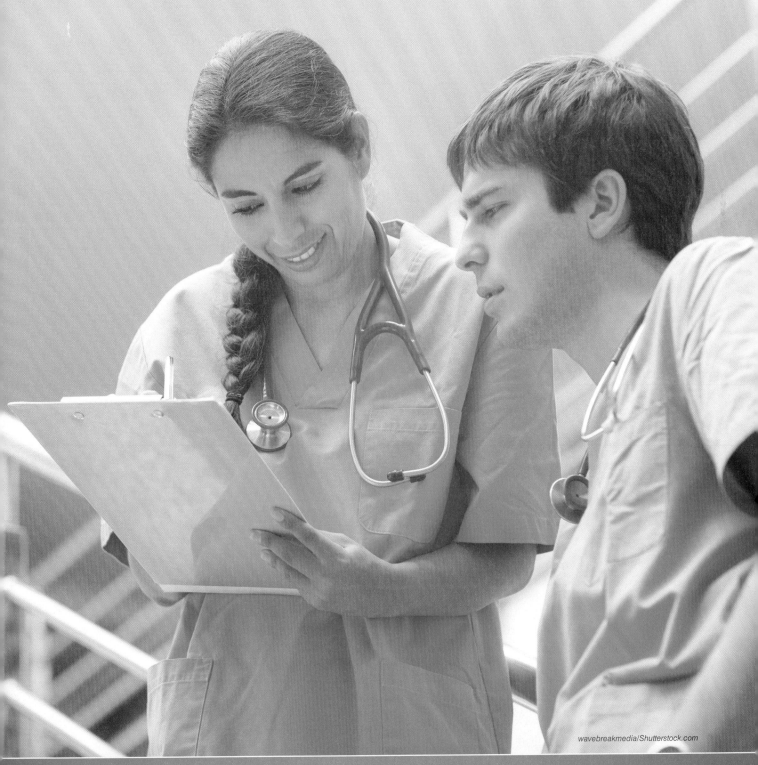

wavebreakmedia/Shutterstock.com

Terms to Know

 Build Vocab

abdominal quadrants	dorsal recumbent position	semi-Fowler's position
acronyms	Fowler's position	Sims' position
anatomical position	knee-chest position	suffix
body cavities	lateral position	supine position
body planes	lithotomy position	Trendelenburg position
combining form	prefix	word elements
combining vowel	prone position	word root

Chapter Objectives

- Recognize that many medical terms have Latin and Greek roots.
- Explain how medical words are constructed.
- Define *word roots, prefixes, suffixes, combining vowel,* and *combining form* and understand how each of these word elements can be used to form medical terms.
- Describe why proper pronunciation and spelling of medical terms are important.
- Identify common abbreviations used in healthcare.
- Identify body cavities, body positions, body directions, planes of the body, as well as abdominal quadrants.

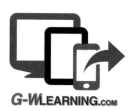

While studying, look for the activity icon to:

- **Build** vocabulary with e-flash cards and interactive games.
- **Assess** progress with chapter and unit review questions.
- **Expand** learning with animations and illustration labeling activities.
- **Simulate** EHR entry with healthcare documents.

G-WLEARNING.com

www.g-wlearning.com/healthsciences/

Has your doctor ever spoken to you using terms that were hard to understand or that you had never heard before? Sometimes it can seem like doctors and healthcare professionals speak a foreign language. Learning the language of medicine, called *medical terminology*, might feel overwhelming at first. However, if you wish to enter the healthcare field, you need to understand the basic rules for forming medical terms.

In ancient times, both the Greeks and Romans advanced the study and practice of medicine. Using the Greek and Latin languages, these early medical professionals named parts of the human anatomy, diseases, and treatments. First used centuries ago, these Greek and Latin terms remain a part of today's medical language (Figure 5.1).

Origins of Medical Terms		
Term	*Origin*	*Definition*
artery	Latin, *arteria*	blood vessel that carries oxygen-rich blood away from the heart
phobia	Greek, *phobos*	irrational fear
vein	Latin, *vena*	blood vessel that carries oxygen-poor blood back to the heart
sperm	Greek, *sperma*	male sex cell that fertilizes the female's egg

Goodheart-Willcox Publisher

Figure 5.1   Greek and Latin medical terms

Building Medical Terms

word elements

parts that are used to form medical terms; include the word root, prefix, suffix, combining vowel, and combining form (word root plus combining vowel)

Medical words are like puzzles, with the **word elements** serving as the puzzle pieces. Each word element offers clues to the function, structure, or processes of the term as a whole. When the word elements are put together correctly, it is possible to determine the definition of the word by first defining each element.

Mastering medical terminology requires extensive review and practice. The time and effort you put into learning these words will pay off once you begin your healthcare career. You do not have to memorize every medical term right away. Instead, you can break down terms into their word elements to determine their overall definitions. In a short time, you will do this automatically when introduced to a new term.

As you develop your medical vocabulary, you should keep in mind the word elements that may be used to form a word. Analyzing these word elements can help you understand each medical term as a whole. The word elements that you will encounter are

1. word root;
2. prefix;
3. suffix;
4. combining vowel; and
5. combining form (word root and combining vowel together).

Extend Your Knowledge ▶ Determining Term Origin

The ancient Greeks were the first to study the field of medicine, including anatomy. They also developed a vocabulary to accompany their studies. When the Romans began studying medicine, they often adopted Greek terms and modified them to fit their alphabet and grammar. After the Romans altered the Greeks' terminology, Latin became the language of science. As a result, most of the medical terminology that we use today derives directly from these Latin roots. In addition, some terminology is derived from Arabic, French, Italian, and Spanish.

Apply It

1. Use a printed or online medical dictionary to find ten medical terms that have Latin origins and ten words that have Greek origins.

2. Find three medical terms with both Greek and Latin origins.

Word Root

The **word root** is the body, or the main part, of the word. Examples of word roots include

- *cardi*, the word root for "heart";
- *nephr*, the word root for "kidney";
- *hepat*, the word root for "liver";
- *arthr*, the word root for "joint";
- *path*, the word root for "disease"; and
- *mast*, the word root for "breast."

word root
the body or the main element of a word

Word Root Characteristics

Every medical term contains a word root. The word root is the foundation of the medical term and gives the word its meaning. In some cases, a medical term may contain two or more word roots. When more than one word root is present in a term, the subsequent word roots follow immediately after the first. Refer to Table A in the reference section at the end of this chapter for a list of common word roots you will encounter when working in the healthcare field.

Check Your Understanding ✓

Table A in the reference section at the end of this chapter provides numerous examples of medical terms formed by common root words. Review these examples and make a note of any terms that are familiar to you. If you are not familiar with a word, look it up in your medical dictionary.

Prefix

prefix
the part of a word that comes before the word root; changes the meaning of the word root

A **prefix** is the part of the word that comes before, or *precedes*, the word root. Prefixes change the meaning of the word root. Some common prefixes are

- *intra-* meaning "within";
- *trans-* meaning "across, through, or beyond";
- *sub-* meaning "under, below";
- *poly-* meaning "many"; and
- *macro-* meaning "large."

Prefix Characteristics

- A prefix attaches to the beginning of a word root and modifies the root's meaning (refer to Table B in the reference section at the end of this chapter). For example, in the term *autoimmune*, the prefix *auto-* means "self." Thus, the prefix signifies the immune response in the body is against itself.
- Not all medical terms include a prefix—it is an optional word element.
- A prefix can be a single letter (*a-*) or a group of letters (*hyper-*).
- A prefix is never the foundation of a medical term.
- When presented by itself, a prefix always ends with a hyphen to show it is just a word element, rather than a complete word. The hyphen disappears when the prefix joins another word element.

Suffix

suffix
the part of a word that is added after the word root to change its meaning

The **suffix** is the word element added after the word root to change its meaning. Examples of suffixes include

- *-ectomy*, the suffix meaning "excision, surgical removal";
- *-itis*, the suffix meaning "inflammation";
- *-logy*, the suffix meaning "study of"; and
- *-gram*, the suffix meaning "record."

Suffix Characteristics

- Every medical term includes a suffix (see Table C at the end of this chapter).
- A suffix is always at the end of a medical term. A suffix attaches to the end of the word root and modifies its meaning.
- A suffix can be a single letter (*-y*) or a group of letters (*-ectomy*).
- A suffix *cannot* be the foundation of a medical term.
- When presented by itself, a suffix always begins with a hyphen to show it is not a complete term. The hyphen is deleted when the suffix joins the word root.

Figure 5.2 includes common suffixes that mean "pertaining to." These suffixes might also be translated as "belonging to," "connected to," or "dependent on something." An example is the word *cutaneous*. When the word root *cutane* is joined with the suffix *-ous*, the newly formed term means "pertaining to the skin."

Combining Vowel

A **combining vowel** is used to join two word roots, or is placed between a word root and a suffix. The most commonly used combining vowel is an *o*; however, there are some rare exceptions in which an *i* or *e* may be used as the combining vowel.

The combining vowel makes the word easier to pronounce. The combining vowel has no impact on the meaning of the word—it exists only to join word elements.

When a word root is combined with a suffix that begins with a vowel, the word root's combining vowel is dropped from the new term. An example of this is the word root and combining vowel *oste/o* (*oste* means bone). When *oste/o* is combined with the suffix *-itis*, the combining vowel *o* is dropped. The word is spelled *osteitis*, meaning "inflammation of the bone."

Combining Form

Books that list medical terms often present the combining vowel and the word root together, such as *oste/o*, *aden/o*, or *hyster/o*. When the word root and the combining vowel are joined, the result is called the **combining form**. Note that the combining form is not a fifth word element. Instead, it is an alternative way of expressing the first and fourth elements (roots/vowels) described above.

Combining Word Elements

Once you are familiar with the word elements, you can put them together to build a medical vocabulary (Figure 5.3).

Example 1: poly/arthr/itis

The term *polyarthritis* is composed of the prefix *poly-*, which means "many"; *arthr*, which means "joint"; and finally, the suffix *-itis*, meaning "inflammation." Together these word elements create the term *polyarthritis*, which is defined as "inflammation of many joints."

Suffixes	
Suffix	*Example*
-ac, -al, -an, -ar	meningococcal (me-NIN-jah-KAHK-al)
-eal	peritoneal (PER-i-toh-NEE-al)
-iac, -ic, -ical	manic (MAN-ik)
-ine	intrauterine (IN-tra-YOO-ter-in)
-ose	sclerose (skle-ROHZ)
-ous	cutaneous (kyoo-TAY-nee-uhs)
-tic	septic (SEP-tik)

Goodheart-Willcox Publisher

Figure 5.2   Suffixes meaning, "pertaining to"

combining vowel
letter used to combine two word roots, or a word root and a suffix; usually an o

combining form
term that describes a word root and a combining vowel together; used to form medical terms

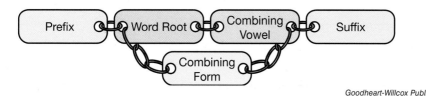

Goodheart-Willcox Publisher

Figure 5.3   Combining word elements allows you to form a variety of medical terms.

It is important to note that not every medical term contains all the word elements. Some terms, for example, might have just a word root, combining vowel, and a suffix.

Example 2: cardi/o/logy

Cardiology is formed by combining the word root *cardi*, meaning "heart"; the combining vowel *o*; and *-logy*, the suffix meaning "study of." Together these word elements create the term *cardiology*, which means "the study of the heart."

Other medical terms have only a word root and a suffix with no combining vowel or prefix.

Example 3: mast/ectomy

The term *mastectomy* is made up of the word root *mast*, meaning "breast," and the suffix *-ectomy*, which means "removal." Combining this word root and suffix gives us the term *mastectomy*, which can be defined as the "surgical removal of the breast."

It is important to learn and recognize the most common prefixes, suffixes, and word roots. Exceptions to general rules of medical terminology can be learned gradually as you become familiar with the basic structures of medical terms.

Singular and Plural Endings

Many medical terms originate from Latin and Greek words, a fact that affects their singular and plural forms. The rules for forming singular and plural forms of some medical terms follow rules of Greek and Latin, rather than rules of the English language.

For example, the heart has a right atrium and a left atrium. We do not call these two parts of the heart *atriums*, but rather *atria*. Other words, such as *biopsy* and *biopsies*, change from singular to plural by following English language rules. Consider each medical term individually when changing from singular to the plural form (Figure 5.4).

Singular and Plural Endings		
Terms Ending in...	**Singular Form**	**Plural Form**
-a	bursa	bursae
-ax	thorax	thoraces
-ex *or* -ix	appendix	appendices
-is	metastasis	metastases
-ma	lipoma	lipomata
-nx	phalanx	phalanges
-on	ganglion	ganglia
-us	nucleus	nuclei
-um	ovum	ova
-y	artery	arteries

Goodheart-Willcox Publisher

Figure 5.4   Singular and plural endings

Pronunciation and Spelling of Medical Terms

Medical terms can be difficult to pronounce, especially if you have never heard the words read aloud before. Even if you have heard a particular word, you might have heard different pronunciations. Another complication is that some words like *abduction* and *adduction* sound alike, but their meanings are completely different.

Clear pronunciation is important for effective communication in the medical environment. Remembering the following tips will help you properly pronounce difficult terms.

- *ch* often sounds like *k* as in "chronic" (KRO-nic)
- *g* usually sounds like *j* when the *g* comes before *e*, *i*, and *y* as in "genetics" (je-NE-tics)
- *i* is pronounced *eye* when it is added at the end of a word to make it plural as in "bacilli" (ba-SIL-eye)
- *pn* sounds like *n*, as though the *p* didn't exist, as in "pneumonia" (nu-MO-ni-a)
- *ps* sounds like *s*, ignoring the *p*, as in "psychiatry" (si-KI-a-tree)

Although the pronunciations of medical terms may vary, there is always only one accurate spelling. A medical dictionary is a valuable tool when determining the correct spelling of a term. Even experienced healthcare workers occasionally use a dictionary.

If just one letter in a word is out of place, the meaning of the word can change. Small errors in spelling can result in serious mistakes. A misspelled word in a doctor's order could cause a patient to receive the wrong medication or treatment. A misspelling could also cause a misinterpretation by an insurance biller, possibly resulting in an unpaid insurance claim.

Remember the importance of clear, appropriate communication when you become a healthcare worker. You need to be comfortable with medical vocabulary so that you can use medical terms specific to the healthcare setting in which you work. When you speak to fellow healthcare workers, you will use medical terms. However, do not assume that your patients and their families understand medical vocabulary. Instead, use common terms so that you will be understood.

Check Your Understanding

Write the correct spelling of these incorrectly spelled terms on a separate sheet of paper. Refer to Table A at the end of the chapter to check your answers.

1. neumonia	4. hepititis	7. narkotic	10. oncolagy
2. gynacology	5. hemitology	8. leucemia	
3. artharitis	6. ileim	9. carcinigen	

Real Life Scenario

Understanding Your Doctor

Jeanette visits her family doctor, Dr. Nolan, to discuss some health concerns. During her visit, the doctor is quite rushed, with a waiting room full of patients. When Jeanette finally sees Dr. Nolan, Dr. Nolan answers her questions using several medical terms she doesn't understand.

Apply It

1. If you were in Jeanette's position, what would you do—leave the office and look up the confusing terms in a medical dictionary or ask Dr. Nolan to explain the terms?
2. Would you consider switching to a new doctor? What factors would influence your decision?

Medical Abbreviations

The healthcare world is a fast-paced environment, and abbreviations may be used to speed up communication (Figure 5.5). Different healthcare facilities may have varying meanings for certain abbreviations. Hospitals often publish a list of acceptable abbreviations that may be used in the facility.

In some cases, abbreviations have caused confusion that leads to incorrect interpretations and results in serious errors. As a result, some healthcare facilities are moving toward restricting or eliminating the use of medical abbreviations.

Some abbreviations are called **acronyms**. An example of a common acronym is AIDS, which means *acquired immunodeficiency syndrome.*

acronyms
words formed from the first letters or parts of other words

Medical Abbreviations and Acronyms			
Abbreviation or Acronym	**Meaning**	**Abbreviation or Acronym**	**Meaning**
ABG	arterial blood gas	cap	capsule
ADL	activities of daily living	CBC	complete blood count
AIDS	acquired immunodeficiency syndrome	cc	cubic centimeter
AM	in the morning or before noon	CCU	coronary care unit
Amb	ambulatory	CHF	congestive heart failure
ASAP	as soon as possible	cm	centimeter
ASHD	arteriosclerotic heart disease	CNS	central nervous system
BID, b.i.d.	twice a day	COPD	chronic obstructive pulmonary disease
BMR	basic metabolic rate	CPR	cardiopulmonary resuscitation
B/P, BP	blood pressure	CSF	cerebrospinal fluid
BS	blood sugar	CT scan	computerized tomography scan
°C	centigrade, Celsius temperature	CVA	cerebrovascular accident
c̄	with	D&C	dilatation and curettage
Ca	calcium	DOA	dead on arrival
CA	cancer	DOB	date of birth
Cath	catheter; catheterization	Dx	diagnosis

Goodheart-Willcox Publisher

Figure 5.5   Common medical abbreviations and acronyms

Medical Abbreviations and Acronyms

Abbreviation or Acronym	Meaning	Abbreviation or Acronym	Meaning
ECG; EKG	electrocardiogram	NPO	nothing by mouth
ED; ER	emergency department; emergency room	OB/GYN	obstetrics/gynecology
EMG	electromyogram	OD	overdose, right eye
ENT	ear, nose, and throat	OR	operating room
FBS	fasting blood sugar	ORTH	orthopedics
FDA	Food and Drug Administration	oz	ounce
Fe	iron	PDR	Physician's Desk Reference
FUO	fever of unknown origin	PID	pelvic inflammatory disease
Fx	fracture	p.o.	by mouth
GB	gallbladder	p/o	postoperative
gm	gram	preop	before surgery
gtt	drop	pt	patient
HBV	hepatitis B virus	q	every
Hgb	hemoglobin	QID, q.i.d.	four times a day
HIV	human immunodeficiency virus	R	respiration, right
ICU	intensive care unit	ROM	range of motion
IV	intravenous	R/O	rule out
kg	kilogram	RT	right, radiation therapy
L&D	labor and delivery	Rx	prescription
L, l	left, liter	$\bar{s}$	without
lab	laboratory	Staph.	*Staphylococcus*
LPN, LVN	licensed practical nurse, licensed vocational nurse	STAT, stat.	immediately
lytes	electrolytes	STI, STD	sexually transmitted infection; sexually transmitted disease
mcg	microgram	T&A	tonsillectomy and adenoidectomy
MD	Doctor of Medicine	TIA	transient ischemic attack
mEq	milliequivalents	TID, t.i.d.	three times a day
mg	milligram	TPR	temperature, pulse, respirations
MI	myocardial infarction	UA	urinalysis
ml	milliliter	URI	upper respiratory infection
mm	millimeter	UTI	urinary tract infection
MRI	magnetic resonance imaging	VD	venereal disease
MRSA	Methicillin-resistant *Staphylococcus aureus*	VS	vital signs
N/A	not applicable, not available	wt	weight

Goodheart-Willcox Publisher

Figure 5.5   Common medical abbreviations and acronyms (continued)

The Joint Commission's "Do Not Use List" includes abbreviations that the Commission recommends organizations stop using (Figure 5.6). This includes eliminating these dangerous abbreviations, acronyms, symbols, and dose designations from the organization's software. The items on this list can cause serious problems if mistaken for an incorrect designation.

The Joint Commission's "Do Not Use List"		
Do Not Use	**Potential Problem**	**Use Instead**
U, u (unit)	mistaken for *0* (zero), the number 4 (four), or *cc*	write *unit*
IU (International Unit)	mistaken for *IV* (intravenous) or the number 10 (ten)	write *International Unit*
Q.D., QD, q.d., qd. (daily)	mistaken for abbreviations in next row	write *daily*
Q.O.D., QOD, q.o.d., qod (every other day)	mistaken for abbreviations in row above	write *every other day*
Trailing zero (X.0 mg)	decimal point is missed	write *X mg*
Lack of leading zero (.X mg)	decimal point is missed	write *0.X mg*
MS	can mean "morphine sulfate" or "magnesium sulfate"	write *morphine sulfate*
MSO_4 and $MgSO_4$	confused for one another	write *magnesium sulfate*

Goodheart-Willcox Publisher

Figure 5.6   The "Do Not Use List" of abbreviations by the Joint Commission

Check Your Understanding ✔

Match each abbreviation with its definition on a separate sheet of paper.

1. prescription	A.	AIDS
2. operating room	B.	BS
3. hepatitis B virus	C.	UA
4. acquired immunodeficiency syndrome	D.	ICU
5. blood sugar	E.	HBV
6. urinalysis	F.	CHF
7. myocardial infarction	G.	Rx
8. congestive heart failure	H.	ECG
9. intensive care unit	I.	OR
10. electrocardiogram	J.	MI

Real Life Scenario — Decoding a Medical Record

Peter is taking his father to see Dr. Wilson to discuss his father's upcoming surgery. With his father's permission, Peter asks to see his father's medical record. Peter reads the following:

Patient found to have a tumor in the colon following a colonoscopy. Biopsy done in pathology found to be a carcinoma, breaking through the colon wall. Surgery to follow in 10 days, with possible colostomy. Patient surgical history includes a T&A in 1970. Patient has chronic UTIs and had a mild MI in 2000.

Apply It

1. Using what you have learned in this chapter, translate this section from the father's medical record. The tables at the end of this chapter, in particular, may be useful.
2. Do you think Dr. Wilson broke the law or acted unethically in giving Peter his father's medical record? To whom can Dr. Wilson show the record? Do some research (including other chapters of this text) to answer these questions.

Using Medical Terminology Appropriately

When you become familiar with medical terminology, be sure to use terminology specific to the healthcare setting. For example, the approved medical abbreviations may vary among healthcare facilities. Remember that patients may not be familiar with this terminology and may become confused when you speak so specifically to them. Do not confuse your patient with technical language.

If you work in a specialty area in a hospital or clinic, learn the vocabulary that is relevant to that specialty. For example, if you are working in orthopedics, a specialty concerned with problems pertaining to the skeletal system, you will have to learn specific terms related to the skeletal system.

Terms for Location and Movement

Special terminology is used to describe the locations and movements of the human body's various parts. It is helpful to understand these terms and how to use them correctly before beginning your healthcare career. Healthcare workers must write detailed reports after examining a patient, and their descriptions and diagnoses must be exact. For example, radiologists must be very specific when reporting what they see in X-rays, and insurance companies want precise details about diagnoses. It is very important that terms related to body cavities, body positions, directions of the body, body planes, and abdominal quadrants become part of every healthcare worker's vocabulary.

Body Cavities

body cavities

spaces in the body that contain organs; the human body is divided into the dorsal and ventral cavities

The human body is divided into several **body cavities**, or spaces that house internal organs (Figure 5.7). Of these body cavities, the dorsal cavity (near the back) and the ventral cavity (near the front) are the two main divisions found in the body.

The dorsal cavity can be subdivided into the spinal and cranial cavities. The cranial cavity is located within the skull and holds the brain, large blood vessels, and nerves. The spinal cavity contains the spinal cord.

The ventral cavity is divided by the diaphragm into the thoracic (chest) cavity and the abdominopelvic cavity. Included in the thoracic cavity are the lungs, heart, major blood vessels, and part of the esophagus. Organs in the upper area of the abdominopelvic cavity (called the *abdominal cavity*) include the stomach, most of the intestines, the pancreas, liver, spleen, gallbladder, and kidneys. The lower part of the abdominopelvic cavity (often called the *pelvic cavity*) contains the bladder, urethra, reproductive organs, parts of the large intestine, and the rectum.

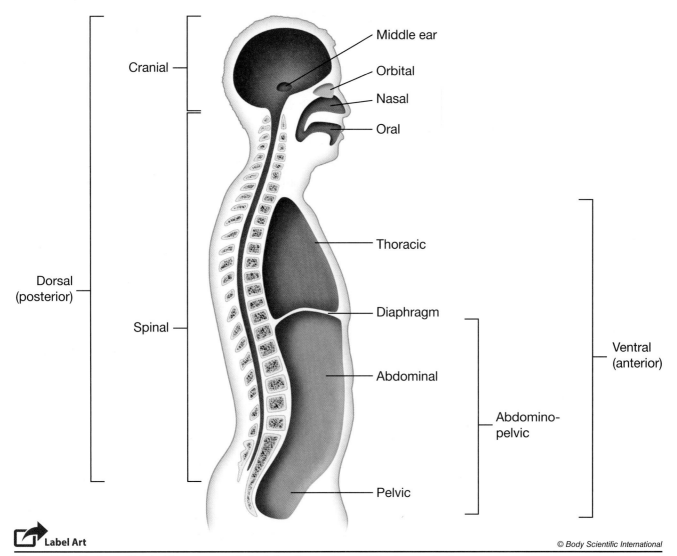

Label Art

Figure 5.7   Body cavities hold organs and help define the anatomy of the human body.

Body Positions

Although the body can assume many positions, there are eleven positions that may be mentioned in clinical exams and treatments (Figures 5.8 and 5.9). Placing a patient in the correct position for treatment, examinations, and comfort measures is important for providing safe and accurate patient care. These eleven positions include the following:

- anatomical position
- prone position
- supine position
- Fowler's position
- semi-Fowler's position
- lateral position
- Trendelenburg position
- Sims' position
- lithotomy position
- knee-chest position
- dorsal recumbent position

Anatomical position is an erect, standing position in which the patient faces forward, with the feet parallel and arms hanging at the side, palms facing forward. This position is often considered the starting point when describing movement and directional terms of the human body. The **prone position** occurs when a patient lies facedown, or on her stomach. The **supine position** calls for a patient to lie faceup, or on his back. A patient sitting in bed with the head of the bed elevated 45° is in the **Fowler's position**. The **semi-Fowler's position** is similar to the Fowler's position, but the patient's head is less elevated. The **lateral position** features a patient lying on her side.

The **Trendelenburg position** involves having the patient lie flat on his back with the head of the table lowered at a 45° angle (head is down). The legs may be bent or extended. The **Sims' position** has the patient on his left side, with the right leg drawn up high and forward, the left arm along the patient's back, and the chest forward resting on the bed. The **lithotomy position** has the patient lying on her back with her feet in stirrups and knees flexed and separated. The **knee-chest position** requires that a patient rest her body weight on her knees and chest. The **dorsal recumbent position** has the patient lying on her back with her knees flexed and separated.

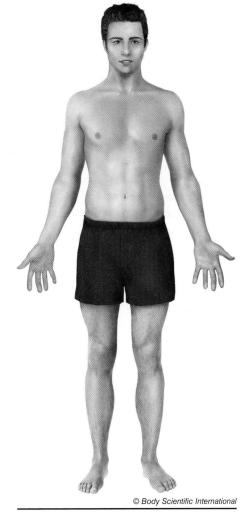

© Body Scientific International

Figure 5.8 Anatomical position is often used as the reference point when describing body movements.

anatomical position
a standing position in which the feet are parallel and the arms and hands are at the sides, palms facing out

prone position
a position in which a patient lies facedown

supine position
a position in which a patient lies faceup

Fowler's position
a position in which a patient lies in bed with the head of the bed elevated 45°

semi-Fowler's position
a position in which a patient lies in bed with the head of the bed elevated at 30°

lateral position
a position in which a patient lies on his or her side

Trendelenburg position
a position in which a patient lies flat on his or her back with the head of the table lowered at a 45° angle

Sims' position
a position in which a patient lies on his or her left side, with the right leg drawn up high and forward, the left arm along the back, and the chest forward resting on the bed

lithotomy position
a position in which a patient lies on her back with the feet in stirrups and knees flexed and separated

knee-chest position
a position in which a patient rests his or her body weight on the knees and chest

dorsal recumbent position
a position in which a patient lies on her back with the knees flexed and separated

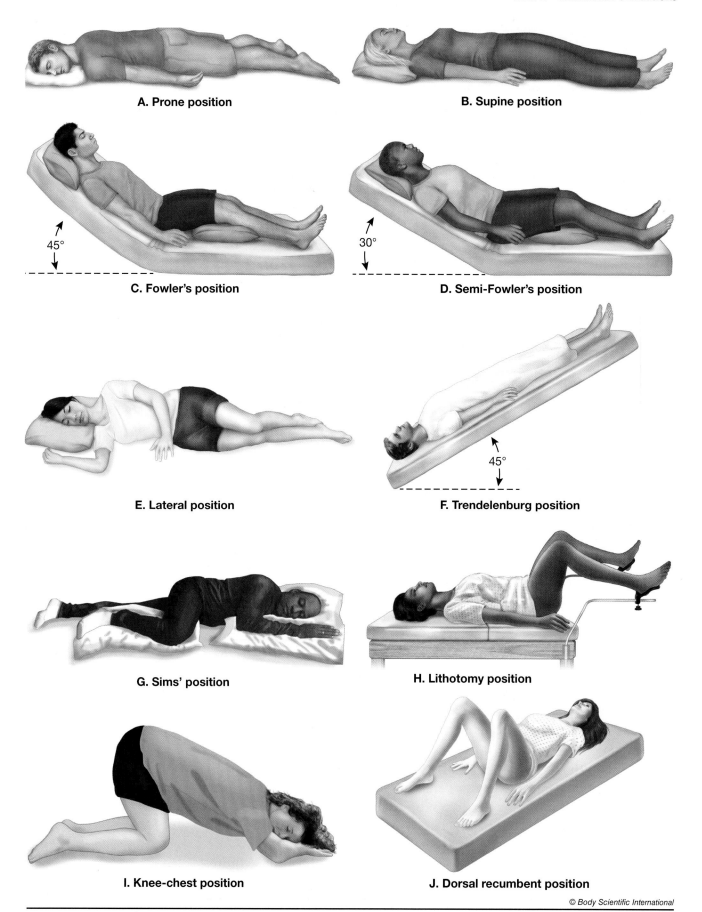

A. Prone position

B. Supine position

C. Fowler's position

45°

D. Semi-Fowler's position

30°

E. Lateral position

F. Trendelenburg position

45°

G. Sims' position

H. Lithotomy position

I. Knee-chest position

J. Dorsal recumbent position

© Body Scientific International

Figure 5.9   Patients are placed in various positions depending on the type of examination or treatment they are to receive.

Did You Know?   **Origins of the Trendelenburg Position**

The Trendelenburg position, named for Doctor Friedrich Trendelenburg, was originally developed for use in surgery. Today this position is used for certain kinds of medical procedures.

When patients are in this position, they lie faceup on a table or bed, and they are angled so that their feet are higher than their head. In the reverse Trendelenburg position, the patient's position is switched so that the head is higher than the feet. This position is often used for head and neck surgery to reduce the flow of blood.

In the past, the Trendelenburg position was used for people in shock and anaphylaxis, but this position is no longer routinely used because it increases the risk of the patient choking on fluids or vomit.

Directional Terms

When working in healthcare, you will often need to describe body directions. These directional terms are often used to describe movements, the relationship between body parts, or the location of a patient's symptom or problem. Directional terms are often used in doctor's orders, medical reports, insurance forms, and medical histories.

When studying the human body, you will often need to describe not only the location of a body part, but also the position of body parts in relation to other areas of the body (Figure 5.10). The front of the human body is called the anterior, or *ventral*, side. The back of the body is the posterior, or *dorsal*, side.

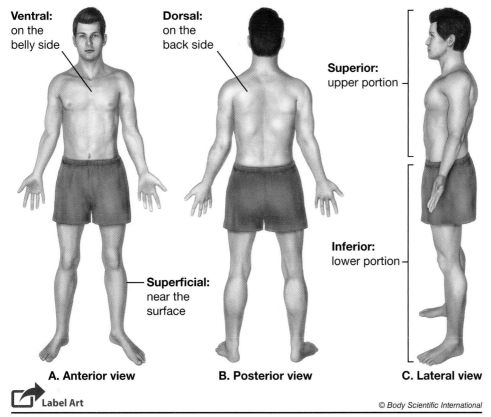

Ventral: on the belly side

Dorsal: on the back side

Superior: upper portion

Inferior: lower portion

Superficial: near the surface

A. Anterior view   **B. Posterior view**   **C. Lateral view**

Label Art   © Body Scientific International

Figure 5.10   Medical terminology used to describe location on the body is often used in health records such as a patient's medical history.

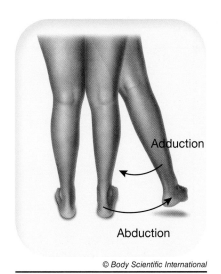

Figure 5.11   Directional terminology such as *adduction* and *abduction* describes the movement of the body.

Other commonly used directional terms include superior, inferior, distal, proximal, medial, and deep. Areas closer to the head are described as *superior*. The *inferior* portion of the body is closer to the feet. The terms *distal* and *proximal* are used to describe the position of the appendages in relation to their point of attachment on the trunk. *Distal* indicates the farthest area from the point of attachment, and *proximal* means closer to the point of attachment. For example, the wrist is distal to the elbow, and the fingers are distal to the wrist. The knee is proximal to the ankle, but the ankle is proximal to the toes. The term *medial* pertains to the middle or midline of the body. In this context, the term *deep* means farther away from the surface.

Directional terms are also used to describe the body's movement (Figure 5.11). For example, the term *abduction* means "movement of the limb away from the body." *Adduction* refers to "limb movement toward the body." *Flexion* (bending) decreases the joint angle, and *extension* (straightening) increases the angle.

Planes of the Body

body planes
imaginary planes, or flat surfaces, that divide the body into sections; include sagittal, coronal, and transverse planes

To document information about their patients, healthcare workers often refer to sections of the body in terms of anatomical planes. These **body planes** are imaginary lines drawn through the upright body (Figure 5.12).

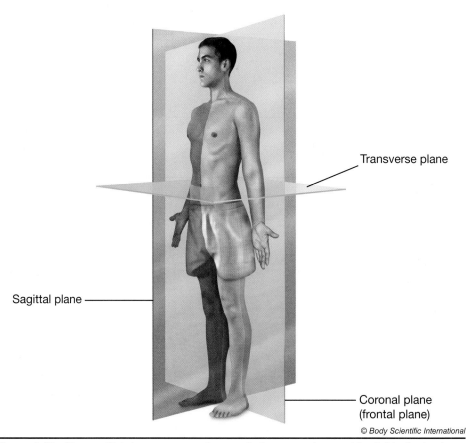

© Body Scientific International

Figure 5.12   The sagittal, transverse, and coronal planes can be used to divide the body and describe movements.

Three commonly identified planes of the body include the sagittal, coronal, and transverse planes. The sagittal plane, a vertical plane, divides the body into *inexact* left and right sides. The midsagittal plane, or *median plane*, divides the body *evenly* into left and right sides. The coronal plane, also known as the *frontal plane*, also divides the body vertically, but into front and back halves. Finally, the transverse plane, known also as the *horizontal plane*, separates the body into upper and lower parts. Planes of the body are often referred to in medical histories, doctors' reports, and insurance forms as part of a detailed description of a patient's condition.

Abdominal Quadrants

The abdominal cavity is large, so it is divided into **abdominal quadrants**. Figure 5.13A illustrates the four quadrants: the right upper quadrant (RUQ), left upper quadrant (LUQ), right lower quadrant (RLQ), and left lower quadrant (LLQ).

abdominal quadrants
the four divisions of the large abdominal area

Each quadrant contains certain vital organs. The right upper quadrant includes the liver and gallbladder. The right lower quadrant contains the appendix. The left upper quadrant contains the stomach, pancreas, and spleen. The right lower quadrant is the location of the descending and sigmoid colon, with the small intestines spread across the right and left lower quadrants.

Healthcare providers will ask a patient where his or her pain is located. Using their knowledge of the abdominal quadrants, they will determine in which quadrant the pain is located. This allows them to understand which organ may be causing the problem. For example, the appendix is located in the right lower quadrant, and pain in that quadrant is often caused by appendicitis.

Another method is to divide the abdomen into nine regions, narrowing the focus even more (Figure 5.13B).

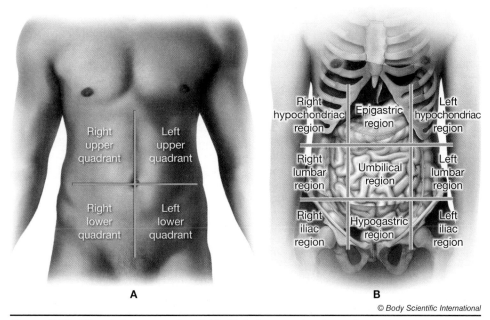

© Body Scientific International

Figure 5.13   The abdomen can be divided into four quadrants or nine regions.

Medical Terminology Reference Tables

Table A Common Word Roots (shown as combining forms)		
Word Root **(shown as combining forms)**	**Meaning**	**Example**
acr/o	extremities	acromegaly (AK-roh-MEG-a-lee)
aden/o	gland	adenopathy (AD-ee-NAHP-a-thee)
albin/o, alb/o	white	albinism (AL-bigh-nizm)
angi/o	vessel	angioma (an-jee-OH-ma)
arteri/o	artery	arteriogram (ar-TER-ee-oh-gram)
arthr/o	joint	arthritis (ar-THRIGH-tis)
audi/o	hearing	audiology (AW-dee-AHL-oh-jee)
aur/o	ear	auriform (AW-ri-form)
bi/o	life	biology (bigh-AHL-oh-jee)
blephar/o	eyelid	blepharitis (BLEF-a-RIGH-tis)
brachi/o	arm	antibrachial (AN-tee-BRAY-kee-al)
bronchi/o	bronchial tube	bronchial pneumonia (BRAHNG-kee-al noo-MOH-nee-a)
bucc/o	cheek	buccal cavity (BOOK-al)
carcin/o	cancer	carcinogen (kar-SIN-oh-jen)
cardi/o	heart	cardiologist (KAR-dee-AHL-oh-jist)
cephal/o	head	cephalogram (SEF-a-loh-gram)
cerebr/o	brain	cerebrospinal fluid (SER-ee-broh-SPIGH-nal)
cervic/o	neck	cervical collar (SER-vi-kal)
chol/e	bile	cholecystic (KOH-leh-SIS-tik)
cholecyst/o	gallbladder	cholecystectomy (KOH-leh-sis-TEK-toh-mee)
chondr/o	cartilage	chondrotomy (kahn-DRAHT-oh-mee)
chrom/o	color	chromatosis (KROH-ma-TOH-sis)
col/o, colon/o	colon	colonoscopy (KOH-lahn-AHS-koh-pee)
cost/o	ribs	costectomy (kahs-TEK-toh-mee)
crani/o	skull	craniotomy (KRAY-nee-AHT-oh-mee)
cutane/o	skin	cutaneous (kyoo-TAY-nee-uhs)
cyan/o	blue	cyanotic (SIGH-a-NAHT-ik)

Table A Common Word Roots (shown as combining forms)		
Word Root *(shown as combining forms)*	**Meaning**	**Example**
cyst/o	bladder	cystogram (SIS-toh-gram)
cyt/o	cell	cytoplasm (SIGH-toh-plazm)
dacry/o	tear	dacryocyst (DAK-ree-oh-SIST)
dactyl/o	fingers; toes	dactylitis (DAK-ti-LIGH-tis)
dent/i	tooth	dentistry (DEN-tis-tree)
derm/o, dermat/o	skin	dermatology (DER-ma-TAHL-oh-jee)
enter/o	intestine	enteritis (EN-ter-IGH-tis)
erythr/o	red	erythrocyte (e-RITH-roh-sight)
esophag/o	esophagus	esophagectomy (eh-SAHF-a-JEK-toh-mee)
fasci/o	band; fibrous	fasciitis (fa-SIGH-tis)
gastr/o	stomach	gastrocele (GAS-troh-sel)
gingiv/o	gum	gingivitis (JIN-ji-VIGH-tis)
gloss/o	tongue	glossospasm (GLAHS-oh-spazm)
gluc/o, glyc/o	sugar; sweet	glycogen (GLIGH-koh-jehn)
gynec/o, gyn/o	woman	gynecology (GIGH-neh-KAHL-oh-jee)
hem/o, hemat/o	blood	hematology (HEE-ma-TAHL-oh-jee)
hepat/o	liver	hepatitis (HEP-a-TIGH-tis)
hist/o	tissue	histology (his-TAHL-oh-jee)
home/o	same; similar	homeostasis (HOH-mee-oh-STAY-sis)
hydr/o	water	hydrophobia (HIGH-droh-FOH-bee-a)
hyster/o	uterus	hysterectomy (HIS-ter-EK-toh-mee)
icter/o	jaundice	icteric (ik-TER-ik)
idi/o	unknown; individual; distinct	idiopathic (ID-ee-oh-PATH-ik)
ile/o	ileum (part of the small intestine)	ileitis (IL-ee-IGH-tis)
kerat/o	cornea; scaly	keratotomy (KER-a-TAHT-oh-mee)
lact/o	milk	lactation (lak-TAY-shuhn)
lapar/o	abdomen	laparotomy (LAP-a-RAHT-oh-mee)

Table A Common Word Roots (shown as combining forms)		
Word Root (shown as combining forms)	Meaning	Example
leuk/o	white	leukemia (loo-KEE-mee-a)
lingu/o	tongue	lingual (LING-gwal)
lip/o	fat	liposuction (LIP-oh-SUHK-shuhn)
lith/o	stone	lithology (li-THAHL-oh-jee)
mast/o	breast	mastitis (mas-TIGH-tis)
melan/o	black	melanoma (MEL-a-NOH-ma)
mening/o, meningi/o	membrane covering the brain or spinal cord	meningitis (MEN-in-JIGH-tis)
mon/o	one; single	monocyte (MAHN-oh-sight)
myc/o	fungus	mycology (migh-KAHL-oh-jee)
myel/o	spinal cord; bone marrow	myelogram (MIGH-eh-loh-gram)
my/o	muscle	myopathy (migh-AHP-a-thee)
narc/o	stupor; sleep	narcotic (nar-KAHT-ik)
nas/o	nose	nasopharynx (NAY-zoh-FAIR-ingks)
necr/o	death	necropsy (NEK-rahp-see)
nephr/o	kidney	nephritis (ne-FRIGH-tis)
neur/o	nerve	neuritis (noo-RIGH-tis)
ocul/o	eye	oculist (AHK-yoo-list)
onc/o	tumor	oncology (ahng-KAHL-oh-jee)
oophor/o	ovary	oophorectomy (OH-ahf-oh-REK-toh-mee)
ophthalm/o	eye	ophthalmologist (AHF-thal-MAHL-ah-jist)
orch/o, orchi/o	testicle	orchiopexy (OR-kee-oh-PEK-see)
orth/o	straight	orthopedics (OR-thoh-PEE-diks)
oste/o	bone	osteoma (AHS-tee-OH-ma)
ot/o	ear	otology (oh-TAHL-ah-jee)
path/o	disease	pathologist (pa-THAHL-ah-jist)

Table A Common Word Roots (shown as combining forms)		
Word Root *(shown as combining forms)*	**Meaning**	**Example**
ped/o (Latin)	foot	pedograph (PED-oh-graf)
ped/o (Greek)	child	pediatrician (PEE-dee-a-TRISH-an)
pharyng/o	throat	pharyngoplasty (fa-RING-goh-PLAS-tee)
phleb/o	vein	phlebotomist (fle-BAHT-oh-mist)
phot/o	light	photolysis (foh-TAHL-i-sis)
pleur/o	pleura (a membrane that encompasses the lungs)	pleurisy (PLOOR-i-see)
pneum/o, pneumon/o	air; lungs	pneumonia (noo-MOH-nee-a)
proct/o	rectum	proctoscope (PRAHK-toh-scohp)
psych/o	mind	psychologist (sigh-KAHL-ah-jist)
pulmon/o	lung	pulmonitis (POOL-moh-NIGH-tis)
pyel/o	renal pelvis	pyelonephritis (PIGH-eh-loh-neh-FRIGH-tis)
py/o	pus	pyogenic (PIGH-oh-JEN-ik)
rhin/o	nose	rhinopathy (righ-NAHP-a-thee)
salping/o	tube	salpingolysis (sal-ping-GAHL-i-sis)
scler/o	hardening	scleroderma (SKLEH-roh-DER-ma)
semin/i	seed	seminal (SEM-i-nal)
seps/o	poison; infection	sepsis (SEP-sis)
somat/o	body	somatogenic (SOH-mat-oh-JEN-ik)
splen/o	spleen	splenomegaly (SPLEE-noh-MEG-a-lee)
thorac/o	chest	thoracotomy (THOH-ra-KAHT-ah-mee)
thromb/o	clot	thrombosis (thrahm-BOH-sis)
trache/o	trachea	tracheostomy (TRAY-kee-AHS-tah-mee)
ur/o, ur/i	urine	urology (yoo-RAHL-ah-jee)
vas/o, vascul/o	vessel	vasoconstriction (VA-soh-kahn-STRIK-shuhn)

Table B Prefixes for Medical Terms		
Prefix	**Meaning**	**Example**
a-, an-	without; lack of; absent	asepsis (a-SEP-sis)
ab-	from; away	abduction (ab-DUK-shuhn)
ad-	near; toward	adrenal (a-DREE-nal)
ante-	before; forward	antenatal (AN-tee-NAY-tal)
anti-	against	antiseptic (AN-ti-SEP-tik)
auto-, aut-	self	autoimmune (AW-toh-i-MYOON)
bi-	two; twice	bicellular (bigh-SEL-yoo-lar)
brady-	slow	bradycardia (BRAD-ee-KAR-dee-a)
contra-	against; opposite	contraception (KAHN-tra-SEP-shuhn)
de-	lack of; down; away from	dehydration (DEE-high-DRAY-shuhn)
di-	two	dimorphic (digh-MOR-fik)
dia-	through; between; complete	diarrhea (DIGH-a-REE-a)
dys-	painful; difficult	dysmenorrheal (DIS-men-oh-REE-al)
ecto-	outside	ectomorph (EK-toh-morf)
endo-	within; inner	endometrium (EN-doh-MEE-tree-uhm)
en-	in; inside	endemic (en-DEM-ik)
epi-	upper; above	epiglottis (EP-i-GLAHT-is)
eu-	good; normal	euphoric (yoo-FOR-ik)
ex-, extra-	out; away from	extrahepatic (EKS-tra-heh-PAT-ik)
hemi-	half	hemiplegia (HEM-ee-PLEE-jee-a)
hyper-	over; above; increased	hyperactive (high-peh-RAK-tiv)
hypo-	under; beneath; decreased	hypotension (HIGH-poh-TEN-shuhn)
inter-	between	intercostal (IN-ter-KAHS-tal)

	Table B Prefixes for Medical Terms	
Prefix	**Meaning**	**Example**
intra-	within; into	intramuscular (IN-tra-MUHS-kyoo-lar)
macro-	large	macrocyte (MAK-roh-sight)
mal-	bad; poor	malabsorption (MAL-ab-SORP-shuhn)
mega-	large	megacephaly (MEG-a-SEF-a-lee)
meta-	change; beyond	metachromatic (MET-a-kroh-MAT-ik)
micro-	small	microscope (MIGH-kroh-skohp)
multi-	many	multi-infarct (in-FARKT)
neo-	new	neoplasm (NEE-oh-plazm)
pan-	all	pangenesis (pan-JEN-e-sis)
para-	alongside; abnormal	paraplegia (PAIR-a-PLEE-jee-a)
peri-	surrounding	pericarditis (PER-i-kar-DIGH-tis)
poly-	much; many	polycystic (PAHL-ee-SIS-tik)
post-	behind; after	postpartum (pohst-PAR-tuhm)
pre-	before; in front of	premenstrual (pree-MEN-stroo-al)
pseudo-	false	pseudotumor (SOO-doh-TOO-mer)
retro-	behind; backward	retrosternal (RET-roh-STER-nal)
semi-	half	semicircular (SEM-ee-SIR-kyoo-lar)
sub-	under; below	subacute (SUB-a-KYOOT)
supra-	upper; above	supraventricular (SOO-pra-ven-TRIK-yoo-lar)
tachy-	rapid	tachycardia (TAK-i-KAR-dee-a)
trans-	across; through	transfusion (trans-FYOO-zhuhn)
ultra-	beyond; excess	ultramicroscopic (UL-tra-migh-kroh-SKAHP-ik)
uni-	one	unicellular (YOO-ni-SEL-yoo-lar)

Table C Suffixes for Medical Terms		
Suffix	**Meaning**	**Example**
-algia	pain	neuralgia (noo-RAL-jee-a)
-cele	hernia	cystocele (SIS-toh-sel)
-cide	kill	germicide (JER-mi-sighd)
-crine	to secrete; separate	endocrine (EN-doh-krin)
-ectomy	removal; excision	hysterectomy (HIS-ter-EK-toh-mee)
-emia	blood condition	leukemia (loo-KEE-mee-a)
-esthesia	nervous sensation	anesthesia (AN-es-THEE-zee-a)
-form	resembling; in the shape of	auriform (AW-ri-form)
-gene, -genic	production; origin	neurogenic (NOO-roh-JEN-ik)
-gram	record	myelogram (MIGH-eh-loh-gram)
-graph	instrument for recording	cardiograph (KAR-dee-oh-graf)
-iasis	abnormal condition	cholelithiasis (KOH-lee-li-THIGH-a-sis)
-ism	process; condition	hyperthyroidism (high-per-THIGH-royd-izm)
-itis	inflammation	appendicitis (a-PEN-di-SIGH-tis)
-lepsy	seizure	epilepsy (EP-i-LEP-see)
-logy	study of	biology (bigh-AHL-oh-jee)
-lysis	breakdown; destruction	hemolysis (hee-MAHL-i-sis)
-mania	obsessive preoccupation	monomania (MAHN-oh-MAY-nee-a)
-megaly	enlargement	splenomegaly (SPLEE-noh-MEG-a-lee)
-meter	measure	thermometer (ther-MAHM-eh-ter)
-oma	tumor	lipoma (li-POH-ma)
-opia	vision condition	amblyopia (AM-blee-OH-pee-a)

Table C   Suffixes for Medical Terms

Suffix	Meaning	Example
-opsy	view of	autopsy (AW-tahp-see)
-orexia	appetite	anorexia (AN-oh-REK-see-a)
-osis	condition; usually abnormal	neurosis (noo-ROH-sis)
-pathy	disease	arthropathy (ar-THRAHP-a-thee)
-penia	too few	leukopenia (LOO-koh-PEE-nee-a)
-phobia	fear	photophobia (FOH-toh-FOH-bee-a)
-plasm	formation	ectoplasm (EK-toh-plazm)
-plasty	operative revision	rhinoplasty (RIGH-noh-PLAS-tee)
-plegia	paralysis	hemiplegia (HEM-ee-PLEE-jee-a)
-rrhage	bursting forth	hemorrhage (HEM-or-ij)
-rrhea	hemorrhage; flow	diarrhea (DIGH-a-REE-a)
-sclerosis	hardening	arteriosclerosis (ar-TER-ee-oh-skler-OH-sis)
-scope	instrument to examine	microscope (MIGH-kroh-skohp)
-scopy	visual examination	microscopy (migh-KRAHS-koh-pee)
-somes	bodies	chromosomes (KROH-moh-sohms)
-spasm	contraction	cardiospasm (KAR-dee-oh-spazm)
-stasis	stoppage	hemostasis (HEE-moh-STAY-sis)
-stomy	new opening	colostomy (koh-LAHS-toh-mee)
-tomy	process of cutting	lobotomy (loh-BAHT-oh-mee)
-type	picture; classification	genotype (JEN-oh-tighp)
-uria	urination; condition of urine	hematuria (HEE-ma-TYOO-ree-a)
-y	process; condition	gastroenterology (GAS-troh-EN-ter-AHL-ah-jee)

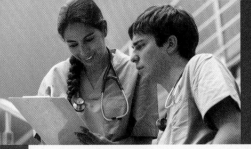

Chapter 5
Review and Assessment

Summary

The healthcare world uses its own language. Familiarizing yourself with medical prefixes, suffixes, word roots, the combining vowels, and the combining forms will help you succeed as a healthcare worker. Proper pronunciation and spelling of medical terms is very important. Using common medical abbreviations is vital to understanding medical terminology. The Joint Commission recommends avoiding the use of certain abbreviations that may be misinterpreted in documentation.

In addition to learning the basic word elements, healthcare providers are often expected to learn terms related to body cavities, positions, directions, and planes as well as abdominal quadrants. Such terms must be used properly to explain the exact location of a symptom or describe a patient's anatomy. Insurance forms require precise language about the patient's medical status.

Mastery of medical terminology takes study, repetition, and drills. Although proper medical terminology must be used when working with other healthcare providers and filling out paperwork, remember that patients are probably not familiar with this language. Do not use medical language when explaining something to a patient. Instead, explain things using terms he or she can understand.

Review Questions

Answer the following questions using what you have learned in this chapter.

True or False Assess

1. *True or False?* Patients will be very impressed with your use of medical terms.
2. *True or False?* The anatomical position is a sitting position.
3. *True or False?* Adduction refers to "limb movement away from the body."
4. *True or False?* The correct abbreviation for calcium is "cm."
5. *True or False?* NPO means "nothing by mouth."
6. *True or False?* The plural form of *thorax* is *thoraces*.

7. *True or False?* The transverse plane divides the body into right and left sides.
8. *True or False?* A combining vowel makes a word easier to spell.
9. *True or False?* Arteriosclerosis means "hardened artery walls."
10. *True or False?* Many medical terms come from Greek and Latin.

Multiple Choice Assess

11. Which of the following accurately describes Sims' position?
    A. the patient on his or her left side, right leg drawn up high and forward
    B. the patient standing with hands over the head
    C. the patient lying on the stomach with the head of the bed lowered 45°
    D. the same as the anatomical position

12. If a body part is closer to the feet than to the head, it is referred to as _____.
    A. distal
    B. proximal
    C. inferior
    D. superior

13. The word elements used in medical terminology include prefixes, suffixes, _____.
    A. combining vowels, combining forms, and vocabulary terms
    B. word roots, combining vowels, and combining consonants
    C. word roots, combining vowels, and combining forms
    D. combining vowels, word roots, and plural forms

14. The suffix _____ means "inflammation."
    A. *-osis*
    B. *-cide*
    C. *-rrhea*
    D. *-itis*

15. When in Fowler's position, the patient is _____.
    A. lying on his or her back, with the head of the bed raised about 45°, and knees elevated
    B. standing erect and facing forward with arms at the sides and palms facing forward
    C. lying faceup
    D. lying on his or her side

16. Which of the following terms means "toward the front"?
    A. posterior
    B. superior
    C. dorsal
    D. anterior

17. The prefix _____ means "bad" or "poor."
    A. *tachy-*
    B. *pseudo-*
    C. *ecto-*
    D. *mal-*

18. Inferior means _____.
    A. "closer to the feet"
    B. "on the belly side"
    C. "close to the head"
    D. "limb movement toward the body"

19. The suffix *-osis* means _____.
    A. "origin"
    B. "formation"
    C. "view of"
    D. "abnormal condition"

20. How many quadrants and regions can the abdominal cavity be divided into?
    A. 6 and 12
    B. 2 and 4
    C. 4 and 9
    D. 4 and 8

21. _____ position is considered the starting point when describing movement and directional terms.
    A. Supine
    B. Prone
    C. Lithotomy
    D. Anatomical

Medical Terms and Abbreviations

Identify the equivalent medical term or abbreviation for each English term or phrase provided.

22. removal of a breast
23. inflammation of the liver
24. red blood cell
25. white blood cell
26. abbreviation for heart attack
27. removal of a gallbladder

Identify the meaning of the following abbreviations.

28. CA
29. Ca
30. CCU
31. FBS
32. OB/GYN
33. CPR

Short Answer

34. Identify the word elements used in medical terminology.
35. Explain the purpose and use of prefixes and suffixes in medical terminology.
36. Why might a combining vowel be dropped when forming a medical term?
37. Why is it critical that all medical terms are spelled correctly in a patient's medical history?
38. Describe anatomical position.
39. What is an acronym?
40. Describe the sagittal, transverse, and coronal planes of the body.
41. What is the "Do Not Use List" created by the Joint Commission?
42. What does the medical abbreviation *CPR* mean?
43. Where is the cranial cavity?

Critical Thinking Exercises

44. Working with a partner, role play a discussion between two healthcare workers. Incorporate medical terms you learned in this chapter into the discussion. Evaluate your ability to communicate using medical terminology.
45. How might the use of abbreviations lead to errors in a healthcare facility?

Chapter 6
Anatomy and Physiology

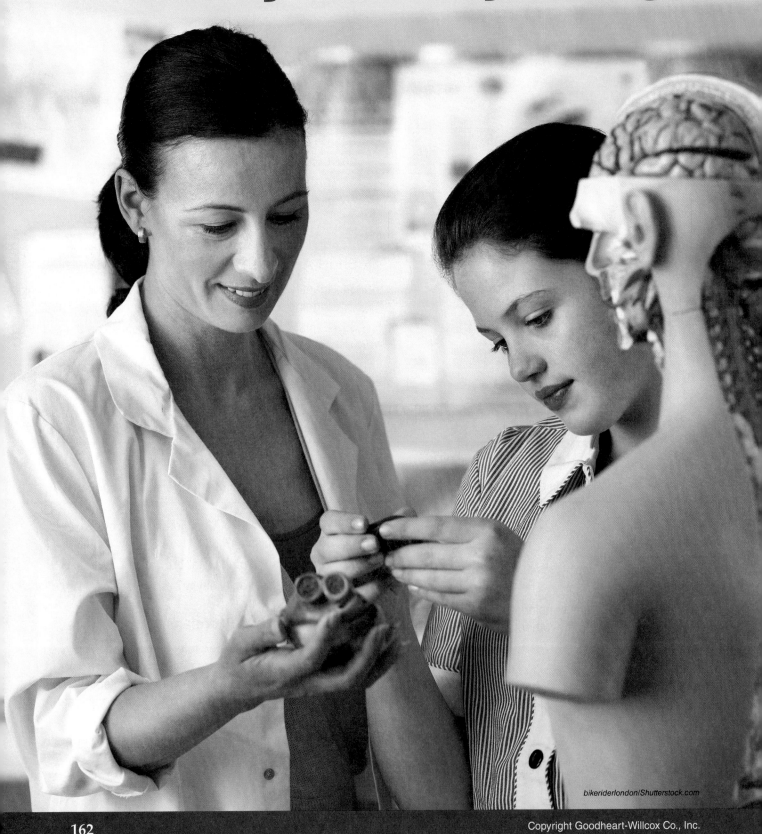

bikeriderlondon/Shutterstock.com

Terms to Know Build Vocab

anatomy
antibody
antigen
bone marrow
cell membrane
central nervous system (CNS)
chromosome
cytoplasm
deoxyribonucleic acid (DNA)
differentiation
endocrine glands
exocrine glands
formed elements

homeostasis
hormones
human reproduction
immunity
joint
ligaments
lymph
lymphocyte
menstrual cycle
metabolism
nucleus
organs
peripheral nervous system (PNS)

pH scale
phagocytosis
physiology
plasma
platelets
puberty
red blood cells
respiration
sexually transmitted infection (STI)
stem cells
tendons
tissues
white blood cells

Chapter Objectives

- Define *anatomy* and *physiology*.
- Identify the six most prominent chemicals in the human body.
- Describe basic parts of the human cell.
- Discuss the importance of the discovery of DNA.
- Identify the importance of homeostasis in the human body.
- Explain the differences between cells, tissues, organs, and body systems.
- Identify the body systems discussed in this chapter, including their main organs and associated diseases.

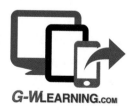

While studying, look for the activity icon to:

- **Build** vocabulary with e-flash cards and interactive games.
- **Assess** progress with chapter and unit review questions.
- **Expand** learning with animations and illustration labeling activities.
- **Simulate** EHR entry with healthcare documents.

G-WLEARNING.com

www.g-wlearning.com/healthsciences/

anatomy
the study of the structure of the body

physiology
the study of the function of the body

Figure 6.1 illustrates components that make up the human body. Each component is critical to understanding how the body functions. **Anatomy** is the study of the structure of the body. **Physiology** involves the study of the function of the body.

Chemical Composition of the Human Body

The composition of the human body is made up of six elements that represent 99 percent of the body's chemicals. These include oxygen, carbon, hydrogen, nitrogen, calcium, and phosphorus. Another almost 1 percent includes five trace elements: potassium, sulfur, sodium, chlorine, and magnesium. All of these chemicals must be present to sustain life.

About 65 percent of the mass of the human body is composed of oxygen, with carbon at almost 19 percent, hydrogen at 10 percent, nitrogen at 3 percent, calcium at 1.5 percent, and phosphorus at about 1 percent.

Cells

The human body is built on a foundation composed of approximately five trillion microscopic cells. Cells vary according to their specific function.

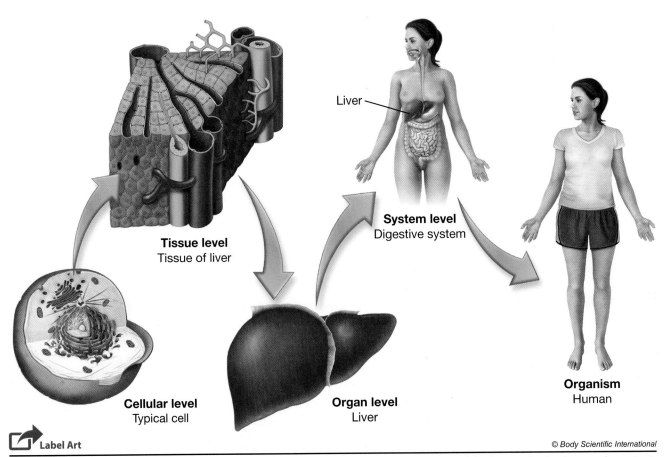

Tissue level
Tissue of liver

Liver

System level
Digestive system

Organism
Human

Cellular level
Typical cell

Organ level
Liver

Label Art

Figure 6.1   From the smallest cell to the most complex organ system, each component of the human body plays an important role in making the body function.

Bone, muscle, skin, and blood are made up of different types of cells, a phenomenon called **differentiation**. Cells can be flat, round, irregularly shaped, or threadlike. All cells can reproduce, use oxygen, utilize nutrients, produce energy, eliminate wastes, and maintain their shape.

As Figure 6.2 shows, the human cell has several components. With the exception of mature red blood cells, all human cells have a **nucleus**. The nucleus is the "brain" of the cell that directs all of its activities. Inside of the nucleus are 23 paired (46 total) **chromosomes** that contain genetic information, or *deoxyribonucleic acid* (DNA).

Every cell is held together by an outer layer called the **cell membrane**. The cell membrane is selectively permeable, meaning it controls what enters and exits the cell. Inside of every cell is the **cytoplasm**, a transparent, gel-like substance that is usually composed of 70–90 percent water and houses all of the organelles, the microscopic functional units of the cell. Structures such as the mitochondria and ribosomes are organelles; each performs a specific function in the cell.

differentiation
process through which cells of the body vary according to their specific function

nucleus
the "brain" of a cell; directs all activities and contains genetic information

chromosome
threadlike structure found in the nucleus of most living cells; carries genetic information

cell membrane
the outer layer of a cell that holds the cell together

cytoplasm
transparent, gel-like substance inside of every cell; cellular activities occur here

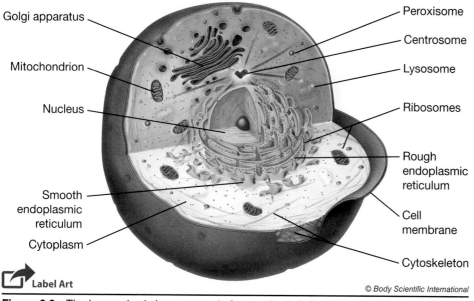

Golgi apparatus — Peroxisome
Mitochondrion — Centrosome
Nucleus — Lysosome
— Ribosomes
Smooth endoplasmic reticulum — Rough endoplasmic reticulum
Cytoplasm — Cell membrane
— Cytoskeleton

Label Art

© *Body Scientific International*

Figure 6.2 The human body is composed of approximately five trillion cells.

Extend Your Knowledge ▶ What's in a Cell?

Organelles are all of the structures within the cell's cytoplasm. Organelles help to carry out the life processes in the cell. With the exception of the cytoplasm and cytoskeleton, the labels in Figure 6.2 all show various organelles in the cell.

Apply It

1. Research the organelles shown in Figure 6.2.

2. Create a table that lists and describes the function of each organelle shown.

deoxyribonucleic acid (DNA)
genetic material shaped like a double helix; part of all living cells

Deoxyribonucleic Acid (DNA)

Deoxyribonucleic acid, or *DNA*, is found in every cell of the human body. DNA is shaped like a twisting ladder composed of chemical base pairs, called a *double helix* (Figure 6.3).

DNA resides on chromosomes in the nucleus of a cell, sections of which are called *genes*. The structure of DNA was not known until James Watson, an American scientist, and Francis Crick, a British researcher, discovered the famous double helix. This was a major scientific breakthrough.

In 2003, the Human Genome Project, an international research initiative, successfully mapped the DNA sequence of a human, known as the *human genome.* Mapping the human genome allows researchers to better understand the genetic factor of human disease. Researchers identified and mapped approximately 20,000 to 25,000 genes located on the DNA helix. This development may enable researchers to discover damaged genes causing genetic disorders and, hopefully, eliminate those disorders.

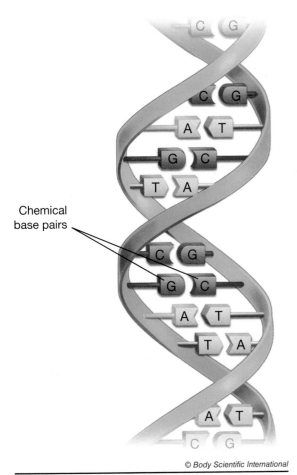

Chemical base pairs

© Body Scientific International

Figure 6.3 DNA is described as the *molecule of life.*

Stem Cells

All cells in the body begin as undifferentiated **stem cells**. Stem cells mature into differentiated cells, meaning that they evolve to function in a particular organ system. For example, white blood cells develop to fight infection, while mature red blood cells carry oxygen and carbon dioxide through the body.

After an embryo develops, adult stem cells can be found throughout the human body. Stem cells have been found in tissues such as the brain, bone marrow, blood, blood vessels, and the skin.

stem cells
cells in the body that evolve into specific cells in a particular organ system

tissues
groups of cells that work together to accomplish a task

Tissue

Just as there are many different kinds of cells in the human body, there is also an assortment of **tissues** of various shapes and sizes. Body tissues are groups of cells that work together to accomplish the same task. There are four types of tissues:

- connective tissue
- epithelial tissue
- muscle tissue
- nervous tissue

Connective Tissue

Connective tissue helps hold body parts together. The most common of all body tissues, connective tissue, is found in bones, organs, muscles, nerves, and skin. Connective tissue holds body parts together by forming fine webs of tissue that provide support and structure.

Connective tissue is composed of collagen fibers and elastic fibers. Collagen fibers are densely packed and arranged in a parallel construction to provide tissue strength. Elastic fibers enable connective tissue to stretch.

Cartilage

One example of connective tissue is cartilage. Cartilage is a flexible connective tissue found in the rib cage, the ear, the nose, the bronchial tubes, and the joints between bones. Cartilage is not as hard and rigid as bone, but it is stiffer and less flexible than muscle.

Epithelial Tissue

Epithelial tissue covers the external and internal body surfaces. The skin consists of epithelial tissue. The linings of internal organs are made of this tissue as well.

Muscle Tissue

Muscle tissue allows the body to move. The three kinds of muscle tissue are skeletal, cardiac, and smooth muscle. Skeletal muscle is attached to bones and facilitates movement by contracting and relaxing. The walls of the heart are composed of cardiac muscle, while the walls of other organs are composed of smooth muscle.

Nervous Tissue

Nervous tissue reaches all parts of the body but is concentrated in the spinal cord and brain. Nervous tissue sends electrical signals or messages throughout the body. Neurons—cells found in nervous tissue—are responsible for generating, sending, and receiving these electrical signals to all parts of the body.

Check Your Understanding ✓

1. What is the difference between *anatomy* and *physiology*?
2. With the exception of mature red blood cells, all cells in the body have a(n) _____.
3. What are the four types of tissues found in the body?
4. Which type of tissue allows the body to move?

Organs

organs
two or more groups of tissues working together to perform specific functions

As tissues are groups of similar cells, **organs** are two or more groups of tissues working together. For example, the stomach is made up of connective, epithelial, muscle, and nervous tissue. Every organ in the human body performs one or more specific functions. Although there is typically only one of each organ, some organs occur in pairs, such as the kidneys or the lungs.

Some organs are called *vital organs*. Vital organs are those without which the human body cannot survive. These organs include the brain, heart, liver, and lungs (you must have at least one functioning lung to live). Organs that you *can* live without are called *non-vital organs*. These include the appendix, gallbladder, and spleen.

The Body Systems

Human body functions are controlled by groups of organs known as *body systems*. A body system consists of organs that work together to accomplish a more complex task than a single organ can perform. For example, the urinary system removes wastes, controls the body's fluid balance, and ensures electrolyte balance in the blood. (Electrolytes are a mixture of sodium, potassium, chloride, and bicarbonate ions that affect metabolic processes of the body.) To accomplish these tasks, the kidneys eliminate wastes and substances that may upset fluid and electrolyte balance. Waste and other substances cannot be removed without the cooperation of the kidneys, bladder, urethra, and ureters.

If one organ is not functioning properly, the entire system, or even the body as a whole, will be affected. An example of this is a poorly functioning heart. When the heart is not functioning properly, insufficient amounts of blood are pumped to the lungs to gather oxygen. This means that the rest of the body does not get proper amounts of oxygen. In this case, the failure of one organ may cause oxygen deprivation throughout the entire body.

Real Life Scenario | Finding an Organ Donor

Kim's kidneys have failed, and her doctor has put her on hemodialysis, a treatment that simulates the work of the kidneys by mechanically filtering waste from the blood. Kim needs a kidney transplant, and both her sister and brother are willing to donate one of their kidneys to Kim. To do so, they must go through a procedure known as *tissue typing* to determine if their tissues are compatible with Kim's, a quality called *histocompatibility*.

Tissue typing examines the antigens found on the surface of cells located in kidney tissue. Antigens are molecules found on cells that react to foreign molecules, triggering a response that can lead to organ rejection.

A donor's antigens must match the recipient's antigens for an organ transplant to be successful.

To test for histocompatibility, blood is drawn and tests are performed on the blood cells to determine compatibility. In Kim's case, her sister was a compatible donor, and Kim received a healthy kidney.

Apply It

1. The only transplant that does not require tissue typing is a corneal transplant. Research corneal transplants and explain why a person receiving a transplanted cornea need not undergo tissue typing.

> ### Did You Know? | Living with One Kidney or Lung
>
> Did you know that you can live successfully with only one lung or one kidney? For example, some people are only born with a single kidney (in this case, the left kidney is often missing). When one organ of the pair is missing, the remaining kidney or lung increases in size and compensates for the loss of the other organ.

Homeostasis

Homeostasis is a self-regulating process by which all biological functions in the body work together to maintain the stability of the organism. Examples of homeostatic processes include controlling body temperature, blood sugar, water balance, and blood pressure and balancing electrolytes. Electrolytes affect the amount of water in the body, the pH of blood (the relative acidity or alkalinity of the blood), muscle function, and other processes. The body systems that are the most involved in maintaining homeostasis are the nervous and endocrine systems.

An example of homeostasis (a word that comes from a Greek phrase that means "staying the same") is the way in which the human body maintains control over body temperature. Normal body temperature stays around 37°C, or 98.6°F. The body is subjected to various factors—hormones, changing inside or outside temperatures, and disease—that can cause body temperature to fluctuate. Body temperature is regulated by a region in the brain called the *hypothalamus*. When body temperature rises significantly, the hypothalamus triggers signals to different organ systems resulting in perspiration, or sweat. As the sweat evaporates, it cools the body. Blood vessels that are close to the skin dilate to release heat.

If body temperature falls below normal ranges, the hypothalamus signals the muscles to begin shivering. Shivering produces heat, warming the body. The blood vessels close to the skin now constrict to reduce heat loss through the skin.

Other examples of homeostatic processes in the body include the kidney removing excess water, salt, and urea from the body. The pancreas secretes insulin if the body needs more glucose to maintain the body's cells. When insulin is deficient or the cells become resistant to it, diabetes occurs. Blood pH must be slightly alkaline to maintain health of the body.

homeostasis
state of internal balance achieved by adjusting the physiological systems of the body

Homeostatic Control Mechanisms

Homeostasis needs three components to succeed:

- **Receptor nerves** that monitor and respond to a change in the environment. The receptor then sends a message to the control center.

- The **control center** that analyzes the information and determines an appropriate response to what might be causing the imbalance in the organism. Then a signal is sent to the effector.

- An **effector**, which could be a muscle, organs, or other structure, that initiates changes to correct the deviation.

Animation   **Negative Feedback**

Most homeostatic mechanisms function by a principle known as *negative feedback*. Conditions that cause a challenge to homeostasis trigger a negative reaction in the opposite direction. An example would be a house's thermostat. The thermostat is set to make sure your house is neither too cold nor too hot. If the thermostat is set at 76°F in the summer, the thermostat will trigger the air conditioner to turn on when the temperature in the house goes over 76°F. When the house cools down, the thermostat will turn off the air conditioner.

Many diseases disturb homeostasis. Inefficiencies of this process lead to an unstable internal environment, increasing the risk of illness.

The Integumentary System

The integumentary system covers and protects the body. Functions of the integumentary system include

- regulation of body temperature;

- production of vitamin D from sunlight;

- excretion of minor amounts of waste materials in sweat; and

- transmission of sensory information for pain, touch, pressure, and temperature.

The integumentary system includes the skin, sebaceous glands, sweat glands, fingernails, and hair.

The Skin

The skin is the largest organ in the body. The average adult body has almost 21 square feet of skin. The skin has three layers of tissue (Figure 6.4):

1. **Epidermis.** The visible layer of skin, the epidermis, lacks blood vessels and nerve cells. Everyday activities such as bathing and moving around cause the body to shed about 500 million cells of the epidermis each day. These cells must continuously replace themselves.

2. **Dermis.** Located below the epidermis, the dermis is a layer of dense, irregular connective tissue. Capillaries, muscles, nerve endings, hair follicles, sweat glands, and sebaceous (oil) glands can all be found in the dermis. This layer helps your skin move with you. Age and frequent suntanning decrease the dermis' firmness.

3. **Subcutaneous.** This layer of skin (the epidermis and dermis are the cutaneous layers) is primarily composed of lipocytes (or *fat cells*), which manufacture and store large amounts of fat. This skin layer is important because it protects deeper tissues of the body, acts as a heat insulator, and stores energy.

Sebaceous Glands. Visible only by microscope, these small glands are responsible for depositing an oily secretion on the hairs that cover the skin. They are found in all parts of the skin covered by hair, with the exception of the soles of the feet and palms of the hands. The acidic nature of these glands helps destroy some pathogens on the skin's surface. The oily secretion of sebaceous glands also keeps the skin from drying out.

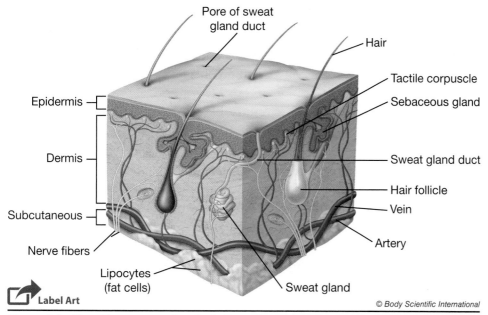

Figure 6.4   The skin covers and protects the entire body.

Sweat Glands. Sweat glands, also referred to as *sudoriferous glands*, play an important role in regulating body temperature. There are two types of sweat glands: *apocrine* and *eccrine*. Apocrine sweat glands secrete sweat at the hair follicles in the groin, anal region, and armpits. Eccrine sweat glands are located all over the skin, but are more prominent on the palms, feet, forehead, and upper lip.

Hair and Fingernails

In addition to contributing to our physical appearance, body hair also serves several important purposes. Body hair helps regulate body temperature, functioning as a sensor to detect skin changes. Hair in the nose helps to filter out dust and other small particles, while the eyelashes protect our eyes from foreign objects.

Both hair and fingernails are composed of the protein *keratin*. As specialized epithelial cells grow out and over the nail bed, they become keratin. The *cuticle* of the nail is a fold of tissue at the nail root. The nails' pinkish color comes from blood vessels beneath them, while the half-moon-shaped area is a result of a thicker layer of cells at the nail's base.

There are many diseases and disorders associated with the integumentary system. Some of these include eczema, dermatitis, psoriasis, and skin cancer. There are also various diseases associated with viruses that affect the integumentary system. These diseases are commonly known as *chicken pox, shingles, cold sores, genital herpes,* and *human papillomavirus (HPV)*.

The Musculoskeletal System

Together, the muscular and skeletal systems form the framework that holds the human body together. While these systems are sometimes considered separately, they are known collectively as the *musculoskeletal system*. The entire musculoskeletal system consists of bones, joints, and muscles.

Bones

The skeleton is composed mainly of bones, but also cartilage and joints. The skeletal system is divided into two sections: the axial and appendicular skeleton (Figure 6.5). The axial skeleton consists of the main trunk of the body, including the skull, spinal column, breastbone, and ribs. The appendicular skeleton includes the extremity bones— the shoulder girdle, arm bones, pelvic girdle, and leg bones.

The skeletal system performs critical functions for the human body. Bones provide an internal support system that enables humans to stand upright, with the ribs supporting the chest cavity. Bones also offer protection for delicate internal organs. For instance, ribs protect the heart and lungs, while the skull protects the brain. Movement is made possible when muscles, attached to bones, contract (shorten) and pull on bones. Bones also provide storage for minerals, such as calcium and phosphorus, and bone marrow. **Bone marrow**, a soft, flexible tissue found inside bones, is responsible for manufacturing blood cells.

bone marrow
soft, spongy, blood-forming tissue found inside bones

There are four types of bones in the human body:

- **Long bones.** These bones are longer than they are wide. Long bones are found in the arms and legs.

- **Short bones.** About the same size in length and width, short bones are mostly found in the ankles and wrists.

- **Flat bones.** These bones are thinner than both short and long bones. They can be flat or curved and are plate-like in appearance. Examples of flat bones include the skull, sternum (or *breastbone*), and ribs.

- **Irregular bones.** These are odd-shaped bones that do not fit into the other bone categories. These bones are needed to connect other bones. Examples of irregular bones are vertebrae (found in the spinal column) and coxal (hip) bones.

Long bones are covered with a tough, fibrous connective tissue called *periosteum*. Periosteum contains blood vessels to provide nutrients to the bone cells. Each bone has bulbous ends called *epiphyses*. The region between two bone ends is called the *diaphysis* or the *shaft*. The diaphysis is hollow and acts as a storage area for bone marrow. Bone marrow comes in two types— yellow and red. Yellow marrow stores fat, while red bone marrow is needed for the production of blood cells.

The human body continues to build new bone tissue throughout a person's life, but it also constantly tears down old bone. *Osteoblasts* are specialized cells that form bones. *Osteoclasts* tear down bone material and help move calcium and phosphate into the blood.

Did You Know?   How Many Bones Are in the Human Body?

The average adult human has 206 bones in her body. An infant can have between 300 and 350 bones at birth. Some of these bones fuse together as the infant grows. When some bones fuse and become one bone (such as the bones that comprise the skull), the total number of bones drops to 206.

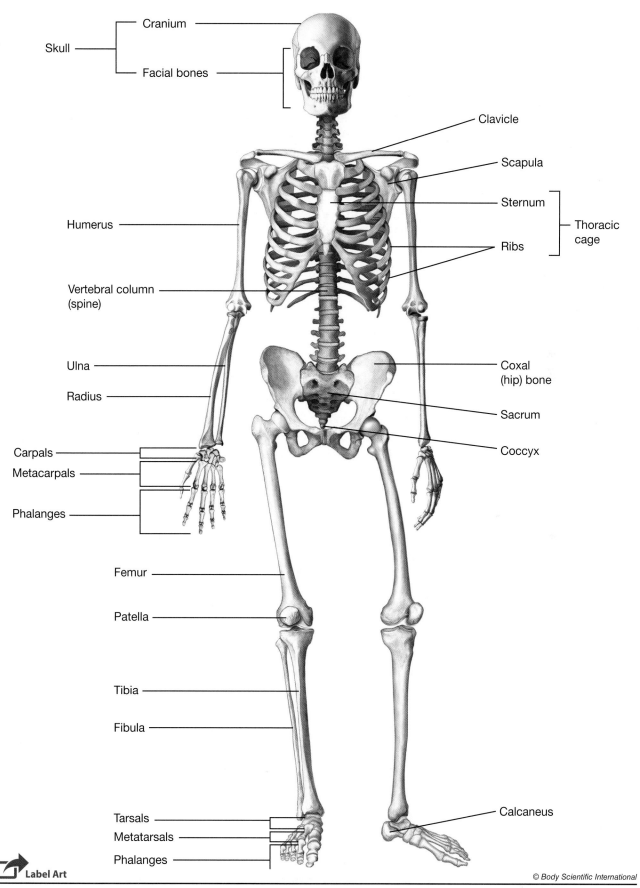

Skull
Cranium
Facial bones

Clavicle
Scapula
Sternum
Thoracic cage
Ribs

Humerus

Vertebral column (spine)

Ulna
Radius

Coxal (hip) bone
Sacrum
Coccyx

Carpals
Metacarpals
Phalanges

Femur
Patella

Tibia

Fibula

Tarsals
Metatarsals
Phalanges

Calcaneus

Label Art

© Body Scientific International

Figure 6.5   The human skeleton is composed of two parts—the appendicular skeleton (tan) and axial skeleton (pink). Bones of the axial skeleton provide support, while the appendicular bones provide movement of the appendages.

About 10 percent of the body's bone tissue is torn down and rebuilt each year. This process of breaking down and rebuilding bone (called *bone remodeling*) continues into a person's 40s with no net gain or loss of bone mass. In later life, bone loss can outweigh bone growth.

Exercise is one of the best ways to slow bone loss and prevent muscle, bone, or joint problems. A moderate exercise program can help the body maintain strength and flexibility and the bones stay strong. A well-balanced diet with adequate amounts of calcium is especially important. Women in particular must be careful to get enough calcium and vitamin D as they age to avoid osteoporosis, a disease characterized by softening of the bones.

Breaks in a bone are called *fractures*. Fractures are common injuries associated with the skeletal system. Four of the common classifications of fractures are greenstick, stress, comminuted, and spiral. Scoliosis, an abnormal lateral curvature of the spine, is another disorder associated with the bones.

 Animation

Joints

joint
physical point of connection between two bones; also known as an articulation

ligaments
tough bands of fibrous tissue that connect bone to bone

tendons
fibrous tissues that connect muscles to bone

Without **joints**, or *articulations*, the human body could not move. When two or more bones come together, a joint is formed. Joints are held together by connective tissue called **ligaments**. Ligaments are tough, white bands that connect bone to bone. **Tendons** attach muscles to bones.

There are several types of joints:

- **Amphiarthroses.** These joints move only slightly; for example, the joints between vertebrae in your spine are amphiarthroses joints.
- **Synarthroses.** Joints that do not move are synarthroses joints. The fibrous joints between the skull bones are an example of synarthroses.
- **Synovial joints.** These joints are covered with a membrane that contains a fluid lubricant, making movement easy. Hip and knee joints are synovial joints.

Joint pain or injury can be attributed to several diseases or disorders. Joint dislocation, arthritis, and bursitis are some conditions related to the joints.

 Animation

Muscles

There are more than 600 individual muscles in the human body. Figure 6.6 shows examples of these muscles. Muscles account for about 40 percent of the total body weight of an adult human. Muscles usually act in groups to help the body and its organs move. There are three types of muscle tissue in the human body:

1. Cardiac muscles cause contractions of the heart.
2. Smooth muscles facilitate movements that we do not control. These are *involuntary muscles* that create movement in the organs and systems of the body, such as the digestive system.
3. Skeletal muscles can move at our will and are also called *voluntary muscles*. These muscles attach to bones and are responsible for the movement of the skeletal system.

Figure 6.7 shows the microscopic anatomy of each of the three types of muscle tissue.

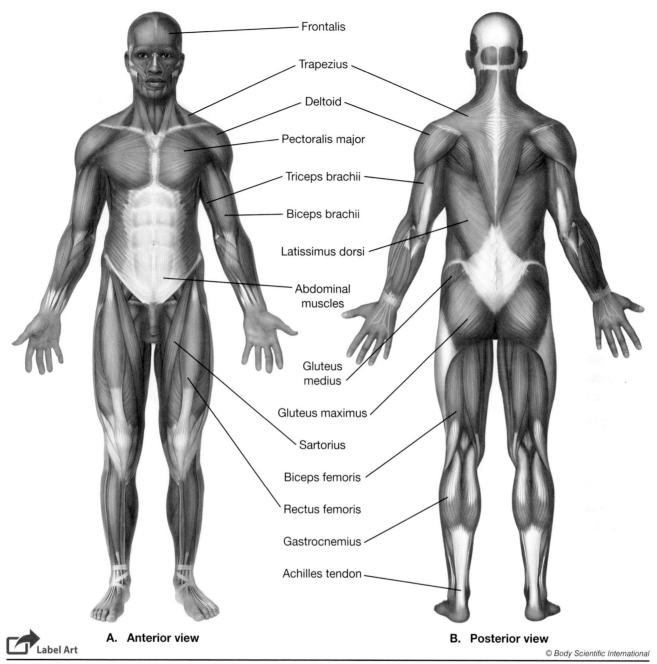

A. Anterior view

B. Posterior view

Label Art

© Body Scientific International

Figure 6.6 There are more than 600 individual muscles in the human body.

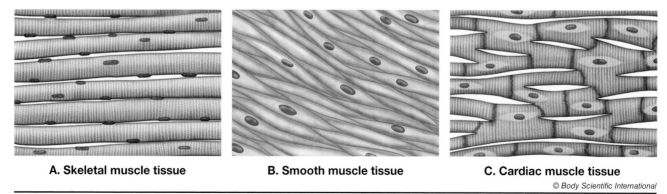

A. Skeletal muscle tissue

B. Smooth muscle tissue

C. Cardiac muscle tissue

© Body Scientific International

Figure 6.7 Microscopic anatomy of muscle tissue

Directional Terms Describing Movement. A variety of different actions or movements performed by muscles are illustrated in Figure 6.8. Many different directional terms must be understood to interpret muscle movement. These terms are often used in doctor's orders, medical reports, insurance forms, and medical histories.

Diseases and Disorders of the Muscular System. Common muscle-related diseases include fibromyalgia and muscular dystrophy. The muscles can also suffer from strain, contusion, cramps, delayed-onset muscle soreness (DOMS), tendinitis, and shin splints.

Check Your Understanding ✓

1. What is homeostasis?
2. Identify four functions of the integumentary system.
3. Identify the four types of bones found in the human body.
4. Explain the different functions of cardiac, smooth, and skeletal muscles.

The Nervous System

The nervous system directs the functions of all other body systems through nerve impulses generated by neurons, or *nerve cells*, located throughout the body. The nervous system is divided into two parts—the **central nervous system (CNS)** and the **peripheral nervous system (PNS)** (Figure 6.9 on page 178).

Dementia, Alzheimer's disease, epilepsy, multiple sclerosis, Parkinson's disease, cerebral palsy, cardiovascular accident (stroke), and meningitis are all diseases or disorders of the nervous system.

Neurons

The CNS and PNS work together to send messages that direct all of our body movements and functions to the brain. These messages are carried to the correct areas of the brain by neurons. All activity in the body is controlled by more than 100 billion neurons located throughout the body.

Neurons produce an electrical impulse that moves down the extension of the nerve cell, or the *axon*. Dendrites extend out from the neuron's cell body and stimulate the neuron by collecting and responding to different types of stimuli. The axon is surrounded by a protective myelin sheath, which affects the rate at which electrical transmissions travel through the neuron. There is a terminal bundle at the end of the axon that sends nerve impulses to neighboring neurons.

The Central Nervous System (CNS)

The central nervous system (CNS) is made up of the brain and the spinal cord. Three thin layers of tissue, called *meninges*, cover and protect the brain and spinal cord. The bones of the spinal column also protect the spinal cord.

central nervous system (CNS)

part of the nervous system that includes the brain and the spinal cord

peripheral nervous system (PNS)

collective term for nerves that lie outside the central nervous system; transmits information from the CNS to all parts of the body

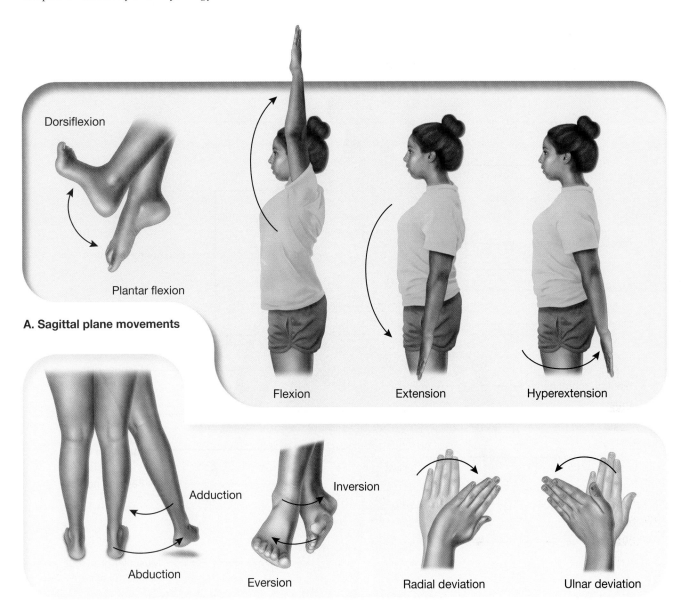

A. Sagittal plane movements

Dorsiflexion

Plantar flexion

Flexion

Extension

Hyperextension

Adduction

Abduction

Inversion

Eversion

Radial deviation

Ulnar deviation

B. Coronal plane movements

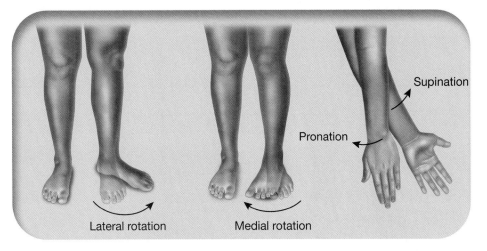

Lateral rotation

Medial rotation

Supination

Pronation

C. Transverse plane movements

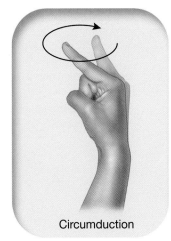

Circumduction

D. Multi-plane movement

© Body Scientific International

Figure 6.8   Directional movement vocabulary of muscles

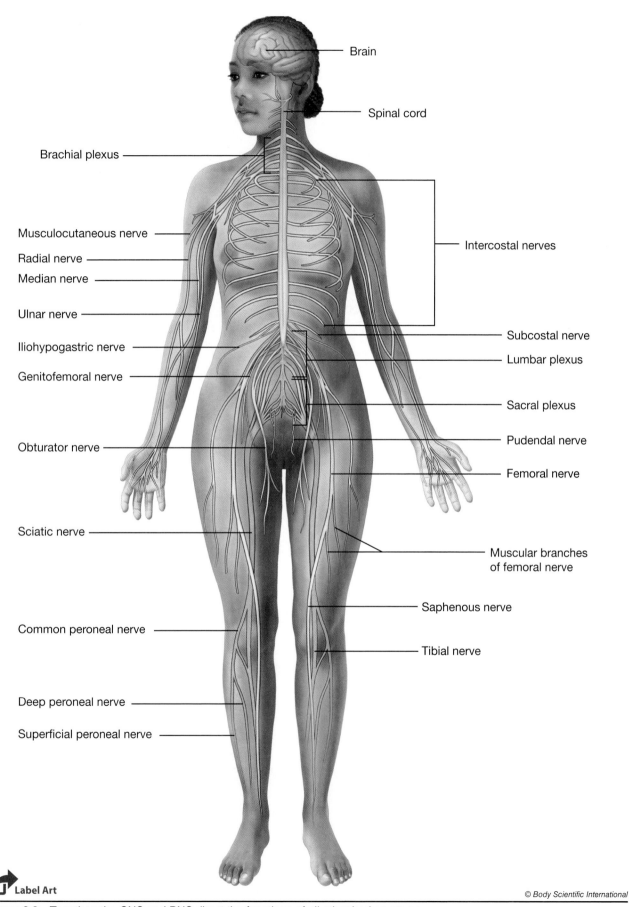

Brain

Spinal cord

Brachial plexus

Musculocutaneous nerve

Radial nerve

Median nerve

Ulnar nerve

Iliohypogastric nerve

Genitofemoral nerve

Obturator nerve

Sciatic nerve

Common peroneal nerve

Deep peroneal nerve

Superficial peroneal nerve

Intercostal nerves

Subcostal nerve

Lumbar plexus

Sacral plexus

Pudendal nerve

Femoral nerve

Muscular branches of femoral nerve

Saphenous nerve

Tibial nerve

Label Art

© Body Scientific International

Figure 6.9　Together, the CNS and PNS direct the functions of all other body systems.

The spinal cord is considered a "super-highway" for information coming to and from the central nervous system. Nerves of the spinal cord convey messages to and from the brain. The thalamus, an important part of the brain, relays sensory messages between the brain and spinal cord. The spinal cord extends from the brain stem and passes through the spinal column. Injury to the spinal cord can result in paralysis and the loss of voluntary muscle function.

Many important structures of the brain contribute to the function of the CNS (Figure 6.10). For example, the hypothalamus—a small gland that works as part of both the CNS and endocrine system—exercises control over the pituitary gland and body functions such as emotions, appetite, body temperature, and sleep.

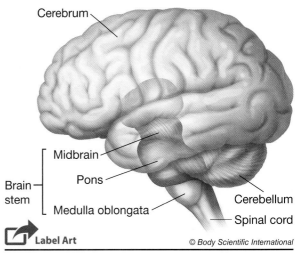

Figure 6.10   As the director of the nervous system, the brain is both structurally and functionally complex.

Cerebrum. The cerebrum is involved in the processing of memory and learning. The cerebrum also controls voluntary movements and interpretation of the senses. Spaces within the cerebrum called *ventricles* contain cerebrospinal fluid (CSF), a watery fluid that bathes the brain and spinal cord and serves as a cushion to help protect them from injury.

Cerebellum. The cerebellum coordinates muscle activity and balance. It receives sensory information from the eyes, inner ears, and other receptors throughout the body, allowing it to constantly monitor and adjust, if necessary, the body's positions and motions.

Brain Stem. The brain stem plays an important role in the CNS. It is a stalk-like structure that connects the cerebrum with the spinal cord.

The brain stem is divided into three sections: the midbrain, the pons, and the medulla oblongata. The midbrain relays sensory information concerning vision, hearing, temperature regulation, sleep, and motor skills to various parts of the CNS. The pons plays a role in regulating breathing. The medulla oblongata contains important centers that regulate vital activities of the body. For example, the medulla oblongata's respiratory center controls breathing, its cardiac center slows the heart when it beats too fast, and the vasomotor center controls blood pressure by narrowing or enlarging blood vessels.

The Peripheral Nervous System (PNS)

While the CNS controls the activity of the brain and spinal cord, the PNS transmits information to all other parts of the body. The PNS contains all of the nerves and ganglia (the junction where two nerves meet) outside of the brain and spinal cord.

Twelve pairs of cranial nerves relay impulses to and from the left and right sides of the brain. These nerves enable the senses of smell, sight, hearing, and taste, as well as facial sensations. They also control eye movements, balance, and communication between the brain and various organs. Thirty-one pairs of spinal nerves carry signals throughout the body.

The Sensory System

The sensory system is a part of the nervous system that consists of sensory receptors such as the eyes and ears, and the senses of taste, smell, and touch. This system's receptors transmit information from internal and external environments to the brain, where it is processed.

The Eyes

The eyes enable one of the most vital senses—vision (Figure 6.11). Each eye (commonly called the *eyeball*) is set into an orbital socket (or *eye socket*) in the skull. Eyelids and eyelashes cover the eye and aid in eye protection. Tears produced in the lacrimal gland help rid the eye of foreign matter that might cause irritation. The white of the eye, called the *sclera*, is the outer lining. The front part of the sclera is called the *cornea*.

The colored portion of the eye is called the *iris*. In the center of the iris is an opening called the *pupil*. Muscles of the iris control the amount of light allowed into the eye through dilation (enlarging) and contraction (shrinking) of the pupil.

Located behind the pupil is the lens, which focuses light rays on the retina. The retina is the innermost coating of the eye, which is filled with specialized nerve endings that sense vision. The nerve endings of the retina send impulses to the optic nerve located at the back of the eye. Once the optic nerve receives a picture, it communicates this information to the brain so the brain can interpret what the eye is seeing.

Cataracts, conjunctivitis (also known as *pink eye*), glaucoma, and macular degeneration are all diseases and disorders of the eye.

The Ears

The ears have two important functions: hearing and maintaining the body's sense of balance, or *equilibrium*. An ear is divided into three main parts—the outer (external) ear, the middle ear (sometimes called the *tympanic cavity*), and the inner (internal) ear (Figure 6.12).

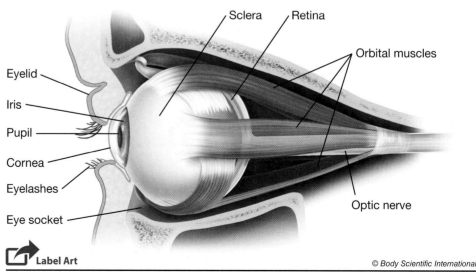

Label Art

© *Body Scientific International*

Figure 6.11 Specialized internal structures of the eye send messages to the brain, creating the sense of sight.

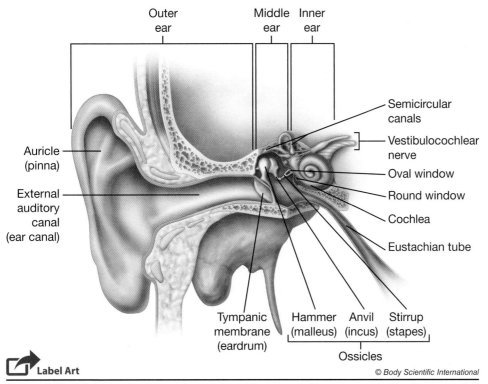

Label Art

© Body Scientific International

Figure 6.12   The complex internal structure of the ear enables a person's hearing as well as his or her balance.

The outer ear is made up of the lobe and the auricle, which is also called the *pinna*. The auricle is the outer portion of the ear that leads to the ear canal, or *external auditory canal*. At the end of the ear canal is the eardrum, or *tympanic membrane*. The tympanic membrane is a very thin membrane, measuring approximately 0.1 millimeters thick. It separates and transmits sound between the outer ear and the middle ear.

The middle ear is a space containing three small bones, which are collectively referred to as *ossicles*. The ossicles include the malleus (*hammer*), incus (*anvil*), and stapes (*stirrup*). These bones transmit and amplify sound waves the eardrum receives from the outside world.

The Eustachian tubes are also part of the middle ear. These tubes work to equalize pressure on both sides of the eardrum. The Eustachian tubes also connect the middle ear and the pharynx, which helps match the pressure in the ear and pharynx with the outside world. This connection causes your ears to pop when the pressure in an airplane cabin changes as the plane starts to land. This connection also allows disease-causing bacteria to travel from the throat to the middle ear via the Eustachian tubes, resulting in a middle ear infection. Ear infections are most prevalent in children.

The inner ear has two membrane-covered outlets into the middle ear—the oval window and the round window. The inner ear houses a snail-shaped organ called the *cochlea*, which contains thousands of hair-like nerve endings that carry sound vibrations through the auditory nerve to the brain. This is the actual process of hearing. Semicircular canals in the inner ear transmit signals to the cerebellum. The cerebellum interprets impulses from these canals to maintain balance with signals coming to the brain from the vestibulocochlear nerve.

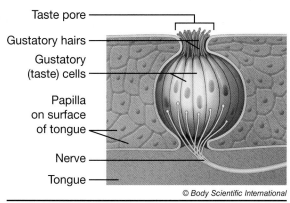

Taste pore

Gustatory hairs

Gustatory
(taste) cells

Papilla
on surface
of tongue

Nerve

Tongue

© Body Scientific International

Figure 6.13   Parts of a taste bud

Deafness, presbycusis (age-related deafness), and tinnitus are disorders of the ear. Various ear infections are also possible, and include external otitis (*swimmer's ear*), otitis media (*middle ear infection*), and labyrinthitis (*inner ear infection*).

Taste, Smell, and Touch

Receptors found in various locations throughout the body contribute to our senses of taste, smell, and touch. These receptors absorb environmental changes and send that information to the brain through nerve impulses. The brain then processes and interprets the messages.

Taste. Taste receptors located in the tongue are called *taste buds* (Figure 6.13). Taste buds are located throughout the interior of the mouth, including on the lips and the sides, top, and back of the mouth. Most are located on the tongue, appearing as tiny bumps known as *papillae*. Each taste bud contains *gustatory cells* that send *gustatory hairs* up through the *taste pores*, which are small openings in the top of the taste bud.

Smell. The sense of smell is made possible by olfactory receptors located in the upper part of the nasal cavity. The olfactory receptor cells connect olfactory hairs, which extend into the nasal cavity and are exposed to odor molecules, with the olfactory nerve. The olfactory nerve sends impulses to the brain, triggering the sense of smell. Figure 6.14 illustrates the nose as the organ of smell.

The nose can detect more than 6,000 different smells. The sense of smell is more sensitive than the sense of taste. However, smell and taste are closely related, as illustrated when a person has a head cold that impairs the sense of taste.

Some diseases that affect our sense of taste and smell include rhinitis, burning mouth syndrome, and oral candidiasis (commonly known as *thrush*).

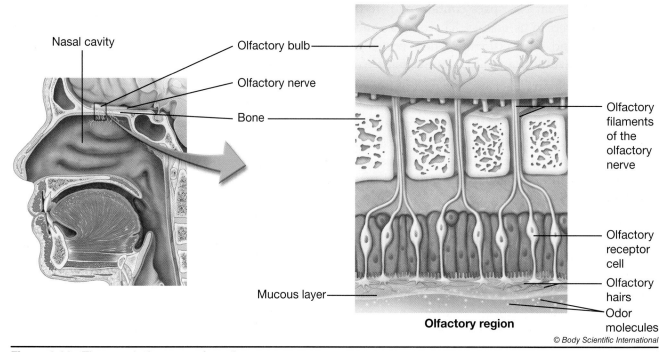

Nasal cavity

Olfactory bulb

Olfactory nerve

Bone

Olfactory filaments of the olfactory nerve

Olfactory receptor cell

Olfactory hairs

Odor molecules

Mucous layer

Olfactory region

© Body Scientific International

Figure 6.14   The nose is the organ of smell

Also, the nasal septum (the structure that divides the right and left air passages) can be deviated or perforated.

Touch. Touch receptors are small, rounded bodies called *tactile corpuscles* found in the skin, the tip of the tongue, and especially the fingertips. Information from these receptors is carried to the spinal cord and up to the brain for interpretation. The sensory information is sorted in the thalamus, then passed on to the postcentral gyrus in the parietal lobe. This is the location of the primary sensory cortex, where the sense of touch is interpreted.

The Endocrine System

The endocrine system contains **endocrine glands** that secrete chemical substances called **hormones** to help regulate body functions (Figure 6.15). The endocrine system affects growth and development, energy balance, reproduction, water and electrolyte balance, and **metabolism**. Your metabolism includes all of the complicated chemical processes by which cells produce energy needed to support and sustain life.

The ductless endocrine glands secrete hormones directly into the bloodstream. Hormones are then carried to the outside of the body or into body cavities. Hormones influence the activities of tissues and cells throughout the body. Every endocrine gland produces or secretes specialized hormones that create a unique response in the body (Figure 6.16).

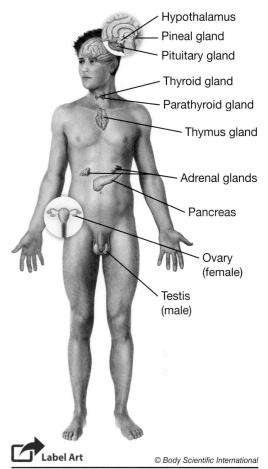

Label Art   © Body Scientific International

Figure 6.15   Endocrine glands are found in various locations throughout the body.

The Endocrine System	
Endocrine Gland	**Function**
Adrenal gland	affects metabolism and growth; monitors electrolyte and fluid balance
Hypothalamus	stimulates or inhibits pituitary secretions; integrates responses from nervous system
Ovaries	contribute to development of female sex characteristics, including the menstrual cycle and reproductive functions
Pancreas	maintains blood glucose levels; islets of Langerhans secrete the hormones glucagon and insulin
Parathyroid glands	maintain blood calcium levels
Pineal gland	releases the hormone melatonin to control sleep
Pituitary gland	regulates and aids in the secretion of essential hormones
Testes	produce testosterone in males
Thymus gland	stimulates the production of T and B cells to aid in the immune response
Thyroid gland	produces thyroxine (T_4) and triiodothyronine (T_3) to regulate the metabolism of proteins, carbohydrates, and fats

Goodheart-Willcox Publisher

Figure 6.16   Functions of the endocrine glands

endocrine glands
glands that secrete chemical substances called hormones, which regulate body functions; part of the endocrine system

hormones
chemicals secreted by endocrine glands to regulate body functions

metabolism
term for the chemical processes, occurring within a living organism, that maintain life

exocrine glands
glands that contain a duct, allowing them to secrete their enzymes directly at the site of action; part of the endocrine system

In addition to endocrine glands, the human body also contains **exocrine glands**. Unlike endocrine glands, exocrine glands contain a duct that allows these glands to secrete their products (enzymes) directly at the site of action, which is either at the surface of the skin or to other organs. Examples of exocrine glands include salivary glands, which produce saliva, and sweat glands.

Some common diseases and disorders of the endocrine system include Addison's disease, Cushing syndrome, hyperthyroidism, hypoglycemia, hypothyroidism, and diabetes mellitus (commonly known as *diabetes*).

Extend Your Knowledge ▶ Diabetes Mellitus

There are two forms of diabetes mellitus—type 1 and type 2. Type 1 diabetes mellitus is also known as *juvenile-onset* because symptoms appear when the patient is a child. Type 2 diabetes is also known as *adult-onset*, as symptoms do not appear until the patient reaches adulthood.

Apply It

1. Using resources in your school's library or on the Internet, find and list the symptoms of type 1 and type 2 diabetes mellitus.

2. Compare the two types of diabetes and identify ways to prevent or manage these endocrine disorders.

3. Describe the difference between a diabetic coma and insulin shock.

Animation

The Respiratory System

Every cell in the human body needs oxygen to survive. The role of the respiratory system is to supply that oxygen to the cells and remove carbon dioxide, a gaseous waste product of the body. This process is referred to as **respiration**, or *breathing*.

respiration
the act of supplying oxygen to the cells and removing carbon dioxide; also called breathing

Oxygen enters the body through the mouth and nose. This process is called *inhalation* (inspiration). The process of forcing air out of the lungs is called *exhalation* (expiration).

The respiratory system is divided into the upper respiratory tract and the lower respiratory tract (Figure 6.17). Components of the upper respiratory tract include the nose, nasal cavity, paranasal sinuses, pharynx, and larynx. The lower respiratory tract includes the trachea and lungs, which house the bronchi, bronchioles, and alveoli. Figure 6.18 lists the various parts of the respiratory system and the function of each.

After oxygen enters the body through either the nose or mouth, it travels through each structure of the respiratory system before arriving at the alveoli. The alveoli are clusters of microscopic air sacs. Oxygen diffuses, or travels through the thin walls of the alveolar sacs to the capillaries that surround the sacs. Red blood cells in the single cell wall of the capillary absorb the oxygen while sending carbon dioxide out of the capillary. Carbon dioxide is sent to the alveoli through the capillary's single-celled walls, to be exhaled by the respiratory system. This process is called *gas exchange*.

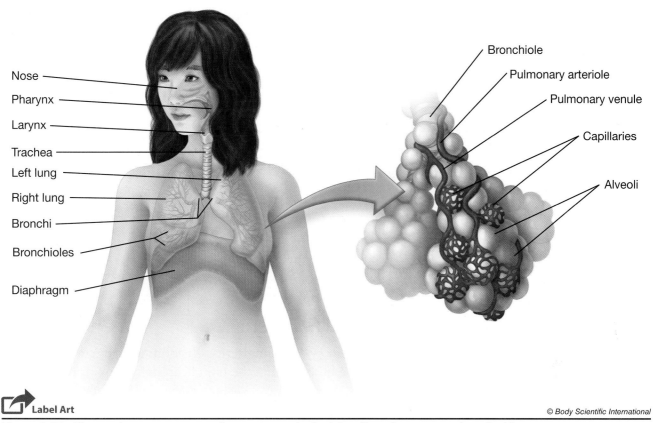

Nose

Pharynx

Larynx

Trachea

Left lung

Right lung

Bronchi

Bronchioles

Diaphragm

Bronchiole

Pulmonary arteriole

Pulmonary venule

Capillaries

Alveoli

Label Art

© Body Scientific International

Figure 6.17 The respiratory system supplies oxygen to the body's cells and removes carbon dioxide.

The Respiratory System	
Structure	*Function*
Alveoli	transport oxygen and carbon dioxide to and from red blood cells in capillaries; main site of gas exchange
Bronchi	air passages located between the trachea and bronchioles
Bronchioles	conduct airflow between the bronchi and alveoli
Diaphragm	moves down (contracts) to promote inspiration; moves up (relaxes) to force air from the lungs during expiration
Epiglottis	a flap that closes and covers the trachea when food or water is ingested to prevent them from entering the lungs
Larynx (voice box)	routes air through vocal cords to produce speech
Lungs	house the structures and tissues that conduct gas exchange
Nasal cavity	filters inspired air; provides sense of smell
Oral cavity (mouth)	inspired and expired air travels through the mouth when the nose is blocked or when someone breathes through his or her mouth
Paranasal sinuses	warm and moisten inhaled air
Pharynx (throat)	passageway that transports air from the nose and mouth to the trachea
Trachea (windpipe)	passageway for air between the pharynx and the bronchi

Goodheart-Willcox Publisher

Figure 6.18 Structures and functions of the respiratory system

The respiratory system is susceptible to several serious conditions and diseases in addition to the common cold and flu. These include asthma, chronic obstructive pulmonary disease (COPD), lung cancer, cystic fibrosis, pneumonia, and tuberculosis.

Check Your Understanding ✔

1. What is the difference between the central nervous system (CNS) and the peripheral nervous system (PNS)?

2. The eyes, ears, and nose are all part of the _____ system.

3. _____ are ductless glands that secrete hormones directly into the bloodstream, while _____ contain ducts that allow for the direct secretion of their enzymes.

4. The respiratory system is divided into the _____ and _____ tracts.

The Cardiovascular System

The cardiovascular system's main responsibility is to circulate, or move blood throughout the body so that the blood can deliver oxygen and nutrients to the body's cells and remove waste materials like carbon dioxide. The blood also transports hormones secreted by the endocrine system. The heart, arteries, and veins are the main organs of this system.

Because of the cardiovascular system's important, life-sustaining role, cardiovascular diseases and disorders are often serious and even life threatening. Heart disease is the leading cause of death in the United States. Some common diseases and disorders of the cardiovascular system include myocardial infarction (heart attack), aneurysm (burst blood vessel), atherosclerosis, heart murmurs, hypertension (high blood pressure), and endocarditis.

The Heart

The normal adult heart beats 72 to 82 beats per minute. This organ is about the size of a clenched fist, weighing 8 to 10 ounces in women and 10 to 12 ounces in men. The heart is located in the thoracic cavity, under the breastbone (or *sternum*).

The heart has four chambers: the upper chambers, or *atria* (plural for *atrium*); and the lower chambers, or *ventricles*. The upper chambers receive blood coming into the heart, while the lower chambers pump blood out of the heart.

The *septum* divides the heart vertically into right and left halves. The interatrial septum separates the right and left atria, and the thick interventricular septum divides the two ventricles. The walls of the septum prevent oxygen-rich blood from mixing with oxygen-poor blood.

The heart consists of three layers. The outer layer, called the *pericardium*, is a double-layered sac. The middle layer, the *myocardium*, is the muscle of the heart. The endocardium, which lines the heart chambers and valves, is the innermost layer of the heart.

Valves of the Heart. The heart has four valves, which ensure that blood flows in only one direction (Figure 6.19). The two atrioventricular valves (*AV valves*) are located between the atria and the ventricles. When these valves open, they allow blood to travel from the atria into the ventricles. If closed, the AV valves prevent blood from flowing backward into the atria as the ventricles contract.

The AV valve on the right side of the heart is called the *tricuspid valve*. On the left side of the heart, the AV valve is called the *mitral valve*, or *bicuspid valve*.

The two valves that separate the ventricles from the lungs and rest of the body are called the *semilunar valves*. One of the semilunar valves is the pulmonary valve, which is located at the opening of the pulmonary artery on the right side of the heart. The aortic valve, the second semilunar valve, is located at the opening of the aorta on the left side of the heart.

Blood Flow through the Heart. To fully understand how the heart performs its critical function, you should understand the step-by-step flow of blood through the heart (Figure 6.20 on the next page). Remember that this process is happening on both sides of the heart at the same time.

1. Deoxygenated blood enters the right atrium from the inferior and superior vena cava.

2. Deoxygenated blood flows through the tricuspid valve into the right ventricle.

3. The right ventricle contracts, forcing the pulmonary valve to open and deoxygenated blood to flow into the pulmonary artery.

4. The right and left pulmonary arteries carry the deoxygenated blood to the lungs.

5. Oxygen-rich blood travels through the pulmonary veins and into the left atrium.

6. The left atrium fills with blood, forcing the mitral valve to open.

7. Oxygenated blood flows through the mitral valve into the left ventricle.

8. The left ventricle contracts, forcing the mitral valve to close and the aortic valve to open.

9. Oxygen-rich blood travels through the aorta to the rest of the body.

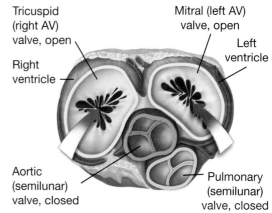

A. Ventricles relaxed

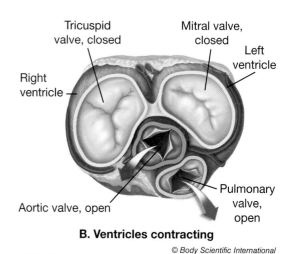

B. Ventricles contracting

© Body Scientific International

Figure 6.19   The four valves of the heart allow blood to flow in only one direction.

Did You Know?   **Heart Statistics**

Every day, the heart beats about 100,000 times, sending approximately 2,000 gallons of blood pumping through the body. The heart performs an incredible job—keeping blood flowing through 60,000 miles of blood vessels to feed the organs and tissues of the body. Any damage to the heart can reduce its efficiency, forcing the heart to work harder to continue supplying the body's much-needed blood.

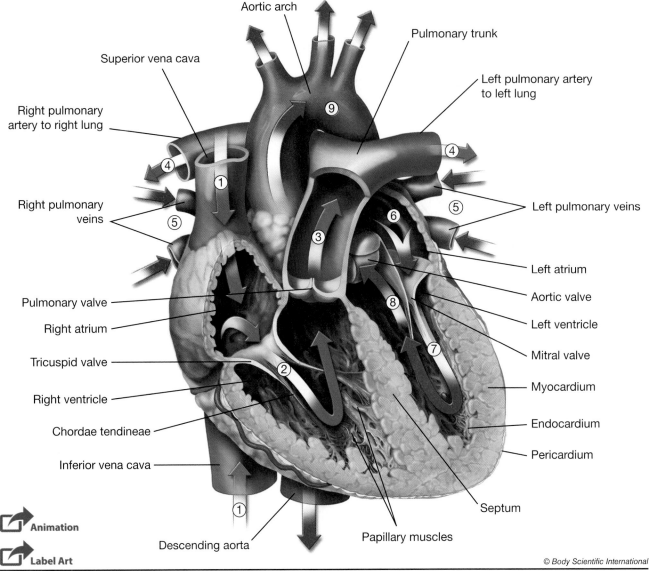

Aortic arch
Pulmonary trunk
Superior vena cava
Left pulmonary artery
to left lung
Right pulmonary
artery to right lung
Right pulmonary
veins
Left pulmonary veins
Left atrium
Aortic valve
Left ventricle
Mitral valve
Myocardium
Endocardium
Pericardium
Pulmonary valve
Right atrium
Tricuspid valve
Right ventricle
Chordae tendineae
Inferior vena cava
Septum
Papillary muscles
Descending aorta

Animation

Label Art

© Body Scientific International

Figure 6.20　As you trace the flow of blood through the heart, note that the blue arrows represent deoxygenated blood, while the red arrows represent oxygenated blood.

Blood Vessels. The heart pumps blood through the blood vessels to all parts of the body. There are three types of blood vessels that transport blood throughout the cardiovascular system. These three types include arteries, capillaries, and veins:

- **Arteries.** With the exception of the pulmonary arteries (which carry oxygen-poor blood to the lungs), all arteries in the body carry oxygen-rich blood away from the heart. Arterial blood is bright red in color because of the oxygen it carries. Arterial walls are thick because they have to withstand the pumping force of the heart. Arteries branch into arterioles, which connect arteries to capillaries. The aorta is the largest artery in the body. Coronary arteries branch off the aorta to supply blood to the walls of the heart. Blockage of a coronary artery may result in coronary artery disease and a heart attack.

- **Capillaries.** Capillaries are microscopic, thin-walled blood vessels. Nutrients pass from the bloodstream to the cells of the body via the capillaries. The body's cells take in oxygen and nutrients from the blood through the thin capillary walls and transfer waste and carbon dioxide to the blood cells in the capillaries.

- **Veins.** Veins are vessels that carry oxygen-poor blood from the capillaries back to the heart. Smaller veins, called *venules*, carry blood from the capillaries to the veins. At that stage, the blood is called *venous blood*. Venous blood is a darker red color than arterial blood. Veins have thinner walls than arteries and valves that help prevent the backward flow of blood. These valves keep venous blood moving forward to the heart.

Components of the Blood. The average adult body contains between four and six quarts of blood. Blood contains many different types of solid cells (known collectively as the **formed elements**), which are suspended in the **plasma**, or liquid portion of blood. Plasma is about 90 percent water with the remaining 10 percent comprised of proteins, electrolytes, nutrients, ions, gases, waste products, and hormones. About 55 percent of blood is made up of plasma, and the other 45 percent is the formed elements. The formed elements consist of red blood cells, white blood cells, and platelets.

Red blood cells (also called *erythrocytes*) are produced in the bone marrow. They live for about 120 days before being broken down by the liver and spleen. Immature red blood cells are rarely seen outside the bone marrow, but mature blood cells appear by the millions in one drop of blood. A red blood cell is shaped like a disk without a hole in the center. Red blood cells contain hemoglobin, a protein that carries oxygen to the body's cells and picks up carbon dioxide from the cells. Hemoglobin contains iron, which is necessary for the body to survive.

White blood cells, or *leukocytes*, are not as numerous as red blood cells and live for about three to nine days. Also part of the immune system, their main function is to fight infection. There are five types of white blood cells: neutrophils, lymphocytes, monocytes, eosinophils, and basophils.

Platelets (*thrombocytes*) are actually fragments of specialized bone marrow cells. Platelets are essential to the formation of blood clots, which stop bleeding. When a cut occurs on the body, platelets form a plug at the site of the cut, beginning the clotting process.

Electrical Activity of the Heart. The conduction system of the heart is responsible for controlling the rate, rhythm, and strength of heart beats, or *contractions*. This system conveys electrical impulses that facilitate proper heart function. Included in the conduction system are two areas of nodal tissue and a network of fibers.

The sinoatrial node, or *SA node*, is located at the top of the right atrium of the heart. The SA node sends out an electrical impulse telling the heart to contract between 60 and 100 beats per minute (bpm).

The SA node fires an electrical impulse that causes the atria to contract. The impulse is also carried to the atrioventricular node (*AV node*). The AV node is a very dense network of fibers that delays the electrical impulse

formed elements
the solid components of blood, including red blood cells, white blood cells, and platelets

plasma
the liquid component of blood

red blood cells
part of the formed elements; contain hemoglobin, which carries oxygen and carbon dioxide to and from the body's cells; also called erythrocytes

white blood cells
part of the formed elements; fight infection in the body; also called leukocytes

platelets
part of the formed elements; play an important role in blood clotting; also called thrombocytes

Animation

briefly (up to a tenth of a second). When the electrical impulse leaves the AV node, it is carried through a collection of conducting fibers called the *bundle of His* and into the ventricular septum. The bundle of His then divides into the right and left bundle branches and forms conduction fibers called the *Purkinje fibers*. The Purkinje fibers transmit the impulse to the ventricles, stimulating their contraction.

Extend Your Knowledge ▶ The Electrocardiogram

When adults have a checkup, they are often given an electrocardiogram (also known as an *ECG* or *EKG*). An electrocardiogram records the electrical activity of the heart. Figure 6.21 is an example of a normal ECG. ECGs are also used to track abnormal heartbeats, called *arrhythmias*. An arrhythmia can occur for a variety of reasons, such as heart beats coming too soon, or flaws in the conduction system of the heart.

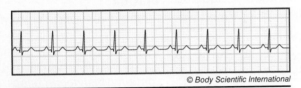

© Body Scientific International

Figure 6.21 An ECG illustrates the electrical activity of the heart. This example shows a normal ECG.

Apply It

1. Each of the following are types of arrhythmias. Research each arrhythmia. Describe each abnormal rhythm, identify the cause of the arrhythmia, and explain whether or not it is life threatening.

bradycardia

tachycardia

atrial fibrillation

premature atrial contractions (PACs)

premature ventricular contractions (PVCs)

ventricular fibrillation (VF)

The Lymphatic and Immune Systems

The lymphatic system and immune system share some of the same structures and functions. Both systems work to prevent and fight disease and destroy any pathogens that find their way into the body.

The lymphatic system helps the body remove and destroy waste products, dead blood cells, pathogens, poisons, cancer cells, and other debris. This system also absorbs fats and fat-soluble vitamins from the gastrointestinal system to deliver nutrients to the body's cells. The immune system facilitates all types of **immunity**, or the ability to resist pathogens.

The lymphatic system is connected to the cardiovascular system by a network of capillaries. As Figure 6.22 shows, the key parts of the lymphatic system include lymphatic capillaries, lymphatic vessels, lymph nodes, lymphatic ducts, tonsils, the thymus gland, and the spleen.

Lymphatic Capillaries

These vessels extend into spaces between body tissues and blood vessels. Lymphatic fluid, called **lymph**, begins as blood plasma that has leaked into tissues from blood vessel capillaries. Lymph contains two types of white blood cells, waste products, and foreign matter from the cells. The lymph travels through the capillaries to lymphatic vessels.

immunity
ability to resist pathogens

lymph
colorless fluid from the body's tissues that carries white blood cells; collects and transports bacteria to the lymph nodes for destruction; carries fats from the digestive system

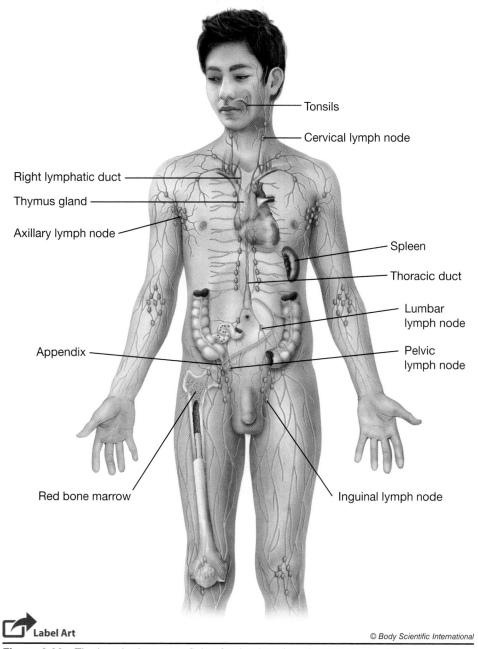

Label Art
© *Body Scientific International*

Figure 6.22   The lymphatic system fights foreign invaders that may cause infection and disease.

Lymphatic Vessels

These vessels, which resemble veins, move the lymph from body tissues to the lymphatic trunks. These trunks deposit lymph into the veins, where it once again becomes plasma—the liquid component of the blood.

Lymph Nodes

Small, bean-shaped lymph nodes lie along the lymphatic vessels. Concentrated in the abdomen, armpits, chest, elbows, groin, and knees, lymph nodes filter bacteria, viruses, and other waste out of the lymph. They also house one type of white blood cells called **lymphocytes**. These cells help the body defend itself from pathogenic microorganisms.

lymphocyte
white blood cell that destroys pathogenic microorganisms

Lymphatic Ducts

There are two main lymphatic ducts—the right lymphatic duct and the thoracic duct. The right lymphatic duct is a vessel that carries lymph from the right side of the body, draining the right arm and the right side of the neck and chest. The thoracic duct drains the rest of the body.

The Spleen

Located behind the stomach, the spleen filters waste products and microorganisms from the blood. The spleen also manufactures two types of white blood cells—lymphocytes and monocytes—to help defend the body against pathogens. The spleen also destroys non-functioning red blood cells and stores red blood cells. Certain infections or traumatic blows to the abdomen may damage the spleen. A person can live without a spleen, but she will be more susceptible to infection than she was before it was removed.

The Thymus Gland

Also part of the endocrine system, the thymus gland is soft and has two lobes. The thymus gland is located beneath the breastbone, at the level of the heart. This gland is large during early childhood and gradually shrinks until it becomes very small in adulthood. The thymus houses T lymphocytes (*T cells*) while they mature. T cells provide immunity and are essential for destroying foreign invaders.

Tonsils

Composed of lymphatic tissue rich with lymphocytes, the tonsils are located at the back of the nasal cavity, above the roof of the mouth. The tonsils are typically large in childhood and shrink during early adulthood. The tonsils filter germs and bacteria that enter the nose and mouth.

On occasion, the tonsils can become overwhelmed by the bacteria they filter, which results in an infection. Infected tonsils become enlarged, make swallowing difficult, and lead to a sore throat and swollen lymph nodes, a condition known as *tonsillitis*. Frequent tonsillitis may be treated by surgically removing the tonsils to prevent further infection.

The pharyngeal tonsil (also called the *adenoid*) lies at the back of the throat and opens into the nasal cavity. The adenoid can also become enlarged and infected.

The Immune System

The immune system is closely linked to the lymphatic system, and the two systems share several organs. The immune system's main job is to defend against intruders, most commonly bacteria and viruses.

The human body has many types of defenses against disease. The skin serves as a physical barrier for pathogens attempting to enter the body. Cilia, tiny hair-like tissues in the nose, also stop infectious invaders. Substances such as gastric juices in the stomach serve as chemical barriers. Specialized white blood cells attack and ingest pathogens in the bloodstream.

Human beings are born with some natural immunity. For instance, people with a healthy immune system are not as susceptible to various bacteria found in the soil. However, these bacteria can harm people with a compromised immune system.

Immunity can also be acquired. Once we have had a certain disease, our bodies are sensitized to that disease. The body may know how to destroy that disease if it attacks again. Vaccinations also produce acquired immunity.

White blood cells (leukocytes) found in the plasma play an important role in the immune system. There are five types of white blood cells (Figure 6.23). These types are classified by the presence of spots, or *granules*, in their cytoplasm. Those with granules are known as *granulocytes* and those without are known as *agranulocytes*.

White Blood Cells		
Type	*Percentage of WBCs*	*Function*
neutrophil 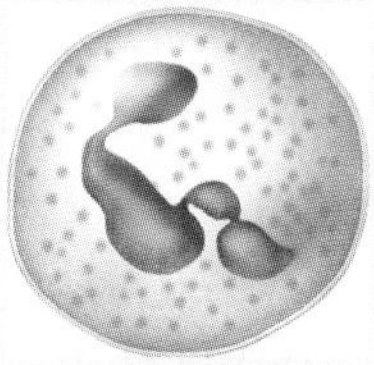	55%–77%	kills bacteria and fungi using phagocytosis
eosinophil 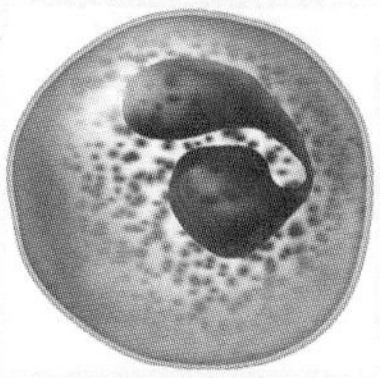	1%–3%	active in the allergic response; destroys parasites
basophil 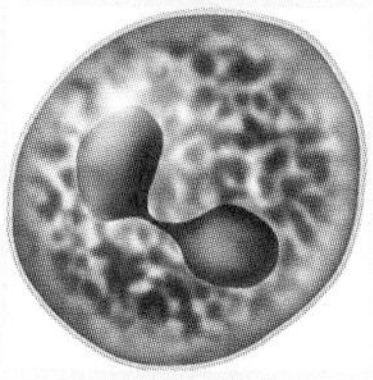	<1%	releases histamine as part of an allergic response
lymphocyte 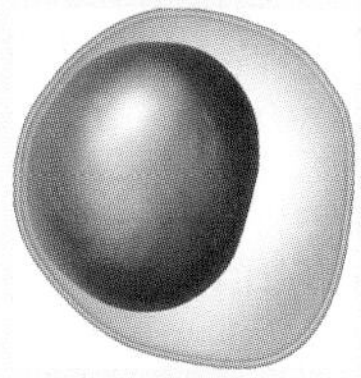	25%–33%	B cells produce antibodies; T cells and natural killer cells fight cancerous tumors and viruses
monocyte 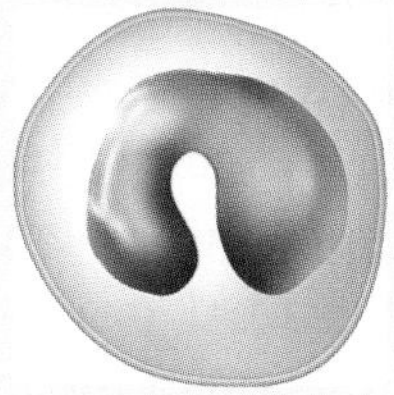	2%–10%	performs phagocytosis; morphs into macrophage that removes dead cell debris and attacks microorganisms

© *Body Scientific International*

Figure 6.23   White blood cells play a major role in the immune response.

Animation

antigen
*any foreign substance,
either outside or inside
the body, that causes the
immune system to produce
antibodies*

antibody
*a protein produced by the
immune system; circulates
in the plasma in response
to the presence of foreign
antigens*

phagocytosis
*process in which white blood
cells surround, ingest, and
destroy a foreign invader*

Antigens and Antibodies. When a potentially harmful foreign molecule enters the body, that molecule is called a foreign **antigen**. Some examples of foreign antigens include microorganisms, splinters, or poison. Our bodies have their own antigens. Other antigens are marked as foreign when they do not match the body's antigens.

A healthy immune system responds quickly to foreign antigens. This response begins when white blood cells produce **antibodies**, which are active in the immune response once foreign antigens are discovered in the body. White blood cells surround, ingest, and destroy the invader as part of a process called **phagocytosis**. Chemicals are released to stimulate inflammation, fever, and the production of pus. Pus is a thick, yellow-white substance composed of white blood cells, dead tissue, and cellular debris. Inflammation, fever, and the presence of pus are all signs that the immune system is working.

There are many diseases and disorders related to the lymphatic and immune systems. Because the immune system is responsible for fighting pathogens, diseases that affect this system can be particularly dangerous. If the immune system is not functioning as it should, the rest of the body systems are at risk for other infections. Allergies, tonsillitis, infected adenoids, and infectious mononucleosis (also called *mono*) are some common diseases related to the lymphatic and immune systems. Untreated tonsillitis can have serious consequences, such as chronic infection and hearing loss. More serious ailments include AIDS, rheumatoid arthritis, leukemias, and lymphomas.

Check Your Understanding ✓

1. What is the difference between an artery and a vein?
2. Describe the function of each of the following components of blood: red blood cells, white blood cells, and platelets.
3. *True or False?* A person can live without a spleen.
4. When are antibodies produced and why?

Animation

The Gastrointestinal System

The gastrointestinal system, also called the *digestive system*, includes many organs working together to ingest and break down food. The gastrointestinal system is responsible for absorbing the nutrients your body needs and disposing of the waste (Figure 6.24).

The process of digestion includes many steps. First, food enters the body via the mouth (*oral cavity*) and is broken down by both mechanical and chemical means. The food travels down the gastrointestinal tract (commonly called the *GI tract*) via the esophagus.

Mechanical breakdown of food is completed by chewing and also through churning in the stomach. Chemical breakdown occurs in the stomach and small intestine, where acids and enzymes (proteins that speed up chemical reactions) break apart food molecules. Nutrients from the food molecules are absorbed primarily in the small intestine. The major function of the large intestine is to absorb water. The feces, or remaining materials not absorbed in digestion, are expelled from the body via the rectum through the anus.

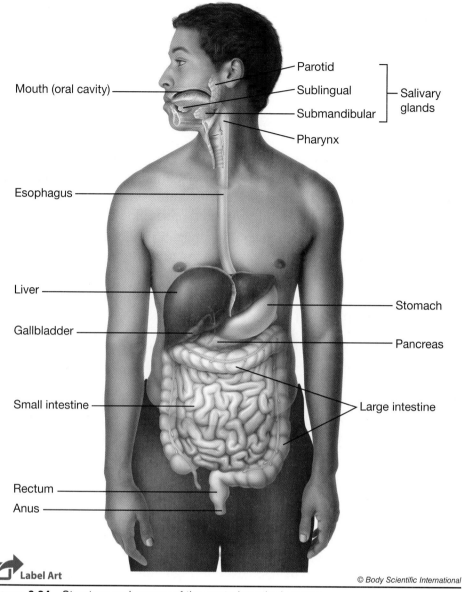

Figure 6.24   Structure and organs of the gastrointestinal system

The Liver and Gallbladder

The liver and gallbladder are accessory, or *supporting*, organs of digestion. The liver has many functions, mostly relating to the body's metabolism—the production and processing of various chemicals. The liver helps maintain a stable, healthy internal environment in the body. The functions of the liver include

- secretion of bile, a brownish-green fluid that helps digest fats;

- monitoring and filtering the blood to remove toxins, destroy old red blood cells, and maintain normal blood concentrations of glucose, fats, and amino acids;

- nutrient breakdown, such as converting carbohydrates to fats; and

- storage of proteins, glycogen (a form of glucose), iron, and vitamins, as well as blood proteins (clotting factors) that are critical in helping the blood to clot.

The liver also has an extensive blood supply, enabling it to accomplish its many tasks.

The gallbladder stores bile secreted by the liver. The gallbladder also delivers bile to the small intestine when it is needed to help break down fats. Humans can live without a gallbladder, but cannot survive without a liver.

The Pancreas

The pancreas is another accessory organ of digestion. Like the liver, the pancreas has both digestive and metabolic functions. The pancreas also makes two important hormones—insulin and glucagon. Insulin lowers blood glucose (sugar) levels, while glucagon raises blood glucose levels.

Cirrhosis of the liver, gastroenteritis, hepatitis, ulcerative colitis, hiatal hernias, and ulcers are all common diseases and disorders of the gastrointestinal system.

The Urinary System

The urinary system filters blood, excretes wastes, and regulates blood pH and volume. The urinary system includes two kidneys, two ureters, a single urethra, and the urinary bladder. Disorders such as kidney stones, chronic kidney disease, and urinary tract infections (UTIs) can cause inflammation or obstruction of the organs in this system. Consequences of these disorders may result in temporary organ malfunction or permanent organ damage.

Urine Production

Urine is produced through three important processes:

1. **Filtration.** The blood is filtered to separate important, beneficial substances—glucose and amino acids—from waste substances—ammonia and certain drugs. This filtering helps identify substances that need to be eliminated as urine.

2. **Reabsorption.** As filtration takes place, beneficial substances such as water, sugar, and salts are moved back into the blood so they can be reabsorbed by the body.

3. **Secretion.** The final step in this process is achieved when the urinary system secretes waste from the body in the form of urine.

Urine Composition

Urine consists mainly of water (approximately 95 percent). It also includes the waste products urea and creatinine; uric acid; and small amounts of enzymes, ions, and other compounds.

When analyzed (using a process called *urinalysis*), certain components found in the urine can signal an abnormality or possible disease. Such components include bacteria, white and red blood cells, abnormal levels of glucose and protein, and yeast.

Structures of the Urinary System

The chief organs in the urinary system are the pair of bean-shaped kidneys (Figure 6.25). Each about the size of a fist, the kidneys are located dorsally to the upper abdomen. The kidneys are a very complex filtration system. As you may recall from the *Suffixes for Medical Terms* table that appears at the end of chapter 5, the word *renal* refers to the kidneys.

Covered by the renal capsule, the interior of the kidney is divided into three parts:

- the cortex (outer layer)
- the medulla (middle layer)
- the pelvis (innermost layer)

Blood is filtered in the cortex of the kidney. Erythropoietin, a hormone necessary for red blood cell production, is produced in the renal cortex. The renal medulla contains a number of triangle-shaped areas called *pyramids*. Urine is collected in the pyramids, which are separated by renal columns. The renal pelvis serves as a funnel for the urine. The pelvis is divided into two or three large collecting cups called *major calyces*, which then branch into several *minor calyces*. Urine continually drains through the pyramids into the calyces.

The major filtering mechanisms in the kidney are called *nephrons*. Blood enters each kidney through a renal artery and leaves through a renal vein. Inside the kidney, the renal artery branches into smaller arteries, which lead to the microscopic nephrons. Each kidney contains about one million nephrons, some in the cortex and some in the medulla.

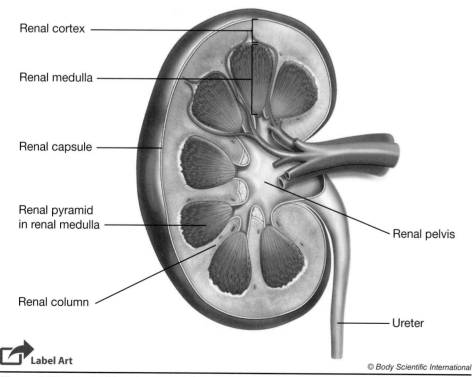

Renal cortex

Renal medulla

Renal capsule

Renal pyramid in renal medulla

Renal column

Renal pelvis

Ureter

Label Art

© *Body Scientific International*

Figure 6.25   Each kidney has approximately one million nephrons, the units that create urine.

The renal pelvis empties into the ureters—two tubes approximately six or seven inches in length that carry urine to the urinary bladder, or *bladder*. The urinary bladder is a hollow, muscular organ that stores urine to be eliminated. The bladder can hold approximately 500 milliliters of urine when moderately full before it empties. The walls of the bladder can stretch and allow the bladder to hold twice as much as it holds when considered full. When the bladder is stretched, nerve endings are stimulated and signal the brain that the bladder is full.

Urine is eliminated from the body by way of the urethra, a tube of smooth muscle with a mucous lining. The female urethra is about 1.5 inches long, whereas the male urethra is 8 inches long. The process of excreting urine is often called *voiding*.

Acid-Base Balance

The kidneys maintain a balance between acids (*acidity*) and bases (*alkalinity*) in the body. All chemicals in the body fall into one of three categories—acid, base, or neutral. *Acidic* and *basic* are terms for the extreme ends of the spectrum. A substance that is neither an acid nor a base is called *neutral*.

pH scale
system for measuring a substance's acidity or alkalinity; ranges from 0 to 14

The level of a substance's acidity or alkalinity is measured on the **pH scale**. The scale ranges from 0 to 14, with acids falling on the lower end of the scale and bases on the upper end. The normal pH of human blood falls in the middle, within a tight range of 7.35 to 7.45.

If the kidneys sense that the blood's pH level is above or below the normal range, buffering agents will be excreted to maintain the acid-base balance. A buffering agent might make the blood more acidic or basic, depending on the pH. The regulation of blood pH is another example of how the body achieves homeostasis.

Common disorders and diseases of the urinary system include acute and chronic kidney failure, cystitis (inflammation of the bladder), kidney stones, various infections of parts of the kidney, incontinence (inability to control when you urinate), and urethritis.

The Reproductive System

The reproductive system allows humans to reproduce, or create offspring. The reproductive system is controlled by hormones and, as a result, shares some organs with the endocrine system.

Hormones play a major role in human reproduction. The pituitary gland is responsible for producing hormones to regulate the maturation and release of gametes (sperm and eggs) in both males and females. In females, the ovaries produce estrogen, progesterone, and other hormones affecting the sex drive and fertility. Testosterone and other hormones produced by cells in the male genitalia are involved in the production of sperm.

puberty
a stage of life beginning between the ages of 8 and 14; indicates sexual reproduction is possible

Unlike other body systems, the reproductive system does not begin to function at birth. Rather, reproductive functions only begin once the system has matured. This maturation takes place during a process called **puberty**. Puberty usually lasts several years, and begins between the ages of 8 and 14 (typically beginning earlier in females than in males). Puberty is an indication that sexual reproduction is possible.

Did You Know? Reproductive System Facts

- The largest cell in the female body is the ovum (or *egg*), found in the ovaries.
- A mature ovum has a life span of 12 to 24 hours.
- In her lifetime, a woman can give birth up to 35 times.
- A female infant is typically born with about 600,000 immature ova in her ovaries.
- The fallopian tubes are only as wide as the head of a pin.
- A healthy male can produce about 500 million sperm each day.
- Sperm live for approximately 36 hours.

The **menstrual cycle** represents a series of changes a female's body goes through in preparation for a pregnancy. About once a month, the uterus grows a new lining, called the *endometrium*. This process prepares the uterus for a fertilized egg. If no egg is present, the uterus sheds its lining. This shedding process is the menstrual period, which causes a discharge that lasts from 4 to 7 days. A female continues to have a menstrual period from the early teen years until approximately the age of 50, when she goes through menopause, or the cessation of bleeding. Some females have longer or shorter menstrual periods, and there is variation in when menopause occurs.

menstrual cycle
the monthly process in which the uterus grows a new lining and then sheds that lining during the menstrual period if a pregnancy does not occur

Human reproduction occurs when the male sex cell (sperm) and female sex cell (ova, or *egg*) unite to create a new human being. This process is known as *fertilization*. After fertilization, a fetus takes approximately 40 weeks to develop, at which point the female will give birth.

human reproduction
process that occurs when the male sex cell and female sex cell unite to create a new human being

The reproductive system is also unique because different structures compose this system depending on your gender (Figures 6.26 and 6.27 on the next page). Because females may become pregnant and give birth, the female reproductive system has more functions than the male reproductive system. Refer to Figures 6.28 and 6.29 on page 201 for a description of the various reproductive structures and their functions.

Common disorders and diseases of the reproductive system include **sexually transmitted infections (STIs)** and reproductive tract infections (RTIs) in both females and males. Various cancers affect the reproductive systems, including ovarian cancer and uterine cancer in women, and testicular cancer in men. Functional problems may also exist, such as male impotence.

sexually transmitted infection (STI)
an infection transferred from one person to another through sexual contact

Check Your Understanding ✓

1. Describe the difference between chemical and mechanical breakdown in the gastrointestinal system.
2. Which organ produces urine?
3. The maturation of the sexual reproductive systems takes place during _____.

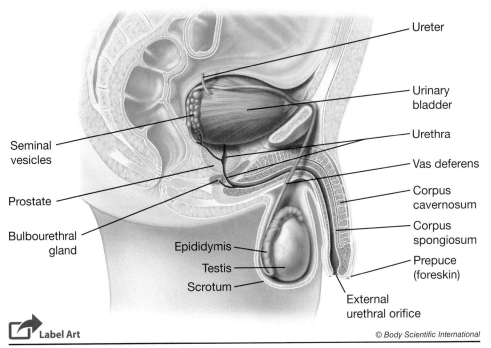

Label Art

© Body Scientific International

Figure 6.26   The male reproductive system

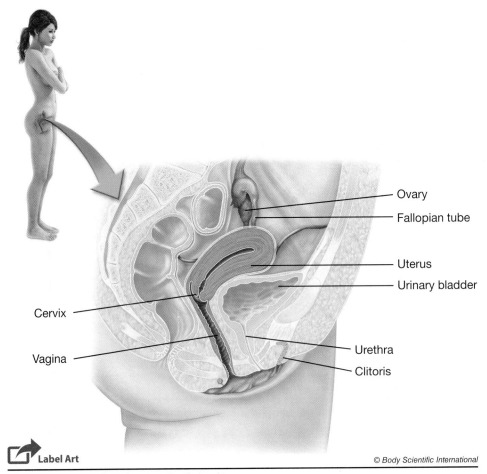

Label Art

© Body Scientific International

Figure 6.27   The female reproductive system

The Male Reproductive System	
Structure	**Function**
Bulbourethral glands	lubricate penis for insertion by secreting small amounts of fluid just before emission of the semen
Corpus cavernosum and corpus spongiosum	sponge-like expandable erectile tissue (capable of being raised to an upright position)
Epididymis	site of sperm maturation and storage; holds the testes in place
Penis	delivers sperm to the female reproductive tract
Prepuce (foreskin)	protects the sensitive glans (head) of the penis
Prostate gland	secretes fluid into the urethra to buffer the acid in urine and the vagina
Scrotum	houses the testes and associated ducts
Seminal vesicles	produce secretions that account for about 60% of the total volume of semen; supply energy for the sperm
Testes	produce sperm and the male sex hormone, testosterone
Urethra	transports sperm and urine out of the body
Vas deferens	carries sperm to the urethra

Goodheart-Willcox Publisher

Figure 6.28   Structures and functions of the male reproductive system

The Female Reproductive System	
Structure	**Function**
Cervix	lower, narrower part of the uterus; allows flow of menstrual blood from the uterus into the vagina, directs sperm into the uterus during intercourse; supports the uterus
Endometrium	receives and nourishes the fertilized ova; thickens and sheds as part of the menstrual cycle
External genitalia	lubricate the entrance to the vagina; produce pleasurable sensations during sex; protect the reproductive tract from infectious agents
Fallopian tubes	bring the ova to the uterus; common site for fertilization
Mammary glands	produce milk in nursing mothers
Ovaries	produce female sex hormones and ova (or *eggs*)
Uterus	receives and nourishes a fertilized egg; houses the fetus during gestational development; expels the fetus using muscular contractions during childbirth
Vagina	passageway for menstrual flow, semen, and the fetus during childbirth; acidic nature of the vagina helps prevent bacterial infections

Goodheart-Willcox Publisher

Figure 6.29   Structures and functions of the female reproductive system

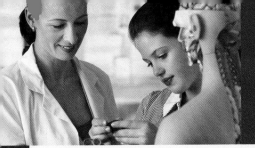

Summary

To understand the human body, it is helpful to study anatomy and physiology. This subject matter focuses on the form and function of the human body. The human body is built on a foundation of approximately five trillion cells. These cells form tissues, organs, and the complex body systems that come together to create a complete organism, or human. Found within each cell is deoxyribonucleic acid, or *DNA*, which contains unique genetic information and can be used to develop treatments and cures for genetic disorders.

The organs of the body work together to accomplish specific tasks a single organ cannot perform alone. These organs are grouped together into body systems based on the process performed. These systems include the integumentary, musculoskeletal, nervous, sensory, endocrine, respiratory, cardiovascular, lymphatic and immune, gastrointestinal, urinary, and reproductive systems. A healthy internal balance among the body systems is achieved through a process called *homeostasis*.

Review Questions

Answer the following questions using what you have learned in this chapter.

True or False

1. *True or False?* DNA is found inside the nucleus of the cell.
2. *True or False?* Multiple sclerosis is a disease of the gastrointestinal system.
3. *True or False?* Physiology is the study of the structure of the body.
4. *True or False?* Capillaries are larger than veins.
5. *True or False?* Eustachian tubes are found in the eye.
6. *True or False?* The skin is the largest organ of the body.
7. *True or False?* The urinary system is the body system most heavily involved in removing carbon dioxide from the body.
8. *True or False?* The aorta divides the heart into two parts.
9. *True or False?* Estrogen and testosterone are hormones involved in the reproductive system.
10. *True or False?* Urine is 70 percent water.

Multiple Choice

11. Which of the following statements is *incorrect*?
    A. Human beings have 23 pairs of chromosomes.
    B. DNA stands for *deoxyribonucleic acid*.
    C. DNA has been called the *molecule of life*.
    D. DNA was discovered in the early 1900s.

12. Which of the following structures is part of the eye?
    A. iris
    B. pupil
    C. retina
    D. All of the above.

13. The _____ is *not* a part of the lymphatic system.
    A. thoracic duct
    B. spleen
    C. heart
    D. thymus gland

14. Basophils, lymphocytes, and _____ are all types of white blood cells.
    A. neutrophils
    B. stem cells
    C. antibodies
    D. cytoplasms

15. Bone marrow can be either red or _____.
    A. blue
    B. yellow
    C. green
    D. orange

16. _____ muscles control voluntary movements.
    A. Coarse
    B. Skeletal
    C. Cardiac
    D. Smooth

17. Functions of the integumentary system include all of the following *except* _____.
    A. vitamin B production from sunlight
    B. regulation of body temperature
    C. excretion of minor amounts of waste material in sweat
    D. transmission of sensory information such as pain, touch, and pressure

18. _____ is a disease of the integumentary system associated with a virus.

   A. A cold sore

   B. Chicken pox

   C. Human papillomavirus (HPV)

   D. All of the above.

19. Which of the following is *not* a part of the respiratory system?

   A. alveoli

   B. lungs

   C. trachea

   D. pons

20. Which of the following is *not* a part of the female reproductive system?

   A. vagina

   B. cervix

   C. ureters

   D. fallopian tubes

21. Which of the following are the most prominent chemicals in the human body?

   A. oxygen, carbon, hydrogen, nitrogen, calcium, and phosphorus

   B. oxygen, nitrogen, sodium, carbon, magnesium, and calcium

   C. oxygen, magnesium, phosphorus, sulfur, and chlorine

   D. oxygen, calcium, phosphorus, potassium, and chlorine

22. Adduction means _____.

   A. movement of a limb away from the body

   B. limb movement toward the body

   C. circular rotation

   D. closer to the feet

23. Plasma makes up _____ of the blood.

   A. 20 percent

   B. 95 percent

   C. 55 percent

   D. 45 percent

24. Which term is *not* a name of a bone fracture?

   A. greenstick

   B. comminuted

   C. critical

   D. spiral

25. Once a month, the uterus grows a new lining. This lining is called the _____.

   A. endometrium

   B. fallopian lining

   C. menstrual lining

   D. None of the above.

Short Answer

26. Describe the pathway of blood through the heart.

27. Which term—anatomy or physiology—has to do with function?

28. What is the function of the pancreas?

29. Which two systems work together to fight disease?

30. What are the differences between arteries, veins, and capillaries?

31. Name three endocrine glands.

32. What is the difference between inspiration and expiration?

33. Name the two sections of the skeletal system.

34. Explain the difference between endocrine and exocrine glands.

35. What does the uterus do if no fertilized egg is present?

36. Name four critical functions performed by the skeletal system.

37. Identify the three formed elements in the blood.

38. Why might urinalysis help identify an undiagnosed disease?

39. Describe the function of platelets.

40. What is homeostasis and why is it important?

Critical Thinking Exercises

41. Identify two body systems whose organs work together to maintain homeostasis. Do some research to identify and summarize both the biological and chemical processes that contribute to homeostasis. Present your findings to the class.

42. Research the layers of the meninges that cover the brain and spinal cord. Describe the characteristics and function of each.

43. Research the Human Genome Project further on the Internet. In your opinion, what is the most promising application of genome mapping? What ethical factors should be considered in the application of this technology?

Chapter 7
Disease

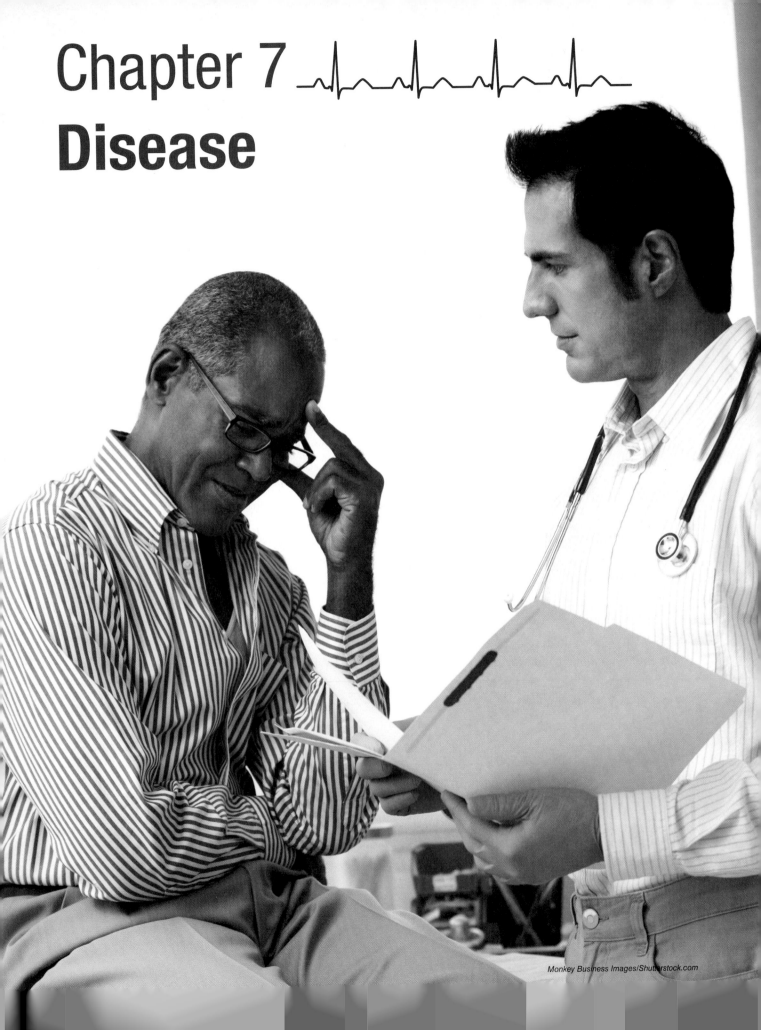

atherosclerosis

autism

body mass index (BMI)

cancer

carcinoma

chemotherapy

chronic disease

communicable disease

dementia

diabetes mellitus

disease

disorder

drug-resistant bacteria

hepatitis

incurable disease

inflammation

malignant

medical specialties

metastasis

monogenic disease

myocardial infarction

neoplasm

noncommunicable disease

post-traumatic stress disorder
  (PTSD)

proteomics

stroke

syndrome

terminal disease

Chapter Objectives

- Define *disease*.
- Explain how a diagnosis of a disease is made.
- Describe classification of diseases by cause.
- List some representative diseases of each cause.
- Identify causes and prevention of heart disease.
- Explain how cancers develop and metastasize.
- Discuss what is meant by *COPD*.
- List various types of trauma caused by accidents.
- Name critical signs of a stroke.
- List signs of Alzheimer's disease.
- Discuss the types of diabetes mellitus.
- Identify several emerging diseases.
- Discuss ways to contain medical costs.

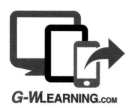

While studying, look for the activity icon to:

- **Build** vocabulary with e-flash cards and interactive games.
- **Assess** progress with chapter and unit review questions.
- **Expand** learning with animations and illustration labeling activities.
- **Simulate** EHR entry with healthcare documents.

What Is a Disease?

disease
any condition that interferes with the normal function of the body

chronic disease
a disease of long duration

incurable disease
a disease that cannot be cured or adequately treated

terminal disease
a disease that eventually ends in death

communicable disease
a disease that is caused by pathogens and can be transferred from one living thing to another

noncommunicable disease
a disease that cannot be passed from one living thing to another, and which is caused by genes, diet, behavior, and other factors

disorder
an abnormality of function; a pathological condition

syndrome
a group of symptoms that together indicate a disease

The term **disease** refers to any condition that interferes with the normal functioning of the body. There are two broad types of disease—infectious disease and non-infectious disease. Infectious disease is caused by pathogens such as bacteria, viruses, fungi, and protozoa. Non-infectious disease includes all other diseases, such as cancer, heart disease, and genetic disease. A disease can be described in several different ways. A **chronic disease**, such as diabetes, has a long duration and progresses slowly. An **incurable disease** cannot be reversed or treated. A **terminal disease** will eventually lead to death.

Diseases can also be either communicable or noncommunicable. A **communicable disease** is caused by pathogens that can be passed from one living thing to another. Examples include influenza and pneumonia. A **noncommunicable disease** is not caused by pathogens and cannot be spread through person-to-person contact. Instead, these diseases are caused by factors such as genes, diet, behavior, and smoking. Examples include heart disease, stroke, cancer, and high blood pressure.

The term **disorder** is often used in conjunction with the term *disease*. Although the terms are sometimes used interchangeably, they do refer to different conditions. While a disease is a process with a specific set of signs and symptoms, a disorder is a condition that causes abnormality of function. For example, a poorly functioning heart valve would be considered a disorder. However, vessels in the heart clogged with cholesterol deposits would be described as heart disease. A **syndrome** is a group of symptoms that indicate a disease, psychological disorder, or other abnormal condition. Figure 7.1 lists common terms related to disease.

Classification of Diseases by Cause

The study of disease and its treatment is one of the most interesting aspects of working in healthcare. There are many ways to classify disease. In this textbook, disease will be classified by cause. Disease classification can be further focused to study autoimmune disease, disease caused by cancer, genetic disease, mental disorders, bacterial disease, sexually transmitted infection, and so on.

Diagnosis

Diagnosis is both an art and a science. Even with the help of diagnostic software, doctors find that diagnosis is often a complex and difficult task. Although it is not always possible to determine what is making a patient ill, diagnosis is one of the most interesting and important roles of the doctor.

A diagnosis is made by studying a patient's medical history, listening to the patient's description of the illness, performing a physical examination, and analyzing the results of any diagnostic tests.

Common Disease Terms		
Term	**Breakdown**	**Definition**
diagnosis	*dia-*, complete; *gnos*, knowledge; *-sis*, state of	act of determining the cause of a disease
prognosis	*pro-*, before; *gnos*, knowledge; *-sis*, state of	prediction of the probable outcome of a disease
idiopathic	*idio-*, unknown; *path*, disease; *-ic*, pertaining to	a disease of unknown cause
epidemic	*epi-*, above; *dem*, people; *-ic*, pertaining to	a disease that spreads rapidly and affects a large number of people
endemic	*en-*, in; *dem*, people; *-ic*, pertaining to	a disease that is prevalent in a particular group of people or region
pandemic	*pan-*, all; *dem*, people; *-ic*, pertaining to	a disease that affects an unusually large number of the population
acute	(no breakdown)	a disease of sudden onset and short duration
chronic	*chron*, time; *-ic*, pertaining to	a long-lasting disease
morbidity	(no breakdown)	a diseased or unhealthy state
comorbidity	(no breakdown)	two or more coexisting diseases
mortality	(no breakdown)	number of deaths in a given population; the condition of being mortal
localized	(no breakdown)	a disease, usually understood to be infectious or malignant, that is confined to a certain area of the body
systemic	*system*, system; *-ic*, pertaining to	a disease that affects a large part or most of the body
benign	(no breakdown)	noncancerous, not threatening
malignant	(no breakdown)	cancerous, growing worse
congenital	*con-*, with; *genit*, reproduction; *-al*, pertaining to	a condition one is born with
hereditary	(no breakdown)	a disease inherited through the genes

Goodheart-Willcox Publisher

Figure 7.1   Common terms related to disease

Common Disease Terms		
Term	*Breakdown*	*Definition*
sign	(no breakdown)	objective finding that can be seen upon observation such as a rash, hair loss, or swelling
symptom	*symptom*, occurrence	subjective findings that are experienced by the patient such as nausea, headache, or dizziness
syndrome	*syn-*, together; *-drome*, to run	group of signs and symptoms appearing together that are typical of a certain disease

Goodheart-Willcox Publisher

Figure 7.1   Common terms related to disease (continued)

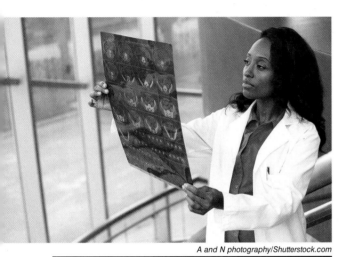

A and N photography/Shutterstock.com

Figure 7.2   X-rays can often help a doctor with a patient's diagnosis.

Diagnostic tests may include orders for diagnostic imaging such as those discussed in chapter 2 (Figure 7.2). Laboratory testing of blood, urine, and other body fluids and visual examinations using a scoped instrument (sometimes with a camera on the end) are diagnostic tests a healthcare provider may perform. For example, a bronchoscopy, or visual examination of the bronchial tubes, may be performed on a patient who has been coughing up blood. This diagnostic test is performed using a bronchoscope.

A variety of treatment options exist, depending on a patient's diagnosis. Some diseases may require surgery. For example, if a biopsy reveals the presence of cancer, surgery is often ordered to remove the diseased tissue. Lung cancer may require a pneumonectomy (lung removal).

Other treatments for various diseases include medications, chemotherapy, radiation therapy, insertion of medical devices, dietary changes, physical therapy, lifestyle modifications, or psychotherapy. Doctors may also recommend incorporating yoga, meditation, or music therapy into a patient's treatment program.

Disease Classifications

Diseases can be classified in different ways, but two of the more common methods include classifying by cause or by the affected body system. Chapter 6 discusses body systems and some representative diseases.

In this chapter, seven classifications of disease by cause will be discussed with examples of each:

- hereditary or genetic
- congenital
- environmental
- nutritional
- infectious
- degenerative
- traumatic

Hereditary and Genetic Disease

Hereditary disease results from abnormalities in the genes that carry a human's genetic information. There are thousands of hereditary diseases—many of which are caused by a flaw in a single gene; these are called **monogenic diseases**. According to the World Health Organization (WHO), about 10,000 monogenic diseases have been identified.

monogenic disease
a disease that is caused by a flaw in one gene

Down Syndrome

One of the most common genetic disorders is Down syndrome, or *trisomy 21* (Figure 7.3). Down syndrome is a condition that occurs when three number 21 chromosomes are present, rather than the usual two. People born with this condition have varying degrees of mental disability. Physically, they may have a flat, broad face; folds of skin on the inner corners of the eyes; stunted growth; poor muscle tone; or atypical fingerprints. Babies born to parents past age 35 are more likely to be born with Down syndrome than babies born to younger parents.

Sickle Cell Anemia

Sickle cell anemia is a common genetic disorder that primarily affects people of African and Mediterranean descent. This hereditary disease occurs when a child receives a sickle cell gene from each parent. Sickle cell anemia causes the red blood cells to take on a sickle, or crescent, shape. The abnormally shaped red blood cells also have a sticky texture. Together, their shape and texture cause these red blood cells to clump together, block capillaries, and restrict blood flow to body tissue (Figure 7.4). Treatments vary based on an individual's symptoms, and often include blood transfusions to replace the sickle-shaped red blood cells with healthy ones.

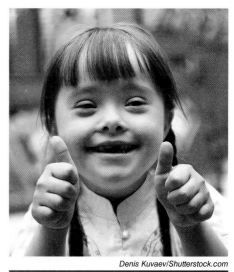

Denis Kuvaev/Shutterstock.com

Figure 7.3 Down syndrome is the most common genetic disorder in the United States.

Congenital Disease

Congenital diseases, or *birth defects*, exist at birth but may not be evident until later. Congenital diseases are often the result of genetic disorders, so hereditary diseases may also be considered congenital. However, some congenital diseases are not considered hereditary. Such congenital diseases are the result of exposing the fetus to harmful substances such as drugs, chemicals, infectious disease, or radiation during development. The fetus is especially vulnerable during the first trimester (the initial three to four weeks of pregnancy). Exposure to rubella (German measles) in a non-immunized mother during the first trimester results in a high incidence of congenital disease.

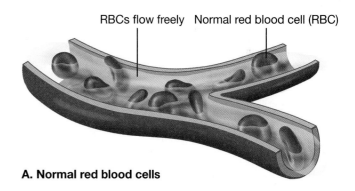

RBCs flow freely   Normal red blood cell (RBC)

A. Normal red blood cells

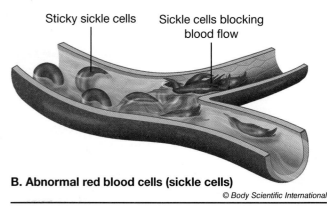

Sticky sickle cells   Sickle cells blocking blood flow

B. Abnormal red blood cells (sickle cells)

© Body Scientific International

Figure 7.4 Sickle-shaped red blood cells can block small blood vessels, halting blood flow.

Fetal Alcohol Spectrum Disorders

Alcohol can harm a baby at any stage during a pregnancy. That includes the earliest stages before a woman even knows she is pregnant. Drinking alcohol can cause a group of conditions called *fetal alcohol spectrum disorders* (FASDs). Effects can include physical and behavioral problems such as trouble with

- learning and remembering;
- understanding and following directions;
- controlling emotions;
- communicating and socializing; and
- daily life skills, such as feeding and bathing.

Cerebral Palsy

Cerebral palsy (CP) is a congenital disease characterized by permanent partial paralysis and lack of muscle coordination. Damage to the central nervous system, primarily during fetal development, can cause cerebral palsy. Conditions in the pregnant woman such as maternal diabetes or *anoxia* (lack of oxygen) can cause cerebral palsy in the fetus. CP can also result from anoxia during birth as a consequence of the umbilical cord wrapping around the baby's neck. Toddlers are also at risk of developing CP if they suffer a brain injury or infection.

Most doctors recommend that women who are planning to get pregnant make an appointment with their obstetrician or primary care doctor to find out what vaccinations are needed. If a mother contracts chicken pox, mumps, measles (especially rubella), hepatitis B, or human papillomavirus (HPV) during her pregnancy, the consequences for the fetus are quite serious. Exposure to these diseases, especially during the first trimester when the fetus is most vulnerable, can lead to congenital diseases.

Environmental Disease

Environmental diseases can result from exposure to air and water pollution, pesticides and other chemicals, the sun, asbestos, and radiation. Factors such as length, amount, and type of exposure as well as individual susceptibility contribute to the development of an environmental disease. Exposure to radiation, lead, pesticides, and other chemical hazards during pregnancy has been linked to birth defects.

Certain cancers are thought to be caused by toxins in the environment. Working with plastics in manufacturing and working around radiation puts people at a greater risk for cancer.

Because they filter the air we breathe, the lungs are particularly vulnerable to environmental diseases. Breathing asbestos has been linked to lung cancer. Secondhand smoke and environmental hazards in the workplace can also damage the lungs. For example, black lung disease is found in coal miners who regularly breathe coal dust. Pottery workers may develop silicosis, a lung disease caused by breathing the silica dust found in clay.

Check Your Understanding ✓

1. What is the difference between the term *disease* and the term *disorder*?
2. Name three disease classifications.
3. What is one example of a congenital disease?
4. Name two effects of fetal alcohol spectrum disorders.

Nutritional Disease

Nutritional diseases are the result of one or more of the following:

1. an inability to consume proper food and nutrients
2. an inability to absorb and utilize nutrients
3. overeating

Malnutrition results from the inadequate intake of nutrients. This condition may result from a variety of causes, including inadequate food availability, fad diets, chronic alcoholism, or chronic illness such as cancer and AIDS. Disordered eating also causes malnutrition. Anorexia nervosa is an eating disorder in which a person fears weight gain, and therefore starves himself or herself to control his or her weight. This voluntary starvation is sometimes accompanied by excessive exercise. Anorexia often leads to extreme weight loss and a weight well below normal for the affected individual's height and age. Bulimia nervosa, another dangerous chronic eating disorder, is characterized by binge eating followed by induced vomiting and the possible abuse of laxatives (see chapter 8).

carcinoma
cancerous tumor derived from epithelial cells

Did You Know? Understanding Skin Cancer

There are three categories of skin cancer—basal cell **carcinomas**, squamous cell carcinomas, and malignant melanoma.

More than 90 percent of skin cancers appear on sun-exposed skin—especially the face, neck, ears, forearms, and hands. A change in color, size, shape, or texture of a mole can indicate skin cancer.

Basal cell and squamous cell carcinomas can cause serious illness and disfigurement, resulting from both the disease and the surgery performed to remove the diseased tissue. Melanomas cause more than 75 percent of all skin cancer deaths. This disease spreads to other organs if left untreated.

In order to avoid skin cancer, stay out of the sun. When spending time outdoors, you should wear sunscreen with a sun protection factor (SPF) of at least 50 (Figure 7.5 inside this box).

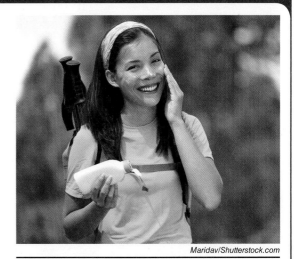

Maridav/Shutterstock.com

Figure 7.5   Depending on a person's sensitivity to the sun, a sunscreen with a higher degree of SPF may be necessary.

Rickets

Rickets is a nutritional disease that occurs in children and adolescents. A prolonged deficiency of vitamin D causes osteomalacia (bone softening). Osteomalacia is characterized by weakening of the bones, which can lead to bone fracture. Vitamin D is essential because it promotes the absorption of calcium and phosphorous from the gastrointestinal tract, which is necessary for bone growth and health.

Obesity

body mass index (BMI)
a method that uses height and weight to determine whether a person is at a healthy weight, overweight, or underweight

Obesity is a medical condition in which a person has too much body fat. A **body mass index (BMI)** of 30 or higher indicates obesity. Body mass index is a measure of body fat based on height and weight that applies to adult men and women.

Obesity is one of the leading preventable causes of death worldwide. The rate of obesity in adults and children has increased in the past 20 years. Some authorities view it as one of the most serious public health problems of the 21st century. In the past, obesity was considered a symbol of wealth and fertility, but it is now generally looked down upon, especially in the Western world. In 2013, the American Medical Association classified obesity as a disease.

The causes of obesity include eating more calories than are burned; lack of exercise; unhealthy food choices and eating habits; a genetic predisposition; certain metabolic disorders, such as low thyroid function; and some medications. Being obese increases a person's chance of developing serious health issues such as heart disease, type 2 diabetes, osteoarthritis, and some cancers.

Losing even 5–10 percent of body weight can delay or prevent some of these diseases. To put this into perspective, an individual who weighs 200 pounds would benefit from losing even 10 or 20 pounds.

Think It Through

Twenty years ago, no state in the United States had an obesity rate above 15 percent. According to the Trust for America's Health, there are now 41 states with obesity rates over 25 percent. Since 1980, the rate of obesity in children and adolescents has almost tripled. What do you think has caused this increase in obesity?

Infectious Disease

In chapter 4, you learned about pathogenic microorganisms and the chain of infection. Infection occurs when pathogenic microorganisms enter the body, overcome the body's normal defenses, and multiply to the point that disease occurs. Bacteria, viruses, rickettsiae, protozoa, and fungi are pathogenic microorganisms that can cause disease. Infectious diseases are also called *communicable diseases* because most can be transmitted from one living thing to another. For example, the common cold is spread to others via virus-filled, airborne droplets produced by coughing or sneezing (Figure 7.6).

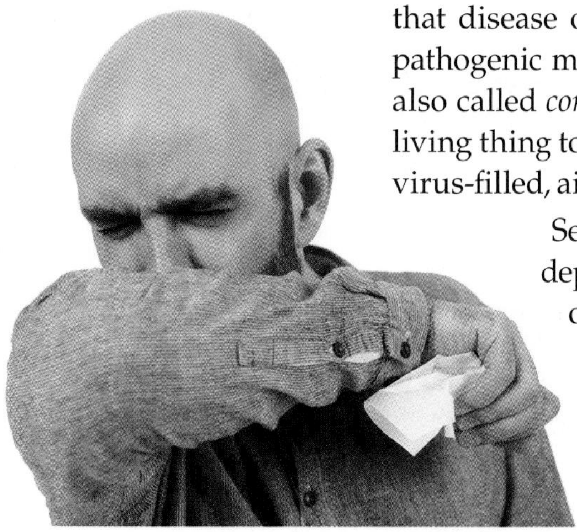

Serious infectious diseases are reported to county and state health departments, who monitor the incidence—or rate of occurrence—of the disease. By monitoring the prevalence of infectious disease, officials can quickly identify epidemics—or widespread growth of the disease. This enables officials to take steps to reduce the disease's impact on the population. Reporting disease cases also alerts officials to new infectious diseases. Organizations such as the National Institute of Allergy and Infectious Diseases (NIAD), the CDC, and WHO collect and share important information about infectious diseases.

kitty/Shutterstock.com

Figure 7.6   Sneezing or coughing into your arm can prevent the spread of communicable diseases.

Extend Your Knowledge ▸ Calculating BMI

Body mass index (BMI) can be used to determine whether a person is at a healthy weight, overweight, or underweight. When a healthcare worker wants to calculate a patient's BMI, he or she must use a specific formula. Different formulas can be used to calculate BMI, depending on whether the English or metric system of measurement is being used. The BMI formulas are as follows:

English system: BMI = weight (in pounds) × 703 ÷ height^2 (in inches)

Metric system: BMI = weight (in kilograms) ÷ height^2 (in meters)

Once you have your BMI calculation, you can determine in which category the patient belongs. A BMI below 18.5 is considered underweight. A BMI from 18.5 to 25 is considered normal or healthy weight. A BMI from 25 to 30 is considered overweight. A BMI of 30 or higher is considered obese.

Because both height and weight are taken into consideration, this is a much more reliable number for determining healthy weight ranges than using weight alone. However, BMI calculations are not perfect. Because muscle and bone weigh more than fat, a particularly muscular patient's BMI may place him or her in the overweight category. Similarly, a patient with an acceptable weight but a higher percentage of body fat than muscle may inaccurately be placed in the healthy range.

Apply It

1. Elizabeth is 1.7 meters tall and weighs 77 kilograms. Calculate her BMI. According to the results, is she underweight, a healthy weight, overweight, or obese?

2. Charlie is 72 inches tall and weighs 155 pounds. Calculate his BMI. According to the results, is he considered underweight, a healthy weight, overweight, or obese?

3. Calculate your BMI. According to the results, where do you fall in the range of underweight to obese?

Hepatitis

Various forms of infectious **hepatitis** are caused by different viruses that affect the liver. Symptoms include fatigue, nausea, poor appetite, belly pain, a mild fever, and yellow skin or eyes (jaundice). There are several types of hepatitis viruses, including the following:

hepatitis
inflammation of the liver

- **Hepatitis A (HAV)** is an acute viral illness that never becomes chronic. The virus can be spread through the ingestion of food or water, especially when food and water is contaminated by human waste (feces) that contains HAV. It is spread among household members and close contacts, often because of poor hand washing. It can also be spread to customers in restaurants and among children in day care centers if hand washing and other sanitary precautions are not observed. Most people who are infected with HAV recover completely and do not experience permanent liver damage. A vaccine is available for HAV.

- **Hepatitis B (HBV)** is spread through contaminated blood by needlesticks and other sharps injuries, intravenous drug use, and sexual contact. Blood transfusions may also spread hepatitis B, but this is rare in the United States because donated blood is screened for diseases, including hepatitis B and C. You can also contract HBV through tattooing, body piercing, and sharing razors if the needles or razors used are contaminated. This serious form of hepatitis can result in severe liver damage and even death. An estimated 6 percent to 10 percent of sufferers with HBV develop chronic HBV infections that last at least six months and often extend to years or decades. These infections leave the infected person at risk for developing liver damage, liver failure, and liver cancer. A vaccine is available for HBV, and it is required for healthcare workers, especially those who work with needles.

- **Hepatitis C (HCV)** is a contagious liver virus that causes symptoms ranging in severity from a mild illness that lasts a few weeks to a serious, lifelong illness that attacks the liver. This virus is spread primarily through contact with the blood of an infected person. HCV can be either acute or chronic. Acute HCV is a short-term illness that occurs within the first six months after someone is exposed to the virus. For most people, acute infection leads to chronic infection. Chronic HCV is a long-term illness that occurs when the HCV remains in a person's body. Hepatitis C can last a lifetime and lead to serious liver problems, including cirrhosis (scarring of the liver) or liver cancer. A vaccine for this virus has not yet been developed.

- **Hepatitis D, E, and G** are also types of viral hepatitis. Hepatitis D (HDV) is also called the *delta virus*. It cannot survive on its own because it requires a protein that HBV makes. It is spread the same way as HBV. Hepatitis E (HEV) is similar to HAV, occurring in Asia and spreading through contaminated water. Hepatitis G (HGV) resembles HCV, but it is not yet recognized as a cause of hepatitis because it is newly discovered.

Treatment of various forms of hepatitis depends on the type and stage of the infection. Treatments for HBV and HCV have advanced over the last several years, and more and improved treatments are being evaluated all the time. Doctors sometimes recommend drug therapy for certain types of hepatitis. Antiviral medications and other treatments have been shown to be effective.

The best way to avoid HBV and HCV is to avoid risky behaviors like sharing intravenous drug needles. You should also observe hand washing and other safety precautions like being careful about food and water contamination. If you stick yourself with a contaminated needle, you must report it immediately to your supervisor (chapter 4), and be sure to get HAV and HBV vaccinations.

Tetanus

Not all infectious diseases are considered communicable. Tetanus is a serious bacterial disease that affects the nervous system, leading to painful muscle contractions, particularly in the jaw and neck muscles. Tetanus can interfere with a person's ability to breathe and ultimately lead to death. Tetanus is commonly known as *lockjaw*. The bacterium that causes tetanus, *Clostridium tetani*, is present in soil and animal feces. Thanks to the tetanus vaccine, cases of tetanus are rare in the United States and the developed world. The incidence of tetanus is much higher in less developed countries. About a million cases occur worldwide each year.

A tetanus bacterial infection (Figure 7.7) may develop after almost any type of skin injury, major or minor, becomes contaminated with the tetanus bacteria. This includes cuts, punctures, burns, and animal bites. In rare cases, a tetanus infection can also occur after an ear infection or a dental infection. Tetanus infections have resulted from heroin injections and can develop after body piercing, tattooing, an insect sting, or even a tiny splinter.

There is no cure for tetanus. Treatment focuses on managing complications until the effects of the tetanus toxin resolve. Fatality is highest in individuals who haven't been immunized, particularly older adults. Booster vaccinations are encouraged every ten years.

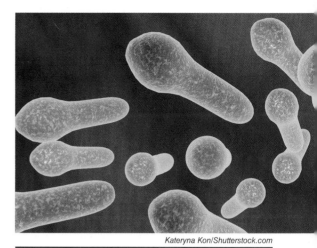
Kateryna Kon/Shutterstock.com

Figure 7.7 The tetanus bacteria (*Clostridium tetani*) can invade your body through a simple cut.

Degenerative Disease

Degenerative diseases, also known as *wear and tear diseases*, are those in which tissues or organs deteriorate over time. This may be due to normal body wear or to lifestyle choices.

Arthritis

Arthritis is a form of joint disorder involving **inflammation** of one or more joints. There are approximately 100 different forms of arthritis. The most common form is *osteoarthritis*, which results from trauma to a joint, an infection, or aging. This degenerative disease causes partial deterioration of the joint cartilage. In some cases, it may also cause abnormal formation of new bone at the joints. Osteoarthritis typically affects the hands, feet, spine, and weight-bearing joints (Figure 7.8). No cure exists for this condition. Staying active, maintaining a healthy weight, and taking certain pain medication can slow the progression of the disease.

Rheumatoid arthritis is an autoimmune disorder that primarily affects joints. It is believed that a combination of genetic and environmental factors causes rheumatoid arthritis. In this condition, the body's immune system attacks the joints, resulting in inflammation and thickening of the joint capsule. It can also affect bone and cartilage. Treatment may include pain medications and steroids to slow the progression of the disease. Surgery to repair and sometimes replace joints can help in certain situations.

inflammation
a localized reaction in which part of the body becomes reddened, swollen, hot, and often painful, especially as a reaction to injury or infection

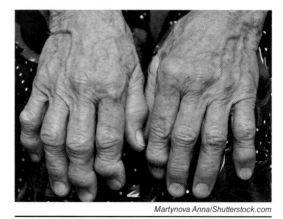
Martynova Anna/Shutterstock.com

Figure 7.8 Arthritis is a painful condition that often affects the hands.

Alzheimer's Disease

dementia
condition characterized by a decrease in mental ability, including loss of memory, impaired judgment, and disorientation

The term **dementia** refers to diseases and conditions characterized by a decline in memory and cognitive abilities that affect a person's ability to perform everyday activities. Alzheimer's disease is the most common form of dementia. This degenerative disease accounts for 50–80 percent of all dementia cases.

Alzheimer's is characterized by confusion; mental deterioration; restlessness, especially near sundown; and the inability to speak and move well. Alzheimer's usually begins at age 65 or older. About 5 percent of cases are called *early onset*, meaning that the disease occurs at a younger age (usually in a person's 40s or 50s).

Alzheimer's disease prevents parts of brain cells from functioning correctly. Two abnormal structures called *plaques* and *tangles* build up inside cells, usually in a predictable pattern. Plaques and tangles can be seen on an MRI scan. The plaques and tangles first develop in areas related to memory before moving to other areas of the brain, destroying nerve cells in their path.

Researchers are working to uncover more details about how Alzheimer's disease develops, how to slow its progression, and how to prevent it altogether. New treatments are rapidly being developed, but there is no cure for this disease.

Trauma

Trauma is any physical injury to the body caused by an accident or violence. Trauma may also be self-inflicted. Blunt force, sharp objects, gunshot wounds, poisons, animal bites or stings, blasts, suffocation, electrical shock, fire, or drowning may all lead to serious changes in the structure and functions of the body systems and, therefore, to traumatic injury.

According to the National Center for Health Statistics (NCHS), traumatic injuries are the leading cause of death for people in the United States under 35 years of age. Motor vehicle accidents and falls are the most common accidents to cause trauma. Safety awareness is an extremely important part of reducing injury and death from trauma.

Check Your Understanding ✓

1. What is body mass index (BMI)?
2. Define the term *communicable disease*.
3. Name three types of hepatitis.
4. What is one example of a degenerative disease?

Leading Causes of Death in the United States

Several diseases are included on the list of the leading causes of death in the United States. This list has remained fairly stable over the last several years, with the included diseases remaining the same. Although some causes on this list are not disease-related, such as accidents and suicide, the diseases that are included are important to understand. As a healthcare worker, these are likely to be the diseases that you encounter the most in your patients.

Heart Disease

Heart disease includes a range of conditions that affect the heart. Conditions in this category include blood vessel diseases (such as coronary artery disease), heart rhythm problems (arrhythmias), and heart defects present at birth (congenital heart defects).

The term *heart disease* is often used interchangeably with the term *cardiovascular disease*. Cardiovascular disease generally refers to conditions that involve narrowed or blocked blood vessels, which can lead to a heart attack, chest pain (angina), or stroke. Other heart conditions, such as those that affect the heart's muscle, valves, or rhythm, also are considered forms of heart disease. Many forms of heart disease can be prevented or treated with healthy lifestyle choices.

Atherosclerosis

Atherosclerosis is the term for the buildup of plaque in the arteries, the most common cause of heart disease (Figure 7.9). This plaque is composed of fats, cholesterol, triglycerides, calcium, and other substances found in the blood.

atherosclerosis
buildup of plaque on the inner lining of an arterial wall over time that causes the arteries to harden and may lead to a myocardial infarction

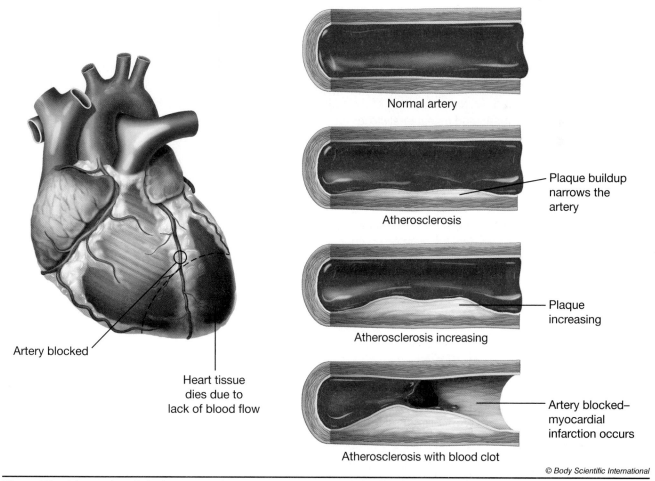

© Body Scientific International

Figure 7.9   Atherosclerosis is the process by which plaque builds in the arteries, eventually causing the artery to harden or become completely blocked. This can lead to the development of a myocardial infarction.

Over time, atherosclerosis causes a hardening of the arteries. Hardened plaque can block an artery, preventing the flow of blood to the heart, brain, kidneys, and other organs. Pieces of unstable plaque may also break loose from the wall of an artery, becoming circulating clots, or *thrombi*. A thrombus can plug another distant artery, potentially causing a sudden event such as a **myocardial infarction** (also known as a *heart attack*) or cerebral vascular accident (CVA), commonly called a *stroke*.

myocardial infarction
heart attack

The key to preventing death from heart disease is to protect the heart and know the warning signs and symptoms of a heart attack. These major signs and symptoms include chest pain or discomfort; pain or discomfort in the upper body, arms, neck, jaw, or upper stomach; breathlessness; nausea; lightheadedness; and cold sweat.

Lowering the Risk for Heart Disease

Lowering your blood pressure and cholesterol can significantly lower your risk of heart disease. This can be achieved by eating a diet that is low in salt, refined sugars, total fat, saturated fat, and cholesterol, but high in fruits and vegetables. You should also avoid smoking and excessive alcohol consumption. Reducing your stress and exercising regularly can also help.

Extend Your Knowledge ▶ Blood Pressure, Hypertension, and Heart Disease

Blood pressure is the force of blood pushing against the walls of the arteries as the heart pumps blood.

Blood pressure is measured as either *systolic* or *diastolic*. Systolic blood pressure is the highest pressure in the arteries and results when the heart muscle contracts and pumps blood out to the body. Diastolic blood pressure is measured when the heart is at rest, filling with blood.

Blood pressure measurements are written with the systolic number above the line and the diastolic number below the line: $^{120}/_{80}$ millimeters of mercury (mmHg).

Prolonged periods of elevated blood pressure can damage the body, leading to a condition called *hypertension*. High blood pressure ($^{140}/_{90}$ is considered above normal) can lead to coronary artery disease, stroke, and kidney damage. People with high blood pressure can control it by living a healthy lifestyle and with medication.

Apply It

1. Why do you think patients with high blood pressure are encouraged to restrict their salt intake? Research to find the answer.

2. Name four lifestyle changes patients can make to lower their blood pressure.

Cancer

cancer
uncontrolled cell growth

neoplasm
a tumor; can be either malignant or benign

Cancer is a disease that occurs when an abnormal growth of cells multiplies rapidly in the body. A **neoplasm** is a tumor that can be either malignant (cancerous) or benign (harmless). Cancer can occur in any part of the body and at any age, and there is a variety of causes.

While a normal human cell replicates itself exactly, stops reproducing when appropriate, and matures, a cancerous cell cannot do these things.

Some unknown glitch in cancerous cells overrides the normal system of replication, maturation, and death. A cancer cell does not stop reproducing, nor is the body able to destroy these cells on its own (Figure 7.10). As a result, the high numbers of cancerous cells damage the part of the body where the cancer is growing.

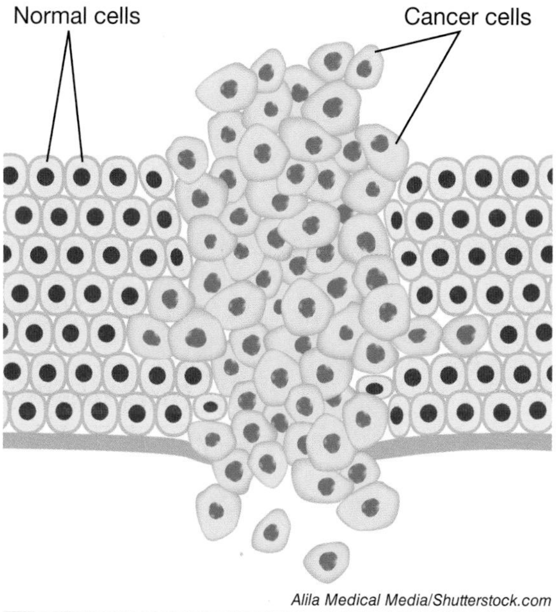

Metastasis

Another unique quality of cancerous cells is their ability to move throughout the body. Normal cells stay together as they grow, keeping the cells in the correct location. Cancer cells, however, can lose the ability to stick together. As a result, cancerous cells may break off the primary tumor and spread throughout the body via the bloodstream. This process, called **metastasis**, allows new, or secondary, cancerous tumors to form in other areas of the body.

Normal cells   Cancer cells

Alila Medical Media/Shutterstock.com

Figure 7.10   Cancer cells in a growing tumor

Common Cancers

Many types of cancer are diagnosed each year, with over 200 types identified. Cancer is a broad term that encompasses a number of **malignant** diseases. Each cancer has its own unique set of possible causes, symptoms, and treatment regimens. Early detection plays a key role in successful cancer treatment.

According to the American Cancer Society, the most common types of cancer are

1. non-melanoma skin cancers;

2. lung cancer;

3. breast cancer;

4. prostate cancer; and

5. colorectal cancer.

metastasis
the spread of cancerous cells from their place of origin to other parts of the body via the bloodstream

malignant
term that describes a life-threatening tumor; also known as cancerous

Signs and Symptoms of Cancer

The American Cancer Society provides a list of the seven warning signs and symptoms of cancer. These signs and symptoms can be remembered by using the acronym **CAUTION**:

1. **Change** in bowel or bladder habits

2. **A sore** that does not heal

3. **Unusual** bleeding or discharge

4. **Thickening** or lump in the breast, testicles, or elsewhere

5. **Indigestion** or difficulty swallowing

6. **Obvious change** in the size, color, shape, or thickness of wart, mole, or mouth sore

7. **Nagging cough** or hoarseness

Other signs and symptoms that should be investigated include

1. white patches in the mouth or white spots on the tongue;

2. unexplained weight loss;

3. fever;

4. fatigue;

5. pain; or

6. skin changes.

Check Your Understanding ✓

1. The text divides heart disease into what three categories?
2. What is another term for chest pain?
3. What disease causes the arteries to harden?
4. How are fruits and vegetables related to heart disease?
5. Name at least two ways in which a normal cell differs from a cancerous cell.
6. What is the term for cancer cells spreading throughout the body?
7. What are the five most common types of cancer?

Treatment for and Prevention of Cancer

There are many different kinds of treatment for cancer. The most common types include surgery, chemotherapy, and radiation. Surgery is often the first option if the tumor can be taken out of the body. Sometimes only part of the tumor can be removed. In that case, radiation, chemotherapy, or both may be used to shrink the tumor before and after surgery.

Doctors may use **chemotherapy** to kill cancer cells (Figure 7.11). The necessary drugs are given through intravenous injection or taken by mouth.

chemotherapy
treatment of a disease with chemical agents

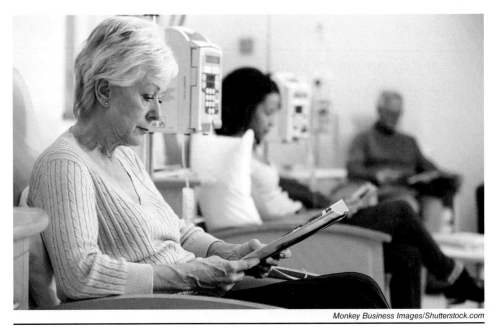

Monkey Business Images/Shutterstock.com

Figure 7.11   Chemotherapy uses drugs to kill cancer cells.

Radiation therapy uses high-energy rays (like X-rays) to kill cancer cells and shrink tumors. The radiation can come from outside the body or from radioactive materials inserted in the tumor. Other cancer treatments include hormone therapy, targeted therapy, immunotherapy, bone marrow transplant, and stem cell transplant. Targeted therapy is a treatment that targets only the cancer cells and causes less damage to normal, healthy cells. Immunotherapy is designed to boost the cancer patient's own immune system to help fight the cancer.

About one-third of all cancer cases are preventable. Certain cancers can be prevented by quitting smoking and reducing alcohol consumption. Other cancers caused by being overweight, obese, or inactive, or having poor nutrition can be prevented through lifestyle changes. Some cancers are related to infectious agents such as human papillomavirus (HPV), hepatitis B (HBV), hepatitis C (HCV), human immunodeficiency virus (HIV), and *Helicobacter pylori* (H. pylori). These may be prevented through behavioral changes and vaccinations.

Many of the more than 3 million skin cancer cases that are diagnosed each year could be prevented by avoiding excessive sun exposure and indoor tanning. Air, water, and soil pollution accounts for 1–4 percent of all cancers. Avoiding exposure to harmful carcinogenic chemicals that might be in drinking water or the air can help prevent these cancers.

Extend Your Knowledge ▶ Transplant Treatment

Bone marrow transplants save thousands of lives each year. Because bone marrow produces blood cells, leukemia (a cancer of the blood) and some lymphomas (cancer of the lymphatic system) can be treated with a bone marrow transplant. Healthy bone marrow is also used to treat several types of bone marrow diseases. Without treatment, both of these diseases can result in death.

The transplantation process begins with large doses of chemotherapy or radiation to destroy the abnormal stem cells in the bone marrow. Healthy marrow is then infused into the patient's bloodstream. If successful, the new bone marrow migrates to the cavities of the large bones, and begins producing normal blood cells.

The donated bone marrow must match the genetic makeup of the patient's own marrow as perfectly as possible. Today, many people are waiting for a bone marrow transplant because a suitable donor cannot be found. Bone marrow registries exist to test potential donors' bone marrow for compatibility with a patient awaiting transplant.

Apply It

1. Research how someone could become a bone marrow donor.

2. Where is bone marrow located in the human body?

3. Research to determine the ideal age range for bone marrow donation.

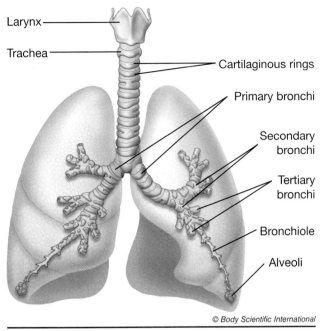

Larynx

Trachea

Cartilaginous rings

Primary bronchi

Secondary bronchi

Tertiary bronchi

Bronchiole

Alveoli

© Body Scientific International

Figure 7.12 Anatomy of a lung

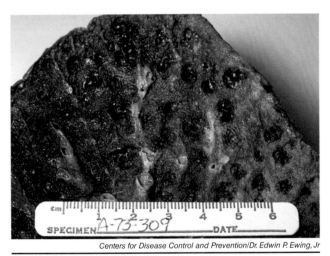

Centers for Disease Control and Prevention/Dr. Edwin P. Ewing, Jr

Figure 7.13 Lung of a smoker with emphysema

Colorectal and cervical cancers can be prevented through screenings that allow for detection and removal of pre-cancerous lesions. Screening also offers the opportunity for secondary prevention by detecting cancer early, before symptoms appear. Early detection usually results in better outcomes and less of a need for extensive, invasive treatment. Some early detection can be done personally through examinations of the breasts, skin, and testicles. Unfortunately, cancer can develop even if a person takes steps toward prevention. In all cases, early detection is the key to the best outcome.

Chronic Lower Respiratory Disease

Chronic lower respiratory disease (CLRD) is a group of lung diseases that cause airflow blockage and breathing-related issues in various parts of the lung (Figure 7.12). CLRD includes diseases such as chronic obstructive pulmonary disease (COPD), bronchitis, emphysema, and asthma. Smoking causes complications for all chronic lower respiratory diseases, especially emphysema (Figure 7.13). Signs and symptoms of CLRD may include difficulty breathing, especially when active; a persistent cough with phlegm; and frequent chest infections.

Recent developments in the treatment of lung disease include inhaled drug treatments for airflow obstruction. In addition, doctors are treating CLRD's related problems earlier in their diagnoses. Quitting smoking and avoiding triggers such as air pollution can slow the progress of CLRD. Oxygen treatments can be administered through a face mask or a small tube that fits in the nose. Surgery is only considered for people with severe COPD that has not improved with other treatment. Patients are encouraged to increase their overall health with regular activity, if possible.

Stroke

stroke

a medical emergency in which blood flow to a part of the brain is cut off

A **stroke**, also known as a *cerebral vascular accident*, is a medical emergency that occurs when blood flow to the brain stops. There are two different types of stroke, an *ischemic stroke* and a *hemorrhagic stroke*. In an ischemic stroke, one of the arteries of the brain is blocked. In a hemorrhagic stroke, an artery in the brain ruptures, causing bleeding in the brain. Within minutes, the brain is deprived of oxygen, causing many problems, including death.

Risk factors for stroke include a family history, high blood pressure, diabetes, and high cholesterol. Excessive alcohol consumption, illegal drug use, obesity, and physical inactivity also increase risk of stroke.

After a stroke, a person might experience paralysis, loss of speech, problems walking, uncontrolled emotional outbursts, depression, or coma. These effects may be temporary if a person experiences a *transient ischemic attack* (TIA), in which there is only a temporary lack of blood flow to the brain. In this case, stroke effects can disappear within one or two hours. However, a more serious stroke can occur following a TIA, and steps for prevention should be taken.

A stroke can be prevented by controlling high blood pressure, lowering cholesterol levels, and quitting smoking. As with all other dangerous diseases, prevention also includes eating a healthy diet, maintaining a healthy weight, getting exercise, lowering alcohol intake, and managing other conditions.

Treatments for a stroke include dissolving the clot with a medication that improves blood flow. This medication must be administered within three hours of the patient's stroke to improve the chances of recovery. Sometimes a surgeon will remove a large blood clot by threading a catheter through an artery in the groin to the blocked artery in the brain. This procedure must be done within six hours of the stroke. The key to minimizing the damage of a stroke is to act immediately when you see or experience signs of a stroke. Call an ambulance so that healthcare workers can start treatment immediately.

Did You Know? **Identifying a Stroke**

The signs of a stroke are easy to identify if you remember the F.A.S.T. tip developed by Methodist Health Systems.

F—Face   Is one side drooping?

A—Arms   Is one arm weak or numb?

S—Speech   Is speech slurred?

T—Time   Time is critical. Call 911 or get to a hospital quickly.

Diabetes (Diabetes Mellitus)

Diabetes mellitus is a disease in which the body is no longer able to carefully control blood glucose, leading to abnormally high levels of blood glucose (hyperglycemia). If levels of blood glucose are elevated for a long period of time, the body's nerves, blood vessels, and tissues in the eyes may become damaged. Most of the food we eat is turned into a simple sugar (glucose) that the body converts into energy. The pancreas, an organ situated near the stomach, makes a hormone called *insulin* that helps glucose get into body cells. Sugar builds up in the blood if the body doesn't have enough insulin, or if it cannot use insulin as it should.

diabetes mellitus
a disease caused by insufficient utilization of insulin resulting in an increased amount of glucose in the blood and urine

Symptoms of diabetes can include the following:

- frequent urination
- excessive thirst
- unexplained weight loss
- extreme hunger
- sudden vision changes
- tingling or numbness in hands or feet
- feeling very tired most of the time
- very dry skin
- sores that heal slowly
- more infections than usual

There are two types of diabetes mellitus. Type 1 diabetes is an autoimmune condition in which the immune system attacks the insulin-producing cells in the pancreas. Researchers are attempting to determine the genes and other factors that cause type 1 diabetes. There is no method of prevention for type 1 diabetes.

Type 2 diabetes, which was previously called *non-insulin-dependent diabetes mellitus* or *adult-onset diabetes*, accounts for about 90–95 percent of all diagnosed cases of diabetes. Type 2 diabetes results from the body's improper use of insulin. Over time, the pancreas can't make enough insulin to keep the body's blood glucose levels normal. This type of diabetes can be treated through healthy eating and an active lifestyle. In addition, oral medications or insulin may be ordered by a doctor. Although medications may not be used at first, they will likely be needed later on because type 2 diabetes typically worsens over time.

Both types of diabetes, but especially type 1, can require continual blood tests to monitor blood glucose levels (Figure 7.14). These tests are done with devices that extract a drop of blood and calculate its glucose level. Eating healthy foods, getting exercise, and losing excess weight can help prevent type 2 diabetes or reduce blood glucose levels.

Influenza and Pneumonia

Influenza (flu) is a highly contagious viral infection that is one of the most serious illnesses of the winter season. A person can have the flu more than once because the

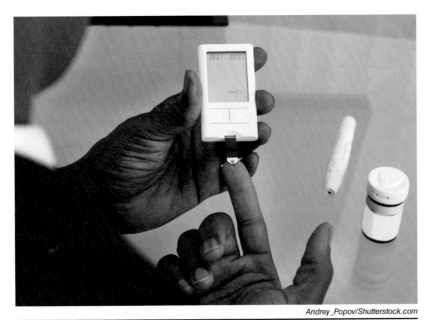

Figure 7.14 People with type 1 diabetes usually have to monitor their blood glucose level using a glucometer, which takes a sample of blood and measures its glucose level.

disease may belong to different strains of viruses. Signs and symptoms of influenza include

- fever;
- headache;
- cough;
- chills;
- sore throat;
- nasal congestion;
- muscle aches;
- loss of appetite; and
- malaise (a general feeling of discomfort).

A serious case of the flu can lead to inflammation of the lungs, which is called *pneumonia*. In this condition, the air sacs of the lungs fill with pus and other liquid, preventing oxygen from reaching the blood. Pneumonia has over 30 different potential causes, including chemicals, bacteria, viruses, and other infectious agents. Signs and symptoms of pneumonia include

- fever;
- wheezing;
- cough;
- chills;
- rapid breathing;
- chest pains;
- loss of appetite;
- malaise; and
- feeling of weakness or ill health.

Vaccinations against flu are available every year. There are also vaccinations against a type of pneumonia called *pneumococcal pneumonia* and *Hemophilus influenza* (given to children). The best way to prevent influenza is to receive a yearly vaccination, wash your hands frequently, quit smoking, eat a healthy diet, and get regular exercise. There are drugs to prevent or lessen the effects of pneumonia and the flu. In addition to these medications, rest and plenty of fluids are important to flu treatment.

Kidney Disease

Chronic kidney disease (CKD) is a condition in which the kidneys are damaged and can't filter blood as well as healthy kidneys. In this condition, waste from the blood remains in the body and can cause other health problems. Kidney disease is most common among adults older than 70 years.

Diabetes and high blood pressure are the most common causes of chronic kidney disease. Common causes of kidney injury include a traumatic injury with blood loss, dehydration (lack of water), severe infection, obstruction of urine flow, and damage from certain drugs or toxins.

Signs and symptoms of kidney disease include appetite loss, a general feeling of fatigue, headaches, itchy and dry skin, nausea, and weight loss. When kidney disease becomes severe, symptoms include the following:

- abnormally dark or light skin
- bone pain
- drowsiness or problems concentrating or thinking
- numbness or swelling in the hands and feet
- muscle twitching or cramps
- breath odor
- easy bruising, or blood in the stool
- excessive thirst
- menstrual periods stop (amenorrhea)
- shortness of breath
- sleep problems
- vomiting, often in the morning

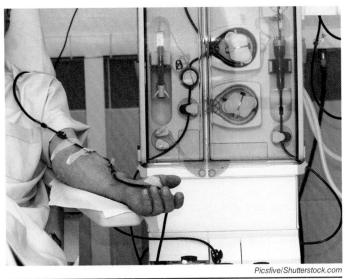

Picsfive/Shutterstock.com

Figure 7.15 Dialysis machines filter the blood when the kidneys can no longer function.

Treatment for kidney disease includes medication to treat high blood pressure and lower cholesterol that builds up with kidney disease. In addition, a diet lower in salt and protein can minimize waste products in the blood. If the damage done to the kidney cannot be controlled and kidney failure occurs, there are two options: a *kidney transplant* and *dialysis* (Figure 7.15). In dialysis, a machine removes waste products and extra fluid from your blood when the kidneys can no longer perform that function.

Kidney disease can be prevented by managing blood pressure, avoiding alcohol and illegal drugs, and taking medication prescribed by a doctor as directed. Certain antibiotics can be dangerous if they are not taken correctly. Additionally, avoiding type 2 diabetes can help prevent kidney disease.

Check Your Understanding ✓

1. Name two breathing-related issues caused by chronic lower respiratory disease.
2. What condition occurs when an artery in the brain bursts?
3. What are three symptoms of diabetes?
4. Will annual flu vaccinations reduce a person's chances of getting influenza?
5. Name three symptoms of severe kidney disease.

Medical Specialties

Because the medical field is so complicated, and there are so many diseases and disorders, doctors often develop a specialty to narrow their focus to a particular body system. This enables them to better treat their patients. **Medical specialties** are often defined by the body system to which they are connected (Figure 7.16).

Healthcare practices that are not directly related to a body system, but nevertheless have a specialty focus, include the following:

- dentistry (dentist): the study and treatment of the teeth and gums
- geriatrics/gerontology (geriatrician): the study and treatment of the elderly
- dietetics (dietician): the study and use of nutrition, nutrients, and diet
- epidemiology (epidemiologist): the study of disease, disease-causing factors, and other public health problems, in an effort to prevent their occurrence or spread
- neonatology (neonatologist): the study and treatment of newborns
- oncology (oncologist): the study and treatment of cancer
- pediatrics (pediatrician): the study and treatment of infants and children
- pharmacology (pharmacologist): the study and use of drugs as medicines
- psychiatry (psychiatrist): the study and treatment of the mind
- radiology and nuclear medicine (radiologist): the use of X-rays, sound waves, and other forms of radiation and energy to diagnose and treat disease

medical specialties
specific areas of medicine that are often named according to a body system

Medical Specialties	
Body System	*Specialty*
integumentary system	dermatologist
musculoskeletal system	orthopedist; orthopedic surgeon
nervous and sensory systems	neurologist; neurosurgeon; otolaryngologist (ENT doctor); ophthalmologist
endocrine system	endocrinologist
respiratory system	pulmonologist
cardiovascular system	cardiologist; cardiac surgeon; hematologist
lymphatic and immune system	immunologist; internist; hematologist
gastrointestinal system	gastroenterologist
urinary system	urologist; nephrologist
reproductive system	obstetrician and gynecologist (OB/GYN); embryologist; urologist

Goodheart-Willcox Publisher

Figure 7.16 Medical specialties by body system

Emerging Diseases and Disorders

According to the World Health Organization, an emerging disease or disorder is one that has appeared in a population for the first time, or which may have existed previously but is now rapidly increasing in incidence or geographic range. These diseases and disorders are becoming more prevalent and, as a healthcare worker, you will likely encounter them during your career.

Autism

autism
mental condition present from early childhood, most often characterized by difficulty communicating, forming relationships, using language, and understanding abstract concepts

Autism is a mental condition that is present from early childhood. This condition is characterized by difficulty in communicating and forming relationships, as well as difficulties with language and abstract concepts. Autism seems to have its roots in early brain development that occurs between the ages of two and three. The prevalence of autism has increased up to 17 percent annually in recent years. This increase is likely a result of improved diagnoses and environmental influences. Autism is four or five times more common in boys than girls. Today, autism is more commonly referred to as *autism spectrum disorder*.

There are many types of autism and many different causes associated with the condition. Scientists have identified several rare gene mutations that may cause autism. Factors that increase a child's risk include advanced parent age at time of conception (both mother and father), maternal illness during pregnancy, and difficulties at birth, particularly periods of oxygen deprivation. Some scientists believe these environmental factors don't cause autism on their own, but increase the risk when combined with genetic factors.

Each person with autism is considered unique, so each patient's treatment plan should be tailored to address specific needs. Treatment can include medication and behavior modification by professionals. Additional medical conditions, such as sleep disturbance, seizures, and gastrointestinal distress, should be addressed as well. Early behavioral intervention involves the child's entire family and a team of professionals, including therapists who come into the home.

Drug-Resistant Bacteria

drug-resistant bacteria
strains of a bacterium that have adapted and are no longer controlled or killed by normal antibiotic treatment

In recent years, the overuse of antibiotics has resulted in strains of bacteria that have developed the ability to resist normal antibiotic treatment. These **drug-resistant bacteria** are created when a doctor doesn't include accurate instructions with an antibiotic prescription, or when a patient does not take all of the pills in an antibiotic treatment. For years, antibiotics have been prescribed for colds, flu, and other viral infections that don't respond to these drugs. Even when antibiotics are used appropriately, they contribute to the rise of drug-resistant bacteria because they don't destroy every germ they target. Bacteria live on an evolutionary fast track, so germs that survive treatment from one antibiotic soon learn to resist others.

The *Staphylococcus* bacterium exists in many forms. *Staphylococcus aureus* is one of the most common causes of hospital-related infections. This bacterium can cause anything from a pimple to a serious blood infection that can lead to organ failure and death. *Staphylococcus aureus* has become resistant to a growing number of antibiotics typically used to treat it. Examples of drug-resistant *Staphylococcus* include vancomycin-resistant *Staphylococcus aureus* (VRSA) and methicillin-resistant *Staphylococcus aureus* (MRSA). These drug-resistant bacteria are no longer controlled or killed by normal antibiotic treatment.

Being hospitalized can put a person at risk of contracting MRSA or VRSA, especially if the person is an elderly patient or has a weakened immune system. Having an invasive medical device such as an intravenous line (IV) or urinary catheter can provide a pathway for these bacteria to travel into the body. In addition, residing in a long-term care facility can increase the spread of these drug-resistant bacteria.

Tuberculosis is a very serious bacterial infection that most commonly affects the lungs. Before the development of antibiotics, tuberculosis was almost always fatal. There are now two forms of drug-resistant tuberculosis: *multidrug-resistant TB* (MDR TB) and *extensively drug-resistant TB* (XDR TB). MDR TB cannot be killed by the two main medications used to treat tuberculosis, known as the *first-line medications*. However, there are second-line medications that can successfully treat MDR TB. The XDR TB bacterium is resistant to the first-line group of drugs developed to treat tuberculosis and one of the three second-line medications.

Post-Traumatic Stress Disorder (PTSD)

As soldiers return from combat overseas and more research is done, cases of **post-traumatic stress disorder (PTSD)** have increased. PTSD is a psychiatric disorder that can occur as a result of experiencing or witnessing life-threatening events, such as military combat (Figure 7.17), natural disasters, terrorist incidents, serious accidents, and physical or sexual assault. Most survivors of trauma return to normal after time to recover. However, some people have stress reactions that do not go away on their own, or even worsen over time. These individuals may develop PTSD.

post-traumatic stress disorder (PTSD)
an anxiety disorder that may develop after exposure to a terrifying event or ordeal in which severe physical harm occurred or was threatened

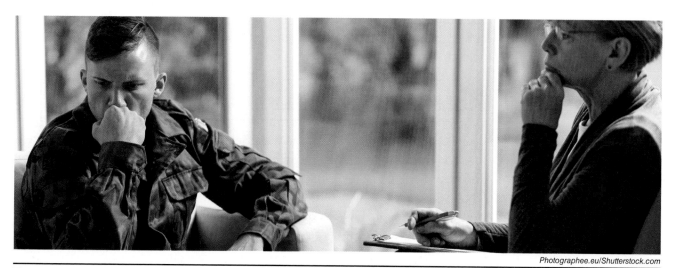

Photographee.eu/Shutterstock.com

Figure 7.17 Talk therapy can be helpful for some people with post-traumatic stress disorder.

People who suffer from PTSD often relive their traumatic experience through nightmares and flashbacks, have difficulty sleeping, and feel detached or estranged. These symptoms can be severe enough and last long enough to significantly impair a person's daily life.

People who have PTSD experience three different kinds of symptoms. The first set of symptoms involves reliving the trauma in some way, such as becoming upset when confronted with a traumatic reminder or thinking about the trauma when trying to do something else. The second set of symptoms involves staying away from places or people that serve as a reminder of the trauma, avoiding other people, or feeling numb. The third set of symptoms includes feeling on guard, irritable, or startling easily.

PTSD can be treated with counseling and psychotherapy, also known as *talk therapy*, and medication such as antidepressants. Early treatment is important and may help reduce long-term symptoms. Unfortunately, many people do not know they have PTSD or do not seek treatment.

Listeriosis

Listeriosis, commonly called *listeria*, is an infection caused by eating *Listeria monocytogenes* bacteria. In recent years, listeria has been responsible for dozens of food product recalls, numerous hospital visits, and even several deaths. Listeria lives naturally in soil and water, which can lead to contamination of vegetables that grow in the ground. Meat from animals contaminated by other animals that carry listeria but don't show any symptoms can also spread listeriosis, especially if the meat isn't properly cooked. Unpasteurized milk is also a common carrier of the bacteria.

Symptoms of listeria include headache, fever, chills, upset stomach, and vomiting. A blood test is the most common way of diagnosing listeriosis. Prevention methods include washing fruits and vegetables with a clean brush for 20 seconds, properly cooking milk, and drinking only pasteurized milk. You should also take care not to use the same knife or cutting board for vegetables after using them to cut meat.

In many cases, those infected with listeria will simply need to let their immune systems fight through the disease. Those with more severe cases, newborns, and those who are pregnant are often prescribed antibiotics to help combat the infection.

Biotechnology Research to Fight Disease

Biotechnology is a large scientific field that uses advances in life science to study or solve problems, including human disease prevention, pathology, and treatment. Chapter 1 discusses *geonomic medicine*, the study of a person's DNA sequences, which tells scientists the kind of genetic information carried in a particular DNA sequence. DNA has become the building block for research tools and diagnostic tests.

Gene Therapies

Researchers are working to develop gene therapies to treat and hopefully cure genetic diseases. Several inherited immune deficiencies have been treated successfully with gene therapy. Gene therapies are being developed to treat different types of inherited blindness, and several promising treatments for cancer are under development. One gene therapy, consisting of a modified version of the herpes simplex 1 virus, has proved effective against melanoma that has spread throughout the body.

Today, researchers are conducting clinical trials to ensure that any gene therapy brought into the clinic is both safe and effective. With the possibility of eliminating and preventing hereditary diseases such as cystic fibrosis and hemophilia, and the capability for curing heart disease, AIDS, and cancer, gene therapy has great potential.

Human Proteomics

Proteomics is a branch of biotechnology that uses techniques from molecular biology, biochemistry, and genetics to analyze the structure, function, and interactions of the proteins produced by the genes of a particular cell, tissue, or organism. Organizing this information into a database will create a resource to advance the diagnosis and treatment of diseases.

proteomics
field of biotechnology concerned with analyzing the structure, function, and interactions of the proteins produced by the genes of a particular cell, tissue, or organism

Cloning

The term *cloning* describes the processes used to create an exact genetic replica of a cell, tissue, or organism. The copied material, which has the same genetic makeup as the original, is referred to as a *clone*. The most famous clone was a Scottish sheep named Dolly. The three types of cloning are gene cloning, which creates copies of genes or segments of DNA; reproductive cloning, which creates copies of whole animals; and therapeutic cloning, which creates embryonic stem cells. Researchers hope to use cloned cells to grow healthy tissue that can replace injured or diseased tissues in the human body.

Did You Know?   Dolly Makes History

In 1996, scientists in Scotland successfully cloned the first mammal—a sheep named Dolly. The donor cell was taken from a mammary gland of Dolly's mother. Therefore, Dolly became the clone of her mother. The successful birth of a healthy clone proved that a cell taken from a specific part of the body could recreate the whole individual. Today, even more animals have been cloned. In fact, a few companies offer the service of cloning a beloved pet.

The conversation surrounding cloning typically prompts questions about whether human cloning is possible or ethical. Only one or two out of a hundred reproductive cloning attempts are successful. Nearly a third of the animals that are born through this process suffer from rare but serious conditions, and many do not live long. The possibility of putting a human life at such risk is considered immoral by many people. Both the American Medical Association and the American Association for the Advancement of Science have urged a ban on human cloning. There is not yet a federal law in place to control the practice. Public opinion is solidly against human cloning.

Stem Cell Research

Stem cells have the remarkable potential to develop into many different cell types in the body during early life and growth. In addition, these cells serve as a form of internal repair system for many tissues, dividing essentially without limit to replenish other cells as long as the person or animal is still alive. When a stem cell divides, each new cell has the potential to either remain a stem cell or become another type of cell with a more specialized function, such as a muscle cell, red blood cell, or brain cell.

All of the organs and tissues in the human body develop from stem cells. Healthy stem cells may be used to generate new tissues, such as skin, for transplant. Scientists hope to use stem cells to develop cellular-level treatments for many diseases and conditions, such as heart disease, diabetes, or degenerative nerve conditions (Figure 7.18).

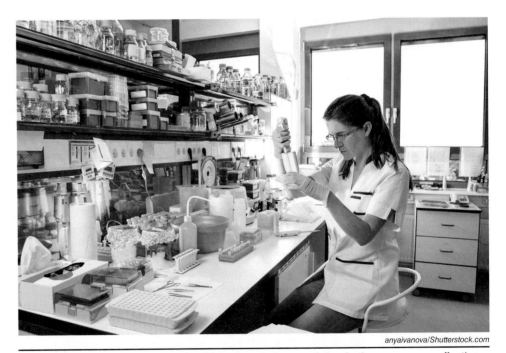

anyaivanova/Shutterstock.com

Figure 7.18 Stem cell research is widely done in hopes of developing new, more effective medical treatments.

As with cloning, there is controversy surrounding stem cells. Originally, stem cell research used embryonic cells left over from in vitro fertilization and abortion. President George W. Bush issued a partial ban on federal funding of stem cell research that used embryos. Today, adult stem cells may be more promising than embryonic stem cells. Much work is still needed before stem cell treatments are successfully developed.

Global Disease Prevention and Cost Containment

It should be obvious after studying this chapter that many, if not most, serious diseases can be avoided by the practice of preventive medicine. Trillions of dollars used to treat disease all over the world could instead be used to prevent such diseases. Diseases make it difficult or impossible for those who have them to work and earn money for their families. Massive disease outbreaks obviously disrupt the economy of affected areas.

Preventing illness is always more cost-effective than treating illness. Some preventive methods include patient education, immunizations, regular physical examinations to detect problems early, and easy access to healthcare services. Patient education is particularly important in terms of encouraging healthy eating, exercise, getting enough sleep, losing weight, and avoiding smoking and excessive drinking.

Other ways of reducing the costs of healthcare include the following:

- avoid duplication of services in healthcare facilities located in close proximity to each other
- have healthcare facilities come together to share specific services
- order supplies and equipment in larger quantities at reduced prices
- perform energy conservation to avoid major electricity, water, and gas expenses

Check Your Understanding ✓

1. What is the more commonly used term for autism?
2. Name one type of drug-resistant bacteria prevalent today.
3. Why have cases of PTSD increased in recent years?
4. Name two conditions that gene therapy might help to treat.
5. What unique characteristic of stem cells makes them so important?

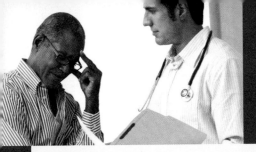

Summary

It is important to familiarize yourself with common diseases and disorders. Understanding the classifications of disease by cause, which include hereditary, congenital, environmental, nutritional, infectious, degenerative, or trauma-related, is helpful. Heart disease is the number one cause of death in the United States. Chronic lower respiratory disease, stroke, diabetes mellitus, influenza and pneumonia, and kidney disease are some of the other leading causes of death in the United States. Cancer is a prevalent disease that can affect all parts of the body. Early detection through recognition of the signs and symptoms of cancer is a key factor in successful treatment.

Because of the vast amount of information in the medical field, many doctors choose to develop a specialty in medicine to better treat conditions and diseases. According to the World Health Organization, several emerging diseases are rapidly increasing throughout the world. Some of these diseases include autism, drug-resistant bacteria, post-traumatic stress disorder (PTSD), and listeriosis. Biotechnology is rapidly making great progress in prevention of many diseases through methods such as stem cell research and gene therapies. While treating these diseases costs millions of dollars each year, cost containment methods are being developed.

Review Questions

Answer the following questions using what you have learned in this chapter.

True or False 📤 Assess

1. *True or False?* An epidemic is a disease that spreads rapidly and affects a large number of people.

2. *True or False?* A common way to classify disease is by cause.

3. *True or False?* Sickle cell anemia is an environmental disease.

4. *True or False?* Communicable diseases are transmitted from person to person.

5. *True or False?* Tetanus is caused by a virus.

6. *True or False?* Black lung disease is an example of an environmental disease.

7. *True or False?* Type 2 diabetes is exclusively treated with insulin injections.

8. *True or False?* Oncologists study and treat cancer.

9. *True or False?* A syndrome is a collection of symptoms.

10. *True or False?* Skin cancer is a congenital disease.

Multiple Choice 📤 Assess

11. The red blood cells of patients with sickle cell anemia take on a(n) _____ shape.
    A. oblong
    B. crescent
    C. rectangular
    D. heart

12. The American Cancer Society lists the seven warning signs of cancer. Which of the following is *not* included in that list?
    A. acne
    B. nagging cough or hoarseness
    C. a sore that does not heal
    D. unusual bleeding or discharge

13. The following treatments are routinely used for treating cancer *except* _____.
    A. chemotherapy
    B. radiation
    C. surgery
    D. cough medicine

14. A(n) _____ is a specialist in nervous system diseases.
    A. nephrologist
    B. endocrinologist
    C. orthopedist
    D. neurologist

15. Which of the following can put you at risk for a stroke?
    A. high blood pressure
    B. obesity
    C. high cholesterol
    D. All of the above.

16. _____ is an autoimmune condition in which the body's immune system attacks the insulin-producing cells in the pancreas.
    A. Type 1 heart disease
    B. Type 2 diabetes mellitus
    C. Pancreatic cancer
    D. Type 1 diabetes mellitus

17. The term *metastasis* means _____.
    A. a stroke
    B. the spread of cancer throughout the body
    C. progressive dementia
    D. type 2 diabetes

18. Which of the following is considered an emerging disease or disorder?
    A. heart disease
    B. post-traumatic stress disorder
    C. Alzheimer's disease
    D. tetanus

19. Which of the following is an example of drug-resistant bacteria?
    A. MRSA
    B. XDR TB
    C. VRSA
    D. All of the above.

20. Which of the following definitions best describes COPD?
    A. a lung disease
    B. a form of cancer
    C. dementia
    D. a heart valve problem

21. A traumatic injury, resulting in serious changes in body structure and function, could result from which of the following?
    A. gunshot wounds
    B. fires
    C. blunt force
    D. All of the above.

Short Answer

22. What causes cerebral palsy?
23. What are the different kinds of skin cancer?
24. What are the causes of obesity?
25. What does atherosclerosis mean?
26. Name two types of arthritis.
27. Define blood pressure.
28. Name four steps you can take to reduce your risk of heart disease.
29. Identify three types of diagnostic tests.
30. What is a congenital disease?
31. Identify the differences between hepatitis A, B, and C.

Critical Thinking Exercises

32. What kinds of cancers are predominant in your area? Where would you find that information?

33. Research a specific type of cancer online. Explain the causes, diagnosis, treatment, and prevention of the cancer.

34. Post-traumatic stress disorder (PTSD) is most often associated with soldiers returning from war. Who else can suffer from PTSD?

35. Research the seven different causes of disease listed in this chapter. Describe a disease in each category that was not discussed in this chapter. Discuss not only the cause of the disease, but also the resulting changes in the body's structure and function.

36. Cooperate and collaborate with team members to research the global impact of disease prevention. Discuss and compare your findings, document your evidence, then express your results and ideas in a clear, concise, and effective written report for your class.

37. Pick a disease to research. Access several creditable websites to identify and retrieve reportable information about that disease. Compile and record the information in a format that will be clear and informative for your classmates. Present your results to the class.

38. Refer to the medical terminology related to disease in Figure 7.1 at the beginning of this chapter. Write a short, imaginary dialogue involving a doctor and a patient in which your characters communicate with each other and use at least five of the terms defined in that figure. If you can work more of the terms into your dialogue, do so.

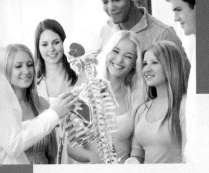

Unit 2
Cumulative Review Assess

Review Questions

Answer the following questions using what you have learned in this unit.

True or False

1. *True or False?* Medical word elements include suffixes and prefixes.

2. *True or False?* Arteries carry oxygen-poor blood back to the heart.

3. *True or False?* Atherosclerosis is the reduction of needed plaque in the arteries.

4. *True or False?* The human body is divided into several body cavities.

5. *True or False?* More than 90 percent of skin cancers appear on sun-exposed skin.

6. *True or False?* Hemoglobin is found within the white blood cell.

7. *True or False?* An acronym is a disease of the digestive system.

8. *True or False?* Type 2 diabetes mellitus can develop because of obesity.

9. *True or False?* The term *flexion* means "increasing the angle between joints."

10. *True or False?* The central nervous system is made up of the brain and spinal cord.

Multiple Choice

11. _____ is a disease of the liver.
    A. Pneumonia
    B. Nephritis
    C. Hepatitis
    D. Leukemia

12. The following are all body positions used in healthcare, *except* _____.
    A. Trendelenburg position
    B. semi-Fowler's position
    C. Sims' position
    D. superior position

13. The human nose can detect more than _____ smells.
    A. 10,000
    B. 700
    C. 6,000
    D. 1,000

14. The word roots *arthr* and *path* mean _____ respectively.
    A. liver and kidney
    B. kidney and heart
    C. joint and disease
    D. disease and liver

15. Which of the following words is spelled correctly?
    A. hepatitis
    B. ileim
    C. narkotic
    D. artharitis

16. Going from smallest to largest blood vessels, which order is correct?
    A. veins, capillaries, arteries
    B. veins, venules, arteries
    C. capillaries, venules, veins
    D. venules, capillaries, veins

17. Which of the following diseases is *not* considered a nutritional disease?
    A. rickets
    B. obesity
    C. bulimia nervosa
    D. tetanus

18. Lymphocytes are _____.
    A. crucial in helping the body fight pathogenic microorganisms
    B. white blood cells
    C. contained in lymph nodes
    D. All the above.

19. Arthritis is considered a(n) _____.
    A. infectious disease
    B. nutritional disease
    C. degenerative disease
    D. environmental disease

20. Which component of the blood is the most plentiful in the body?
    A. red blood cells
    B. white blood cells
    C. platelets
    D. plasma

Short Answer

21. Name four diseases caused by a virus.

22. What is bone marrow and where is it located?

23. What is the difference between the terms *adduction* and *abduction*?

24. What are body planes? Identify the three most common body planes.

25. Identify the four chambers of the heart.

Critical Thinking Exercises

26. Contact your local public health department to find out what diseases are currently of greatest concern in your area. How do your results compare with the Centers for Disease Control and Prevention (CDC) national focus on disease prevention? Were your results similar to the CDC's focus? vastly different? Why do you think that might be the case?

27. Identify four diseases that can be avoided by vaccination. Have any of these diseases made a resurgence in recent years? If so, what reasons can be attributed to this resurgence?

28. With a partner, take turns posing in different body positions used for treatment and examination to provide safe and accurate patient care. Guess what positions you each present.

Career Exploration

Athletic Trainer

An athletic trainer works to prevent injuries, including sports-related injuries. He or she treats people of all ages. Athletic trainers work with team physicians, physical therapists, coaches, and exercise physiologists to treat not only sports injuries, but exercise injuries not related to sports, as well. Employment is usually at a high school, college, or even at professional level sports. Athletic trainers can also be employed in sports medicine clinics.

A bachelor's degree is required for this profession. Most states also require state licensure. In Alaska, West Virginia, and the District of Columbia, licensure is voluntary but recommended. One of the requirements for licensure is to pass the National Athletic Trainers' Association (NATA) certification examination.

The field of sports medicine is booming, being one of the fastest rates of growth of any healthcare field. The US Department of Labor projects a rate of growth of 20% or higher for athletic trainers in the coming years.

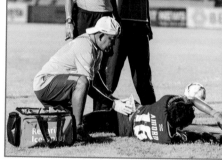

Jakkrit Orrasri/Shutterstock.com

Related Careers

Aerobics exercise instructor
Certified health fitness specialist (HFS)
Conditioning coach
Doctor of osteopathic medicine (DO)
Exercise physiologist
Kinesiotherapist (RKT)
Medical doctor (MD)
Occupational therapist (OT)
Personal trainer (CPT)
Physical therapist (PT)
Sports nutritionist

Further Research

1. Research one of the related careers listed above using the *Occupational Outlook Handbook* and other reliable Internet resources. What is the outlook for this career? Are workers in demand, or are jobs dwindling?

2. Review the educational requirements for this career. What classes would you need to take to pursue a related degree?

3. What is the salary range for this job?

4. What do you think you would like about this career? Is there anything about it you might dislike? Compare the job you have chosen to research to the description of an athletic trainer. Which job appeals to you more? Why?

Unit 3

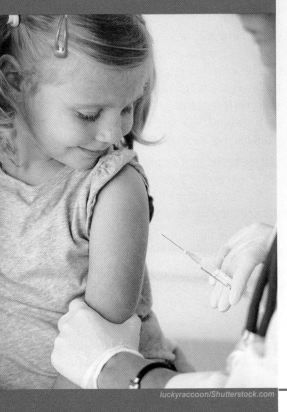

luckyraccoon/Shutterstock.com

Critical Concepts in the Healthcare World

Chapter 8:   Health and Wellness

Chapter 9:   Lifespan Development

Chapter 10: Healthcare Technology

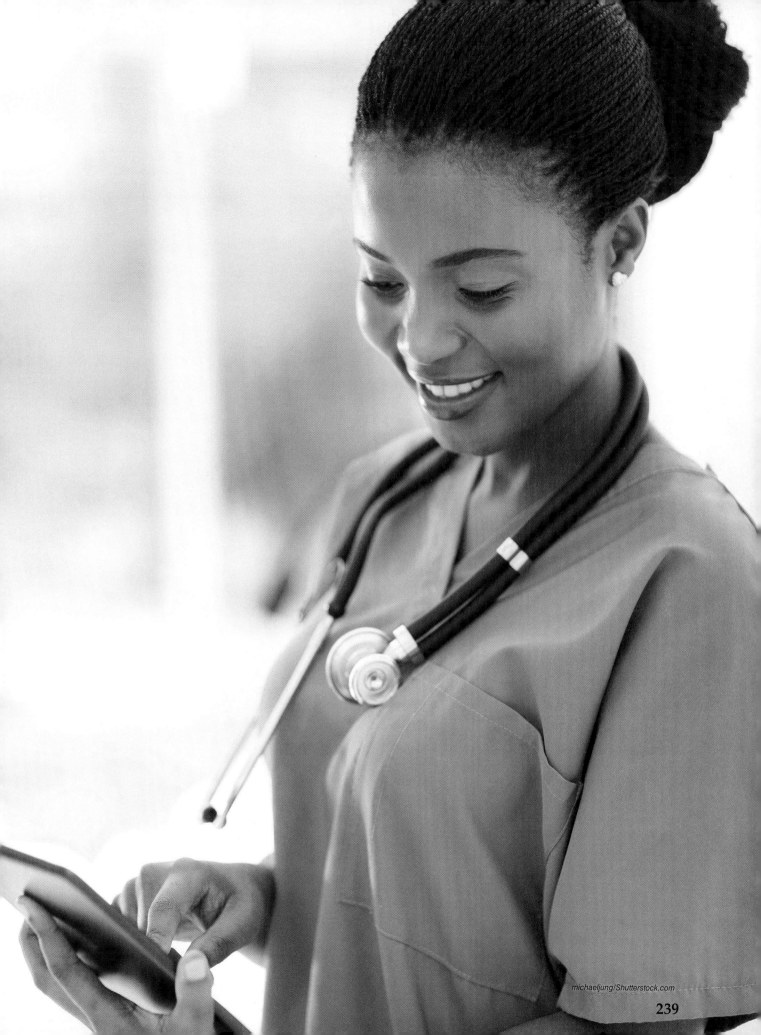

Chapter 8
Health and Wellness

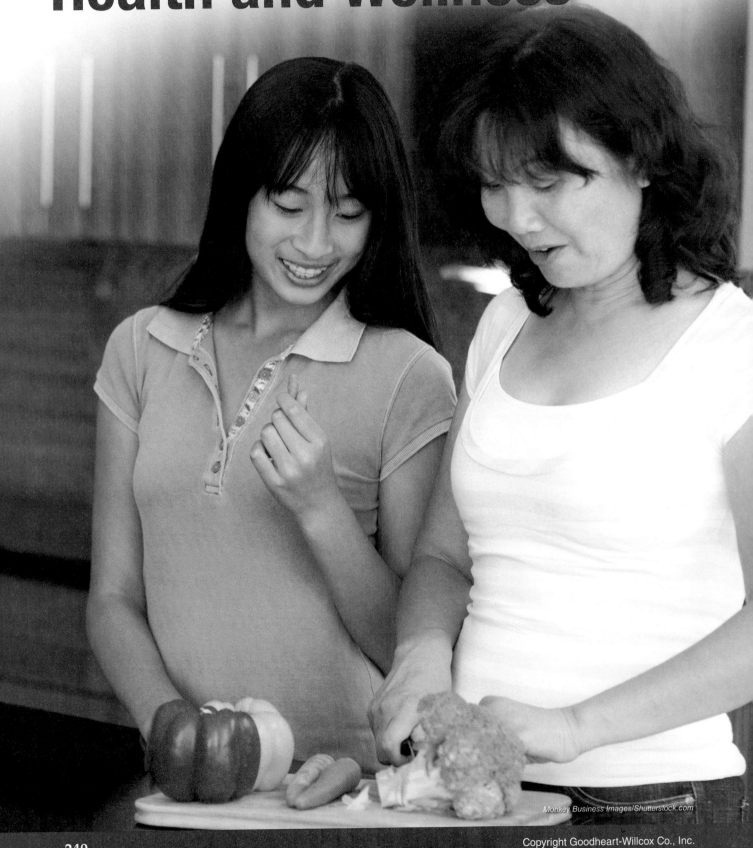

Terms to Know Build Vocab

addiction	complementary and alternative medicine (CAM)	holistic health
aerobic exercise		self-esteem
anorexia nervosa	depression	stress
bipolar disorder	emotional intelligence (EI)	substance abuse
body image	endorphins	suicide
bulimia nervosa	euphoria	suicide cluster
	health literacy	suicide contagion

Chapter Objectives

- Explain the concept of holistic health.
- Identify ways to maintain physical health, as well as the benefits of regular exercise, a healthful diet, and adequate sleep.
- Explain strategies for maintaining positive mental and emotional health.
- Identify several risk factors associated with depression and suicide.
- Explain the concept of body image.
- Discuss the causes, symptoms, and treatments for anorexia nervosa and bulimia nervosa.
- Identify how having relationships can impact one's health both positively and negatively.
- Discuss spiritual health.
- Describe healthy strategies for managing stress.
- Identify some wellness strategies for preventing disease.
- Discuss how community health officials help promote good health.
- Explain the importance of health literacy.
- Identify complementary and alternative medicine (CAM) practices.

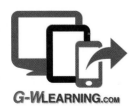

While studying, look for the activity icon to:

- **Build** vocabulary with e-flash cards and interactive games.
- **Assess** progress with chapter and unit review questions.
- **Expand** learning with animations and illustration labeling activities.
- **Simulate** EHR entry with healthcare documents.

www.g-wlearning.com/healthsciences/

In 1946, the World Health Organization (WHO) Constitution defined health in the following way, "Health is a complete state of physical, mental, and social well-being, and not merely the absence of disease or infirmity." This definition remains in the WHO Constitution today. Australian Aboriginal people define health similarly: "Health does not just mean the physical well-being of the individual but refers to the social, emotional, spiritual, and cultural well-being of the whole community." In Western culture, good health encompasses a healthy body, mind, and spirit, and being an active part of one's community.

holistic health

a wellness approach that advocates for treating the patient as a whole, rather than just the symptoms of disease, because the body works as a combination of physical, emotional, mental, and spiritual health

Today, the concept of **holistic health** emphasizes the body working as a combination of mental, emotional, physical, and spiritual health to maintain optimal wellness through daily living. Holistic health practices treat not just a disease, but the entirety of the patient. Wellness is focused on functioning well in spite of infirmity or disease.

Working toward your career goal will require that you develop effective methods of maintaining your health. You will be dealing with the demands of school—studying for exams, writing papers, meeting deadlines, and preparing presentations—while also juggling family responsibilities and planning for the future. Understanding health and wellness benefits you as a person, but it also enables you to provide better care to your patients during your healthcare career.

Physical Health

aerobic exercise

exercise that requires the heart to deliver oxygenated blood to working muscles

Maintaining your physical health requires effort to keep your body functioning well. There are six main areas to focus on to keep the physical body healthy:

1. Eat a healthy diet.

2. Maintain a reasonable weight.

3. Exercise regularly and be sure to incorporate **aerobic exercise** such as running or swimming into your routine (Figure 8.1). It is recommended that teens get rigorous aerobic exercise for about an hour a day at least three days a week and regular, more moderate activity during the rest of the week.

4. Try to get adequate sleep every night.

5. Use healthy stress management strategies.

6. Avoid substance abuse.

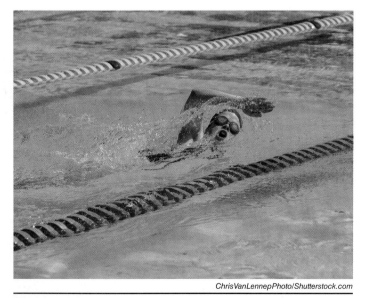

ChrisVanLennepPhoto/Shutterstock.com

Figure 8.1 Many health benefits are associated with aerobic exercise, including increasing your stamina, strengthening your heart and immune system, and achieving or maintaining a healthy weight.

Maintaining your physical health also plays a large role in promoting mental and emotional health. All aspects of your health are interrelated.

Maintain a Healthy Diet

Eating healthful foods gives your body the energy it needs. Taking in the proper nutrition can reduce health problems such as depression, headaches, fatigue, and insomnia. The United States Department of Agriculture (USDA) helps educate people on healthy eating by publishing a nutrition guide called MyPlate (Figure 8.2). MyPlate helps consumers adopt healthful eating habits by encouraging them to build a healthier plate with the proper balance of food groups.

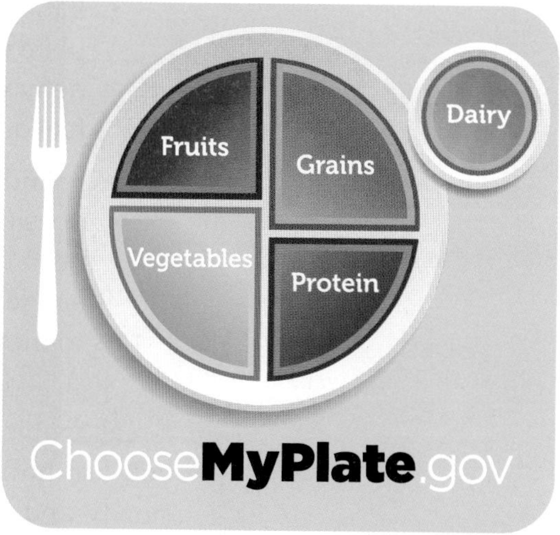

The USDA's dietary guidelines include an emphasis on eating fruits, vegetables, whole grains, and fat-free or low-fat milk and milk products (Figure 8.3). Consuming proteins from sources such as lean meats, poultry, fish, beans, eggs, and nuts is encouraged. It is also best to limit your intake of saturated fats, *trans* fats, cholesterol, salt (sodium), and added sugars.

If you wish to lose weight, fad diets may result in initial weight loss, but the loss is often temporary. Incorporating the following habits can lead to lasting weight loss and maintenance:

- **Don't skip breakfast.** Breakfast provides the energy you need as you begin your day.

- **Slow down as you eat.** Chewing slowly may give your body time to recognize when you are full. People who eat quickly often consume more calories because they do not give their stomach time to signal their brain that they are full.

- **Are you really hungry?** Ask yourself this question when you are tempted to eat. Are you eating because you are bored? Are you eating because the food is available, or are you really hungry?

- **Eat greens, fiber, and lean proteins first.** Vegetables contain fiber that can fill you up and, when raw, provide a satisfying crunch. Fill up on fiber and lean proteins, which give you energy without excess fat. Nuts and seeds can be satisfying as well, and provide protein.

- **Say no to late-night snacks.** Your metabolism slows down when you sleep, which means you begin to store fat, rather than burn it.

- **Eat healthy snacks.** Try to eat every three or four hours to avoid binge eating. Healthy snacks may include a piece of fruit, a handful of almonds, avocado with cottage cheese, edamame, a protein bar (200 calories or under), or a hard-boiled egg.

United States Department of Agriculture (USDA)

Figure 8.2   Developed by the USDA, MyPlate is a visual reminder of a healthy eating style intended to help you make positive decisions about the foods and beverages you consume.

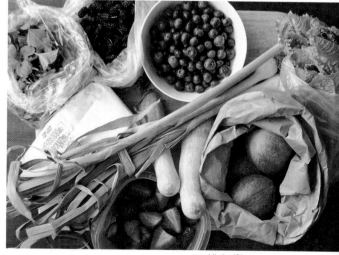

v.schlicting/Shutterstock.com

Figure 8.3   Eating healthful foods gives your body the energy it needs.

- **Eat moderate portions.** Cut down on portion size by using a salad plate instead of a dinner-sized plate, for example. Don't completely deny yourself your favorite foods, as this can lead to bingeing if you feel deprived.

- **Avoid soda.** Diet and regular sodas have both been linked to obesity, kidney damage, and certain cancers. Regular sodas have been linked to elevated blood pressure. Sugary sodas are the biggest single source of empty calories in the American diet, and they add to the obesity epidemic in the United States.

You will have more energy and enjoy better health if you maintain a reasonable weight for your height, body frame, and age. Eat only when you are hungry, not because you are depressed, bored, or worried. Eat slowly and try not to eat on the run, which may cause you to overeat. If you are overweight, talk to your doctor about how to lose weight without trying fad diets or fasting. You should also speak to your doctor if you find yourself exhibiting signs of disordered eating, which impacts all aspects of health.

Exercise

Exercise and physical activity can help you feel better, have fun, and improve your physical health. The health benefits of aerobic exercise are numerous. Regular aerobic exercise involves raising your heart rate above its normal level for at least 20 minutes a day, three or four days a week. Aerobic exercise reduces stress, strengthens the immune system and heart, reduces excess fat, and increases stamina. The key is to start slowly, building up gradually until you are able to maintain a consistent exercise schedule.

There are many benefits of establishing a regular plan for exercise:

1. **Exercise can control weight.** When you exercise, you burn calories. If you don't have time for a daily workout, be active throughout the day in simple ways, such as walking fast to class, taking the stairs whenever possible, and putting more energy and effort into physical education classes.

2. **Exercise can help protect the body from negative health conditions.** Exercise keeps the body flexible; improves balance; boosts high-density lipoprotein, or *HDL* (good cholesterol); helps with weight control; and has many other benefits.

endorphins
hormones secreted within the brain during exercise that reduce the sensation of pain or stress

3. **Exercise improves your mood.** Physical activity stimulates various chemicals in the brain, such as **endorphins**, that may leave you feeling happier and more relaxed. Exercise can boost your confidence and improve your self-esteem by helping you feel better about your appearance.

4. **Exercise improves energy.** Regular physical activity can improve muscle strength and boost endurance. Exercise delivers oxygen and nutrients to tissues, making your cardiovascular system work more efficiently.

5. **Exercise helps you sleep better.** Regular physical activity can help you fall asleep faster and deepen your sleep. However, exercising too close to bedtime may leave you feeling too energized to sleep.

6. **Exercise can be fun.** Exercise can give you a chance to unwind and perhaps enjoy the outdoors (Figure 8.4). Exercising with family and friends in a social setting helps you connect with people you love. Find an exercise you enjoy. If you get bored, try something else.

Don't Skimp on Sleep

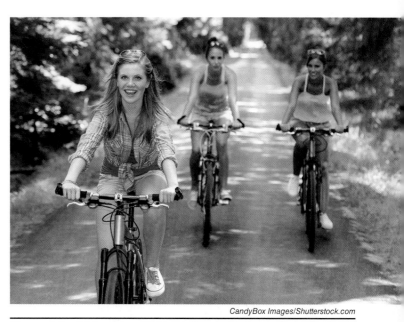

CandyBox Images/Shutterstock.com

Figure 8.4   A bike ride with friends is not only beneficial for your physical health, it may also improve your mental and emotional health by boosting your mood.

Getting a good night's sleep makes you feel better. But the importance of being well rested goes far beyond boosting your mood or banishing under-eye circles. Adequate sleep is a key part of a healthy lifestyle, benefiting your heart, weight, mind, and more. A Stanford University study found that football players who slept at least 10 hours a night for seven to eight weeks improved their sprint time, experienced less daytime fatigue, and had more stamina. Studies also show that getting too little sleep is associated with a shorter life span, as well as an increased chance of developing diabetes, heart disease, hypertension, and stroke. A good night's sleep has many benefits.

Improve Memory

Sleep can help improve memory, which can be beneficial to your studies. One example is studying medical terminology. Imagine you are studying medical abbreviations before you go to sleep. While you are sleeping, your brain can strengthen memories or skills learned when you were awake. This is a process called *consolidation*.

Increase Creativity

Getting a good night's sleep may result in more creativity as well. During sleep, your brain strengthens components of your memory that help to enhance the creative process. Sleep assists the brain in recognizing unrelated ideas and memories, making connections among them that increase the odds that a creative idea or insight will surface. After sleep, people are 33 percent more likely to make connections among distantly related ideas. This may improve your ability to analyze the novel you are reading in English class, helping you make connections among seemingly unrelated ideas and themes.

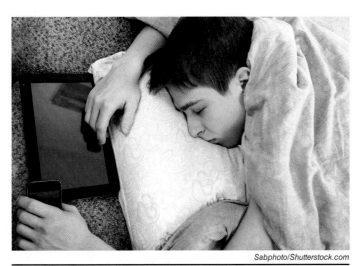

Sabphoto/Shutterstock.com

Figure 8.5 Experts suggest turning off your electronic devices at least 30 minutes before going to bed. Using devices such as a tablet or smartphone right before sleeping will not only make it harder for you to fall asleep, it can prevent you from getting quality sleep.

Sleep Deprivation in Teens

Teenagers are often sleep deprived. Studies show that most teenagers need between nine and nine-and-a-half hours of sleep. Teens need significantly more sleep than adults to support their rapid mental and physical development. Less sleep affects mood, behavior, and academic performance.

It is critical to maintain a regular sleep schedule. Engaging in certain activities, such as watching television, playing computer games, going on the Internet, or using your smartphone at bedtime makes it harder to fall asleep (Figure 8.5). With homework, participation in clubs or athletics, early start times for classes, and other demands, getting enough sleep is almost impossible, but careful planning could help your sleep schedule.

Lack of sleep can result in ADHD-like symptoms in children and teenagers. Tired students can be hyperactive, inattentive, and impulsive in class. Lack of sleep can cause or increase depression as well.

Take Naps

A power nap can boost your memory and creativity, as well as increase your energy levels. Naps can help pick you up and make you work more efficiently, if you plan them right. Naps that are too long or too close to bedtime can interfere with your regular sleep. Consuming caffeine close to bedtime can hurt sleep as well.

Check Your Understanding ✓

1. Do you have time to exercise regularly?
   A. If not, how could you make time?
   B. What kind of exercise do you get?
2. How much sleep do you get each night?
   A. Does it feel like you get enough sleep?
   B. Do you ever nap?
   C. Do you need caffeine to stay awake?
   D. Do you fall asleep in class?
   E. Why do you think teenagers need more sleep than adults?
3. What is your daily diet like each day?
   A. Do you have time for breakfast?
   B. Do you eat fast food at least once a week? If more, how much more?

Mental and Emotional Health

As you learned earlier in the chapter, holistic health emphasizes the body working as a combination of mental, emotional, physical, and spiritual health to maintain optimal wellness through daily living. Strong mental and emotional health can be described as a state of well-being in which the person is realistic about his own abilities, has coping strategies for the normal stresses and challenges in life, is able to work effectively, and can contribute to his community.

It is difficult to separate mental, emotional, and physical health as they are interrelated. Nutrition, exercise, and getting adequate sleep certainly may seem specific to maintaining your physical health, but these activities are also connected to your emotional and mental health. People with good mental and emotional health often have a positive outlook and feel good about themselves (Figure 8.6).

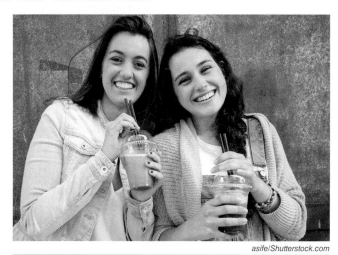

asife/Shutterstock.com

Figure 8.6   Developing strong, positive friendships can affect your self-esteem and improve your mental and emotional health.

Mental and emotional health describes your internal life, including your feelings and thoughts. **Self-esteem** is shaped by what you think and feel about yourself. Your self-esteem is highest when you see yourself as the person you would like to be. Doing something well, such as earning an A on a challenging exam, may raise your self-esteem. People who have positive self-esteem have an easier time handling conflicts, resisting negative pressures, and making friends. Positive self-esteem may help you laugh and smile more and have a generally optimistic view of the world and life.

self-esteem
the personal level of satisfaction about oneself and one's abilities

Your emotions include moods and feelings that you experience throughout the day. Emotions can conflict. You might feel positive about your geometry teacher on Monday, but after not doing well on an exam, you may feel that the teacher was unfair in her grading. Emotions can be wonderful when you experience joy, gratitude, and love. However, when you also experience loneliness, anxiety, jealousy, stress, or depression, it can be hard to handle those emotions. Learning how to manage your ups and downs, especially as a teenager, can be quite challenging.

Think It Through

On a scale of 1 to 10, how would you rate your self-esteem? What could you do to improve your self-esteem?

Negative emotions may sometimes appear seemingly out of nowhere. Identifying why you suddenly feel a certain way is the first step in working through these emotions. Covering up how you feel and holding onto negative emotions can cause these emotions to be expressed in a nonproductive way, such as yelling at someone who is not the object of your frustration. Look for support if your emotions become too much to handle. Look to good friends who have a positive outlook to help you work through these feelings. Learn to cope with problems instead of holding on to them.

Unfortunately, challenges such as poor self-esteem, inability to cope with problems, and lack of emotional control can lead to serious mental health issues.

emotional intelligence (EI)
the measure of one's ability to be aware of, control, and express one's emotions and to maintain successful interpersonal relations

> ## Extend Your Knowledge ▶ Emotional Intelligence
>
> **Emotional intelligence (EI)** is the measure of one's ability to be aware of, control, and express one's emotions. It is also the capability to successfully maintain interpersonal relationships. Many researchers believe that EI matters more than your intellectual quotient (IQ) when it comes to your health, happiness, and success in life. There are three parts to emotional intelligence:
>
> 1. emotional awareness, which means being able to identify your own emotions and the emotions of others
> 2. the ability to calmly perform tasks like problem solving and productive thinking
> 3. the ability to manage your emotions instead of having continual angry outbursts
>
> ### Apply It
>
> 1. Do you know someone who cannot control his emotions? someone who is continually angry and blaming others for his problems? Describe that person. What do you think his EI might be?
> 2. Would you say that you have a high EI? What traits do you possess that add to your EI? If you think you have a low EI, what do you have to work on to make it higher?

Addiction and Substance Abuse

addiction
a physical or psychological need for a habit-forming substance, such as drugs or alcohol, or an activity, such as shopping

Addiction is the physical and psychological need for a substance or behavior. There are many types of addiction. Common addictions include alcohol, drugs, food, the Internet, video games, gambling, nicotine, and even shopping. Addictions can seriously interfere with your health, relationships, and work.

People who experiment with drugs, alcohol, or nicotine may continue to use these substances for a variety of reasons. They may like the way the substance makes them feel. Social pressures from friends, family, or the media may also contribute to their use of these substances. The use of illegal drugs and alcohol, or the misuse of prescription medication despite the harmful effects, is called **substance abuse**.

Risk Factors for Addiction and Substance Abuse

substance abuse
the use of drugs or alcohol, or a misuse of prescription medication

No single factor can predict whether or not a person will develop an addiction or abuse drugs or alcohol. Risk factors for addiction and substance abuse are affected by many things. Some people are genetically predisposed to alcoholism and other addictions because of the way their bodies process (or do not process) certain chemicals. Chemical changes in the brain can leave people addicted to alcohol or drugs after using them for some time.

People with mental health problems may be more likely to develop substance abuse problems. In some cases, drugs and alcohol can be used to self-medicate.

Attempting to treat mental health problems with drugs and alcohol is not only dangerous, but it may worsen existing mental health problems.

A person's environment may also contain risk factors. Peer pressure, physical and sexual abuse, and stress are some factors that may influence a person's use and abuse of harmful substances. A family history of substance abuse may also increase a person's chance of developing substance abuse problems of their own.

Developmental stages in a person's life can affect addiction vulnerability. The earlier drug or alcohol use begins, the more likely it is to progress into serious abuse. Adolescent brains are still developing in areas that affect decision making, judgment, and self-control. This development can lead to more risk-taking behaviors, including trying drugs.

Effects of Addiction and Substance Abuse

The use and abuse of drugs, alcohol, and tobacco products, among other addictions, are associated with many negative health consequences. Smoking has been connected to several serious health problems, including various forms of cancer and heart disease. Alcohol is not easily metabolized by the body and can do serious damage to the liver as well as brain cells. Drug abuse increases a person's chance of contracting an infectious disease, such as hepatitis or HIV, which may be caused by sharing needles. It can also lead to overdose or death. Addiction to food can cause obesity, which has been linked to various health problems, including diabetes.

Addiction and substance abuse have other far-reaching consequences, including legal troubles, trouble staying in school or holding down a job, homelessness, and strained relationships with family and friends (Figure 8.7).

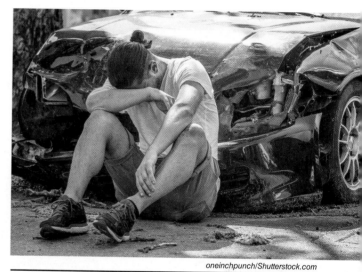

oneinchpunch/Shutterstock.com

Figure 8.7   Driving while under the influence of drugs or alcohol may lead to a variety of negative consequences including personal injury, injuring others, trouble with the law, and financial trouble.

Overcoming Addiction and Substance Abuse

In some cases, it can be challenging to identify when experimentation develops into addiction and abuse. People who use a substance regularly often develop a tolerance to it, meaning they have to use more and more of it to feel the same effects. This increased use often leads to dependence (requiring the substance to function) and addiction.

Few addicts are able to recognize when they have crossed that line. The frequency of use or the amount of drugs being taken can often indicate a drug-related problem. The first step in conquering addiction may be taken when the person realizes her substance abuse is interfering with her schoolwork, health, or relationships. Seeking support, guidance, and expert advice on how to overcome addiction and substance abuse problems is the next step. Therapy, medical interventions, 12-step programs, or even in-patient programs can be of great help.

Professional Ramifications of Alcohol and Drug Use

A serious addiction will almost always interfere with the goal of entering the healthcare profession. Smelling of alcohol, behaving as if you are "high" at work, being inattentive, and making mistakes with patients while under the influence are all grounds for being fired. Healthcare facilities must comply with industry standards for substance abuse. This may involve random and routine drug testing of all healthcare workers. The most common method of drug testing, urinalysis, can be done at the workplace (if you work in a health unit, for example), a doctor's office, or any other site selected by the employer. Urinalysis can identify evidence of recent alcohol, prescription drug, and illegal drug use.

Healthcare workers who come to work under the influence of drugs and alcohol put their patients, visitors, and coworkers at risk. Workplace accidents are more likely to occur, and it is impossible to provide quality care when under the influence of these substances. Workplace alcohol use and drug abuse are also associated with crime (workplace violence or inventory theft, for example) and lost time at work due to low productivity and high incidence of tardiness and sick days.

Strategies for Preventing Addiction and Substance Abuse

There are positive things that people can do to avoid addiction or substance abuse:

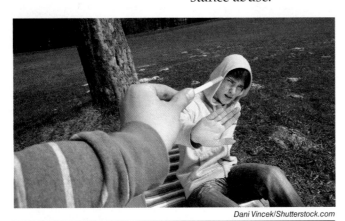
Dani Vincek/Shutterstock.com

Figure 8.8 Practicing your refusal skills will make it easier to avoid tobacco, drugs, or alcohol if you are ever pressured to use these substances.

- **Stand up to peer pressure.** The biggest reason that teens start using drugs, alcohol, or tobacco is because they feel pressure from their peers to do so. Some people find themselves doing things in a group that they normally would not do, just to fit in. If you find yourself continually surrounded by a group of people who do not have your best interests in mind, it is time to find a new group of friends. Practice refusal skills and plan ahead of time to avoid giving in to dangerous situations (Figure 8.8). True friends will support your decision to not engage in these risky behaviors.

- **Deal effectively with stress.** Continual exams, pressure to be the best at sports, worrying about getting into the "best" college, and maintaining a romantic connection are all stressors felt by many teenagers. There are effective and healthy ways of handling the stress of these pressures. Exercise, read a good book, or sign up for volunteer work. Relieving your stress in a healthy way can help you avoid substance use.

- **Assess your risk factors.** Recognize the risk factors for addiction and substance abuse in your life. Does your family have a history of addiction and substance abuse? Do any of your close friends use drugs? Being aware of such factors can help you overcome the temptation to use.

- **Seek help for mental health problems.** Self-medication can be a tempting option for those suffering from mental health problems. Seek professional help if you are suffering from mental health problems such as anxiety, post-traumatic stress disorder, or depression before such challenges lead to substance abuse and addiction.

- **Keep balance in your life.** Find activities to engage in that keep you busy and fulfilled. Set achievable goals for yourself and work to make them happen. Exercise on a regular basis. Make friends who respect your limits and your values and can share in your activities.

Depression

It is not unusual for people to occasionally feel sad or get "the blues." Teenagers, especially, may have strong emotional reactions because they are experiencing a stage of life with many physical, emotional, psychological, and social changes. Occasional bouts of sadness, however, are different from **depression**, which is a medical condition characterized by feelings of hopelessness, worthlessness, or a general disinterest in daily life. For most people, feelings of sadness pass over time, but that is often not the case for people suffering from depression.

Adolescent depression is increasing at a fast rate. Recent surveys indicate that as many as one in five teens suffer from clinical depression. A family history of depression can increase the risk for depression. This is a serious problem that calls for prompt, appropriate treatment. A related mental illness is called **bipolar disorder**, formerly known as *manic-depression*. This form of depression alternates between periods of **euphoria** and depression.

depression
mood disorder causing a persistent feeling of sadness and loss of interest

bipolar disorder
mental disorder characterized by alternating periods of euphoria, or an elevated mood, and depression

euphoria
emotional and mental condition in which a person experiences intense feelings of well-being, happiness, and excitement

---

Did You Know?   Beating Depression through Exercise

It's a scientific fact that exercise helps treat or prevent depression. Many studies have shown that moderate exercise can have a significant effect on depression.

A study conducted at the Cooper Research Institute in Dallas, Texas, shows that as few as three hours of regular exercise a week can reduce levels of depression. Participants who walked 35 minutes a day for six days a week reduced their symptoms of mild to moderate depression by 47 percent. Exercise was as effective as the leading antidepressants in reducing depression.

Aerobic exercise, in particular, improves blood flow and oxygen to the brain. This type of vigorous exercise has the added benefit of releasing endorphins. However, many people feel that they can't maintain continual aerobic exercise. It has been shown that even gardening can help with depression. Walking with a friend can yield several benefits such as being out in nature, having social contact, reducing stress, and treating depression (Figure 8.9).

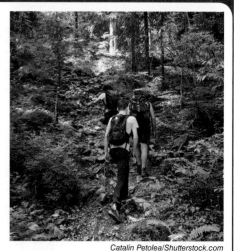

Catalin Petolea/Shutterstock.com

Figure 8.9   Hiking with friends is an activity that may yield several health benefits.

Depression may be difficult to diagnose. If the following symptoms of possible depression last more than two weeks, ask for help:

- poor performance in school
- withdrawal from friends and activities
- sadness and hopelessness
- lack of energy, enthusiasm, or motivation
- agitation, anger, and rage
- overreacting to criticism
- inability to satisfy ideals
- poor self-esteem and crippling guilt
- indecision
- changes in sleep patterns
- substance abuse
- problems with authority
- suicidal thoughts

There are several ways to treat depression. Psychotherapy is one option that helps patients explore painful feelings and teaches coping mechanisms (Figure 8.10). If psychotherapy is not enough, some healthcare providers will prescribe antidepressants, or medication used to treat depression. Family therapy, support groups, and inpatient treatment are other options that may help.

Suicide

suicide
intentionally ending one's life

Sometimes depression can become so severe that the person considers ending his or her life. Each year, over 5,000 people from 15 to 24 years of age commit **suicide**. Suicide is the third leading cause of death in adolescents and the second leading cause of death among college-age youth. Predicting who is at risk of committing suicide is challenging.

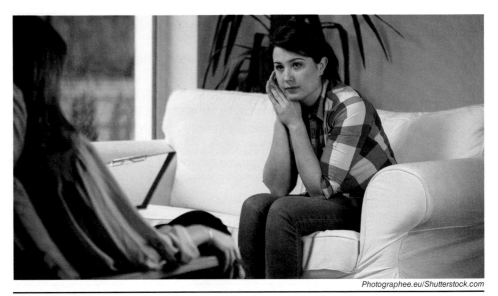

Photographee.eu/Shutterstock.com

Figure 8.10   Many resources exist to help treat depression, including therapy.

Risk Factors

Personal, social, and environmental risk factors all contribute to suicide. One predictive factor is whether a person has attempted suicide previously. Someone who has made a previous attempt is more likely to try again. Other risk factors include a history of mental disorders and a history of substance abuse.

Teenagers may experience a great deal of stress, confusion, self-doubt, pressure to succeed, financial concerns, and other worries. Change within the family, such as divorce or the formation of a new family of stepparents and stepsiblings, can be very unsettling and create more self-doubt. Suicide may appear to be a solution to these problems.

Teenagers who are bullied by their peers are at greater risk of thinking about and attempting suicide (Figure 8.11). Teens whose families suffer financial hardships, long-term issues of abuse and neglect, or addiction problems can also have an increased risk of suicide. If you hear one of your friends threaten suicide, take the threat seriously and immediately seek assistance from a teacher, counselor, or your parents about how to handle the situation.

Many of the signs of suicidal feelings are similar to those associated with depression, but more severe. A person considering suicide may simply say, "I want to kill myself," or "I won't be a problem to you much longer." She might also give away favorite possessions, "getting her affairs in order" by cleaning her room and throwing away her important belongings.

Unfortunately, hearing about someone else's suicide may increase the risk of other people thinking about or attempting suicide. Copycat suicides are caused by **suicide contagion**. When one person in a community or group commits suicide, other people in that community or group may copy the suicide. This is called a **suicide cluster**.

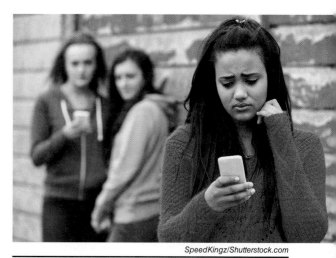
SpeedKingz/Shutterstock.com

Figure 8.11 Cyberbullying, or bullying that takes place electronically, can make the victim feel anxious, depressed, and as if they cannot escape their attackers. Victims of cyberbullying should tell a trusted adult about the attacks as soon as possible and avoid reacting to the bully.

suicide contagion
term for the copying of suicide attempts after hearing about another person's suicide

suicide cluster
multiple suicides that occur within a community during a relatively short period of time

---

Real Life Scenario — Depression and Suicide Threats

Ashley's lifelong friend Sadie has seemed sad lately. Ashley understands why Sadie is feeling this way. Sadie's parents have divorced, her sister has left for college, and Sadie's boyfriend recently broke up with her. Sadie has recently gained weight and has told Ashley she is ashamed of her body.

Ashley includes her friend in activities, invites her for sleepovers, and tries to be a good friend. However, Sadie is isolating herself and does not want to be social. This both worries Ashley and hurts her feelings.

One day at school, Sadie confides that "I wish I were dead. Life is too hard!"

Apply It

1. How can Ashley tell if Sadie's statement is serious?
2. What would you advise Ashley to do after hearing Sadie's comment at school?
3. What are Ashley's options if she decides to act upon Sadie's possible suicide threat?

The Survivors

Those who commit suicide leave survivors (parents, siblings, friends, other relatives) devastated for the rest of their lives. Survivors may suffer guilt because they did not realize the extent of the victim's suffering. They may feel rejected and abandoned by the victim. Suicide deaths are sudden, and the loved ones are unable to prepare themselves for such a catastrophic loss.

Getting Help

If you ever find yourself contemplating suicide or hurting yourself, take your feelings very seriously. Immediately talk to an adult you trust. This person can help you find a mental health professional who can help. You can also call 911 and ask for a number of a suicide hotline to reach a trained counselor. Remember, suicide is a permanent solution to a temporary problem that can be solved.

Body Image and Eating Disorders

How do you feel about your body overall? Are you thin enough? Are you too skinny? Is there a part of your body that you would like to change? How you feel about your body and appearance helps form your **body image** (Figure 8.12).

Although men and boys can have poor body images, women and girls are more apt to have negative images of their bodies. Women are often defined by their physical appearance. Women in the media are often criticized about their hair, clothes, and other superficial aspects of their appearance. Family and friends can influence a person's body image by emphasizing the importance of body weight and body shape. Teenagers may feel that they won't fit in if they are too thin or too fat or if their nose is too big, and so on. Every day, the media bombards us with images of "perfect" women, who are usually thin, have a beautiful complexion, and long, shiny hair.

It has been suggested that the preference for a thin female body is not shared across all ethnic groups. Different groups may have different values and preferences when it comes to ideal weight and appearance. Some research suggests that African-American women and girls do not embrace the Caucasian preferences of a very thin female body. African-American girls and women tend to prefer a heavier weight and are less preoccupied with weight and dieting. The thin ideal is not universal.

If a person has serious body image problems, she might be at a normal weight but see an obese person looking back at her in the mirror. Each year thousands of teens develop eating disorders, or problems with weight, eating, or body image. Eating disorders include more than just going on a diet to lose weight or exercising every day. They are extremes in eating behavior and ways of thinking about eating.

The most common eating disorders are **anorexia nervosa** and **bulimia nervosa** (commonly known as *anorexia* and *bulimia*). Other food-related disorders include avoidant or restrictive food intake disorder, binge eating, and food phobias.

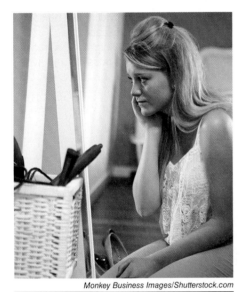

Monkey Business Images/Shutterstock.com

Figure 8.12   Your body image is defined by how you *think* you look, not how you actually look. A person who would be considered fit and attractive by others but still feels negatively about her appearance has a poor body image.

body image
a person's thoughts and feelings about how he or she looks

anorexia nervosa
an eating disorder characterized by low weight, fear of gaining weight, and food restriction

bulimia nervosa
an eating disorder characterized by bingeing and purging

Anorexia Nervosa

People with anorexia have a strong fear of weight gain and a distorted view of body size and shape. They often strive for perfection and hold themselves to very high standards (Figure 8.13). Unfortunately, their view of a "perfect" body is distorted, leading them to adopt extreme eating restrictions. As a result, they eat very little and often become dangerously underweight. Food intake is restricted by dieting or fasting. The person may also exercise excessively.

The starvation associated with anorexia takes a heavy toll on the body. People with anorexia often experience hair loss; the development of soft hair that covers the body (lanugo); inability to concentrate; anemia (insufficient numbers of red blood cells); swollen joints; brittle bones; and a drop in blood pressure, pulse, and breathing. Women or girls with anorexia often do not menstruate. Anorexia can also cause organ failure, infertility, and heart and brain damage. The effects of anorexia can remain long after the person has recovered and gained weight. For example, people who suffered from anorexia at a young age are more likely to develop osteoporosis and bone fractures later in life.

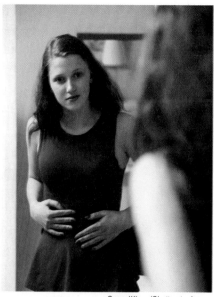

SpeedKingz/Shutterstock.com

Figure 8.13   A person suffering from anorexia nervosa may have a distorted body image and obsess over perceived "flaws" in his or her body weight or shape.

Bulimia Nervosa

People with bulimia nervosa binge eat, eating excessively in one sitting, and then compensate in extreme ways by purging (vomiting) and exercising excessively (Figure 8.14). These efforts are all made in an attempt to prevent weight gain. This disorder can be harder to detect than anorexia because many bulimics are average weight, or even overweight.

Frequent vomiting and a lack of nutrients can cause many health problems in people with bulimia, including constant stomach pains; damage to the stomach and kidneys; lack of menstruation in women and girls; dehydration; and loss of electrolytes, which can cause a heart attack. Stomach acid in vomit can also lead to tooth decay, tearing and bleeding in the esophagus, and burning of the throat or mouth. Studies show that those suffering from bulimia also have a tendency to engage in other destructive behaviors, such as alcohol or drug abuse.

Treatment for and Recovery from Eating Disorders

The emotional pain of having an eating disorder can take its toll. People with an eating disorder may feel exhausted from constantly monitoring their food intake and exercise. It can be hard for them to concentrate on much else. They may become withdrawn and less social.

Fortunately, eating disorders can be treated. Mental health professionals, doctors, and dietitians are often involved in a person's treatment and recovery. Therapy or counseling is very important. Family and friends should form a support network for someone working to overcome an eating disorder, helping them to regain weight and develop a positive body image.

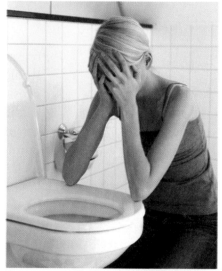

TunedIn by Westend61/Shutterstock.com

Figure 8.14   Binge eating often leaves a person feeling out of control. One way a person with bulimia may attempt to regain control is to follow bingeing by purging, or vomiting. Many people with bulimia describe feelings of guilt and self-hatred after a binge-purge cycle.

Recovering from an eating disorder can be a long process. Working to improve self-esteem and body image, and to change thoughts and attitudes about eating and food, are important steps to take in recovery. In some cases, the body is able to recover from the damage caused by the eating disorder, but there may be lifelong effects. Unfortunately, many people who have suffered from an eating disorder in the past experience relapses, or recurrence of their disease.

Social Health

Social health involves forming healthy personal relationships with others. It also includes a person's relationship to his or her community. As people grow and mature, they develop social skills that enable them to form and maintain relationships. These relationships can help improve mental and emotional health, academic performance, and the development of successful adult relationships. Teenagers who lack strong social health and positive relationships may exhibit a tendency to be delinquent, committing illegal or immoral actions, and may have psychological problems.

Social support is positively linked to good health and longevity; social isolation has been shown to predict a shortened life span. For example, marriages that are full of conflict have been linked to poorer health than happy marriages. Having people in your life who listen to you when you need support makes you feel good; this, in turn, positively influences your health.

A healthy social life is good for your long-term health. For example, blood pressure and heart rate tend to rise when a person is stressed. However, recent studies show that when a person is accompanied by a friend or loved one, stressful situations have a lesser effect on blood pressure and heart rate. Other studies have found that people who enjoy successful friendships have stronger immune systems than those who do not have a healthy social life. The immune response is thought to be affected by stress hormones, so a strong social life (which helps eliminate stress) may improve immune function, helping people resist infections and better fight off the cold virus.

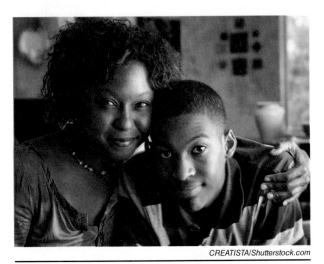

CREATISTA/Shutterstock.com

Figure 8.15 Developing positive relationships with parents and other family members can have a long-lasting effect and impact future relationships.

Family

Positive family relationships are strongly associated with healthy social development. If you have a good relationship with your parents or a strong parental figure, you can learn critical social skills such as conflict resolution and intimacy. The positive relationships family members enjoy with others may also serve as an example to you and influence your friendships and romantic relationships (Figure 8.15).

Family relationships serve unique functions that set them apart from other relationships. Families typically provide for the physical needs of members, making sure all family members have food, clothing, and a place to live. They are also responsible for members' health and well-being, and should schedule regular dentist and doctor appointments. Rules are often set with the goal of keeping all family members safe and healthy.

Families can also help members meet mental and emotional needs, such as love, self-esteem, and emotional support. Your family members celebrate your special occasions and can also give you advice about challenges you face. Families should educate and socialize children. Your family teaches you language, and some pass down important cultural and religious values. Families also have unique traditions, and encourage cooperation, sharing, and compromise.

Healthy Relationships with Others

Enjoying successful relationships with others not only contributes to your happiness, but also increases your energy and improves your overall health. Finding the time to develop these relationships will be beneficial to your health and well-being.

Friends and family can help us think through problems, brainstorm ideas, overcome boredom, and bring us joy and laughter. Establishing healthy relationships with others will also create a support system of people who will provide encouragement when you have a bad day or become overwhelmed at school. Neglecting relationships because you are busy at school and work can make it challenging to maintain healthy relationships.

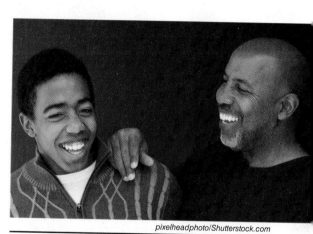

pixelheadphoto/Shutterstock.com

Figure 8.16 Developing relationships with trusted adults outside of your family builds a strong support system and helps you relate to people of all ages, which will be beneficial when you begin your healthcare career.

A teenager's relationships with adults outside the family can promote social development (Figure 8.16). Respected older adults can teach social skills, model behavior, and give positive or negative reinforcement. Trustworthy adults can give advice, emotional support, and companionship, and serve as real-life examples of positive social relationships. Once you begin your healthcare career, you will be working with people who are a variety of ages. It is important to be able to relate to people of all ages.

Successful relationships with your peers also promote the development of social skills. Interactions with your peers can help you learn to compromise, express empathy, and understand other perspectives. Positive peer relationships can discourage aggression, emotional distress, and antisocial behavior.

While some people enjoy social activities, others are less prone to be socially active at times. Social health doesn't have to mean being continually involved with large groups. It does mean developing meaningful relationships with family and friends. Social health is about giving and receiving support from loved ones, friends, and your community.

Dealing with Conflict and Abuse

Unfortunately, not all relationships are loving or supportive. Just as healthy relationships can have a positive effect on your overall well-being, conflict and abuse can negatively affect all aspects of your health and wellness. Conflict is a normal part of everyday life, but when minor conflict escalates, it can destroy relationships and become a serious source of stress.

Abuse of any kind is unacceptable and can lead to serious physical, emotional, and mental health issues. Abuse may have physical consequences such as broken bones; poor nutrition; and stress, bringing on high blood pressure, heart disease, and other disorders. Unhealthy relationships may also affect a person's mental and emotional well-being, leading to fear, anger, depression, trust issues, or trouble developing healthy relationships later in life.

One specific type of abuse you may witness as a healthcare worker is elder abuse. Elder abuse occurs when older individuals are victims of abuse in their homes, long-term care facilities, or other living situations. Elder abuse is usually committed by a caregiver or a family member. The following are examples of elder abuse:

- physical abuse
- neglect, or failing to provide for the person's basic needs (Figure 8.17)
- sexual abuse
- ignoring calls for help
- stealing money or other valuables

If you witness any signs of abuse in your healthcare facility, report it immediately.

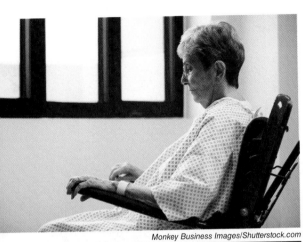

Monkey Business Images/Shutterstock.com

Figure 8.17 Neglecting a patient or failing to provide for her basic needs is one form of elder abuse found in healthcare facilities.

Community Connections

It is important to think of yourself as a member of your community. By connecting with the community, you are never alone. You have a place to go and people to talk with when you need it. There are several ways you can become involved in your community.

Volunteer work allows you to help others, which makes you feel better about yourself. Service projects are a great opportunity to give back to your community by volunteering at homeless shelters, soup kitchens, nursing homes, or child care centers. You may have a chance to talk with people from different cultural backgrounds, who have different religious or spiritual beliefs and political values. Being involved in the community will help you become independent, develop new skills, and help others. This is great preparation for succeeding in the job world.

Each healthcare facility is a community of its own, filled with patients, visitors, and healthcare workers. You must be able to work within that community and appreciate its diversity and challenges. Forming positive relationships among all members of a healthcare facility creates an environment where health and wellness can be promoted and achieved. A sense of community might contribute to patients' comfort and confidence that their healthcare is going to be provided by a group of competent healthcare professionals. When these professionals work well together, it is easier for them to achieve their common goal of optimizing patient health and wellness. This healthcare community, if large enough, can also offer great health outreach through vaccination clinics, family planning information, and free healthcare.

Spiritual Health

The term *spirituality* means different things to different people. Each person's path to exploring spiritual health is personal and unique. For some, spirituality is the religion of their family, while others think spirituality is harmony with nature, a notion of a higher power, or other interpretations. One thing most people agree on is that it is good to have peace and harmony in your life. Continual conflict negatively impacts both your health and your relationships. Achieving a calm and confident state will serve you well as a healthcare worker, promoting a sense of peace with your patients.

The term *meditation* refers to a broad variety of practices that includes techniques designed to promote relaxation and harmony with your environment (Figure 8.18). Meditation can also mean resting your mind from all the worries of your life. People can do this by watching a sunset, gardening, touring an art museum, or holding a baby. It is important to just enjoy time away from all your cares. When feeling angry and frustrated, you should be able to take time out to relax before saying or doing something you might regret. When you are on the job, if you feel angry with a coworker or with your supervisor, taking time out to cool off and try to feel some peace will be invaluable for maintaining good relationships.

As with other aspects of maintaining good health, developing good spiritual health contributes positively to all other aspects of health and wellness, including physical, mental, and emotional health.

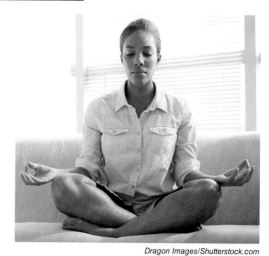

Dragon Images/Shutterstock.com

Figure 8.18 Meditation may help you relax, serve as a stress reliever, or help improve your sense of spiritual health.

Think It Through

Review Figure 8.19. How many of the listed stressors have you experienced? How did you manage the stress you experienced?

Managing Stress

Everyone experiences daily **stress** throughout life (Figure 8.19). Sometimes, situations can introduce multiple sources of stress. High levels of stress can impact all aspects of your health. The chemicals that your body produces when you are experiencing stress can weaken the immune system.

stress
the body's physical, mental, and emotional response to change, trauma, or challenging situations

Common Stressors	
Life-Altering Events	***Daily Stressors***
• death of a family member or a friend • divorce or separation in the family • personal injury • change in health of family member • job loss (either your own or that of a family member) • moving • starting classes at a new school	• losing important items • concern about physical appearance • fight with family or friends • too much homework • tests and quizzes at school • peer pressure • jealousy • breakup with significant other

Goodheart-Willcox Publisher

Figure 8.19 Stressors will come and go throughout your life. How you handle life-altering events and daily stressors will impact your health.

This can leave the body more open to infection. An overwhelmed student may lose focus and even give up on educational and career goals because the stress of school is too much to handle. Learning to manage and prevent stress can help reduce the impact of stress on your overall health and personal goals.

Each person responds differently to stress. What may be stressful to one person may not be to another. One student might think the world is ending after earning a C in a course, while another is happy with a C. A third student might be motivated to turn the C into a B by studying harder.

Real Life Scenario   Role Playing

You will likely encounter many stressful situations during your career in healthcare. How you handle such situations will be important for both your personal health and the health of your patients.

Apply It

1. Imagine you are a registered nurse in an emergency department. Ricky, your patient, has just been badly hurt in a motorcycle accident. The doctor assigned to Ricky is with another patient at the moment, and your job is to try to calm Ricky down. He is scared and in a lot of pain. How can you help Ricky? He cannot have pain medication until he has been thoroughly examined by a doctor.

2. Working in groups of two, role play the following scenario with a classmate. Your best friend has been feeling down lately and today she does not want to get out of bed. Her mother asks you to visit and see if you can help her. What might you do or say in this situation?

3. Working in groups of two, role play the following scenario with a classmate. You are a medical student who is assigned to the night shift at University Hospital. You are asked to speak with Mr. Knight, who has just learned he has cancer and is very frightened. What do you say to Mr. Knight?

Personality Types

Reactions to stress often depend on personality types. Some people (*type A personalities*) are ambitious, organized, impatient, and sometimes take on more than they can handle. Others (*type B personalities*) are generally patient, relaxed, easygoing, and are not plagued by a sense of urgency. A third personality type (*type C personalities*) is described as suppressing emotional expression, denying strong emotional reactions, having trouble coping with stress, and feeling hopeless or helpless.

Most people have some qualities belonging to each personality type. Depending on a person's personality, he or she will react to stress in various ways.

Attitude

When considering how a person may cope with stress, attitude may be a more important factor than personality. Those who approach problems as challenges to overcome are more likely to react positively when faced with stressful situations. Research has found that positive outcomes are more related to your reaction to stress than to the types of stressors in your life.

Strategies for Stress Management

It is important to recognize the signs of too much stress. Frustration, irritability, and depression are common emotional reactions to stress. Headaches, upset stomachs, and fatigue are physical indications that you have too much stress in your life (Figure 8.20). After identifying the source of these symptoms, take a deep breath, relax, and sort out what is causing your stress.

You cannot avoid stress and, in fact, some stress in your life can motivate you to perform well and achieve your goals. Adopting some of the following strategies will help you work through stress and achieve a positive outcome.

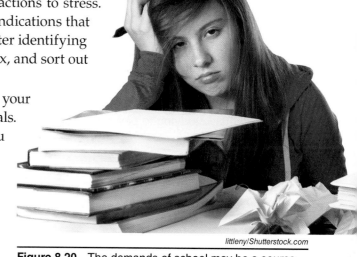

littleny/Shutterstock.com

Figure 8.20 The demands of school may be a source of stress in your life, leaving you feeling physically ill, fatigued, or overwhelmed. Adopting healthy stress management strategies may improve your health.

- **Stay healthy by eating a nutritious diet, staying physically fit, and getting plenty of sleep.** A balanced diet will give you energy to complete tasks required for effective studying. Physical exercise produces endorphins, and exercise can also help to control weight. A well-rested person can be more productive than someone who has not gotten enough sleep.

- **Avoid substance abuse.** Some people feel that alcohol and other drugs will relieve stress. However, such substances only mask stress symptoms. Eventually, substance abuse will add new stressors to your life, creating physical, mental, and emotional health problems. Substance abuse can also ruin healthy relationships and may lead to fights, accidents, and even arrests.

- **Learn how to relax.** Set aside time for enjoying leisure activities. Everyone has a different way of relaxing. You might like to listen to music, read a good novel, or exercise. Some people may find relaxation techniques such as yoga, deep breathing, and meditation to be helpful.

- **Adopt positive strategies for effective time management.** Maximize the time you have set aside for studying. Having a good balance of work, school, and life will make you happier, healthier, and a more effective student.

- **Reach out to your support system.** Family members, friends, school counselors, social workers, religious leaders, teachers, and psychologists can all help you deal with stressful situations. In return, you can support them when they are in need.

- **Be positive about your abilities.** Remember your strengths and have a positive attitude. Avoid dwelling on failures or negative qualities; doing so will only leave you feeling discouraged and more stressed. If you are confident in yourself, you will find it easier to work through a stressful situation.

It is impossible to completely avoid stress, but finding ways to manage stress is important to your overall health and wellness.

Disease Prevention

In addition to practicing physical, mental, emotional, social, and spiritual wellness on a daily basis, there are some additional measures you can take to reduce your chances of acquiring a disease. As you learned in chapter 7, there are two types of disease—communicable diseases, which are caused by pathogens, and noncommunicable diseases, which are caused by factors such as genetics, diet, behavior, or smoking. Adopting various strategies can help you prevent both types of disease.

Preventive Care

Regular visits to your doctor, dentist, and optometrist can help you stay healthy and prevent certain diseases. Yearly physical examinations (more frequent if you have a chronic problem) will allow your doctor to monitor your health and ensure your immunizations are up to date. You will have your height and weight measured at each visit because your doctor wants to see how these change over the years. Blood pressure measurements will also be taken at these appointments, and your doctor may also ask you to monitor your blood pressure frequently if it is elevated.

Your doctor may also collect blood or urine samples to monitor your cholesterol and blood glucose levels and to screen for certain diseases or disorders. You will be asked about any health problems you might be having, and your doctor may recommend a mental health screening, if needed.

In addition to regular physical exams, you should visit the dentist every six months and the optometrist every year. Dental cleanings and exams will help you maintain your oral health and allow your dentist to identify and treat any problems. Your optometrist will assess the health of your eyes and identify any vision problems. If you wear glasses or contact lenses, regular exams are recommended to keep your prescription up to date.

Avoiding the Spread of Disease

Infectious diseases can be transmitted, or spread, through a variety of methods, including contact with infected objects or people, through the air, by animals, and due to improper food sanitation.

If you do become sick, visit your doctor for treatment as soon as possible. If you are prescribed antibiotics, use them exactly as instructed. Report to your doctor any worsening infection that isn't better after taking an antibiotic. When sick, allow yourself time to heal and recover. Avoid spreading colds and the flu. When coughing or sneezing, cover your mouth and nose with your upper arm, not your hands (Figure 8.21). Wash your hands often, especially during flu and cold season. Hand washing is universally acknowledged to be the most important method of preventing many infectious diseases.

Be cautious around wild and domestic animals that aren't familiar to you. They can transmit pathogens that cause various diseases, including rabies, which can be fatal if not treated properly. Insects such as mosquitoes and ticks can transmit serious diseases including malaria, West Nile virus, and Lyme disease.

Be careful what you eat, making sure it is prepared properly. Cook meat thoroughly to kill any pathogens and wash your hands thoroughly after handling raw meat. Avoid nonpasteurized drinks, which have been linked to outbreaks of *E. coli*. Refrigerate and freeze perishables. Wash vegetables and fruits thoroughly.

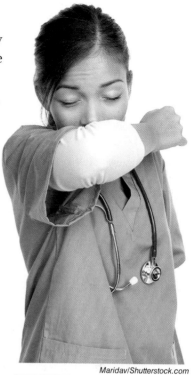

Maridav/Shutterstock.com

Figure 8.21 Sneezing into one's arm is more hygienic than sneezing into the hands because dirty hands more easily spread those germs to other surfaces or people.

Adopt Good Health Practices

Practice good posture to reduce the incidence and levels of back and neck pain. Make sure to report to your doctor any pain that is severe or persistent, such as knee pain or headaches.

Adopt strategies to manage your stress. As you learned earlier in the chapter, high levels of stress can cause numerous health problems. Your doctor can help recommend techniques to control your stress.

Avoid risky behaviors connected with addiction, driving carelessly, participating in dangerous sports activities, and becoming sexually active.

Check Your Understanding ✓

1. What are three signs that someone might be depressed?
2. List four strategies for dealing effectively with stress.
3. Explain the three main personality types.
4. What is meant by *social health*?
5. What is the difference between anorexia nervosa and bulimia nervosa?
6. Why is it important to cook meat thoroughly?

Community Health Resources

Community health resources address a wide variety of health promotion and disease prevention issues with the goal of promoting health and wellness. These efforts may include offering educational programs, giving vaccines (Figure 8.22), and providing preventive care, among other initiatives, such as the following:

- providing primary care services such as checkups
- providing some mental health services such as psychological counseling
- treating and providing information about chronic diseases such as HIV
- treating and providing information about sexually transmitted infections
- treating other infectious diseases
- treating minor injuries
- providing information and treatment for adolescent health
- providing information and materials for reproductive health

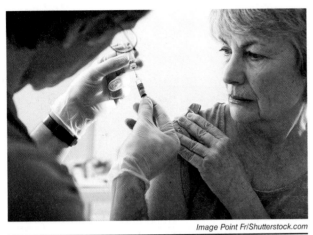

Image Point Fr/Shutterstock.com

Figure 8.22   Community health centers often offer free vaccines.

Many communities do not have access to quality healthcare, especially in rural areas. Ensuring that all people have equal access to high-quality healthcare to help them live healthy, productive lives should be a core goal of all healthcare systems. Where you live affects whether or not you have access to the best quality healthcare the United States can offer. There is a wide gulf in access to and the quality of care between people with low incomes and the rest of society.

Among low-income adults age 50 or older, just 22 percent to 42 percent received preventive care. In all states, low-income adults age 50 and over were less likely to receive preventive care than were higher-income adults. Low-income adults had a much higher rate of being uninsured.

Community health resources are incredibly important to low-income individuals. It is critical for healthcare professionals to promote a healthy community. Healthcare professionals need to create partnerships with organizations that seek to improve the health of people and the communities in which they live.

Community hospitals can provide low- or no-cost screenings for diseases such as diabetes and breast cancer. These hospitals can also provide free lectures on subjects such as substance abuse, nutrition, heart health, and prenatal care.

Community health centers can provide free vaccinations and other services for people who cannot afford a health plan and do not qualify for Medicaid. The Affordable Care Act has put in place comprehensive health insurance reforms that are designed to improve access, affordability, and quality in healthcare for Americans. Community health centers often invite families to sign up for and take advantage of health services at their center.

Extend Your Knowledge ▶ Healthcare Access

Access to comprehensive healthcare services is critical for achieving optimal health and wellness. People may not have access to healthcare for a variety of reasons, including limited healthcare services in the community, the high cost of healthcare, or a lack of health insurance.

With these barriers, health needs are not met and preventive services are not available. This often leads to unnecessary health crises that could have been avoided. Populations that do not have access to proper medical care tend to have shorter life spans than those who do have access to healthcare.

Underserved populations that exist in the United States include racial and ethnic minorities. Many of these individuals cannot afford services, and they may experience language barriers, inadequate healthcare facilities, lack of insurance, and lack of transportation. Older adults may have challenges such as lack of transportation to facilities, high cost of

services (even with Medicare coverage), and lack of an advocate to help with confusing paperwork. Rural areas far from cities can be underserved by medical services and often have transportation challenges.

Apply It

1. What do you think can be done to get more medical services into rural areas? Brainstorm ideas with a partner.

2. What other effects might poor access to healthcare have on a population?

3. Research healthcare access in two other countries and compare your findings to healthcare access in the United States. Do individuals in other countries have better access to healthcare than most Americans? Do they have worse access? How does healthcare access affect the general population of these countries?

Health Literacy

Health literacy is defined as the degree to which an individual has the capacity to obtain, communicate, process, and understand basic health information and services to make appropriate health decisions. Many people do not know how their bodies work. Others have no idea why they take pills that are prescribed to them. Some do not ask for explanations about diagnoses they are given or ask for second opinions. Understanding the services available to you, your doctor's diagnosis and treatment plans, and how your medical care impacts your overall health and wellness show that you possess health literacy (Figure 8.23).

Health literacy means that a person can navigate the healthcare system by locating providers and services. A person who understands and engages in self-care and who can manage a chronic disease is knowledgeable enough to make important decisions about his health.

Health literacy also means understanding mathematical concepts. An example of this is a patient who can understand cholesterol and blood sugar levels and respond appropriately. This patient can read nutrition labels, choosing healthy options. Comparing health plans and prescription drug coverage requires you to calculate premiums, copays, and deductibles.

health literacy
an individual's ability to obtain, communicate, and understand basic health information and services, allowing him or her to make appropriate health decisions

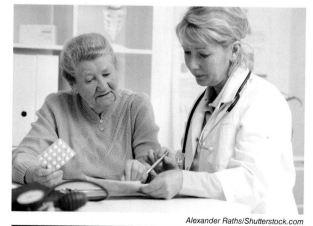

Alexander Raths/Shutterstock.com

Figure 8.23 Asking healthcare providers questions enables patients to make informed decisions about their treatments, prescriptions, and medical insurance benefits.

In addition to basic health literacy skills, a person should have knowledge of various health topics. Lacking knowledge or having misinformation about the body can lead to serious health challenges. People should have an understanding of how to prevent disease, such as washing your hands frequently. Without basic health literacy, a person may not understand the relationship between lifestyle factors, such as exercise and diet, and reducing various health risks.

Even if you have a great deal of health literacy, it can be challenging to keep up with rapid changes in medical science. What information you have gained during your school years can often become outdated or incomplete. Keep up to date!

Limited English proficiency can be a barrier for accessing health information and services. Medical jargon and terminology can feel like a foreign language even to English speakers. As someone who wants to work in healthcare, you may face the challenge of using language that your patient understands to explain important medical information. You may need a translator when working with patients who have limited English proficiency.

According to the National Assessment of Adult Literacy, less than 20 percent of adults in the United States are health literate. About 14 percent of adults have some health literacy but not enough to make informed choices about their healthcare. Low literacy has been linked to poor health outcomes, higher rates of hospitalization, and less frequent use of preventive services.

The populations most at risk for poor health literacy include older adults, racial and ethnic minorities, people with less than a high school degree or GED certificate, people with low income levels, nonnative English speakers, and people who are too sick to advocate for themselves.

Healthcare professionals and public health systems must work together to ensure that health information and services can be understood and used by all. With an education in healthcare, you can be a part of the effort to improve health literacy in your community. It is also your task to become more health literate so that you can make smart decisions about your own health.

Alternative Health Practices and Therapies

The most common healthcare therapies in the United States are part of Western, or *conventional*, medicine. These therapies are based on evaluating the physical signs and symptoms of the patient. Then, a diagnosis is made and a treatment plan is determined. However, there is a growing trend in the use of alternative medicine instead of conventional medical therapies. Alternative medicine describes medical products and practices that are not part of standard care.

Alternative medicine sometimes falls outside of the system of medical regulation (Figure 8.24).

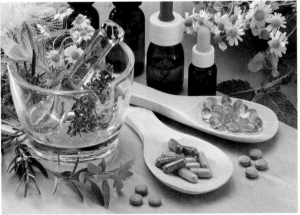
Pat_Hastings/Shutterstock.com

Figure 8.24 Herbal supplement manufacturers are not legally required to seek approval from the Food and Drug Administration (FDA) before selling their products.

Some states license and credential a variety of alternative medicine professions, but others do not. Sometimes it is hard to judge which providers are qualified and which are not. Be sure to thoroughly investigate alternative medicine providers before scheduling your visit.

There have recently been major trends toward using **complementary and alternative medicines (CAM)**, sometimes called *integrative health*. This is the use of a combination of complementary therapies (treatments that are used along with conventional medicine) and alternative methods. For example, some healthcare facilities now use both medicines and CAM therapies to treat chronic pain, encouraging stress reduction and relaxation techniques (Figure 8.25).

When you work in healthcare, you may encounter different cultural beliefs about how to treat an illness or disease. Alternative medicines are an important part of cultural practices for some ethnic groups. Some patients do not want mainstream medicine forced on them.

It may be challenging to find insurance coverage for CAM therapies. Wellness rebates can be received from some insurance companies for therapies such as massage, acupuncture, or yoga. Other alternative therapies may not be covered.

complementary and alternative medicine (CAM)
health practices used in place of or in conjunction with traditional Western medicine; also known as integrative health

Specific Complementary and Alternative Medicine (CAM) Practices	
Acupuncture	An ancient Chinese therapy that involves the insertion of very thin needles into specific points along the pathways of the body to stimulate and balance the flow of energy (*qi*). This belief is based on the concept that illness and pain occur when the *qi* is blocked.
Aromatherapy	The use of selected fragrances and oils from roots, bark, plants, and flowers to relieve muscle tension, tension headaches, or backaches; lower blood pressure; and create a soothing effect.
Reiki	Ancient Japanese and Tibetan art based on the idea that disease causes an imbalance in the body's energy field. Also called the *healing touch*, gentle hand pressure is applied to the body's *chakras* (energy centers) to harness and balance the life energy force, help clear blockages, and stimulate healing.
Homeopathy	The use of very small doses of drugs made from natural substances to produce symptoms of the disease being treated; based on the belief that these natural substances will stimulate the immune system to heal the body.
Hypnotherapy	Inducing a trance-like state so a person is receptive to suggestion; hypnotherapy is used to encourage desired behavior changes such as losing weight or stopping smoking.
Reflexology	Ancient art based on the concept that the body is divided into 10 zones that run from the head to the toes; illness or disease of the body causes deposits of calcium or acids in the corresponding part of the foot. The therapy includes applying pressure to specific points on the foot so energy is directed toward the affected body part. This is used to promote healing and relaxation; improve circulation; and treat asthma, sinus infections, irritable bowel syndrome, kidney stones, and constipation.
Yoga	Hindu discipline that uses concentration, specific positions, and ancient ritual movements to maintain the balance and flow of life energy; used to increase spiritual enlightenment and well-being and to develop an awareness of the body to improve coordination, relieve stress, and improve muscle tone.
Naturopathy	All natural therapies such as special diets, lifestyle changes, and supportive approaches to promote healing and treat illness; surgery and medicines are avoided.

Goodheart-Willcox Publisher

Figure 8.25   Complementary and alternative medicines (CAM) may be used on their own or along with conventional medicines to treat a variety of diseases and/or conditions.

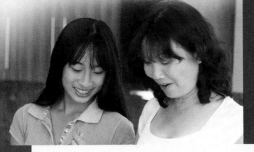

Chapter 8
Review and Assessment

Summary

Holistic health emphasizes the body working as a combination of mental, physical, and spiritual aspects to maintain optimal wellness through daily living. Maintaining physical health requires eating a healthy diet, maintaining a healthy weight, exercising, getting a good night's sleep, and avoiding addictions and substance abuse. Staying mentally and emotionally healthy means not only taking care of your physical body, but also maintaining positive self-esteem, avoiding destructive behaviors, recognizing the signs of depression, and asking for help if you have suicidal thoughts.

Social health involves establishing healthy relationships with others, as well as having connections to your community. Spiritual health is working to have peace and harmony in your life, without continual conflict challenging your good health.

Disease prevention is another important part of maintaining your overall health and wellness. Yearly physical exams, keeping immunizations up to date, allowing yourself time to heal, and using antibiotics as directed will help prevent disease.

Community health resources are available to ensure that as many people as possible have access to healthcare. These resources often educate people on important health practices, helping them to achieve health literacy. As a future healthcare worker, you must also become health literate, allowing you to advocate for your own health and provide quality care for your future patients. You may be responsible for imparting important medical knowledge to your future patients.

Increasingly, people are using complementary and alternative medicines (CAM) to achieve good health. Be aware that some of these therapies are not regulated and must be thoroughly researched before using.

Many health and wellness strategies are available to help you achieve optimal well-being. Understanding challenges to achieving health and wellness will not only benefit you personally, but can also be applied during your future career in healthcare.

Review Questions

Answer the following questions using what you have learned in this chapter.

True or False Assess

1. *True or False?* Holistic health only refers to dieting successfully.
2. *True or False?* Taking naps is not a good idea.
3. *True or False?* The USDA symbol for nutritional balance is a plate.
4. *True or False?* A diet rich in lean protein from eggs, nuts, and fish is beneficial for your health.
5. *True or False?* Insurance coverage covers all alternative health practices.
6. *True or False?* Most people in the United States are health literate.
7. *True or False?* Periods of euphoria are associated with bipolar disorder.
8. *True or False?* You should use antibiotics exactly as prescribed.
9. *True or False?* Exercise can improve your mood.
10. *True or False?* People can die from eating disorders.

Multiple Choice Assess

11. To be _____ is to feel overwhelmed by change and challenging situations.
    - A. motivated
    - B. fatigued
    - C. stressed
    - D. irritated
12. A healthful diet is one that includes _____.
    - A. lean proteins such as poultry, fish, beans, and nuts
    - B. an emphasis on fruits and vegetables
    - C. limited intake of saturated fats, sodium, and sugar
    - D. All of the above.

13. Which of the following is considered a life-altering event?

    A. the death of a relative

    B. moving

    C. too much homework

    D. A and B only.

14. You should go to the dentist every _____.

    A. year

    B. six months

    C. two years

    D. three months

15. A person who is ambitious, organized, and impatient is said to have which type of personality?

    A. type C personality

    B. type A personality

    C. type B personality

    D. None of the above.

16. In which country did acupuncture originate?

    A. Japan

    B. India

    C. China

    D. United States

17. Which of the following are types of eating disorders?

    A. anorexia nervosa

    B. bulimia nervosa

    C. restrictive food intake disorder

    D. All the above.

18. Aerobic exercise should be accomplished for 20 minutes a day for at least _____.

    A. 7 days a week

    B. 5–6 days a week

    C. 1–2 days a week

    D. 3–4 days a week

19. Which of the following statements is *not* true?

    A. Exercise improves energy.

    B. Exercise helps you sleep better.

    C. Exercise gets harder as you do it more.

    D. Exercise can be fun.

20. The USDA's dietary guidelines recommend the following foods *except* _____.

    A. fried foods

    B. lean meats

    C. whole grains

    D. poultry

Short Answer

21. List three risk factors associated with suicide.

22. Explain the difference between suicide contagion and suicide clusters.

23. Explain the three personality types listed in this chapter.

24. List three benefits of a good night's sleep.

25. What are three examples of alternative medicine?

26. Explain health literacy.

27. List five strategies for disease prevention.

28. Why is it important for healthcare facilities to test employees for drug use?

29. Define *holistic health*.

30. Explain the benefits of positive relationships among community healthcare workers.

Critical Thinking Exercises

31. What steps do you take to remain healthy? In what ways are you doing a good job? What could you do to improve your health?

32. How do you handle stress? What do you do to reduce stress?

33. Research and analyze the effects of access to quality healthcare.

34. Research wellness strategies for the prevention of disease. Include information on alternative health practices and therapies used in your community. Make a decision to incorporate one of the strategies into your lifestyle. Evaluate the impact of your decision and develop a list of modifications based on your current outcomes.

35. Research the role of the Food and Drug Administration in relationship to health and wellness.

36. How up to date are you in regards to current medical breakthroughs? Name three recent medical discoveries.

37. Evaluate both the positive and the negative effects of relationships on your physical and emotional health.

Chapter 9
Lifespan Development

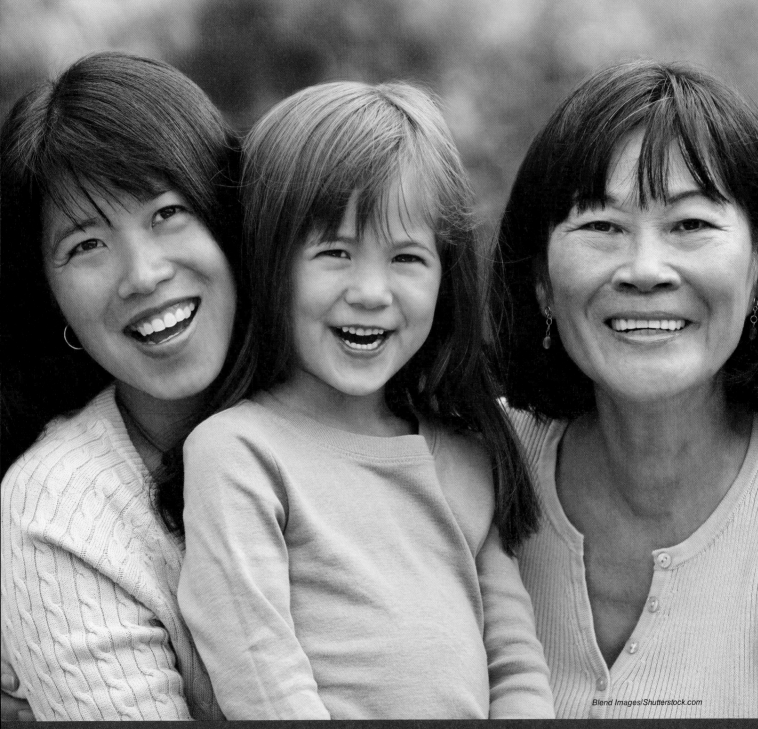

Blend Images/Shutterstock.com

Terms to Know

 Build Vocab

adolescence

Apgar scale

bonding

Brazelton Neonatal Behavioral
   Assessment Scale

fetal alcohol syndrome (FAS)

geriatrics

gerontology

gestation

infant

Maslow's hierarchy of needs

neonate

palliative care

prenatal

preschoolers

preteens

rooting reflex

startle reflex

sudden infant death syndrome
   (SIDS)

toddlers

Chapter Objectives

- Explain the significance of Maslow's hierarchy of needs.
- Identify four types of growth and development that occur in every life stage.
- Discuss the following human life stages: prenatal; infancy; early, middle, and late childhood; adolescence; early, middle, and late adulthood; and death.
- Describe medical specialties related to life stages.

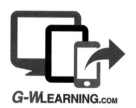

G-WLEARNING.com

While studying, look for the activity icon to:

- **Build** vocabulary with e-flash cards and interactive games.
- **Assess** progress with chapter and unit review questions.
- **Expand** learning with animations and illustration labeling activities.
- **Simulate** EHR entry with healthcare documents.

www.g-wlearning.com/healthsciences/

From the moment of conception until death, humans pass through many stages in which they experience continual change. Most life changes occur as a result of biology and psychology. Of course, some changes may also result from personal choices and accidental happenings. Most growth and developmental stages are shared among all people.

This chapter presents an overview of the important stages that humans go through in their lifetime. These include prenatal; infancy; early, middle, and late childhood; adolescence; early, middle, and late adulthood; and death. Throughout these stages, there are certain significant needs that must be met, as described by Maslow in his "hierarchy of needs." Each stage has its own medical specialty to treat specific needs of the stage.

Human Growth and Development

The scientific study of lifespan development is important not only to psychology, but also to areas such as biology, anthropology, sociology, education, and history. Students who are interested in a career in healthcare are encouraged to take several science classes. The most relevant courses include anatomy and physiology, which covers the form and function of the human body (see chapter 6). A class that covers lifespan development is just as important.

Healthcare workers must be aware of the various stages of human growth and development to better meet their patients' needs and provide quality healthcare. Human growth and development begins at conception and ends at death. Each stage of life brings unique challenges and changes.

Maslow's Hierarchy of Needs

Maslow's hierarchy of needs
a theory of human needs developed by American psychologist Abraham Maslow

In 1943, American psychologist Abraham Maslow proposed that healthy humans have a certain number of needs. These needs are arranged in a hierarchy, or an organized system of ranking people or things. **Maslow's hierarchy of needs** is often represented as a five-level pyramid. The base of the pyramid represents the most basic human needs. If these basic needs are not met, the higher-level needs toward the top of the pyramid may not be realized (Figure 9.1).

Four Types of Growth and Development

Throughout the stages of life, every person encounters four types of growth and development:

- physical (body growth)
- mental (development of the mind)
- emotional (feelings)
- social (interacting and relating to others)

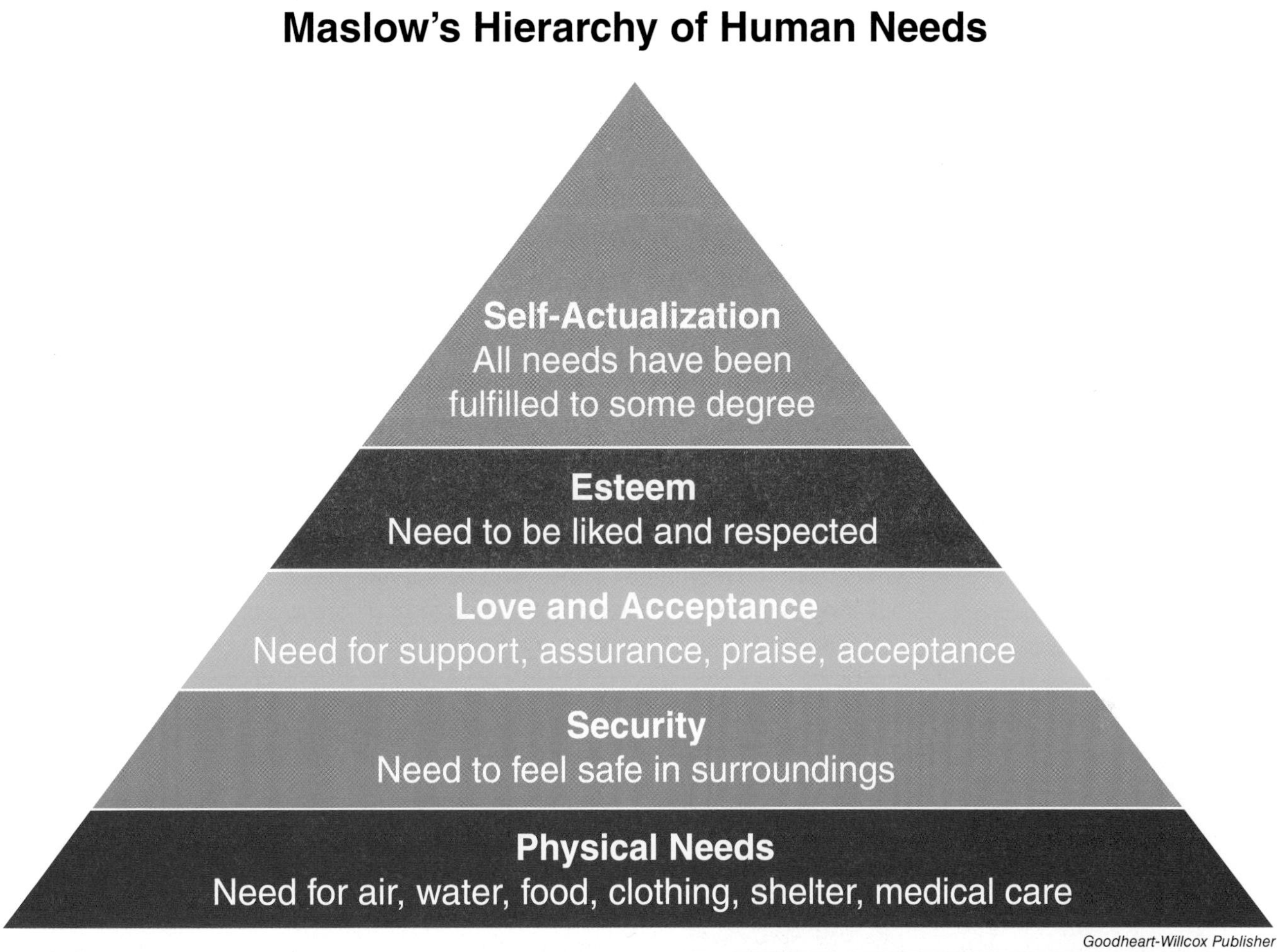

Maslow's Hierarchy of Human Needs

Self-Actualization
All needs have been
fulfilled to some degree

Esteem
Need to be liked and respected

Love and Acceptance
Need for support, assurance, praise, acceptance

Security
Need to feel safe in surroundings

Physical Needs
Need for air, water, food, clothing, shelter, medical care

Goodheart-Willcox Publisher

Figure 9.1 Maslow believed that basic needs must be mastered before an individual can progress up the pyramid to the higher-level needs. Which of these needs do you feel are fulfilled in your own life right now?

Each type of change occurs during every life stage. Growth and development varies greatly among all individuals. Physical bodies, mental development, and social interaction may grow at different rates. For instance, emotional maturity differs from person to person, and social interaction can range from extreme shyness to dramatic extroversion. Teenagers' bodies may be physically mature, but teens may still have childlike tendencies. Senior citizens can have bodies that limit mobility but minds that are very much alive. An elementary student can have a superior mind but will not participate in class due to debilitating shyness.

The Stages of Life

There are many different ways to classify the stages of human life. Each stage presents its own challenges. For our purposes, the following stages are discussed: prenatal, infancy, childhood (early, middle, and late), adolescence, adulthood (early, middle, and late), and death.

Animation

Prenatal: Fertilization until Birth

prenatal
the life stage before birth; during or relating to pregnancy

The **prenatal** stage spans the period from fertilization until birth (Figure 9.2). During the first eight weeks of development, the fertilized egg is in the embryo stage. The fetus stage, which lasts until birth, comes next.

Prenatal development occurs during approximately forty weeks of pregnancy. Pregnancy is divided into *trimesters*, or three-month periods. During the first trimester, the fetus' liver and bones begin to form, kidneys produce urine, and the lower trunk muscles develop. In the second trimester, the ribs and major body systems develop. Before the third trimester, survival outside the mother is difficult. Growth and organ development are rapid during the third trimester.

gestation
the period between fertilization and birth; also known as pregnancy

Did You Know?   Prematurity and Development

Babies born before 24 weeks of **gestation** have poor rates of survival and are considered premature. Those who do survive may endure a great deal of suffering and health problems in the long term. There are of course exceptions, but delivering before 30 weeks of gestation is risky.

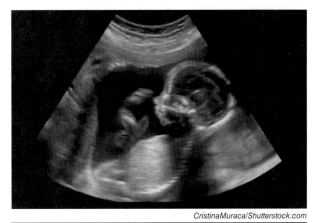

CristinaMuraca/Shutterstock.com

Figure 9.2   A fetus' growth and development can be monitored throughout pregnancy using ultrasounds. What might a doctor be looking for on a sonogram?

Having a Healthy Pregnancy

Regular medical care and checkups are very important during pregnancy. These checkups can verify the health of the mother as well as the healthy development of the baby. It is recommended that women schedule a checkup once a month for weeks 4 through 28, twice a month from weeks 28 through 36, and once a week from week 36 to birth.

During pregnancy, women should avoid alcohol consumption, smoking, and most drugs, including over-the-counter and prescription drugs not given by an obstetrician. Secondhand smoke should also be avoided. Women are strongly encouraged to eat a healthy, well-balanced diet during their pregnancy.

It is recommended that women take extra *folic acid* (a B vitamin) before and during pregnancy, as it promotes healthy brain and spinal cord development. Pregnant women are also encouraged to take prenatal vitamins. In addition to folic acid, these vitamins contain iron, iodine, and calcium.

Problems with Prenatal Development

In the great majority of cases, pregnancy and birth go well. However, there can be complications during pregnancy. These complications, which can affect the developing baby, include the following:

- **Genetic Disorders.** Some problems may be passed down through family genes. Prenatal testing can determine the possibility of such problems before pregnancy. Others can be detected during pregnancy. Some genetic disorders can be treated, and others cannot (Figure 9.3).

Genetic Disorders			
Name	*Description*	*Effects*	*Treatment*
Cystic fibrosis	Caused by two faulty genes that interfere with the respiratory, digestive, and reproductive systems. The body cannot easily process mucus, which creates blockage within the body.	Digestive, reproductive, and respiratory issues. Effects range from mild to severe.	No cure exists, but treatments are available and vary depending on symptoms. Treatments may include medications, exercise, and dietary supplements.
Down syndrome	Caused by an extra chromosome.	Severe cognitive disability and delayed language development. Effects are not uniform.	Possible surgery; specialized learning programs.
Fragile X syndrome	Caused by a faulty gene. The X chromosome is unstable (fragile) and usually breaks.	Effects range from short attention span to a learning disability to severe cognitive disability.	Treatments vary, but may include specialized education and therapy.
Huntington's disease	Caused by an abnormal gene that provides instructions for producing a protein called *huntingtin*, which is suspected to play an important role in nerve cells in the brain.	Loss of some physical control, memory, and ability to rationalize. Often leads to depression and death from complications.	There is no cure, but medication is available to treat symptoms. Physical activity is also recommended.
Phenylketonuria (PKU)	Caused by two mutated genes that prevent the body from processing phenylalanine, an amino acid.	If undetected, can cause permanent internal damage and cognitive disability.	When detected early, a modified diet can prevent physical and cognitive damage.
Sickle cell anemia	Caused by a recessive gene that alters the shape of the red blood cell. Affected cells are bowed instead of circular and do not properly carry oxygen throughout the body.	Effects range from no effect to chronic illness to early death.	Blood transfusions, penicillin, and proper medication.
Spina bifida	Caused by incomplete development and formation of the spine.	Partial to complete paralysis, fluid buildup in the skull.	Corrective surgery, physical therapy, and a modified diet.
Tay-Sachs disease	Caused by a recessive gene. The body is unable to break down certain types of fats, which build up in the system and can block neural transmissions.	Cognitive and physical deterioration that usually leads to early death.	No cure exists, but a modified diet and medication can ease symptoms.

Goodheart-Willcox Publisher

Figure 9.3   Genetic disorders

Real Life Scenario   Pregnancy Advice

Gabriella and José are having their first child. They are in their early twenties and are unsure what to expect. They both come from large families with many aunts, grandmas, mothers, and big sisters. Everyone wants to give the couple advice about Gabriella's pregnancy. Advice they have been given includes the following:

- Don't travel by plane.
- You are "eating for two."
- You must lie on your left side at night.
- Don't drink coffee.
- Don't exercise.

- Exercise is good for you and the baby.
- Avoid all seafood.
- You can drink in moderation.
- If you carry low, it's a boy.
- Eat sensibly, not dieting.

Apply It

1. Which pieces of advice are myths and which are based on common sense?
2. How do you handle advice that you know probably isn't correct or accurate?

- **Mother's Age.** A woman's age can affect her pregnancy. Teen mothers may experience preterm labor and deliver babies with low birth weights. Older women (past age 35) may give birth to babies with birth defects and abnormalities. This may be due to longer exposure to environmental toxins or the age of the fertilized egg. Studies show that the father's age may also be a factor in pregnancy complications.

- **Illness.** If a woman has an infectious illness, this can cause an infection in the fetus. For example, if a women contracts rubella (German measles) during the first three months of her pregnancy, it can cause infant blindness. Some infections can be treated with antibiotics if detected and treated early.

- **Environmental Factors.** Exposure to harmful substances during pregnancy can cause adverse effects. These substances can include chemicals, medications, alcohol, illegal drugs, and cigarettes. Pregnant women should check with their doctors on what items to avoid.

fetal alcohol syndrome (FAS)

term that describes conditions such as cognitive disabilities resulting from prenatal exposure to alcohol

Did You Know?   Fetal Alcohol Syndrome (FAS)

Fetal alcohol syndrome (FAS) occurs when women drink alcohol during pregnancy. Some researchers refer to FAS as *FASD*, which stands for *fetal alcohol spectrum disorders*, an umbrella term for a range of disorders. These disorders range from mild to severe, often causing physical and mental birth defects.

When a pregnant woman drinks alcohol, some alcohol passes to the fetus. The developing fetus cannot process alcohol as an adult can, so the alcohol is more concentrated in the fetus, preventing nutrition and oxygen from reaching vital organs.

People born with FAS may experience problems with their vision, hearing, memory, attention span, and their learning and communication abilities. While these problems can differ among individuals, the damage is often permanent.

Infancy: Birth until One Year

Infancy is the time between birth and the first birthday. During the first month of life, the baby is considered a **neonate**. After these first 30 days, the baby is called an **infant** until the first birthday (Figure 9.4).

Immediately after birth, babies are covered with blood and a thin, white coating called the *vernix caseosa*. A baby's head may be temporarily misshapen as he or she passes through the birth canal. The baby is tested with the **Apgar scale** one minute after birth and then again at five minutes after birth. This scale rates the baby's heart and respiratory rates, muscle tone, responsiveness, and body color. The doctor rates each condition on a scale of 0 to 2, with 2 being the best. The **Brazelton Neonatal Behavioral Assessment Scale** measures a baby's reflexes and responses to sounds, touch, and light. The ability to soothe the baby and catch its attention is also observed.

Babies are born with *reflexes*, which are involuntary movements or actions that occur spontaneously. When something is placed on the roof of their mouth, babies' reflexes to suck are triggered. When the side of their mouth is stroked, babies move toward a bottle or their mother's breast. This is called a **rooting reflex**.

Babies also have a **startle reflex**, which can be triggered when the baby is disturbed by a sudden noise or jolt. This reflex causes the limb and neck muscles to contract, producing the startle. Triggers for this reflex can include the noise of a vacuum, a telephone ringing, being touched while asleep, other children screaming, loud crowds, and turning on the television or radio. This reflex usually disappears at about six months old. Although all babies have reflexes, they may exhibit reflexes at different times.

At birth, a baby's neck muscles are not strong enough to support the head. The neck must be carefully supported with care until the baby can support the head on its own. During infancy, brain development occurs at a rapid pace. Care must be taken to protect a baby's head from falls or other head injuries. A baby should never be shaken, which can cause brain swelling and possible brain damage.

The infancy stage brings dramatic and rapid changes. The baby begins to roll over, crawl, walk, and grasp objects. Mental development brings responses to cold, hunger, and pain through crying. The baby also begins to recognize surroundings and people. Emotionally, the baby is able to show anger, distrust, happiness, and excitement. During infancy, the baby is dependent on others for all of its needs.

Good nutrition is particularly important during infancy. Like adults, babies need to eat well-balanced diets. However, a baby's needs are quite different from an adult's. Newborns are just learning to suck and swallow, so their nutrition must come in liquid form. Breast milk is ideal for at least the first six months. Adoption, health issues, and medication may prevent a mother from breastfeeding, so she may choose to feed her baby formula. It is important to select a formula that meets nutritional requirements.

neonate
term that describes a baby from birth to one month

infant
term that describes a child from thirty days after birth until the first birthday

Apgar scale
a measure used to determine the health of a newborn based on heart and respiratory rates, muscle tone, responsiveness, and body color

Brazelton Neonatal Behavioral Assessment Scale
a test given to a newborn that measures reflexes and responses to sounds, touch, and light

rooting reflex
the natural inclination of newborns to turn their head toward a food source when the side of their mouth is stroked

startle reflex
the natural inclination of a baby's limb and neck muscles to contract in response to a loud noise or jolt

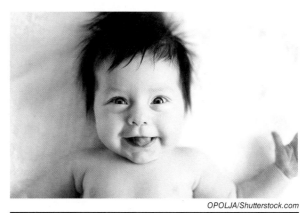
OPOLJA/Shutterstock.com

Figure 9.4 Infancy lasts from birth until the first birthday. What rapid changes occur during infancy?

Extend Your Knowledge ▶ Sudden Infant Death Syndrome (SIDS)

sudden infant death syndrome (SIDS)
unexpected death that occurs for unknown reasons during the first few months of a baby's life

Sudden infant death syndrome (SIDS) can occur in infants under the age of one. There are no warning signs before SIDS occurs. The baby can appear healthy and normal when put to bed, making the death truly unexpected. The exact cause of SIDS is unknown, but researchers have found correlations with the baby sleeping on its side or stomach, overheating, and exposure to cigarette smoke. There is also a possible connection with low birth weight, as well as infections, genetic disorders, and heart problems.

The most effective methods of preventing SIDS are putting a baby on its back to sleep, using a firm mattress, avoiding loose bedding, keeping the sleeping environment cool, and avoiding exposure to tobacco smoke. In the United States, the incidence of SIDS has decreased in the last twenty years.

Apply It

1. Research to determine the worldwide occurrence rate for SIDS.
2. What does the latest research say about possible causes of SIDS?

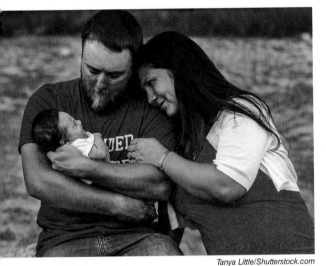

Tanya Little/Shutterstock.com

Figure 9.5 Bonding is important for parents and the infant.

bonding
the act of developing an emotional connection between a parent or caregiver and a baby

Between 6 and 12 months, babies can begin eating solids. Solid foods should be introduced one at a time and always in small amounts. Parents may begin to notice food intolerances at this time.

Sleep is very important to an infant's growth and development. Typically, babies sleep for about three hours, wake for one, and then repeat the pattern. Eating and sleeping patterns are not necessarily consistent. As babies grow, their stomachs are able to hold more food, and they may adapt to the rhythms of the household. Throughout infancy, babies may take two naps a day.

Bonding is the emotional connection that a parent or caregiver develops with a baby. It is particularly important at the infant stage, although bonding can occur throughout life. Bonding occurs when the caregiver spends time with the baby and becomes confident in meeting the baby's needs (Figure 9.5).

Check Your Understanding ✓

1. What is on the bottom level of Maslow's hierarchy of needs?
2. What are two things a pregnant woman should avoid?
3. How can a woman's age affect her pregnancy?
4. What are two important infant reflexes?
5. What is a baby's typical sleeping pattern?

Early Childhood: One to Six Years

Early childhood is defined as the time between one year and six years (Figure 9.6). Children in this stage, who are between one and three years of age, are called **toddlers**. A toddler needs constant attention. Most toddlers walk by fifteen months and can run easily, throw a ball, and scribble with a crayon by the age of two.

By their second birthday, most toddlers weigh about 27 pounds and are about 3 feet tall. At this time, most toddlers also have all of their primary teeth except the second molars. By their third birthday, toddlers weigh around 32 pounds and are about 38 inches tall.

Toddlers can fall and get up several times an hour. Toddlers are able to open cabinets and get into bottles that may contain harmful or poisonous liquids. As a result, toddlers must be monitored constantly. Active exploration is typical of toddlers, so they must have a safe environment that is childproofed. Childproofing measures include the following:

- placing sharp objects out of reach

- ensuring that medicine, kitchen, and other cabinets have childproof locks

- installing child protection gates at tops and bottoms of staircases

- being aware of new safety regulations and product recalls for cribs, car seats, and more

- making sure all doors and windows are closed or safely locked

toddlers
term that describes children between the ages of one and three

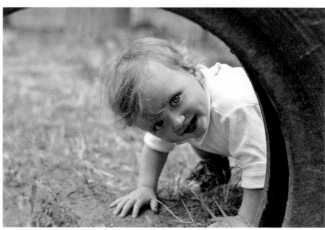

Denis Omelchenko/Shutterstock.com

Figure 9.6 Toddlers are curious about their world. What specific safeguards can ensure that a toddler explores in a safe environment?

During early childhood, physical development is slower than in infancy. Mental development includes verbal growth, a short attention span, asking questions, and recognizing letters. Children develop self-awareness and often know the effect they have on others. Children can become impatient and frustrated when trying to do something beyond their capabilities. Younger children may be self-centered but typically become more sociable as they grow and develop. Children also develop strong attachments to their parents during this stage.

By age three, most children have made significant progress with toilet training. However, they still have accidents, and they need to be reminded to use the toilet throughout the day. The progress of toilet training varies among children.

Children who are between three and five years old are often called **preschoolers**. During this period, boys and girls appear slimmer as the trunks of their bodies lengthen and body fat lessens. Their bodies are more muscular, and most preschoolers are capable of learning many coordinated activities. Fine-motor skills begin to improve, and by four years old, most children can attempt activities such as copying alphabet letters, building a block tower, and dressing and undressing.

preschoolers
term that describes children between the ages of three and five

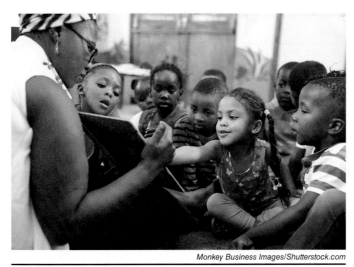

Monkey Business Images/Shutterstock.com

Figure 9.7   Reading to preschoolers encourages them to learn to read on their own.

One way to help prepare children to read and increase their vocabulary is by reading books to them. Most children can recognize some letters of the alphabet during this time. By age five, many children can identify all letters of the alphabet and write their name. Of course, there is a great deal of variety in the progress each child makes in this area. Increasingly, children are reading by age 5 (Figure 9.7).

Many children between three and five years of age are enrolled in preschool programs. There are movements in the country to provide free preschool education to all three to five year olds. Research shows that attending preschool may give children an advantage when they go to kindergarten.

Preschoolers are active in the world, and this means they are often exposed to illnesses. Their immune systems are still developing and are not as strong as adults' immune systems. Most children receive vaccinations to help prevent illnesses, but these children can still become ill.

Middle Childhood: Six to Ten Years

The period of time from six to ten years of age is the middle childhood stage. Physical development at this stage is slow and steady. Muscle coordination becomes well developed, and some children master physical activity requiring complex motor-sensory coordination. Mentally, these children are developing quickly, as much of their life revolves around school. Reading and writing skills advance, and abstract concepts like loyalty, values, honesty, and morals become understood. Typical growth in height averages between two and three inches a year. At this age, many children show signs that their bodies are changing.

Emotional development brings greater independence and a more defined personality during this stage. Children are talkative, imaginative, and develop a sense of humor. Each child is an individual with varying personality attributes. Today, most children in this age range are familiar with computers (Figure 9.8). Many schools use computers for instruction. At this age, some children are beginning to be active on social media, although some parents do not allow it.

Obesity is on the rise in children from six to ten years old. Some children lead sedentary lives, spending most of their time inside watching TV or playing computer games. They may eat junk food as a snack instead of fruits and vegetables. Obesity during childhood is a serious concern because it can lead to diseases throughout life such as high blood pressure, high cholesterol, and type 2 diabetes.

Children in this age range may become involved with sports. Team sports can be beneficial because they allow children to gain experience interacting with others and to improve their motor skills. Sports also provide outdoor exercise.

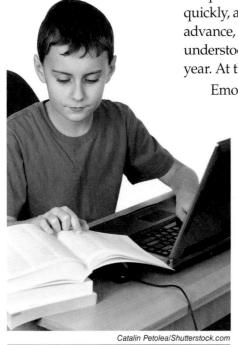

Catalin Petolea/Shutterstock.com

Figure 9.8   In middle childhood, children may begin working with computers and exploring the Internet. What were your first experiences with computers as a child?

Late Childhood: Ten to Twelve Years

Preadolescence is often defined as the years from age 10 to age 12. Children in this age group are sometimes referred to as **preteens** (Figure 9.9). Many preteens begin to replace fear with the ability to cope. Socially, preteen activities become more group-oriented and the opinions of others become more important. Preteens need reassurance, parental approval, and acceptance from their peers.

By age 10 to 12, sexual maturation and changes in body functions can lead to emotional ups and downs. These changes can cause restlessness, anxiety, and periods during which the preteen is difficult to understand. By this age, many children can better understand abstract concepts such as loyalty, honesty, and values. Preteens also may begin to develop an awareness of the opposite sex. Dependency on parents begins to lessen during this time, and preteens may spend less time at home.

preteens
term that describes children between the ages of 10 and 12

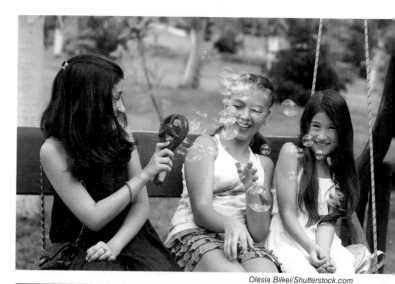

Olesia Bilkei/Shutterstock.com

Figure 9.9   Activities become more group-oriented as an individual enters late childhood. Preteens tend to seek the approval of their friends and peers.

Adolescence: Twelve to Twenty Years

Adolescence can be full of excitement and exploration. It is also a time for tremendous physical and psychological changes that can cause anxiety and conflict.

Physical development during this stage is accelerated. Puberty leads to the development of secondary sexual characteristics. Both boys and girls experience the growth of underarm and pubic hair. Girls' breasts begin to develop and their hips widen, while boys experience muscle growth and facial hair development. Girls also begin to menstruate, and boys produce sperm and semen (the fluid that contains sperm). Hormones surge, weight control may become an issue, and acne may influence teenagers' physical appearance and social interactions.

Mental development during this stage may include reasoning, abstract thinking, and critical thinking. Adolescents may not see the connection between behavior and consequences, leading them to make potentially bad decisions. In this stage of life, teenagers must learn to make good decisions and accept responsibility for negative actions.

A teenager's emotions can be stormy and may cause conflict with those around them. The use of alcohol and/or drugs can occur at any life stage, but it frequently begins during adolescence. Reasons for drug abuse may include stress relief, peer pressure, escape from problems, experimentation, the need for instant gratification, and possibly hereditary traits. During this stage, teenagers may also develop concern for the welfare of others. This may lead to involvement in community service projects.

adolescence
the stage of life following the onset of puberty during which a young person develops from a child into an adult

Real Life Scenario   Teenage Rebellion

Judith and her husband Ken wonder why their sweet, loving daughter Sophie is changing. At age fourteen, Sophie is not interested in spending time with her parents. She even announced that she doesn't want to go on the family vacation this year. Sophie spends more and more time in her room, texting her friends and playing loud music. Recently, Ken sent Sophie back to her room to change out of an outfit that he felt was inappropriate for school.

Apply It

1. Should Sophie's parents be worried about her recent attitude changes? Explain your reasoning.
2. When, if at all, do you think parents should become concerned about teen behavior? Give two or three specific examples of teen behaviors that you believe should cause parents to be concerned.

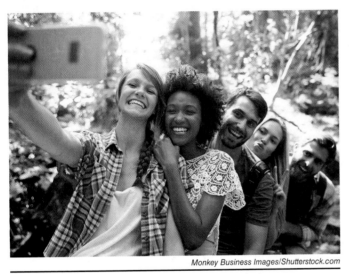

Monkey Business Images/Shutterstock.com

Figure 9.10 Friendships play an important role in an adolescent's development.

Social development revolves around a teenager's peers, who hold great influence (Figure 9.10). Adolescents often feel enormous pressure to look good. Body image is often influenced by flawless, unrealistic examples presented in the media. As a result, eating disorders can be a problem among adolescents. Chapter 8 includes a more in-depth discussion of eating disorders. Bullying, a common problem among adolescents, can lead to hurt feelings and dangerous behaviors, including suicide.

As a healthcare provider, dealing with teenagers can be a challenge. Establishing a rapport with an adolescent requires adopting a nonjudgmental attitude, listening to what the teenager has to say, involving the teenager in decisions, and answering questions as honestly as possible.

Toward the end of adolescence, teenagers hopefully feel more comfortable with who they are and begin to focus on who they might become as an adult.

Check Your Understanding

1. During what age range are children considered toddlers?
2. What mental developments occur during middle childhood?
3. Which age group is referred to as *preteens*?
4. Name two developments associated with puberty.
5. Why might teenagers begin to abuse drugs or alcohol?

Early Adulthood: Twenty to Forty Years

When an individual reaches early adulthood, physical development has been completed. Muscles are fully developed, and coordination is at its peak.

Young adults often experience many transitions in their lives as they choose careers and achieve independence, which can be a challenge. Moving from a familiar, comfortable environment to a new location can be stressful and intimidating. Early adulthood can also be exciting for those who are happily establishing their adult identities and feeling free to manage their own lives. Some young adults pursue additional education so they may progress in their chosen careers.

Many individuals find a partner and start a family during this life stage. However, this stage in life is very different now than it was in the past, when people got married in their late teens or early twenties. Economic strains may result in young adults living at home until their late twenties. This may cause young adults to delay the start of their own families, and they may not have children until their thirties or even early forties (Figure 9.11). Young adults do not experience many health problems.

Socially, young adults may spend more time with friends who have similar ambitions, interests, and life paths. Career decisions may dictate a young adult's lifestyle choices. Women can choose a career that wasn't available to their mothers or grandmothers. Men may stay at home with the children or choose positions that were traditionally filled by females. Traditional gender roles continue to be in flux for this age group. This is an exciting life stage for most young adults.

Middle Adulthood: Forty to Sixty-Five Years

People in middle adulthood, often called *middle age*, are active and productive but may begin to notice signs of aging. Middle-aged adults may experience thinning or graying hair, wrinkles on their skin, weakening muscles, hearing loss, changes in eyesight, and weight gain. Women experience *menopause*, or the end of menstruation, which causes decreased hormone production and physical and emotional changes. Men also experience a slowing of hormone production.

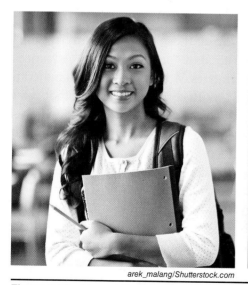
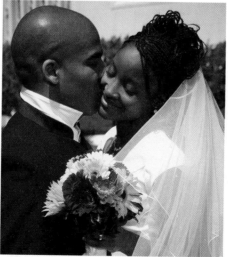
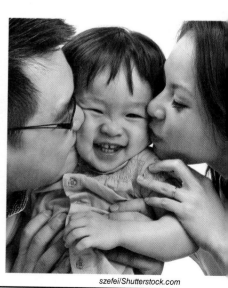

arek_malang/Shutterstock.com   *Alan Bailey/Shutterstock.com*   *szefei/Shutterstock.com*

Figure 9.11   Many milestones, such as obtaining a college degree, getting married, and having children, may occur during early adulthood.

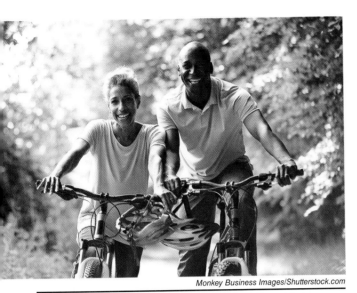
Monkey Business Images/Shutterstock.com

Figure 9.12 Many people find middle adulthood to be a rewarding, active period of their lives.

Middle-aged adults continue to develop mentally, often becoming confident decision makers and troubleshooters. At this stage in life, many people seek more education, sometimes graduating from college with a new degree or starting a new career. By this time, individuals have often gained an understanding of life and have learned to cope productively with stresses.

Emotionally, middle adulthood can bring satisfaction and contentment. As children become more independent, they leave their parents with more personal time to spend together (Figure 9.12). However, the fear of aging, the loss of youth and vitality, and stresses of older children and aging parents can cause feelings of depression, anxiety, and even anger. Divorce rates are high in this age group, as couples who have stayed together to raise children decide to separate.

The term *midlife crisis* was coined in the 1980s to describe a period between the ages of forty and fifty when some men and women realize their own mortality. The burden of unrealized goals, an unfulfilling career, and the appearance of aging-related physical changes may cause personal crises. Children leaving home can cause an individual to reevaluate his or her role in the family. This phenomenon does not appear throughout all cultures, meaning that the "culture of youth" in Western societies might account for this "crisis."

geriatrics
the care of aging people

The health of many middle-aged people is still fairly good, but signs of future problems can appear. These signs may include high cholesterol, arthritis, diabetes, and other issues resulting from obesity and lack of exercise.

Late Adulthood: Sixty-Five Years and Up

During these years, all body systems begin to show signs of aging. Advances in **geriatrics**, a branch of medicine concerned with problems associated with old age, have successfully extended this stage of life for many people. Travel, volunteerism, and social activities can enhance late adulthood (Figure 9.13). Many individuals do not show physical signs of aging until their seventies or eighties. Mental ability can vary among older adults. Some people in their nineties remain alert and oriented, while some younger people may already show signs of decreased mental ability.

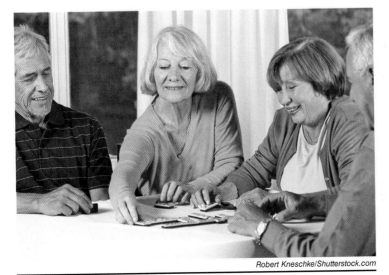
Robert Kneschke/Shutterstock.com

Figure 9.13 Many retirement communities offer a variety of activities that help residents form friendships and enjoy their later years.

Alzheimer's disease and atherosclerosis, which can occur in late adulthood, are discussed in chapter 7.

In late adulthood, wrinkles and age spots begin to appear, and the skin begins to dry. Muscles lose tone and strength, and the bone disease osteoporosis can lead to an increased incidence of bone fracture, especially of the hip. Memory loss can occur during this stage, but many people remain mentally active. A decline in the function of the nervous system can lead to hearing loss, declining vision, and intolerance for temperatures that are either too cold or too hot.

Emotional development during this stage can vary greatly among individuals. Some people slip into depression due to loss of identity after retirement or the death of a spouse and friends. Older adults often feel depressed when facing the reality of their own eventual death as well. Physical infirmities can lead to increased dependence on others, which is very difficult for most people. These infirmities may mean a person must move to a retirement community or assisted-living facility. Today, many retirement communities offer a broad range of life-affirming activities.

Emotional stability varies greatly among individuals in late adulthood. Some people can cope with the stresses of getting old, while others become lonely, frustrated, and depressed. In general, how a person has dealt with stresses throughout his or her entire life will dictate the way stress is handled in late adulthood.

For many aging people, grandchildren become very important in their daily lives. Interacting with young people can bring back positive memories of childhood and raising children (Figure 9.14). However, grandparents are increasingly raising their grandchildren on their own. Nationwide, there are millions of children living in households headed by grandparents. Some common reasons for this phenomenon include parental abandonment, divorce, teenage pregnancy, mental or physical illness, substance abuse, abuse and neglect, and incarceration.

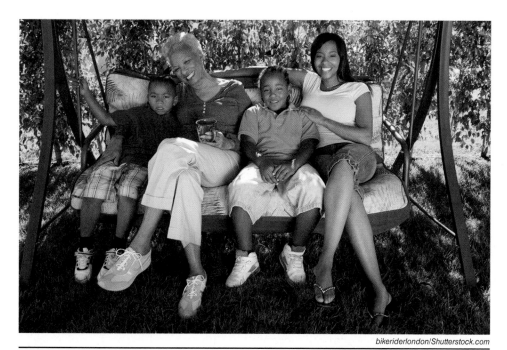

bikeriderlondon/Shutterstock.com

Figure 9.14   Grandchildren can bring great joy to grandparents.

This situation can place great stress on older adults, especially if they have limited financial resources, making it difficult to provide adequate housing, food, and clothing. In addition, grandparents may have limited energy and physical health problems that make becoming a parent again challenging. Raising grandchildren can also cause anxiety and depression in older adults. Fortunately, there are support groups for grandparents who are put into the role of parent at this stage in life.

gerontology
the study of the aging process

Gerontology is a vast field that includes the study of various biological, physical, and mental changes in older people. Geriatrics focuses on the care of aging people, while gerontology is the actual study of the aging process. Subjects such as biology, sociology, psychology, and therapy are the main areas included in gerontology.

People are living longer, and the number of older adults is increasing, along with the diversity of older adults' needs and interests. In addition, many states predict dramatic workforce shortages in industries that provide services to the aging population. Therefore, the demand for professionals with expertise in aging is growing rapidly, and career opportunities in gerontology and geriatrics are numerous and varied.

Death and Dying

Death is the final stage of growth. Death is often accompanied by grief—either the person's own grief at the loss of life, or the grief of the person's family and friends. Dr. Elisabeth Kübler-Ross (1926–2004), a Swiss-American psychiatrist, observed that there are five stages of grief. The stages may not occur in a strict order, and some people may not progress through them all. Some people may fall back to a previous stage. These stages include the following:

1. **Denial.** The person refuses to believe death is coming. *"There must be some mistake. I bet the lab mixed up my lab tests. I can't be dying."*

2. **Anger.** Feelings of negativity develop and may be directed at a person's own illness or body. Individuals may also experience feelings of resentment toward others. *"I am a good person. Why me? Why not my neighbor, who is such a terrible person? Why is my body doing this to me?"*

3. **Bargaining.** A person wants more time, and proposes deals or exchanges (usually with a higher power, family members, or their doctor) to extend life. *"God, if you take away my cancer, I will read the Bible every day and be such a better person."*

4. **Depression.** Struggling with the loss of life can cause people to become sad, withdrawn, and disinterested in activities. *"I don't see any reason to get out of bed."*

5. **Acceptance.** The reality of death is understood and accepted. If a person reaches this stage, death can be a peaceful experience. *"I am at peace with my death. I want my family and friends around me during the last stages."*

In the decades after Dr. Elisabeth Kübler-Ross first shared these findings, her concepts have been largely accepted by the public. Research continues to examine and build upon the findings of Kübler-Ross.

Research in this field has brought about many changes in the way the dying are treated. For instance, hospice services are now widely available. Hospices operate with a philosophy that focuses on bringing comfort, self-respect, and tranquility to the dying. The dying are often given **palliative care**, which relieves and prevents the suffering of patients in their last stages. This service is available to terminally ill patients in their homes as well as in hospice facilities.

Providing supportive care when families and patients require it the most can be one of the greatest satisfactions a healthcare worker can experience. Many people initially think that they cannot be around the dying, but with experience, healthcare workers can find ways to deal with their feelings and learn to embrace the role of supportive friend to patients and their families.

Death is a part of life. By understanding the process of dying and learning about the needs of the dying, the healthcare worker can provide special care to patients, and possibly to his or her own family members when the time comes.

palliative care
term for measures taken to treat symptoms and pain even though the treatment will not cure a disease; use of comfort measures

Check Your Understanding ✓

1. How is the early adulthood stage different now from how it was in the past?
2. What is meant by the term *midlife crisis*?
3. Name three reasons why older adults may have to raise their grandchildren.
4. Name the five stages of grief.
5. What is gerontology?

Specialties Related to Life Stages

Each stage of human life brings with it very specific needs. In the past, a family doctor treated all stages. Today, specialties have developed to concentrate on the needs that arise during each stage of life. Figure 9.15 illustrates many specific specialties related to life stages.

Medical Specialties	
Life Stage	*Specialties*
Prenatal	obstetrician; perinatologist; medical geneticist
Infancy	pediatrician; neonatologist; neonatal nurse
Early childhood	pediatrician; pediatric nurse
Late childhood	pediatrician; pediatric nurse
Adolescence	sports medicine professionals; endocrinologists; dermatologists; psychologists
Early and middle adulthood	internists; specialists such as neurologists, cardiologists, or gynecologists
Late adulthood	internist; geritrician; hospice physician; hospice nurse

Goodheart-Willcox Publisher

Figure 9.15 Medical specialties related to life stages

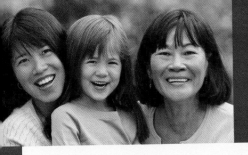

Chapter 9
Review and Assessment

Summary

The study of lifespan development and the concepts described in Maslow's hierarchy of needs will help healthcare workers effectively meet the needs of their patients. The stages of growth and development include prenatal, infancy, early childhood, middle childhood, late childhood, adolescence, early adulthood, middle adulthood, and late adulthood. Most pregnancies go well, but problems can occur with prenatal development. Among those problems are genetic disorders, such as cystic fibrosis and sickle cell anemia, and environmental factors such as fetal alcohol syndrome.

In each stage of life, there will be physical, mental, emotional, and social challenges and changes. Death and dying are studied as the final life stage. There are many professional specialties that focus on specific life stages, such as pediatrician, dermatologist, and hospice nurse.

Review Questions

Answer the following questions using what you have learned in this chapter.

True or False Assess

1. *True or False?* Maslow's hierarchy of needs describes four types of human growth and development.
2. *True or False?* The term *neonate* refers to a baby up to one year old.
3. *True or False?* Geriatrics is a branch of medicine specializing in problems associated with old age.
4. *True or False?* An embryo and a fetus are the same.
5. *True or False?* Normal gestation for a human being is about 40 weeks.
6. *True or False?* Fetal alcohol syndrome can cause permanent damage to a fetus.
7. *True or False?* Mental ability deteriorates at the same rate among older adults.
8. *True or False?* Children are generally quiet, reserved, and not sociable.

9. *True or False?* Most toddlers can learn to read.
10. *True or False?* Dr. Kübler-Ross outlines five stages of grief.

Multiple Choice Assess

11. Which of the following statements are correct?
    A. A hospice facility serves the terminally ill.
    B. People can receive hospice care in their own homes.
    C. Hospice care often includes palliative care, or relief from pain.
    D. All of the above.
12. Which of the following is *not* a stage of grief?
    A. acceptance
    B. denial
    C. anger
    D. questioning
13. Which of the following is *not* true of infants?
    A. Infants have a startle reflex.
    B. An infant's neck muscles are not able to support the head at first.
    C. Breast milk is ideal for at least the first eighteen months.
    D. Many infants begin eating solid foods at six months.
14. Which of the following statements is correct?
    A. All people sixty-five and older have significant mental problems.
    B. Travel is not recommended for seniors.
    C. Seniors live longer today and can be active into their nineties.
    D. Older adults need to be placed in a care home when they turn sixty-five.
15. Which of the following is *not* a type of growth and development every person experiences throughout his or her life?
    A. emotional
    B. physical
    C. spiritual
    D. social

16. Human growth and development begins at _____ and ends at _____.
    A. birth, death
    B. birth, late adulthood
    C. conception, death
    D. None of the above.

17. When does a person typically begin noticing signs of aging?
    A. early adulthood
    B. late adulthood
    C. middle adulthood
    D. All of the above.

18. Early childhood is considered to be from _____ to _____ years old.
    A. 1, 4
    B. 2, 6
    C. 1, 6
    D. 1, 5

19. In Maslow's hierarchy of needs, _____ needs are the most basic.
    A. entertainment
    B. safety
    C. food
    D. self-respect

20. Which specialty focuses on the prenatal life stage?
    A. obstetrician
    B. pediatrician
    C. geriatric specialist
    D. cardiologist

21. _____ is on the rise in children ages six to ten.
    A. Acne
    B. Declining eyesight
    C. Obesity
    D. Bulimia

22. Preteen emotional ups and downs result from _____.
    A. increased carbohydrate intake
    B. sexual maturation
    C. pressure to get into a good college
    D. loss of appetite

23. Adolescents often develop which of the following?
    A. reasoning
    B. critical thinking
    C. abstract thinking
    D. All of the above.

Short Answer

24. List four characteristics of toddlers.

25. What is the difference between a neonate and an infant?

26. Name the four types of growth and development experienced throughout life.

27. Name four specialties related to different life stages.

28. List four physical changes that can occur in adolescence.

Critical Thinking Exercises

29. As you consider the path of your future healthcare career, is there a particular life stage you would like to focus on? Explain your choice.

30. How would you construct your own "hierarchy of needs" at this stage of your life?

31. How many stages of life are represented in your immediate family?

32. What is meant by *palliative care*? Role play techniques for helping patients and family members during stressful situations.

33. Discuss aspects of adolescence that set it apart from all other life stages.

34. With a classmate, role play a situation in which you are a healthcare worker assisting an elderly patient with severe hearing and eyesight loss. Practice your verbal and nonverbal skills in communicating typical messages to the patient. Also simulate a situation in which you must communicate with the patient even though there are language barriers.

35. As you know from your reading, dealing with teenagers can be a challenge for healthcare workers. Working with a classmate, assume that you are an adult healthcare worker caring for a teenager in a healthcare facility. Imagine a real world situation in which you have a conversation with the patient. Demonstrate communication skills that will help you build and maintain a healthy relationship with the teen. Switch roles with your partner. Discuss ways in which you could improve your skills.

36. After reading about late adulthood, inspect your home looking for potentially unsafe conditions for a senior citizen. Report to the class on the unsafe conditions you observe.

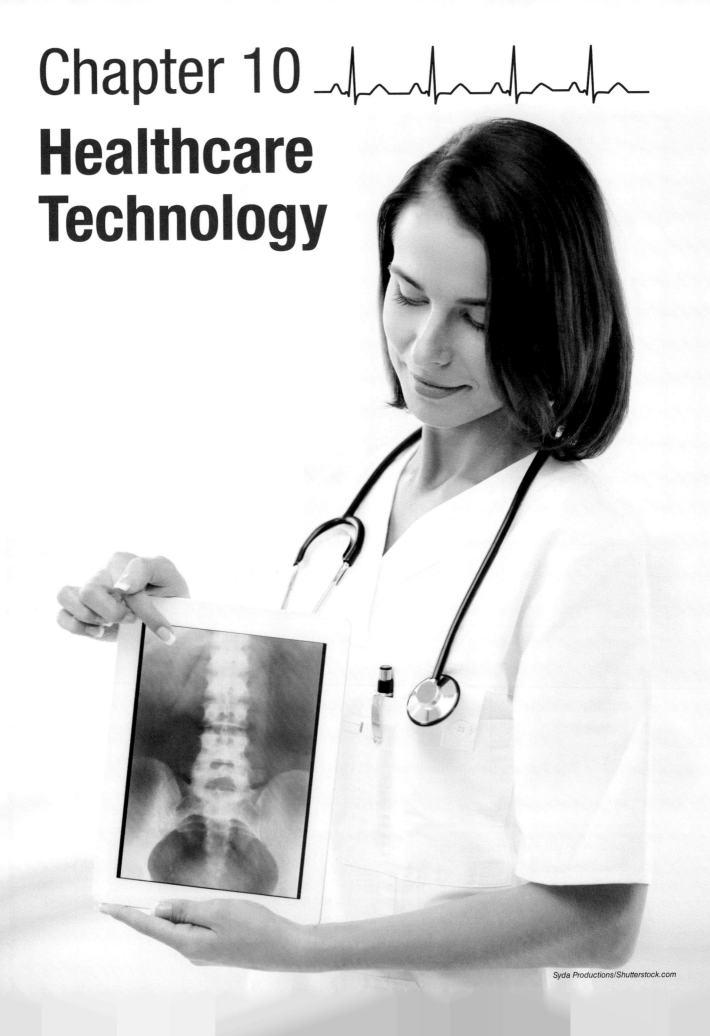

Chapter 10
Healthcare Technology

Terms to Know 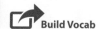 Build Vocab

biopharmaceuticals

biotechnology

cloning

computer on wheels (COW)

electronic medical record (EMR)

genetic engineering

handoff reports

healthcare simulation

Health Information Technology for Economic and Clinical Health (HITECH) Act

prosthesis

telemedicine

Chapter Objectives

- List several uses of computers in healthcare facilities.
- Discuss ways of keeping patient information confidential in healthcare computer systems.
- Explain the difference between an electronic health record (EHR) and an electronic medical record (EMR).
- Explain the process by which information is documented or corrected in an electronic health record.
- List several technologies that remotely gather patient health information.
- Identify smartphone applications used to obtain healthcare information.
- Identify technologies used in diagnostic services.
- Discuss healthcare developments made possible by biotechnology.
- Explain how future healthcare professionals can use simulators as a learning tool.

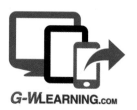

G-WLEARNING.com

While studying, look for the activity icon to:

- **Build** vocabulary with e-flash cards and interactive games.
- **Assess** progress with chapter and unit review questions.
- **Expand** learning with animations and illustration labeling activities.
- **Simulate** EHR entry with healthcare documents.

www.g-wlearning.com/healthsciences/

No matter which healthcare occupation you choose, technology will play a vital role in your future career. Whether you work as a front office medical assistant, nursing assistant, physical therapist, or doctor, technology will be important for your profession (Figure 10.1). Today, medicine and information technology have become increasingly connected, impacting students, healthcare providers, and patients.

Advances in technology have allowed for many improvements in the methods used and quality of healthcare delivered, including monitoring vital signs of critically ill patients, creating three-dimensional pictures of patients using sophisticated radiology scans, and helping doctors make accurate diagnoses. Diagnostic imaging includes complex machinery that enables doctors to assess the severity of a patient's problems, sometimes without resorting to surgery. Biotechnology allows healthcare professionals to solve problems that were not solvable in the past, such as genetic abnormalities in a fetus that can be corrected by surgery. The use of computer applications and other technological innovations in modern medicine has only just begun.

Along with this amazing healthcare technology come several important issues to consider. Serious confidentiality concerns and ethical considerations are being raised as new technology continues to stream into healthcare facilities. Students training for a career in healthcare must be aware of privacy and ethical concerns. Electronic health records (EHRs) present new, exciting ways of communicating patient information to doctors, but they can also raise serious confidentiality concerns. Smartphone applications can impart valuable information to healthcare consumers, but they must be used appropriately in a healthcare facility. These concerns must be addressed even as healthcare workers enjoy the benefits of new technological advances.

Healthcare Computer Systems

Regardless of your position in healthcare, you will almost always use a computer to complete your tasks. Healthcare facilities usually have large

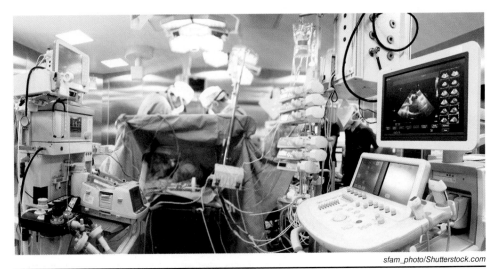

Figure 10.1   Modern operating rooms have the latest technology. What are some examples of technology that could help surgeons?

computer systems that require some on-the-job training. You may also be assigned a username to access computer files and, when you do, you will need to create a unique password. You can refer to Background Lesson 3 for more general information about computers and the Internet.

When you are able to input and find information in the computer system, you will be able to perform such duties as

- ordering supplies and keeping inventories;
- entering treatment notes;
- researching data on the Internet;
- scheduling appointments and tests for patients;
- ordering tests and prescriptions for the pharmacy;
- receiving and entering test results;
- processing patient discharges;
- performing financial calculations; and
- submitting insurance to payers and billing patients.

Working with computers can be challenging, especially when faced with complex technical language found in computer manuals. Understanding such language can be difficult, but you must be able to follow step-by-step instructions written by highly technical specialists. It is important to ask a supervisor if there is any question in your mind about how to proceed.

Computer on Wheels (COW)

As healthcare providers move throughout the healthcare facility, mobile technology can help them do their job more efficiently. In many healthcare facilities, particularly hospitals, healthcare workers use computers that can be rolled to a patient's bedside or into an examining room. These are called **computers on wheels (COWs)**. The user is able to access and enter patient information while also having direct patient contact. These computers on wheels are wirelessly connected to the main computer system of the facility. In some facilities, COWs are being replaced by tablets.

computer on wheels (COW)
a mobile computer used to access and enter patient information while moving around the healthcare facility; often rolled into a patient's hospital room

Tablets

Tablets are another mobile option for accessing and entering patient information. Today, tablets have become indispensable in healthcare facilities. A nurse can use a tablet to enter vital information at the patient's bedside (Figure 10.2). The tablet can be connected wirelessly to a small keyboard or the touch screen keyboard can be used. The tablet is connected wirelessly to the nurse's station, allowing the information entered to be made available to other healthcare providers using the computer system.

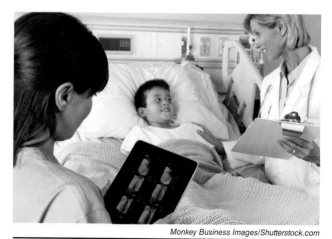

Monkey Business Images/Shutterstock.com

Figure 10.2   A nurse can use a tablet computer to record information at a patient's bedside.

Protecting Patient Confidentiality

Patients expect that their medical records, diagnoses, test results, and personal information will be kept confidential when they visit a healthcare facility. As you learned in chapter 3, healthcare professionals have a legal and ethical duty to keep patients' medical information private.

HIPAA

The Health Insurance Portability and Accountability Act of 1996 (HIPAA) was passed by Congress to protect the confidentiality of a patient's medical information. The HIPAA regulations apply to information in patients' electronic or paper medical records. HIPAA was designed to streamline the insurance coverage and reimbursement process while safeguarding healthcare records and protected health information. The 2003 Privacy Rule of HIPAA gave individuals rights over their personal health information and set rules and limits on who could look at and receive such information.

The HITECH Act

Health Information Technology for Economic and Clinical Health (HITECH) Act *legislation passed to improve healthcare through increased use of health information technology (HIT)*

Passed in 2009, the **Health Information Technology for Economic and Clinical Health (HITECH) Act** was intended to improve healthcare through the increased use of health information technology (HIT). The act was intended to encourage the use of electronic health records (EHRs) to ensure that providers have complete and accurate information. Providers could share patient information electronically, allowing different providers to coordinate care and potentially achieve diagnoses sooner. This should help reduce the cost of healthcare. Funds were provided to doctors and healthcare organizations to help them implement electronic health records and develop or improve existing health information systems.

Threats to Patient Information

Protecting the security of patient information includes watching carefully for threats to computer systems and protecting precious patient data. There are two main threats that affect healthcare computer systems:

1. threats to the accuracy of patient data
2. threats to the confidentiality of patient data

Threats to Accuracy

One of the most common threats to patient data is human inputting errors. Data can be entered incorrectly or even placed in the wrong patient's medical record. Human beings make mistakes. Sometimes these errors may disclose confidential information to the wrong person. In electronic health records, errors must be corrected immediately by attaching an item to the record that corrects the error. You must electronically sign the item with the date and your credentials. If you make a mistake, admit it immediately.

Did You Know? Confidentiality and the Hippocratic Oath

The doctor's duty to keep patient information confidential dates back at least to the earliest codes of medical ethics. The Hippocratic Oath, for example, requires the doctor to promise, "What I may see or hear in the course of the treatment or even outside of the treatment in regard to the life of men, which on no account one must spread abroad, I will keep to myself holding such things shameful to be spoken about."

To avoid making errors when documenting care, take extreme care to enter proper results into the healthcare facility computer. Continually check and recheck information before you post test results online, send a fax, or leave results on a telephone answering machine. (A patient must give permission for a healthcare provider to leave a voice message containing any personal information.)

The use of **handoff reports** at the end of each shift illustrates the importance of careful, accurate documentation of patient information. Healthcare workers use handoff reports after each shift to inform the incoming shift of the current status of every patient. These reports are retrieved and reviewed when transferring and discharging a patient.

handoff reports
reports used during a shift change or change in the level of patient care to explain a patient's current situation

The Joint Commission on Accreditation of Healthcare Organizations reviews the quality of care provided by healthcare organizations on a regular basis. The Commission has identified the handoff time as a key time when medical errors might occur. That is why it is critical that healthcare workers compile and record data with the utmost care according to industry standards.

Threats to Confidentiality

Healthcare facilities rely on physical security, software programs, and educated employees to protect private information stored in the hospital computer systems. Computers may be placed where it is hard for outsiders to access them. Passwords and firewalls are used. Remember to never share your password with anyone. Despite these efforts, breaches in confidentiality do occur.

Curiosity may motivate an employee without a need to know to access a patient's electronic health record. Many healthcare computer systems are equipped with monitoring software that records the usernames of those who have accessed patient information. Unwarranted access to patient information is grounds for discipline and possible termination of employment.

Computer hackers have been known to access information in healthcare facilities and disrupt entire systems. These actions are considered crimes, and efforts are increasingly being made to establish laws against such illegal entry into confidential information. Facility information technology (IT) specialists continually work to put into place systems that make it more difficult for hackers to commit such crimes.

Confidentiality does not apply in situations such as gunshot wounds, suspected child abuse, and intoxication-related accidents. In these cases, a healthcare provider may be required by law to divulge a patient's medical information to law enforcement authorities. Both state and federal laws exist to uphold these exceptions.

Check Your Understanding ✓

1. Why might a healthcare facility release confidential patient information without the patient's permission?
2. How are tablets used in healthcare?
3. What is the HITECH Act?
4. What is one of the most common threats to the accuracy of a patient's medical information?

Electronic Health Records (EHRs)

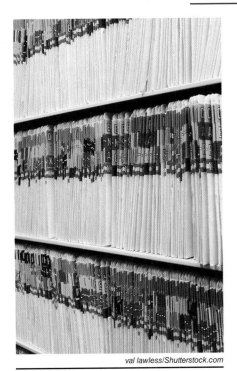

val lawless/Shutterstock.com

Figure 10.3 Traditional paper medical records required frequent filing, superb organization, and took up a great deal of space in the healthcare facility.

When care is given to a patient, it needs to be charted. Charting is the documentation in a patient record (chart) about the care that was delivered. The primary purpose and responsibility of charting is to provide timely documentation with accurate and concise information. It gives healthcare providers the information they need to make appropriate and effective decisions. It is also important to know that any patient health record is a legal document.

In the past, documentation was entered into paper charts kept in files in medical offices or in charts in acute or long-term care facilities. When patients were discharged from hospitals, for instance, these charts or records were stored in large rooms in departments called *medical records* (Figure 10.3). Many times, the charts were incomplete or difficult to retrieve, particularly if the patient had a long-standing medical history or was admitted to a variety of different healthcare facilities.

Today, instead of paper charts, many healthcare facilities use technology to store and retrieve health information, making organizing and storing paper records no longer necessary (Figure 10.4). As you learned in chapter 2, an electronic health record (EHR) is now used as the digital record that contains information about patients and includes their entire medical history and all of their healthcare experiences. Working with electronic records requires special training.

Benefits of Electronic Health Records	
Improved efficiency and reduced medical costs	• reduce time spent on paperwork • reduce duplication of medical tests
Improved care coordination	• gives every provider access to the same information about a patient • up-to-date medication and allergy lists facilitate prescribing among physicians
Improved patient outcomes	• improved patient compliance through automated reminders for routine screening • example: reliable point-of-care information and reminders notifying providers of important health interventions
Improved quality and convenience	• accurate coding and billing facilitated by legible documentation • example: e-prescriptions sent electronically to the pharmacy

Goodheart-Willcox Publisher

Figure 10.4 Benefits of electronic health records

Using an EHR makes information available instantly, displaying all medical and healthcare information from all providers who have given care to the patient. One benefit of the EHR is that this information can be shared among healthcare providers and facilities, and it can literally travel with the patient. Another benefit is that these records are environmentally friendly because they eliminate the vast amount of paper used with paper record keeping.

An EHR includes information about doctor's visits, hospital stays, and consultation by social workers or therapists. Specific healthcare data such as demographics, medical history, diagnoses, medications, allergies, progress notes, immunization dates, laboratory test results, and X-ray images, as well as insurance and billing data, is also stored. This information may have come from a variety of healthcare facilities such as hospitals, pharmacies, or workplace clinics. The goal is for the EHR to contain, in one place (such as with the patient's primary care provider), all medical and healthcare records. This allows for more coordinated, patient-centered care, eliminating duplication and offering smooth transition from one healthcare facility to another.

For example, a pharmacist can enter medication details into a patient's record, which can then be recorded on the permanent medical record, keeping an accurate account of the drugs and dosages ordered (Figure 10.5). When done in hospitals, this is usually called a medication administration record (MAR). When an EHR system is fully functional, a patient could go to her own EHR to view personal lab results to see changes when she complies with a prescribed treatment.

An **electronic medical record (EMR)** typically uses the same technology as an EHR, and many people use the terms interchangeably. Technically, however, there is a difference. The EMR contains information from a *single* medical practice or even a single visit to a particular facility; whereas, the EHR is the patient's complete health record. EMRs help track information over time, identify when screenings or checkups are due, and provide trends in treatment progress and response.

There are many advantages to using electronic records. Researchers have found that using electronic medical records has reduced medical errors. This is due to the fact that handwritten instructions may be difficult to read, potentially causing errors. The use of electronic record keeping has become so important that the Centers for Medicare & Medicaid Services (CMS) has instituted an EHR Incentive Program. The program gives healthcare providers and facilities a financial incentive to adopt, implement, upgrade, or demonstrate use of certified EHR technology. This technology is meant to help achieve health and efficiency goals such as proper electronic data capture and information sharing. One must be aware of and carefully follow the policies involving electronic medical records, including requirements from national, state, and local entities.

electronic medical record (EMR)
a digital record that contains information from a single medical practice or even a single stay in one healthcare facility

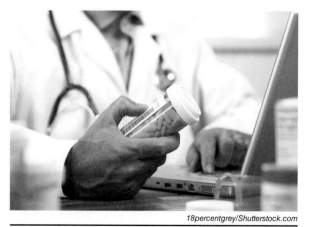

18percentgrey/Shutterstock.com

Figure 10.5 Using electronic medical records allows a pharmacist to record prescriptions directly into a patient's permanent record. What is this called in a hospital?

Guidelines for Documentation in Electronic Medical Records

The following are guidelines to use when documenting in electronic medical records. Remember documentation must be timely, complete, and accurate. When you begin working in healthcare, you may find that your facility has additional guidelines and policies to follow when using their EMR system.

1. Check that you are charting in the correct record.

2. Read the prior notes before you write your own to ensure continuity.

3. Identify the time. You may be using a 12- or a 24-hour clock depending on healthcare facility preference. If you are using a 12-hour clock, be sure to note if the time is a.m. or p.m. If you use a 24-hour clock, you will only need to identify the time. For example, if you are charting at 12 p.m. using the 24-hour clock, the time will be 1200. If you are charting at midnight, the time will be 2400.

4. Think and chart in the same sequence that care was delivered. If you gave a bed bath before you helped the resident walk, document in that order.

5. Chart only what you observed, heard, did, and how the patient responded. Do not give any of your own opinions or interpretations. Use quotation marks when charting subjective information, such as if the patient tells you "I feel so depressed today."

6. Always document any response or behavior that is not typical.

7. Use simple descriptive terms but avoid words such as "normal," "good," or "adequate."

8. Use commonly accepted abbreviations.

9. Sign your full name using a digital signature and include your title.

Correcting the Electronic Medical Record

EMRs are not without problems. For example, because the information is electronic, it can easily be changed. Policies and procedures should be in place to ensure that errors in medical information are closely monitored and handled properly to maintain correct and confidential patient data. The following are guidelines to follow when correcting an error in an electronic medical record:

1. Make sure there really is an error before you continue. If the error is not your error, consult the person who entered the error and encourage him or her to amend the problem.

2. If the error is yours, add an addendum (an item added on to the record that corrects the error) to the original electronic document that then provides the corrected information. *Do not* remove the original information or rewrite it. Make sure the new entry is clearly identified as an addendum on the document.

3. If you failed to enter information, enter a "late entry" where you will insert the missing information. Then add the missing details.

4. Once you correct an error or enter missing information, you must authenticate the information, or prove that it is real. Digitally sign the entry with your full name and credentials. Also include the time and date.

5. Ensure that the original document is retrievable. Remember that medical records are legal documents and must be stored and accessible at all times.

6. When you gain employment in healthcare and are expected to work with EMRs, make sure you are clear on organizational policies and procedures concerning electronic records. Each organization has policies and procedures on how to handle errors in EMRs. Ask questions if you are not clear.

Gathering Patient Health Information Remotely

In the past, the only way for a healthcare provider to get information about a patient's health or condition was by physically examining the patient in person. Today, technological advances have created various ways of collecting important health data from patients remotely, or from a distance.

Telemedicine

Telemedicine uses video, audio, and computer systems to provide healthcare services. Telemedicine uses telecommunication and information technologies to provide clinical health at a distance. It helps eliminate distance barriers, and it can improve access to medical services that would often not be available in rural communities. Telemedicine is also used to save lives in critical care and emergency situations.

telemedicine
a field of medicine in which communication and information technologies are used to provide patients with medical care at remote locations

Patients can now receive care from doctors or specialists far away without having to travel for a visit. Today's technology also allows healthcare providers in multiple locations to share information and discuss patient issues as if they were in the same office. Remote patient monitoring through mobile technology reduces the need for outpatient visits.

Telemedicine can ensure remote prescription verification and drug administration oversight, potentially reducing the overall cost of medical care. It can also help medical education by allowing students and employees to observe experts in their fields and share best practices more easily (Figure 10.6).

Patient Monitoring

Many doctors now use electronics to interact with and monitor their patients. Healthcare providers often have a website that allows patients to schedule appointments, ask quick medical questions, renew prescriptions, and view test results.

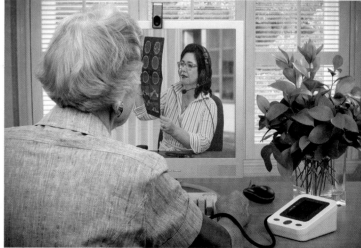

verbaska/Shutterstock.com

Figure 10.6 Through telemedicine, patients can receive treatment from offsite doctors. What are two specific uses of telemedicine?

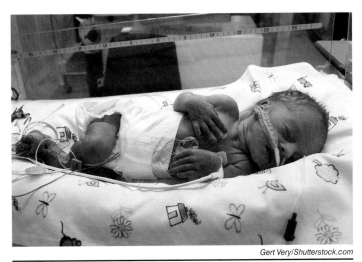

Figure 10.7   Premature babies can be monitored with sophisticated technology to continually measure the baby's vital signs.

The Internet also offers tools for disease management. For instance, electronic home monitoring equipment can send data to the doctor. Studies show that about 20 percent of office visits per year could be eliminated by online communication between doctors and patients.

Patient monitors are utilized in a wide range of inpatient and outpatient environments (Figure 10.7). A patient monitor can be used to keep track of a patient's health status by recording vital signs, glucose levels, heart activity, and so on. Patient monitors typically consist of one or more sensors, a display, processing components, and communication links for displaying or recording the results elsewhere through a monitoring network. These monitors are used in the healthcare facility as well as remotely when a doctor wants to monitor a patient at home or in other locations.

Patient monitors have become vital to care in operating and emergency rooms, as well as in intensive care and critical care units. Additionally, patient monitors have proven valuable for respiratory therapy, recovery rooms, outpatient care, transport, radiology, catheterization labs, gastroenterology departments, the hospital nursery, and many other applications.

Wearable Medical Devices

There are several wearable medical devices that are now available. These devices are often designed to prevent medical crises by identifying signs and symptoms before a condition worsens. These devices also help keep down the cost of medicine by providing critical information that would normally require continual doctor visits. Wearable medical devices can be worn on the wrist, under the skin, embedded in clothing (there is a t-shirt that monitors vital signs), included in a wireless headset to monitor brain function, and even contained in the insole of a shoe. Some specific wearable medical devices include the following:

- **A reusable biosensor patch.** The biosensor is embedded in a disposable patch. It includes technology that can keep track of heart rate, breathing, temperature, and steps, and even detects body position in case the patient falls. It can be connected to any mobile device for monitoring by a doctor or other healthcare provider.

- **A smart device that helps the patient quit smoking.** This device is attached to the patient's skin and is embedded with sensors that indicate cravings for a cigarette and nicotine. Then it will deliver medication to the patient so that the body's craving can be lessened or stopped.

- **Smart contact lenses to monitor diabetes.** When worn by a diabetic, these contact lenses measure the glucose levels in a patient's tears. This information can be uploaded to smartphones and easily monitored by patients and doctors. These contact lenses offer a noninvasive way for diabetic patients to track their blood glucose levels.

- **Cloud-based technology that monitors vital signs.** A patient's vitals are monitored by a device, which sends information to an application, or *app*, on the patient's smartphone. This device is draped across a patient's neck and has two sensors that attach to the chest to monitor and record heart rate, respiration, blood pressure, oxygen, movement, and temperature.

- **A smart bra that tracks breast health.** Sensors in the bra keep track of conditions and rhythms in breast tissue to alert patients and doctors to the possibility of cancer. A companion app displays information that has been recorded and also has a coaching and information section about optimum breast health.

Smartphone and Tablet Applications

There is an application (app) for practically everything, including healthcare information. Doctors can access patient medical information, disease management programs, prescription history, X-rays, or lab tests with their smartphones.

Apps are also available to provide patients with the healthcare information they need. Not all apps provide reliable information, so the Food and Drug Administration (FDA) screens and clears certain mobile apps for reliable use. When using any app, make sure you evaluate the source and quality of information just as you would with a website.

Consumers can use their smartphones to research healthcare pricing and obtain information about providers. Individuals are able to choose a doctor in their network based on each provider's ratings. Smartphone users can also use apps to follow a diet plan, keep track of prescriptions, set reminders for taking their medications, or manage a disease such as diabetes.

> **Think It Through**
>
> How often do you use your smartphone? What sort of apps do you have on your phone? Are any of your apps related to healthcare?

Telephone Systems

Many doctors continue to use landline telephone systems to provide clinical advice, monitor the effects of certain treatments, help patients monitor themselves, discuss results of tests, relay lab results, and handle prescription renewals. Automated telephone systems provide patients with lists of options for directing calls. Automated call systems can remind patients of appointments and notify them of normal test results.

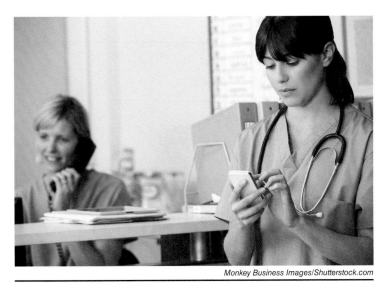

Figure 10.8   Advanced landline telephone systems are used alongside mobile phones in many hospitals to improve call response time and the quality of patient care.

The latest telephone technology is also being used in many healthcare facilities today (Figure 10.8). Most healthcare workers will be using telephone systems, some relatively simple, but others requiring comprehensive training to operate properly. Up-to-date phone systems now function wirelessly using transceivers (a combination of a transmitter and a receiver) located throughout the hospital.

In this type of telephone system, messages are quickly sent to the appropriate caregiver within seconds. Paging systems are built into these telephone networks to locate healthcare workers in and out of the facility without using overhead paging on the facility intercom. If a call is not answered quickly, it is routed to a different extension of the hospital so the caller is not kept on hold for long periods of time.

Some systems monitor the phone traffic in each area of the hospital. Staffing can be adjusted to provide the most efficient method of handling calls and messages.

E-mail

The use of e-mail (electronic mail) in a healthcare facility presents serious challenges. One challenge is remaining compliant with HIPAA laws about maintaining confidentiality in e-mail correspondence. A facility's failure to comply with HIPAA regulations can result in heavy fines.

Security measures must be taken when any confidential information is put into an e-mail message. A secure e-mail network must be established, which can be quite expensive for a small facility. Even interoffice e-mails must be secured to follow HIPAA requirements.

With any electronic communications, the patient's confidentiality must be the healthcare worker's first consideration. This is one of the most important ethical and legal considerations to understand before beginning a healthcare career. Evolving technologies present many challenges to maintaining confidentiality. As a result, facilities and employees must continually work to protect patient information.

Texting

Texting offers healthcare providers numerous advantages for clinical care. It may be the fastest and most efficient means of sending information in a given situation, especially with factors such as background noise, lack of access to a computer, and many e-mails crowding inboxes.

However, text messages can stay on a mobile device indefinitely, exposing privileged information to theft or loss. Anyone who has access to the smartphone on which the text resides may have access to all messages without a password.

There are many policies in healthcare facilities today that prohibit texting confidential information. Many workplaces provide training on the appropriate procedures for work-related texting. Texting friends and family while at work is strictly prohibited in most facilities.

Check Your Understanding ✓

1. Identify three wearable devices that can be used to monitor a patient.
2. How do you correct an electronic medical record?
3. How are smartphones used in the healthcare industry?
4. What challenges does e-mail present to the healthcare community?
5. What is the difference between an electronic health record (EHR) and an electronic medical record (EMR)?

Diagnostic Technology

In hospital departments such as radiology, the clinical laboratory, and cardiology, highly sophisticated and complex machinery is used. Much of this equipment helps diagnose patient illness. In the past, exploratory surgery may have been used to make a diagnosis. Today, new diagnostic technology often replaces invasive exploratory surgery.

The Clinical Laboratory

The clinical laboratory is full of many complex machines used to run tests for diagnostic purposes. One of the most advanced machines in a clinical laboratory is an automated cell counter such as a Coulter counter. The Coulter counter performs multiple examinations on small blood specimens in just seconds. Red and white blood cells and platelets are counted, the sizes of red blood cells are measured, and several other determinations are made. These tests would have taken technologists hours to complete by hand. Other sophisticated computerized equipment can analyze and produce up to a hundred different blood chemistry results on multiple specimens in minutes (Figure 10.9).

Operating and troubleshooting these machines takes much training. The operator must recognize when a machine is not functioning at peak performance.

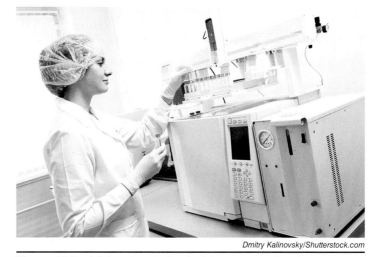

Dmitry Kalinovsky/Shutterstock.com

Figure 10.9 A laboratory technologist can use a chemistry analyzer to test blood and other patient samples. How does this save time in a laboratory?

Real Life Scenario   Keeping Up with Technology

Dorothy has been a clinical laboratory technologist at a small hospital for 25 years. When she started her career, almost all testing was done by hand. Dorothy enjoyed the hands-on aspects of her job. Combining chemicals to run tests, measuring reagents (substances used to create a chemical reaction), and using her experienced judgment for test results was satisfying.

Today, Dorothy must continually learn new technology for the machines that she uses to run tests. Dorothy does not feel comfortable with all the changes she is facing, including troubleshooting complex machinery. Dorothy feels like her years of experience are no longer valuable now that her job is defined by technology.

Apply It

1. Dorothy is at the top of the salary schedule and does not want to give up her position. What do you recommend Dorothy do about her job dissatisfaction?

2. Does a career heavily dependent on ever-changing technology interest you? Why or why not?

Diagnostic Imaging

Gone are the days when simple X-ray machines were responsible for all of a hospital's diagnostic imaging. Today, advanced technology plays a significant role in diagnostic imaging. Technicians are trained to operate highly sophisticated, computerized machines such as the PET machine, CT machine, and MRI machine.

Many other departments in the healthcare facility operate complex technology, including intensive and cardiac care units and surgical units. People in these units require extensive training and supervision because new technologies are continually being developed. Healthcare providers working with new technology must be able to learn new procedures quickly.

PET Scans

A positron emission tomography (PET) scan is done with a computerized machine that scans the body. A small amount of radioactive material called a *tracer* is given to the patient through an IV. The tracer travels through the blood and collects in tissues and organs, making them visible on the PET scan. A PET scan can show how tissues and organs are functioning.

CT Scans

The computerized axial tomography (CT) scan is a medical imaging procedure that allows an organ to be seen in a cross direction. This helps doctors find problems (often tumors) without the use of invasive surgery.

MRIs

Magnetic resonance imaging (MRI) is a test that uses a magnetic field and pulses of radio wave energy to make pictures of structures and organs inside the body (Figure 10.10). MRIs are especially useful when imaging the brain, muscles, heart, and tumors.

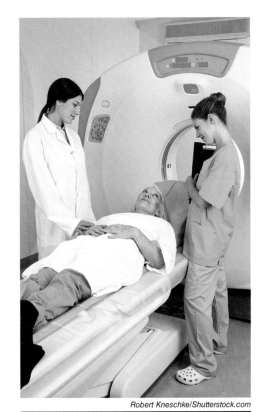
Robert Kneschke/Shutterstock.com

Figure 10.10 An MRI machine uses a magnetic field and pulses of radio wave energy to create pictures of structures and organs inside the body.

Quality Improvement for Diagnostic Machinery

As you learned in chapter 4, quality improvement (QI) is a system for evaluating services based on predetermined criteria. In the case of diagnostic machinery, QI is necessary to ensure diagnostic test results are accurate.

Whether performing tests by hand or with machinery, diagnostic technicians must make sure everything is running properly and that reagents being used are free from contamination. Diagnostic machinery manufacturers provide sample specimens with known test results. These samples can be used to calibrate or measure the machine for accuracy. If the sample does not generate the known result, then something is wrong with the machine. Troubleshooting must be done to fix the problem before the machine can be used.

All quality assurance results are recorded carefully and analyzed during laboratory inspections. Technicians operating advanced machinery must be skilled in both using the machines and testing them for quality assurance purposes. Quality assurance is essential—even sophisticated machines can malfunction.

Biotechnology

Technology that uses biological processes, organisms, or systems to manufacture products intended to improve the quality of human life is called **biotechnology**. Biotechnological advances in the world of medicine have restored, extended, and improved our lives, and will continue to do so in the future.

Biopharmaceuticals

New and exciting advances are being made today in the development of drugs and vaccines (Figure 10.11). Biotechnology and **biopharmaceuticals** may eventually help us eliminate certain diseases, alleviate pain, and extend our life span. In addition to studying new drugs in clinical trials, scientists are now identifying the previously unknown causes of many diseases. The Human Genome Project endeavored to find breakthroughs in treatment and possible cures. Biotechnology is making it possible for scientists to design new drugs that are products of **genetic engineering** (adding new DNA to an organism).

Approved biopharmaceuticals are now treating or helping prevent strokes. Other findings are making a difference in the treatment of multiple sclerosis, heart attacks, leukemia, hepatitis, lymphoma, kidney cancer, cystic fibrosis, and many other diseases. There are now over 900 biopharmaceuticals and vaccines in development to target more life-threatening diseases such as cancer and diabetes.

Gene Therapy

As you learned in chapter 7, gene therapy is a biotechnological technique for correcting defective genes that cause disease. Gene therapy replaces a defective gene with normal genes.

biotechnology
technology that uses biological processes, organisms, or systems to develop products intended to improve the quality of human life

biopharmaceuticals
prescription drugs that are produced as a result of biotechnology

genetic engineering
the manipulation of genetic materials to eliminate undesirable traits or to ensure desirable traits

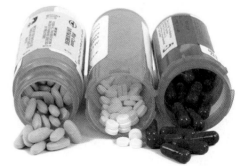

Brian Chase/Shutterstock.com

Figure 10.11 Biopharmaceuticals provide advanced treatment for many diseases and disorders. Which diseases might be treated through biopharmaceuticals?

There are thousands of genetic (hereditary) diseases—most of which are caused by a single gene defect. The defective single genes (or multiple genes) for several genetic disorders have been isolated.

Gene therapy is a new technology that has considerable room for growth. Further development of gene therapy will cost millions of research dollars. Ideally, this investment will enable doctors to effectively treat, or even eliminate, genetic disease.

Extend Your Knowledge ▶ Bone Marrow Transplants

Bone marrow donation is a method of collecting blood-forming cells for bone marrow transplants. Bone marrow donation is a surgical procedure that takes place in a hospital operating room. Doctors use needles to withdraw liquid marrow (where the body's blood-forming cells are made) from both sides of the back of a donor's pelvic bone. The donor is given anesthesia and feels no pain during the donation. After donation, the liquid marrow is transported to the patient's location for transplant.

The National Marrow Donor Program (NMDP) is a nonprofit organization that helps doctors locate matching donors. The NMDP registers people who would be willing to donate bone marrow.

Apply It

1. Would you be willing to donate bone marrow? Why or why not?

2. Research to determine how transplanted bone marrow affects the body's cells.

3. Research the difference between a bone marrow transplant and a stem cell transplant.

---

prosthesis
an artificial device that replaces a missing part of the body such as a limb

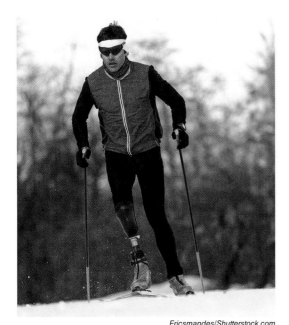
Ericsmandes/Shutterstock.com

Figure 10.12 Prosthetic limbs make it possible for people to enjoy physical activities such as skiing.

Advances in Prosthetics

A **prosthesis** is an artificial replacement for a missing body part. Common prosthetics include limbs, eyes, teeth, hips, and knees (Figure 10.12). Some prosthetics serve a functional purpose, such as helping a person walk, while others are purely cosmetic. Prosthetics have been used throughout history. A prosthetic toe was discovered in an Egyptian tomb. Today, the science behind prosthetic limbs is advancing thanks to developments in biotechnology.

Some prosthetics are powered by batteries, enhancing the function of the artificial limb. Researchers at Vanderbilt University have been working on a mini rocket-powered prosthetic. Instead of battery packs, this limb is fueled by a pencil-sized, rocket-powered engine designed to mimic the system that propels the space shuttle into orbit. A rocket-powered arm would be able to move faster and carry heavier loads than a non-motorized prosthesis.

Bionic limbs are prosthetics whose performance is improved by incorporating electronic devices within the prosthesis. The first bionic lower limb prosthetic enabled the knee and ankle joints to operate together. This was a breakthrough for people who have had their legs amputated above the knee. Microprocessors in the prosthesis are programmed to interpret the person's intended movements and make them happen.

Bluetooth technology is also being used to advance prostheses. In the case of double-leg amputees, Bluetooth is used by the prosthetic legs, allowing them to communicate with one another. This enables the amputee to establish a regular gait and pace as he walks.

Lasers in Surgery

Several types of treatment use lasers (light beams) that have the advantage of focusing on a target with incredible precision. The heat of the laser beam *cauterizes*, or seals off, smaller blood vessels such as those in the skin. This results in less bleeding at the surgical site. Because cells in human tissue are poor heat conductors, tissues close to the laser site are not affected by the laser beam. The surgeon can operate on tiny areas without disturbing the surrounding organs and tissues.

Some laser uses in medicine include

- reshaping the cornea of the eye to correct a vision problem;
- the removal of plaque from arteries, called *laser angioplasty*;
- the removal of moles, warts, scars, birthmarks, and even tattoos;
- performing pediatric circumcisions; and
- the removal of decay in teeth.

Robotic Surgery

Robotic surgery is a technique in which a surgeon uses computer-assisted, robotic equipment to perform an operation. During robotic surgery, the surgeon uses a computer to remotely control surgical instruments attached to a robot. The patient is generally put to sleep while the surgeon sits nearby at a computer station and directs the movements of a robot.

Robotic surgery is much less invasive than traditional surgery. Small cuts are made to insert the robotic equipment. A thin tube with a camera attached allows the surgeon to view the surgical area on a monitor. As the surgeon conducts the procedure, the robot mimics the surgeon's hand movements.

A variety of procedures can be performed using robotic surgery, including

- coronary artery bypass;
- gallbladder removal;
- hip replacement;
- hysterectomy; and
- mitral valve repair in the heart.

Cloning

cloning
the creation of an organism that is an exact genetic copy of another; a clone has identical DNA to its parent

The latest bioengineering developments have allowed scientists to clone various organisms, or living things. **Cloning**, as you learned in chapter 7, is the creation of an organism that is an exact genetic copy (has the same DNA) of another. Identical twins, born from a fertilized egg that has split in two, are natural clones and have matching DNA. No human beings are known to have been artificially cloned, but scientists have successfully cloned many plant varieties, reptiles, and other mammals.

Many scientists believe cloning offers possibilities for treating incurable diseases. This type of cloning, called *therapeutic cloning*, does not advocate the birth of human clones. Therapeutic cloning is performed for the purpose of medical treatment. Potential uses for therapeutic cloning include growing skin, perhaps for burn victims. Therapeutic cloning might also be used to create nerve cells for someone suffering from brain damage.

Cloning is currently a very controversial subject. The ethical issues related to cloning must be considered; the use of cloning technology is up for serious debate.

Artificial Organs

Scientists are using biotechnology to explore many healthcare improvements and advancements. Artificial organs such as lymph nodes and kidneys are being developed. Artificial lymph nodes could replace diseased nodes or be used to boost the immune system in people who have diseases such as cancer or HIV. Manufactured kidneys would shorten the wait for those who need a kidney transplant. This life-saving surgery would benefit patients with chronic kidney disease because they wouldn't have to wait for a compatible donor. Organ transplantation requires that the organ recipient take anti-rejection drugs for the rest of his or her life. The danger of the organ being rejected by its new host is always present with live organ transplants. It is hoped that artificial organs will not trigger rejection. Artificial organs could make transplantation easier and more common.

Check Your Understanding ✓

1. What is biotechnology?
2. What is a bone marrow transplant?
3. What is therapeutic cloning?
4. Name three uses of surgical lasers.

Healthcare Simulations

Healthcare simulation provides a bridge between classroom learning and real-life clinical experience. A simulator is a machine used to show what something looks like, or to practice a healthcare procedure as part of training (Figure 10.13). Simulator exercises include a range of activities that are all focused on the same purpose—improving the safety, efficiency, and effectiveness of healthcare services. Simulators establish a learning environment in which students can practice necessary skills without risking patient health and safety.

Thanks to advances in computer technology, simulators are widely used in medical and nursing schools, veterinary colleges, and allied health programs. Some facilities are also setting up simulation laboratories with operating rooms, intensive care units, and other areas normally found in healthcare facilities.

Examples of simulations include virtual reality scenarios in which students can interview patients, establish a diagnosis, and practice basic surgical skills. These situations are all possible thanks to the complex, computer-generated environment.

Fully computerized, whole-body mannequins are often part of a simulation. These computerized patients respond to certain medications, and they can be used for hands-on procedures such as practicing CPR, drawing blood, assisting in childbirth, and inserting chest tubes and IVs.

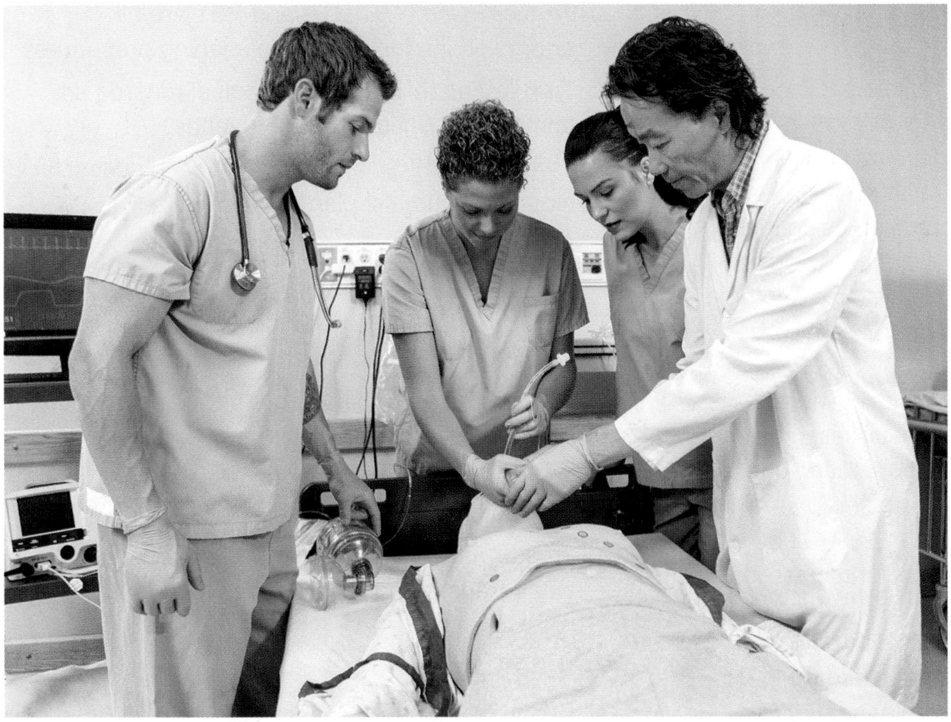

healthcare simulation
the use of learning tools to show what a medical emergency looks like or how a healthcare procedure is performed

Tyler Olson/Shutterstock.com

Figure 10.13   Healthcare students practice inserting a breathing tube as part of a simulation.

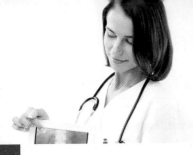

Summary

Regardless of where you work in a healthcare facility, you will be utilizing computer technology in one way or another. If you work with patient information, one of your primary responsibilities will be to ensure that patients' electronic health records (EHRs) are accurately maintained and that their personal information is kept confidential.

Healthcare facilities must do everything they can to protect their computer systems' accuracy and privacy. There are many practices to adopt to protect patient privacy. Electronic health records (EHRs) are replacing cumbersome paper records. EHRs offer greater convenience than paper records, making it possible for doctors to easily access the patient information they need, even if it was recorded in another healthcare facility. However, EHRs pose an additional risk to patient confidentiality. There are steps healthcare workers must take to prevent electronic records from getting into the hands of unauthorized persons.

Several technologies, such as telemedicine, gather patient health information for doctors in a remote location. Smartphone apps can make it possible for patients and their healthcare providers to access medical information using their smartphones or other computer systems. Along with smartphones, advanced telephone systems and other communication technology have improved the quality of patient care in many facilities.

Highly complex diagnostic technology is also found throughout many healthcare facilities, making way for new careers as technicians operating complex machines. This equipment also saves time by making diagnoses quickly and accurately.

Biotechnology is opening doors for many advances in healthcare. Some of these include advanced surgery techniques, electronic devices designed to improve a person's health and wellness, and cutting-edge therapies targeted at treating currently incurable diseases. Developing many of these technologies, specifically in the field of biotechnology, will cost billions of dollars, and some will raise serious ethical issues.

Along with exciting advances in biotechnology comes the development and improvement of simulators that allow students to practice key skills without putting the patient at risk. Simulators have become a valuable training tool for many future healthcare professionals.

The healthcare industry is becoming increasingly driven by technology—this is an exciting time to be entering the field!

Review Questions

Answer the following questions using what you have learned in this chapter.

True or False Assess

1. *True or False?* Maintaining confidentiality of patient records is the duty of all members of the healthcare team.

2. *True or False?* Computer manuals can be written in confusing technical language.

3. *True or False?* MRI, CT, and PET are all abbreviations for diagnostic imaging procedures.

4. *True or False?* Electronic medical records are immune to confidentiality breaches.

5. *True or False?* Scientists have been successful in cloning mammals, plants, and reptiles.

6. *True or False?* Robotic surgery is performed without any human guidance.

7. *True or False?* Telemedicine is a method of providing medical care at a distance.

8. *True or False?* Apps on your phone can contain valuable medical information.

9. *True or False?* You cannot correct an electronic medical record (EMR).

10. *True or False?* Handoff reports are only used when transferring a patient between units.

Multiple Choice Assess

11. Which of the following is a skill required for documentation?

   A. taking care to be accurate in your reporting

   B. reading prior notes

   C. using accepted abbreviations

   D. All of the above.

12. _____ are created by a machine that scans the body for tracer material, which helps show how tissues and organs are functioning.

A. CT scans

B. MRIs

C. PET scans

D. All of the above.

13. Healthcare simulations are used _____.

A. only in medical schools

B. for educating patients about upcoming procedures

C. widely in many schools for training healthcare workers

D. for demonstrating procedures for the general public

14. Which of the following steps should you take when entering information into an electronic health record?

A. Ask your supervisor to enter the information.

B. Don't worry about spelling.

C. Check to see that you are putting information into the right patient's record.

D. Leave the patient record open after finishing entering information.

15. Sending an e-mail in a healthcare facility can be a challenge because _____.

A. it could reveal confidential information

B. you could be fined if confidential information sent through e-mail got into the wrong hands

C. e-mail systems must be secure

D. All of the above.

16. Which of the following is a benefit of HITECH?

A. reduced need for detailed patient information

B. increased ability to share patient information

C. fewer doctors needed to treat patients

D. All of the above.

17. Confidentiality does not apply to any of the following *except* _____.

A. diseases of the reproductive system

B. suspected child abuse

C. intoxication-related accidents

D. gunshot wounds

Short Answer

18. What organization registers bone marrow donors?

19. Which is likely to contain more information, an EHR or an EMR?

20. How does robotic surgery differ from traditional surgery?

21. Name four uses of a computer in a healthcare facility.

22. Name two advantages of using a laser in surgery.

23. Explain how and when handoff reports are created and retrieved.

24. Name two wearable devices that patients might use remotely.

25. What are biopharmaceuticals?

26. What is a prosthesis?

27. What is the purpose of the HITECH Act?

Critical Thinking Exercises

28. What healthcare technology interests you the most? Why?

29. Would you consider donating your organs in the event of a fatal accident? Have you checked the organ donor box on your driver's license? Do you have objections to being an organ donor?

30. Research a controversy resulting from advances in biotechnology. This research may require that you interpret complex technical material. Report your findings to the class in language they can understand.

31. What types of information are integrated into an EHR?

32. One of the goals of HITECH is to contain or reduce healthcare costs. Research healthcare systems globally to compare the use of electronic health records and the effects of EHRs on cost containment.

33. Under the supervision of your teacher, collaborate with a team of classmates to simulate the use of electronic communication devices, such as those discussed in this chapter, in healthcare settings. Discuss the results with your classmates, and then repeat the simulations. Did your skills improve?

34. After researching various document formats and industry standards for compiling and recording health data, create a data management system for a new health clinic. Present your proposal to the class.

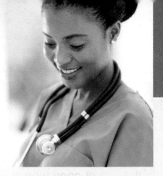

Unit 3
Cumulative Review

Review Questions

Answer the following questions using what you have learned in this unit.

True or False

1. *True or False?* The Apgar scale measures a person's blood alcohol level.

2. *True or False?* Gerontology is the study of genetics.

3. *True or False?* Regular visits to your doctor can help you prevent certain diseases.

4. *True or False?* Early childhood is defined as a time between one and six years old.

5. *True or False?* One goal of the HITECH Act was to decrease the use of health information technology (HIT).

6. *True or False?* Holistic health emphasizes the body working as a combination of only mental and emotional health to achieve optimal wellness.

7. *True or False?* A PET scan uses a small amount of radioactive material given to the patient.

8. *True or False?* A person with a type C personality is generally described as ambitious, organized, and impatient.

Multiple Choice

9. Which of the following are examples of reportable information kept in a patient's EHR?
   A. immunization dates
   B. patient insurance and billing information
   C. laboratory test results
   D. All of the above.

10. Which of the following are significant risk factors for addiction?
    A. genetic predisposition
    B. mental illness leading to self-medicating
    C. peer pressure
    D. All of the above.

11. If you discover an error in an EMR, you should _____.
    A. consult the person who entered the error
    B. create an addendum
    C. authenticate the corrected information by digitally signing the entry
    D. All of the above.

12. How might a relationship affect a person's physical health?
    A. The presence of a friend can decrease blood pressure during a stressful situation.
    B. A strong social life may improve immune function.
    C. Relationships with frequent conflict may negatively impact one's health.
    D. All of the above.

13. A prosthesis is _____.
    A. an artificial body part
    B. a technology for correcting defective genes
    C. a biopharmaceutical
    D. a vaccine

14. Which of the following is *not* a level of Maslow's hierarchy of needs?
    A. safety
    B. esteem
    C. mental development
    D. self-actualization

15. Acupuncture, reflexology, reiki, and yoga are all considered to be _____.
    A. Western medicine
    B. conventional medicine
    C. complementary and alternative medicines (CAMs)
    D. None of the above.

16. Which of the following does *not* belong in an EMR?
    A. any patient behavior that is not typical
    B. the time care is given
    C. commonly accepted abbreviations
    D. your personal opinion

17. Physical activity has many benefits, including
_____.

    A. releasing mood-enhancing endorphins

    B. improving sleep quality

    C. protecting the body from negative health conditions

    D. All of the above.

Short Answer

18. What is *health literacy*?

19. Explain how relationships with others may impact a person's emotional health, both positively and negatively.

20. How do positive relationships among healthcare professionals promote a health community?

21. What role does telemedicine play in today's healthcare world?

22. What is the difference between HIPAA and the HITECH Act?

Critical Thinking Exercises

23. What alternative health practices or health therapies are available in your area? Identify three providers and the services they offer. Then brainstorm a list of possible health conditions that could be treated with the use of each type of health practice or therapy.

24. How does access to quality healthcare play an important role in the overall health of a community? Research the effects of readily available healthcare in a community. How might a community be affected by poor access to healthcare?

25. Imagine you are an experienced healthcare provider who has been asked to train a new employee on entering information into an electronic medical record (EMR). Explain the steps he should follow and any guidelines he should know before creating an entry in the EMR.

Career Exploration

Registered Health Information Technician (RHIT)

Registered health information technicians, also known as *medical records technicians*, organize and manage health information data by carefully and accurately entering the information into electronic health records. Their role is to ensure that patient information is accurate, thorough, accessible, and secure in both paper files and electronic systems. They use various classification systems to code patient information for insurance purposes, to compile databases, and to maintain patients' EHRs.

An RHIT must understand the ethical, legal, and regulatory requirements of handling sensitive patient information. RHITs are employed in a variety of healthcare facilities, law and insurance firms, or vendors of health products.

An associate's degree is required to become an RHIT. Advancement to management positions is possible with the completion of additional education. A certification exam is required to become registered, and is administered by the American Health Information Management Association (AHIMA).

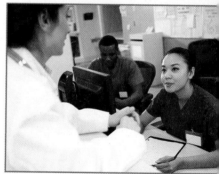

Monkey Business Images/Shutterstock.com

Further Research

1. Research one of the related careers listed above using the *Occupational Outlook Handbook* and other reliable Internet resources. What is the outlook for this career? Are workers in demand, or are jobs dwindling?

2. Review the educational requirements for this career. What courses would you need to take to pursue a related degree?

3. What is the salary range for this job?

4. What do you think you would like about this career? Is there anything about it you might dislike? Compare the job you have chosen to research to the description of an RHIT. Which job appeals to you more? Why?

Related Careers

Billing and collection specialist

Business and billing office administrator

Health records clerk

Health service manager

Healthcare information manager

Medical billing specialist

Medical processor

Medical transcriptionist

Unit 4

Healthcare Skills

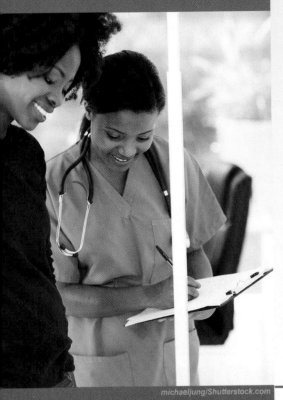

michaeljung/Shutterstock.com

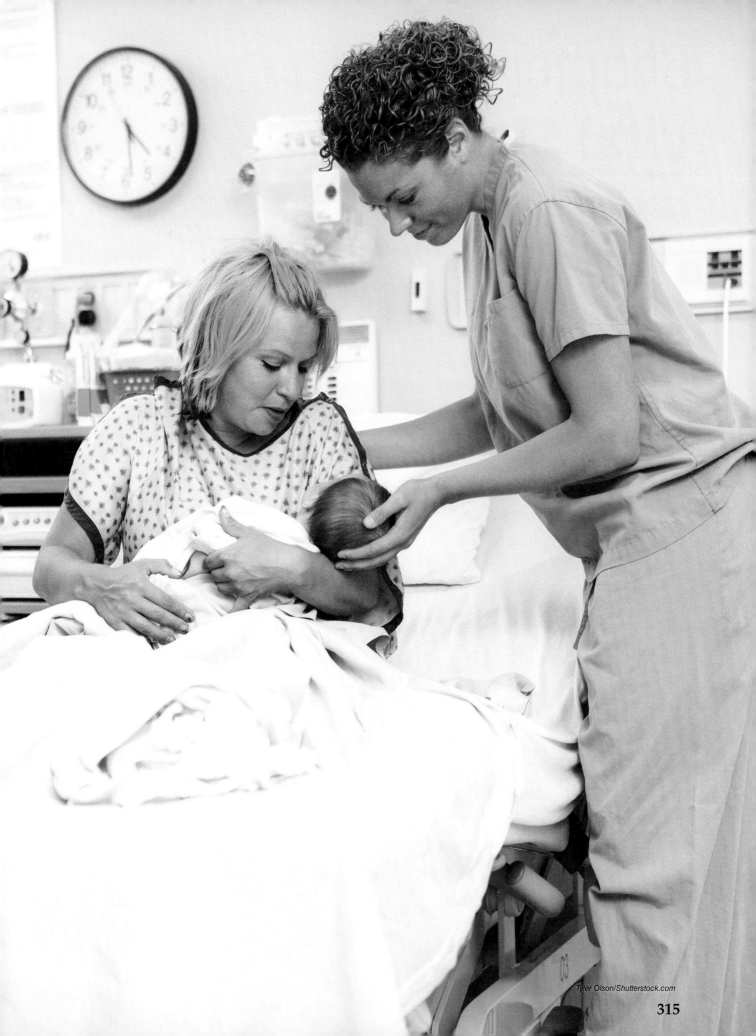

Tyler Olson/Shutterstock.com

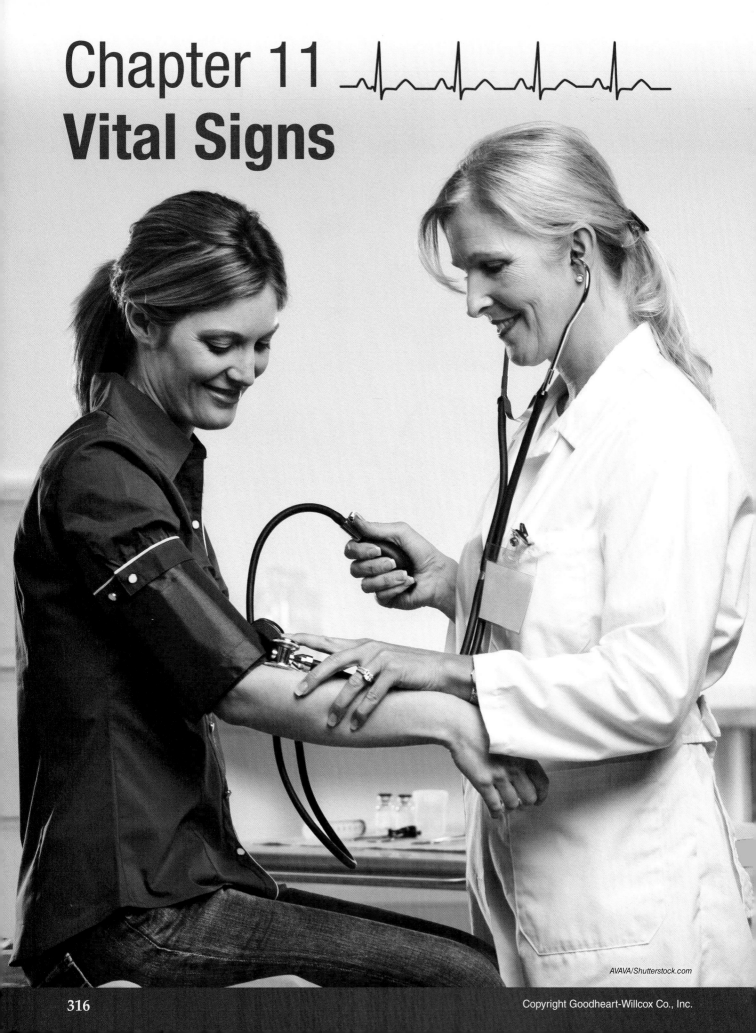

Chapter 11
Vital Signs

Terms to Know

Build Vocab

anus	edema	probe
apical pulse	exhalation	pulse oximeter
apnea	Fahrenheit (°F)	radial pulse
aural	hypertension	sphygmomanometer
axillary temperature	hyperventilation	stertorous breathing
bradycardia	hypotension	stethoscope
bradypnea	hypothermia	systolic pressure
carotid pulse	hypoventilation	tachycardia
Celsius (°C)	hypoxia	tachypnea
diastolic pressure	ideal body weight (IBW)	temporal artery temperature
digital	inhalation	tympanic temperature
dyspnea	intravenous (IV)	

Chapter Objectives

- Discuss the importance and purpose of taking vital signs.
- Explain the bodily processes associated with each vital sign.
- Identify the normal and abnormal range for each of the vital signs.
- Identify the locations where a temperature and pulse can be taken.
- List the types of equipment needed to take each vital sign.
- Discuss the important considerations and guidelines for taking, measuring, and recording each vital sign and height and weight.
- Demonstrate the procedures for taking and measuring vital signs.

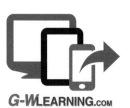

While studying, look for the activity icon **to:**

- **Build** vocabulary with e-flash cards and interactive games.
- **Assess** progress with chapter and unit review questions.
- **Expand** learning with animations and illustration labeling activities.
- **Simulate** EHR entry with healthcare documents.

G-WLEARNING.COM

www.g-wlearning.com/healthsciences/

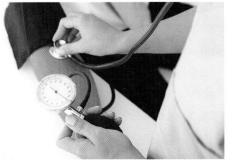

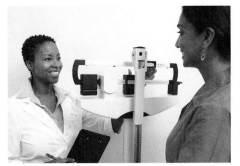

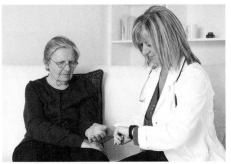

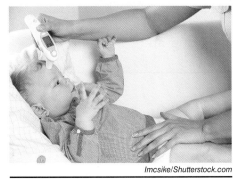

Figure 11.1 Healthcare workers evaluate vital signs to understand a patient's health status and identify the possible occurrence of a disease, disorder, or injury.

Vital signs are a patient's body temperature, pulse, respirations, and blood pressure. These signs are considered *vital* because they are essential to body functions. When vital signs are taken, a patient's height and weight may also be measured and recorded (Figure 11.1). If vital signs are not within the normal range, they give healthcare workers information about a patient's health and may indicate the presence of a disease, infection, or injury.

Understanding Vital Signs

Understanding and learning how to take vital signs—body temperature, pulse, respirations, and blood pressure—are important skills for a healthcare worker to master. Vital signs can help doctors diagnose particular diseases, determine treatments and medications, and evaluate how well these treatments and medications are working. For example, a high temperature is one way of knowing if someone has an infection. Once treatment starts, if the temperature starts to lower, it typically means the body is able to fight the infection and the patient is beginning to get better.

Taking vital signs is essentially the same process for children and adults; however, the method and normal ranges are different. For example, you would use a rectal thermometer for a newborn but an oral thermometer for an adult. With children, there is the additional challenge of keeping them still long enough to obtain an accurate measurement.

Vital signs are usually taken when you visit a doctor's office, or once a day in long-term care facilities (or more frequently when necessary). However, a patient who is very ill in the hospital may have them taken hourly. Vital signs may also be taken if there is a complaint of dizziness, nausea, or pain. Each vital sign has a well-established guideline for adults and children to identify whether they are in a normal range.

Temperature

Taking a patient's temperature means that you are measuring his or her body heat. A temperature is shown in degrees (°). While a patient's body temperature can change over the course of a day due to the dilation and expansion of blood vessels, pyrexia (*fever*) is caused by the body heating up to try to protect itself. Finding out that a temperature is above the normal range gives healthcare workers important information about whether there may be an infection, some other disease process, an injury, or a possible reaction to a medication.

Body temperature is regulated by the hypothalamus, which is located in the brain. It is the body's control center, or internal thermostat. The hypothalamus resets the body to a higher temperature when it becomes aware an infection or illness is present. The heat generated is one of the defenses used by the body against toxins causing the infection or illness.

Temperature is measured using a **Fahrenheit** scale, indicated by using an *F*, or by the **Celsius**, or *centigrade* scale, indicated by using a *C* (Figure 11.2). Chapter 16 explains how to convert between these two types of measurement.

Where to Take a Temperature

There are several different locations where body temperature can be taken:

- oral (taken under the tongue, or *sublingually*)
- rectal (taken in the **anus**)
- axillary (taken under the armpit)
- tympanic (taken in the ear)
- temporal arteries (taken on the forehead)

Oral temperatures are the most common method, but this method is not appropriate for a patient receiving oxygen, for some patients who may be agitated or comatose, or children younger than four years of age.

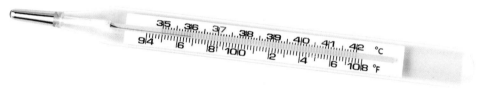

catshila/Shutterstock.com

Figure 11.2 Manual thermometers may feature both a Fahrenheit (°F) and Celsius (°C) scale.

Fahrenheit (°F)
the English system of measurement used for temperature; the freezing point of water is 32°F and the boiling point is 212°F

Celsius (°C)
the metric measurement used for temperature; the freezing point of water is 0° and the boiling point is 100°

anus
the opening at the end of the gastrointestinal (GI) tract, where solid waste leaves the body

Think It Through

When was the last time you had a high temperature? How high was it and why did you have it? How did you feel? What did you do about the high temperature? How long did it take for it to go away?

Extend Your Knowledge ▶ **Taking Vital Signs Should Be a Positive Experience**

Taking vital signs should always be a positive experience for the patient. Be aware that for some patients it may be a new or even an upsetting experience. For example, people from different cultures or generations may feel frightened and wonder what is being done. They may also be worried about the results. Be sure to move slowly and patiently and provide thorough and accurate explanations about what you are doing. If the patient does not speak English, ask someone to interpret, if possible.

Apply It

1. What can you do to ensure that taking vital signs is a positive experience for a patient rather than one that may be frightening or worrisome?

2. After you have completed this chapter, make a list of vital signs procedures that might frighten or concern patients.

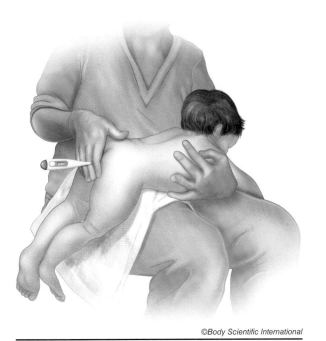

©*Body Scientific International*

Figure 11.3 Rectal temperatures are most commonly used with infants.

temporal artery temperature
temperature taken on either side of the head, where the temporal arteries are located

axillary temperature
temperature taken in the axilla, or armpit

tympanic temperature
temperature taken in the ear

hypothermia
a body temperature below 95°F

Taking the temperature of infants and small children is often done rectally or at the temporal arteries. When taken rectally, the thermometer is inserted one inch or less into the anus and held in place for three to five minutes (Figure 11.3). Rectal temperatures should not be taken if the patient has diarrhea, rectal bleeding, and certain heart conditions, or if the patient cannot follow directions or hold still.

When taking an oral temperature, you must also be aware of whether a patient has recently eaten or had something to drink. If this has occurred, you should wait at least 15 minutes (or follow your facility policy) before inserting the oral thermometer.

Rectal and **temporal artery temperatures** provide more accurate measurements than other temperature sites. As a result, temporal artery temperatures are used more frequently in medical offices. They are also often used for babies and children, as they can be easier to take than rectal temperatures.

When taking an **axillary temperature**, you should note if the patient has recently washed under his arms or put on deodorant. Doing so can affect the reading. If this has happened, wait 15 minutes before taking the temperature.

Tympanic temperatures are more difficult to measure because the thermometer must be properly placed in the ear to receive an accurate reading. Always check that you are using the best and safest location to take a temperature for each patient.

A patient's temperature may change slightly (by 1°F) during the day due to exertion, how much she eats or drinks, or the external temperature. The normal, or average, temperature for an adult is 98.6°F (37°C), although the average range is 97.0°F (36.5°C) to 99°F (37.2°C). The average rectal temperature is approximately 1° higher than an oral temperature, and axillary and temporal artery temperatures can be 1° lower. **Hypothermia**, while not seen often, is a body temperature below 95°F.

Average temperature ranges also vary based on the patient's age and the type of thermometer used (Figure 11.4).

Did You Know? **A Child's Temperature Is Usually Higher and More Variable**

The following temperatures represent the top end of the "normal" ranges for children, by location:
- measured orally (mouth): 99°F (37.2°C)
- measured rectally (anus): 100.4°F (38°C)

- measured in an axillary position (armpit): 99°F (37.2°C)
- measured in the ear (tympanic) or on the temporal artery (forehead): 99.6°F (37.56°C)

Average Ranges of Body Temperature			
Thermometer	*Birth to Two Years*	*Three to Eleven Years*	*Twelve Years and Older*
Oral	Should not be taken	97.0°F–99.5°F (36.1°C–37.5°C)	97.6°F–99.6°F (36.4°C–37.5°C)
Rectal	97.0°F–100.4°F (36.1°C–38.0°C)	97.9°F–100.4°F (36.6°C–38.0°C)	98.6°F–100.6°F (37.0°C–38.1°C)
Tympanic	Should not be taken	98.0°F–99.6°F (36.7°C–37.5°C)	98.6°F–100.4°F (37.0°C–38.0°C)
Axillary	97.5°F–99.3°F (36.4°C–37.4°C)	96.6°F–99.0°F (36.0°C–37.2°C)	96.6°F–98.6°F (35.9°C–37.0°C)
Temporal Artery	98.3°F–100.3°F (36.8°C–37.9°C)	97.8°F–100.1°F (36.5°C–37.8°C)	97.2°F–100.1°F (36.2°C–37.8°C)

Goodheart-Willcox Publisher

Figure 11.4 Temperature ranges, used to determine a patient's health status, vary according to a patient's age and the thermometer used.

Types of Thermometers

Several different types of thermometers are used today. Some are filled with a liquid, which is usually colored alcohol. These are considered non-digital, or *manual*, thermometers. Some have liquid crystals on a plastic strip (usually disposable) that change color to indicate different temperatures, while others are electronic and use digital displays. Healthcare facilities may use any one of these types of temperature devices. No matter what device is used, all types of thermometers have the same purpose. Therefore, it is best to learn them all.

Did You Know? Mercury Thermometers—a Thing of the Past

The first type of clinical thermometer was the mercury thermometer, invented by physicist Daniel Gabriel Fahrenheit in Amsterdam in the early 18th century. The thermometer was originally made of glass with a small bulb at its base filled with pressurized liquid mercury. The stem of the thermometer was a hollow tube with a calibrated temperature scale. Mercury was used because it is a chemical element that rises and falls in response to temperature changes.

When using the thermometer and reading the calibrated temperature scale, one could then determine how hot or cold a person was. This type of thermometer was used for many years. However, in recent years, it has been replaced by mercury-free thermometers because mercury is a toxic substance. Should a mercury thermometer break, releasing its mercury, it could have significant negative effects on a person's health, possibly causing blindness, memory loss, and deafness, among other symptoms.

Non-Digital Thermometers

Non-digital thermometers can be used for oral, rectal, or axillary temperatures. Figure 11.2 shows a non-digital thermometer. These thermometers are tubes filled with a liquid (colored alcohol) that expands and moves up or down when exposed to heat. The bulb at the end of the thermometer is the part inserted into the body. The bulb on the rectal thermometer is different from the oral thermometer—it is more thick and broad. Each thermometer is marked with a colored dot—blue for oral or axillary, and red for rectal.

It is important to correctly place the thermometer and leave it in for the prescribed amount of time. Use the following guidelines based on your thermometer:

digital
an electronic readout of numbers

probe
a long, thin medical instrument with a blunt end used for exploration into body cavities

- oral temperatures: insert the thermometer under the tongue, close the patient's mouth completely, and leave the thermometer in for three minutes

- rectal temperatures: the thermometer should be placed one inch or less into the anus for three to five minutes

- axillary temperatures: lower the patient's arm completely and leave the thermometer under the armpit for five minutes or more

Do not shake the thermometer when removing it. A non-digital thermometer is read by looking at the thermometer's scale. Be sure the scale is visible so you can determine where on the scale the liquid ended up, thus denoting the patient's temperature.

Digital Thermometers

Digital thermometers are used for oral, rectal, or axillary temperatures. They are handheld, have a digital display, and are connected to an electronic unit (Figure 11.5). Instead of a bulb, they have a **probe**. A fresh probe cover should be placed on the probe and discarded after each use (Figure 11.6). Once the probe is inserted, a digital display of the temperature reading will usually appear within 20 to 60 seconds. These probes are often marked by color—blue for oral or axillary, and red for rectal.

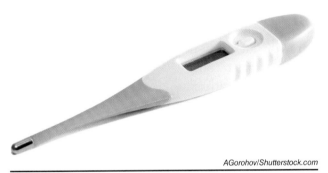

AGorohov/Shutterstock.com

Figure 11.5   Commonly used in both healthcare facilities and homes, digital thermometers such as this one record oral, rectal, or axillary temperatures.

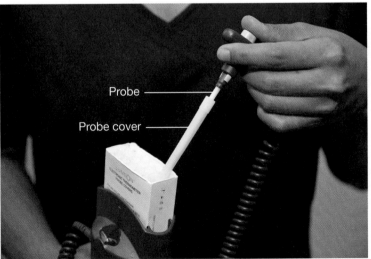

Probe
Probe cover

Wards Forest Media, LLC

Figure 11.6   Place a disposable probe cover on the thermometer before every use.

Note: All procedures are to be practiced in a simulated laboratory setting under your teacher's supervision. Procedures should be performed only after they have been observed by a teacher and he or she has determined that your demonstration is competent.

Procedure 11.1   Oral Temperature—Digital 📲 Expand

Rationale

When a body temperature is outside the normal range, it can be a sign of a health condition or disease, or the result of an injury.

Preparation

1. Assemble the following equipment:
   - a digital thermometer
   - the appropriate probe attachment—the *blue* probe is used for an oral temperature
   - disposable probe covers
   - disposable gloves
   - pen and pad, or a form for recording the temperature
2. Wash your hands to ensure infection control.
3. Explain in simple terms what you are going to do, even if the patient is unable to talk or is disoriented.
4. Be sure the patient has not eaten, had something to drink, smoked, or chewed gum for at least 15 minutes prior to taking the oral temperature.

The Procedure

5. Provide privacy. Screen around the patient, close the curtains, or close the door to the room, if appropriate.
6. Position the patient comfortably.
7. Let the patient know how long the thermometer will be in place. Instruct the patient to not talk while the reading is being taken.
8. Put on disposable gloves.
9. Place the disposable probe cover over the *blue* probe. Start the thermometer and wait for it to show it is ready.
10. Have the patient open his mouth and lift his tongue. Slowly insert the covered probe into the mouth until the tip of the probe is at the base of the mouth—under the tongue and to one side (Figure 11.7). Have the patient lower his tongue and close his mouth.
11. Hold the probe in place in the mouth until you hear or see the signal (Figure 11.8). This indicates the reading is completed.
12. Remove the thermometer from the mouth and read the temperature on the display screen.

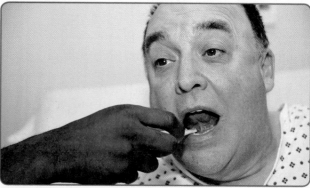

Figure 11.7   *Wards Forest Media, LLC*

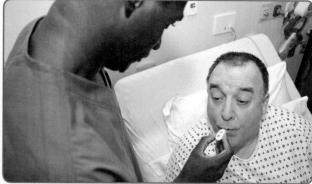

Figure 11.8   *Wards Forest Media, LLC*

13. Do not touch the used probe cover with your bare hands. Dispose of the probe cover safely in the wastebasket or per facility policy.
14. Clean the probe with alcohol and return the probe to its storage compartment on the thermometer.
15. Remove your gloves and wash your hands. Record the temperature on a pad or form so it is not forgotten.
16. Return the thermometer to a charging location per facility policy.

Follow-up

17. Make sure the patient is safe and comfortable.
18. Wash your hands to ensure infection control.

Reporting and Documentation

19. Communicate any specific observations, complications, or unusual responses to the appropriate provider. Also record this information in the patient's chart or EMR.
20. Use your facility's standard policy and forms to record the temperature.

Procedure 11.2 | Rectal Temperature—Digital

Rationale

When a body temperature is outside the normal range, it can be a sign of a health condition or disease, or the result of an injury. The decision to use a rectal thermometer is based on the need for accuracy, and the age and condition of the patient. For example, rectal temperatures can be more accurate than oral for young children.

Preparation

1. Assemble the following equipment:
   - a digital thermometer
   - the appropriate probe attachment—the *red* probe is used for a rectal temperature
   - disposable probe covers
   - disposable gloves
   - water-soluble lubricating gel
   - tissues or toilet paper
   - pen and pad, or a form for recording temperature
   - sheet or drape
2. Wash your hands to ensure infection control.
3. Put on disposable gloves.
4. Explain in simple terms what you are going to do, even if the patient is unable to talk or is disoriented.

The Procedure

5. Provide privacy. Screen around the patient, close the curtains, or close the door to the room, if appropriate.
6. Lock the wheels of the bed and raise it to a comfortable working level, or help the patient to a prepared examining table.
7. Place the disposable probe cover over the *red* probe. Start the thermometer and wait for it to show it is ready.
8. Apply enough water-soluble lubricating gel (about the size of a quarter) on tissues or toilet paper for comfortable entry.
9. Use the tissue or toilet paper to lubricate the end of the covered probe.

10. Assist the patient into a side-lying or lateral position. Have the patient bend the upper leg up to her stomach as far as possible. Help, if needed.
11. If the patient is covered by a drape or top sheet, fold it back to expose the buttocks. Expose only the area necessary for the procedure. Keep the rest of the patient covered to protect her privacy.
12. With one hand, gently raise the upper buttock to expose the anal area.
13. With the other hand, gently insert the rectal probe one inch or less into the anus.
14. Hold the probe in place until you hear or see the signal. This indicates the reading is completed.
15. Remove the thermometer and read the temperature on the digital display screen.
16. Dispose of the probe cover safely in the wastebasket or per facility policy.
17. Wipe the lubricant from the patient and discard the tissue or toilet paper.
18. Clean the probe with alcohol and return the probe to its storage compartment on the thermometer.
19. Remove your gloves and wash your hands to ensure infection control. Record the temperature on a pad or form so it is not forgotten.
20. Return the thermometer to a charging location per facility policy.

Follow-up

21. Lower the bed and make sure the patient is safe and comfortable.
22. Wash your hands to ensure infection control.

Reporting and Documentation

23. Communicate any specific observations, complications, or unusual responses to the appropriate provider. Also record this information in the patient's chart or EMR.
24. Use your facility's standard policy and forms to record the temperature.

Procedure 11.3   Axillary Temperature—Digital

Rationale

When a body temperature is outside the normal range, it can be a sign of a health condition or disease, or the result of an injury. While not as accurate as other locations, the axilla (*armpit*) is one to consider if others are not easily accessible.

Preparation

1. Assemble the following equipment:
   - a digital thermometer
   - the appropriate probe attachment—the *blue* probe is used for an axillary temperature
   - disposable probe covers
   - disposable gloves, if appropriate
   - a towel
   - pen and pad, or a form for recording temperature
2. Wash your hands to ensure infection control.
3. Explain in simple terms what you are going to do, even if the patient is unable to talk or is disoriented.

The Procedure

4. Provide privacy. Screen around the patient, close the curtains, or close the door to the room, if appropriate.
5. Help the patient remove any clothing to expose his upper arm area.
6. Dry the axilla with the towel.
7. Place the disposable probe cover over the *blue* probe. Start the thermometer and wait for it to show it is ready.
8. Place the covered probe in the center of the axilla.
9. Place the patient's arm across his chest while holding the probe in place (Figure 11.9).
10. Hold the probe in place in the axilla until you hear or see the signal. This indicates the reading is completed.
11. Remove the thermometer from the axilla and read the temperature on the display screen.
12. Do not touch the probe cover.

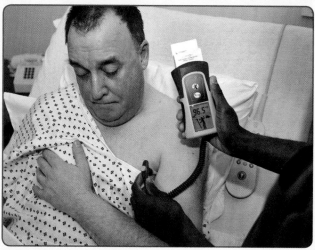

Figure 11.9   *Wards Forest Media, LLC*

13. Dispose of the probe cover safely in the wastebasket or per facility policy.
14. Clean the probe with alcohol and return the probe to its storage compartment on the thermometer.
15. Remove your gloves and wash your hands to ensure infection control. Record the temperature on a pad or form so it is not forgotten.
16. Return the thermometer to a charging location per facility policy.
17. Assist the patient in replacing and securing his clothing.

Follow-up

18. Make sure the patient is safe and comfortable.
19. Wash your hands to ensure infection control.

Reporting and Documentation

20. Communicate any specific observation, complications, or unusual responses to the appropriate provider. Also record this information in the patient's chart or EMR.
21. Use your facility's standard policy and forms to record the temperature.

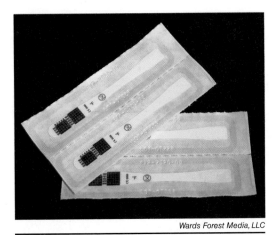

Wards Forest Media, LLC

Figure 11.10 Disposable oral thermometers are considered to be more sanitary than traditional thermometers.

aural
of or relating to the ear or the sense of hearing

Disposable Oral Thermometers

There are also disposable oral thermometers (Figure 11.10). These thermometers may be used to reduce the risk of cross- or re-infection. They are plastic or paper and are discarded once used. The dots found on the thermometer change color to show the change in body temperature.

Tympanic Thermometers

A tympanic thermometer measures the temperature of **aural** blood vessels. It determines whether a patient has a fever by measuring the temperature on the tympanic membrane, or *eardrum*. Tympanic thermometers are usually battery-operated and handheld with a digital display found on the handle (Figure 11.11).

Placement of the thermometer is very important to get an accurate reading. Be aware if there is too much wax in the ears, as excess wax can interfere with the reading. Do not use this type of thermometer if the patient has a sore ear or ear infection, or if they have had ear surgery.

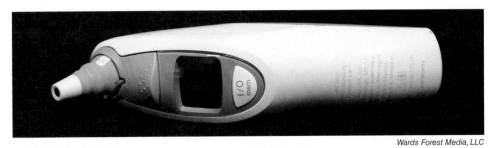

Wards Forest Media, LLC

Figure 11.11 A tympanic thermometer is inserted into the ear and measures the temperature of the tympanic membrane, or *eardrum*.

Procedure 11.4   Tympanic Temperature—Digital

Rationale

When a body temperature is outside the normal range, it can be a sign of a health condition or disease, or the result of an injury. Tympanic (*ear*) thermometers are another option for taking temperatures. Placement is most important for an accurate reading.

Preparation

1. Assemble the following equipment:
   • a digital tympanic thermometer
   • disposable plastic tympanic covers
   • disposable gloves, if necessary, or per facility policy
   • pen and pad, or a form for recording the temperature

2. Wash your hands to ensure infection control.
3. Put on disposable gloves.
4. Explain in simple terms what you are going to do, even if the patient is not able to talk or is disoriented.

The Procedure

5. Provide privacy. Screen around the patient, close the curtains, or close the door to the room, if appropriate.
6. Check the lens of the tympanic thermometer to make sure it is clean and intact.
7. Position the patient's head so that the ear being used for the procedure is directly in front of you.

Procedure 11.4   Tympanic Temperature—Digital (continued)

8. Place the disposable plastic cover on the tympanic thermometer.

9. For an adult or child, pull the outer ear up and back to open the ear canal (Figure 11.12). For an infant, pull the ear straight back.

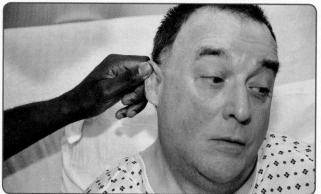

Figure 11.12   *Wards Forest Media, LLC*

10. Gently insert the probe-covered tympanic thermometer into the ear until it seals the ear canal (Figure 11.13).

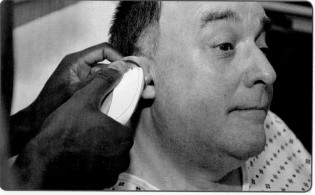

Figure 11.13   *Wards Forest Media, LLC*

11. Start the thermometer.

12. Hold the probe in place in the ear until you hear or see the signal. This indicates the reading is completed.

13. Remove the tympanic and read the temperature on the digital display screen.

14. Do not touch the used plastic tympanic cover.

15. Dispose of the plastic cover safely in the wastebasket or per facility policy.

16. Clean the tympanic thermometer with alcohol and store it according to the facility policy.

17. Remove your gloves and wash your hands to ensure infection control. Record the temperature on a pad or form so it is not forgotten.

18. Return the thermometer to a charging location per facility policy.

Follow-up

19. Make sure the patient or resident is safe and comfortable.

20. Wash your hands to ensure infection control.

Reporting and Documentation

21. Communicate any specific observations, complications, or unusual responses to the appropriate provider. Also record this information in the patient's chart or EMR.

22. Use your facility's standard policy and forms to record the temperature.

Temporal Artery Thermometers

Temporal artery thermometers use the surface temperature of the temporal artery to determine the presence of a fever. This type of temperature is often more accurate than an oral temperature because it is not affected by what a patient eats or drinks. Temporal artery thermometers measure the temperature of arteries on either side of the head using a handheld, infrared scanner with a digital display (Figure 11.14). The device is swept across the forehead to read the patient's temperature.

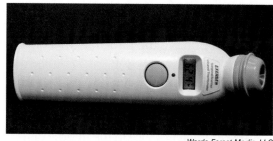

Wards Forest Media, LLC

Figure 11.14 Due to their accuracy and ease of use, temporal artery thermometers are often used on infants and other young patients.

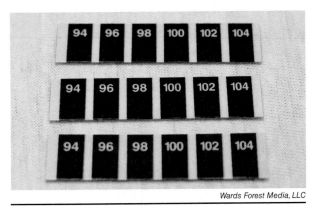

Wards Forest Media, LLC

Figure 11.15 Forehead thermometer strips are a disposable alternative to a temporal artery thermometer.

A forehead thermometer strip is sometimes used to measure a patient's temperature at this location (Figure 11.15). The strips contain heat-sensitive liquid crystals that change color to reflect different temperatures.

The type of thermometer you use when working in healthcare will depend on what is available at your healthcare facility. You will follow a specific procedure for taking, measuring, and recording a temperature. When recording a temperature, identify the type of thermometer used and report any irregularities to the appropriate provider.

Procedure 11.5 | Temporal Artery Thermometer

Rationale

When a body temperature is outside the normal range, it can be a sign of a health condition or disease, or the result of an injury. The temporal artery thermometer, used on the forehead, is another way to take a temperature. This thermometer is less invasive than others because it does not need to enter a body cavity.

Preparation

1. Assemble the following equipment:
   - a temporal artery thermometer
   - a pen and pad, or a form for recording the temperature
2. Wash your hands to ensure infection control.
3. Explain in simple terms what you are going to do, even if the patient is unable to talk or is disoriented.

The Procedure

4. Read the manufacturer's instructions for using the temporal artery thermometer. The facility may also provide more specific training.
5. Position the patient comfortably.
6. Assist or have the patient turn so that his forehead is facing you.
7. Start the thermometer and wait for it to show it is ready.
8. Place the probe on the temporal artery thermometer device in the middle of the patient's forehead (Figure 11.16A). Then slowly move the thermometer across the forehead toward the ear, stopping in front of the ear (Figure 11.16B).

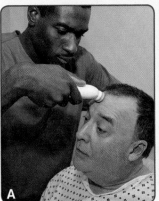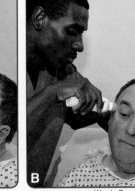

Figure 11.16   Wards Forest Media, LLC

9. When you see or hear the signal, this indicates the temperature is complete.
10. Wash your hands and record the temperature on a pad or form so it is not forgotten.
11. Clean and store the temporal artery thermometer according to the facility policy.

Follow-up

12. Make sure the patient is safe and comfortable.
13. Wash your hands to ensure infection control.

Reporting and Documentation

14. Communicate any specific observations, complications, or unusual responses to the appropriate provider. Also record this information in the patient's chart or EMR.
15. Use your facility's standard policy and forms to record the temperature.

Check Your Understanding ✓

Imagine you are working in a healthcare facility and today you will be taking the temperature of each patient on your unit. Answer the following questions.

1. Name the five different types of temperature and the body locations where you can take each type.
2. Give two reasons why you would select one location over another.
3. Identify the considerations you will need to be aware of to ensure patient safety, infection control, and accurate readings.
4. Discuss the similarities and differences among the procedures for the different locations.

radial pulse
the pulse located on the thumb side of the wrist

apical pulse
the pulse located at the bottom left portion of the heart

carotid pulse
a pulse taken at either of the two main arteries located on each side of the neck

Pulse

When you take a pulse, you are feeling the pressure of the blood against the wall of an artery as the heart beats (contracts and relaxes). The pulse is very important to know because it tells you how well the cardiovascular system is working. It is particularly important if a patient has a heart or respiratory condition.

Pulse Locations

There are several locations where an artery comes close enough to the surface of the skin for a pulse to be felt (Figure 11.17). These arteries are the temporal; carotid; apical; brachial; radial; femoral; popliteal; and dorsalis pedis, which is found on the top of the foot on the dorsalis pedis artery.

There are three pulse locations that are most commonly used:

1. **radial pulse**
2. **apical pulse**
3. **carotid pulse**

Of these three, radial and apical pulses are the ones used most often. The radial pulse is located on the radial artery at the wrist (thumb side of the hand). Two fingers are gently placed on the radial artery to take the pulse.

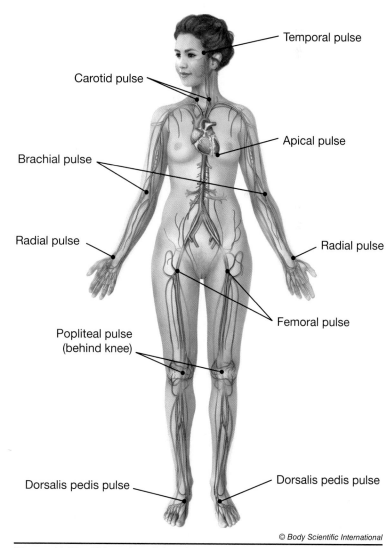

© Body Scientific International

Figure 11.17 Although radial and apical pulses are most commonly taken, there are several locations throughout the body where a pulse can be felt and recorded.

intravenous (IV)
existing or taking place within, or administered into, a vein or veins

stethoscope
a medical device used to listen to body sounds such as breathing, heartbeats, and lung and bowel sounds; composed of two earpieces connected by flexible tubing with a diaphragm at its end

If the patient has an **intravenous (IV)** catheter in one arm, do not use that arm when taking the pulse.

The apical pulse is located at the bottom left of the heart and is usually taken at this location when it is difficult to count a radial pulse and if a patient is unconscious. This pulse is taken by using a **stethoscope**. The carotid pulse may also be used when a patient is unconscious, such as during CPR.

Parts of a Stethoscope

A stethoscope is composed of two earpieces; rubber or plastic tubing; a brace, which connects the tubing to the earpieces; a diaphragm, which magnifies the sound; and a bell, which can detect fainter sounds (Figure 11.18). Always disinfect the earpieces, diaphragm, and bell before use by rubbing them lightly with antiseptic or alcohol wipes. Also wipe the tubing if it has come in contact with the patient or bed linen.

Using the Stethoscope

Before using the stethoscope, be sure the earpieces are firmly in place in your ear canals. They should fit snugly and block out any outside sounds. Once the earpieces are in place, tap lightly on the diaphragm. You must be able to hear these sounds clearly to use the stethoscope. If you don't, rotate the diaphragm and try again. If it still does not work, try this process again with a different stethoscope.

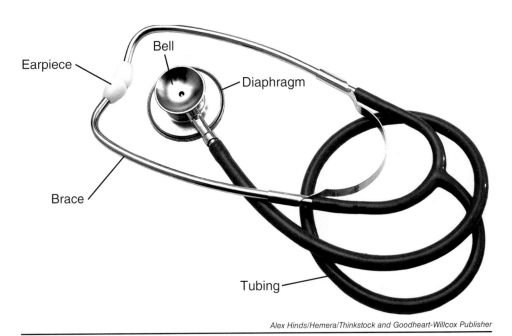

Alex Hinds/Hemera/Thinkstock and Goodheart-Willcox Publisher

Figure 11.18   The parts of a stethoscope

Real Life Scenario — A Young Athlete Gets His Pulse Checked

Your friend Joe likes to participate in sports. Last week he went to the doctor for a physical and found out that his pulse was at 56 beats per minute. The doctor told Joe that he should have his pulse checked again in a month.

Apply It

1. Is Joe's pulse considered in the normal range for an athlete? Why or why not?
2. What term is used to describe Joe's pulse rate?
3. Why do you think the doctor will want Joe to have his pulse checked again?

Pulse Rate Measurements

Pulse rate is measured by "feeling" or "hearing" the pulse and counting the number of beats in one minute using a watch with a second hand. Pulse rate is reported per minute such as *a pulse of 72 beats per minute* or *72 bpm*.

A pulse is taken when a patient is breathing normally and resting (sitting in a chair or in bed).

The average range or normal resting pulse rates are found in Figure 11.19.

Pulse rate can be affected by activity, medication, sleep patterns, and diseases or health conditions. For instance, during exercise, the average person's pulse rate can range from 90 to 120 beats per minute. In contrast, if the person is an athlete, the resting pulse can be as low as 40 to 60 beats per minute. This is because an athlete's body is healthy and in condition, so the heart does not have to work as hard to pump blood.

When a pulse is slow (less than 60 beats per minute), it is called **bradycardia**. When a pulse is fast (100 beats or more per minute), it is called **tachycardia**.

When taking a pulse, it is important to remember that you are not only counting the number of beats felt, but also determining the rhythm (pause between beats felt) and the quality of the pulse. A pulse can be strong; weak; or thready, which means it is hard to feel. For example, a pulse may be reported as *82 bpm and strong*.

The pulse is recorded using a form provided by the healthcare facility. Any irregularities of the pulse must be reported to the appropriate provider.

bradycardia
a slow pulse of less than 60 beats per minute

tachycardia
a fast pulse of over 100 beats per minute

Average Resting Pulse Rates Per Minute	
Adults	60–100 bpm
Teenagers	60–100 bpm
Children	70–120 bpm
Infants	120–160 bpm

Goodheart-Willcox Publisher

Figure 11.19   Average resting pulse rates vary by age.

Procedure 11.6   Counting and Recording a Radial Pulse

Rationale

Counting a radial pulse is the most common method of measuring heart rate and its quality. A pulse not within a normal range may indicate a health issue, medical condition, or disease.

Preparation

1. Assemble the following equipment:
   - a watch or clock with a second hand (digital watches cannot be used)
   - pen and pad, or a form for recording the pulse rate
2. Wash your hands to ensure infection control.
3. Explain in simple terms what you are going to do, even if the patient is not able to talk or is disoriented.

The Procedure

4. Provide privacy. Screen around the patient, close the curtains, or close the door, if appropriate.
5. Have the patient sit or lie down. Select the hand and arm you will be using to take the pulse. Remember, if there is an intravenous (IV) catheter in the arm, do not use that arm to take the pulse.
6. Position the hand and arm so they are well supported and resting comfortably.
7. Locate the radial pulse by placing the middle two fingers of your hand toward the inside of the wrist on the radial, or thumb side (Figure 11.20).

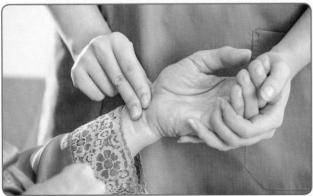

Figure 11.20   Tyler Olson/Shutterstock.com

8. Do not use your thumb to feel for the pulse. The thumb has its own pulse and can cause confusion with the pulse you are taking.
9. Press your fingers gently until you feel the pulse. Note the rhythm and quality.
10. Start taking the pulse when you note the position of the second hand on your watch (Figure 11.21). Count pulse beats for one full minute. (Some facilities allow counting the pulse for 30 seconds and multiplying the results by two. Follow the facility policy.) Counting for one full minute is more accurate and should be done if the pulse rhythm seems weak or irregular.

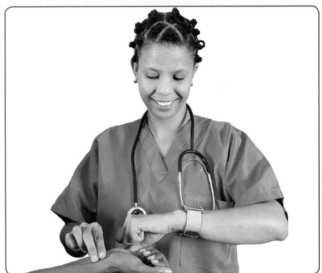

Figure 11.21   michaeljung/Shutterstock.com

11. When completed, write down the pulse.

Follow-up

12. Make sure the patient is safe and comfortable.
13. Wash your hands to ensure infection control.

Reporting and Documentation

14. Communicate any specific observations, complications, or unusual responses to the appropriate provider. Also record this information in the patient's chart or EMR.
15. Use your facility's standard policy and forms to record the pulse.

Procedure 11.7 — Counting and Recording an Apical Pulse

Rationale

Counting an apical pulse (located at the apex, or narrowest point, of the heart) is usually done when you want more information about the heart rate than what a radial pulse provides, or if it is not possible to take a radial pulse. A pulse outside of the normal range may indicate a health issue, medical condition, or disease.

Preparation

1. Assemble the following equipment:
   - a stethoscope
   - antiseptic wipes
   - a watch with a second hand (digital watches cannot be used)
   - a pen and pad, or a form for recording the apical pulse rate
2. Wash your hands to ensure infection control.
3. Explain in simple terms what you are going to do, even if the patient is not able to talk or is disoriented.

The Procedure

4. Provide privacy. Screen around the patient, close the curtains, or close the door to the room, if appropriate.
5. Have the patient sit or lie down.
6. Clean the earpieces and diaphragm of the stethoscope with an antiseptic wipe.
7. Warm the diaphragm of the stethoscope by rubbing it in the palm of your hands.
8. Place the earpieces in your ears.
9. Uncover the left side of the patient's chest. Avoid any overexposure.
10. Place the diaphragm on the left side of the chest, under the breast, or just below the left nipple (Figure 11.22).

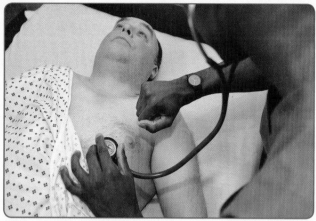

Figure 11.22   *Wards Forest Media, LLC*

11. If the heartbeat is difficult to hear, have the patient turn slightly to the left.
12. Note the position of the second hand on your watch. Count the heartbeats for one full minute. Note the rhythm and quality.
13. Re-cover the patient's chest.
14. Immediately record the pulse rate so it is not forgotten.

Follow-up

15. Make sure the patient is safe and comfortable.
16. Wash your hands to ensure infection control.

Reporting and Documentation

17. Communicate any specific observations, complications, or unusual responses to the appropriate provider. Also record this information in the patient's chart or EMR.
18. Use your facility's standard policy and forms to record the pulse.

Check Your Understanding ✓

1. Identify the eight different locations where a pulse can be taken.
2. How is taking a radial pulse similar to taking an apical pulse? How are they different?

Respiration

inhalation
breathing in; also called inspiration

exhalation
breathing out; also called expiration

The rate of respiration is the measurement of a patient's breathing cycle, which is **inhalation** followed by **exhalation**. Respiration rate helps determine the level of the blood oxygenation, or how well oxygen is being supplied to the body cells. Knowing a patient's respiration rate helps determine if they are breathing in a normal range. This provides information about conditions such as asthma, heart disease, and even infections.

Measuring Respirations

The method used to determine rate of respiration is to record the number of full breaths (the breathing cycle) taken in one minute (Figure 11.23). This is typically done by counting respirations for 15 seconds and multiplying by four. Some healthcare facilities require the healthcare worker to count for 30 seconds and then multiply by two. This is done using a watch with a second hand.

It is best to count the respiration rate immediately after the pulse is taken so the patient is breathing as he normally would. Switch from taking the pulse to counting respirations without mentioning the change to your patient. A patient who knows his respirations are being counted may subconsciously alter his breathing, giving the healthcare worker an inaccurate result.

Understanding Respiratory Rates

A normal adult respiratory rate is 12 to 20 breaths per minute. Infants and children breathe much faster. Infants can breathe from 30 to 60 breaths per minute and children, 18 to 30 breaths per minute.

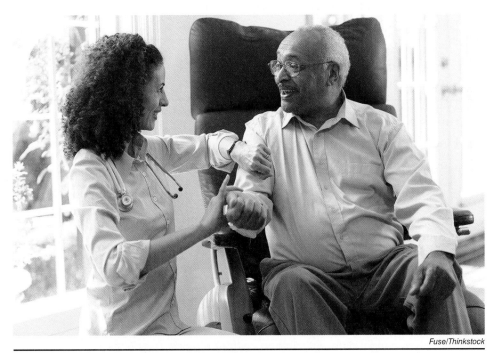

Fuse/Thinkstock

Figure 11.23   By observing the rise and fall of a patient's chest over the course of a specific period of time, this healthcare worker is able to determine the patient's respiration rate, which is an important indicator of health status.

Observing how well the patient is breathing (regularity, expansion of the chest, and depth of respiration) is just as important as the rate (counting breaths). Note the following:

- Is the breathing regular or irregular?
- Is the patient experiencing **hyperventilation** or **hypoventilation**?
- Is the breathing shallow (called **tachypnea**), deep and labored (called **dyspnea**), or unusually slow (called **bradypnea**)?
- Is the breathing noisy like snoring (called **stertorous breathing**)?
- Are there periods of no breathing at all (called **apnea**)?

Using a Pulse Oximeter

Another way to measure how well oxygen is being used in the body is to determine the oxygen's saturation in the blood, or how well it is being carried to the body tissues. This is done with a device called a **pulse oximeter**. This device is often used when a patient is receiving oxygen to measure the oxygen's effectiveness.

A pulse oximeter is applied to the finger (or sometimes the earlobe or toe). It uses infrared light that passes through the body tissue of the finger. A pulse oximeter's digital display will show the amount of oxygen in the blood as a percentage (Figure 11.24). A normal reading is 95 percent to 100 percent oxygen in the blood. A reading below 85 percent is considered too low and is called **hypoxia**. The notation used for recording a pulse oximeter's reading is SpO2 for the saturation level of oxygen in the blood.

There are minimal risks involved in using a pulse oximeter. If the probe is not properly placed, it may result in an inaccurate reading. The skin around and under the probe may also become irritated.

Respirations (rate, regularity, and depth) and pulse oximeter percentages are recorded using a form provided by the healthcare facility. Any irregularities must be reported to the appropriate provider.

hypoventilation
breathing too slowly

hyperventilation
breathing too quickly

tachypnea
rapid, shallow breathing due to the lungs only partially filling

dyspnea
difficult breathing usually observed as shortness of breath

bradypnea
an unusually slow rate of breathing, typically under 12 breaths per minute

stertorous breathing
breathing that sounds like snoring

apnea
lack of breathing

pulse oximeter
a medical device usually applied to the fingertip to indirectly measure the amount of oxygen saturation in the blood

hypoxia
a lack of adequate oxygen

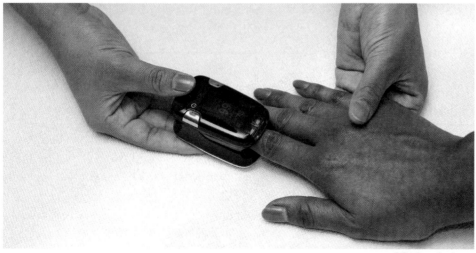

©iStock.com/praisaeng

Figure 11.24   Pulse oximeters are often used in emergency medicine to monitor the patient's oxygen levels.

Think It Through

Have you ever hyperventilated? If so, what do you think caused you to hyperventilate? Were you ill or did something frighten you? Maybe you were feeling stressed or anxious? How did it feel to breathe fast? What did you do to stop it?

Procedure 11.8 | Counting and Recording Respirations

Rationale

Counting respirations means measuring the number of inhalation and exhalation cycles of the lungs. A respiration rate that falls outside the normal range may indicate a health issue, medical condition, or disease.

Preparation

1. Assemble the following equipment:
   - a watch or clock with a second hand (digital watches cannot be used)
   - a pen and pad, or a form for recording the respiration rate
2. Wash your hands to ensure infection control.

The Procedure

3. Provide privacy. Screen around the patient, close the curtains, or close the door to the room, if appropriate.
4. Have the patient sit or lie down.
5. The best time to count respirations is immediately after counting the pulse rate. It is best not to tell patients you are counting their respirations. When people are aware that their breathing is being observed, they may alter their breathing pattern.
6. Whichever pulse was taken (radial or apical), keep your fingers on either the wrist or the stethoscope on the chest while counting respirations.

7. Begin counting respirations when the chest rises. Each rise and fall of the chest counts as one respiration. Note the regularity and depth of respirations, the expansion of the chest, and if there is any pain or difficulty breathing.
8. Note the position of the second hand on your watch. You will need to record the respirations for one full minute. (Some facilities allow counting respirations for 15 seconds and multiplying by four, and others allow counting for 30 seconds and multiplying the results by two. Follow the facility policy). Counting for one full minute should be done if the respiration is irregular.
9. Notify the appropriate provider immediately if the patient complains of pain or difficulty breathing.
10. When completed, record the respiration rate.

Follow-up

11. Make sure the patient is safe and comfortable.
12. Wash your hands to ensure infection control.

Reporting and Documentation

13. Communicate any specific observations, complications, or unusual responses to the appropriate provider. Also record this information in the patient's chart or EMR.
14. Use your facility's standard policy and forms to record the respiration rate.

Check Your Understanding ✓

1. What approach should you take to be sure you are accurately counting a patient's respirations?
2. Besides counting a patient's respirations, what else should you be observing?
3. Suppose you find that a patient's breathing is very slow, labored, and noisy. What terms will you use to describe this patient's respiration?

Blood Pressure

Blood pressure is a measure of the force of the blood pushing against the body's arterial walls. Measuring blood pressure is important. If a patient has blood pressure that is too low, called **hypotension**, it can mean the body is not getting enough oxygen and nutrients. Conversely, **hypertension** (blood pressure that is too high) may place too much pressure on the walls of the arteries. This pressure may cause a stroke or other circulatory problems. High or low blood pressure can also be a sign or cause of certain diseases or conditions such as coronary heart disease, kidney damage or failure, various injuries, or dizziness.

hypotension
a condition in which blood pressure is too low

hypertension
a condition in which blood pressure is too high

Did You Know?   **High Blood Pressure by the Numbers**

The Centers for Disease Control and Prevention recently reported that 67 million American adults (31 percent) have high blood pressure. This means about one in every three adults has hypertension. However, approximately one-half (47 percent) of those with high blood pressure have their condition under control.

Measuring Blood Pressure

There are two pressure levels measured as the heart beats. The first is the **systolic pressure**, in which the heart muscle contracts and pushes blood through the artery. The second is the **diastolic pressure**, which occurs when the heart muscle immediately relaxes. These are measured using a stethoscope and a **sphygmomanometer**. (To break down this term: *sphygmo* = pulse; *mano* = pressure; *meter* = measure.)

Both pressures are measured and recorded in millimeters of mercury (mmHg) as a fraction, such as 120/80. The systolic pressure, which is the higher number, is the first beat heard and measured (120 in the example). The diastolic pressure is the lower number and is the last beat heard and measured (80 in the example). The average range of normal blood pressure for adults, children, and infants can be found in Figure 11.25.

systolic pressure
part of a blood pressure reading that is taken when the heart muscle contracts and pushes blood through the artery

diastolic pressure
part of a blood pressure reading that is taken when the heart muscle relaxes

sphygmomanometer
a specialized manual or digital medical device used to measure blood pressure; also called a vital sign machine

Average Blood Pressure Measurements		
Age	*Systolic Pressure*	*Diastolic Pressure*
Adult	100–130	60–90
Teenager	94–134	64–84
Children	100–120	60–74
Infant	70–90	50–64

Goodheart-Willcox Publisher

Figure 11.25   Average blood pressure measurements vary by age.

Factors Affecting Blood Pressure

Blood pressure can vary for several reasons:

- **Diet.** Diets high in salt and fat may lead to higher blood pressure.

- **Weight.** Being overweight can lead to higher blood pressure.

- **Exercise.** Systolic pressure may be higher if you do not exercise or if you exercised right before it was taken.

- **Race.** African-American individuals tend to have high blood pressure more often, and at an earlier age, than Caucasians or people of Hispanic descent.

- **When the reading is taken.** Blood pressure may be lower in the morning than later in the day. If blood pressure is taken after a meal, it may be higher than if it was taken before the patient ate.

- **Position.** Blood pressure may be higher if a patient is lying down, and lower when the patient is standing up. If someone stands up too quickly, he may experience orthostatic hypotension, in which the blood pressure can drop too quickly, causing the patient to feel dizzy or faint.

- **Cigarettes and alcohol.** Both of these substances can increase blood pressure.

- **Drugs or medications.** Some drugs (both prescription and illegal drugs) will affect blood pressure and may make it higher or lower than it otherwise would be.

- **Stress, fear, or pain.** Blood pressure may be higher if a patient is experiencing any of these feelings.

Think It Through

What three strategies or steps can you personally take to be sure you feel prepared to perform a blood pressure measurement?

Taking a Patient's Blood Pressure

Blood pressure can be taken manually or electronically, depending on the equipment that is available. Both ways are considered accurate; however, the use of an electronic device reduces potential human error as long as the device is regularly checked for accuracy. The equipment may be movable, on a wall mount, or part of a vital sign machine.

When taking a patient's blood pressure, there are several essential factors to consider, including equipment checks, making sure your patient is relaxed, and whether you are feeling prepared to perform the procedure. It is important to recheck a blood pressure reading if you are not sure the measure is accurate due to your own skill, possible faulty equipment, a change in the patient's normal blood pressure, or the first occurrence of a high or low blood pressure for that patient.

When taking a manual blood pressure measurement, you will need a stethoscope and a sphygmomanometer. Before beginning, check that your stethoscope is in working order.

There are three main types of devices used to measure blood pressure (Figure 11.26):

1. **Manual aneroid sphygmomanometer**: has a round dial and a needle that points to the numbers and is movable. You will need to use a stethoscope when using this device.

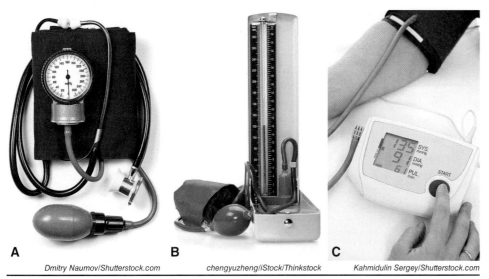

Figure 11.26   A stethoscope must be used with the aneroid sphygmomanometer (A) and mercury manometer (B), but not with an electronic sphygmomanometer (C).

2. **Manual mercury manometer**: has a column of mercury that rises and falls; these can stand alone or be mounted on a wall. You will need to use a stethoscope when using this device.

3. **Electronic sphygmomanometer**: has a digital display and is found in many healthcare facilities. You will not need a stethoscope when using this device.

No matter what type of device you are using, be sure it is in working order before taking a blood pressure measurement.

A sphygmomanometer has two parts: the measuring device and the cuff. When applying a blood pressure cuff, check that it is the right size. Cuffs come in various sizes—pediatric, small adult, adult, and large adult (Figure 11.27). If the cuff is too small or too large, the blood pressure reading will not be accurate. The inflatable part of the cuff should cover two-thirds of the distance from the elbow to the shoulder.

Have patients relax or rest for a few minutes before taking their blood pressure. This helps you get a reading that is most normal for that patient. The blood pressure reading may not be accurate if the patient has just been exercising, is in pain, is feeling anxious, or has recently had physical therapy. If possible, wait at least 30 minutes before taking a routine blood pressure measurement.

Taking blood pressures can be most challenging when you first start to do them early in your healthcare career. Practice helps build confidence and will improve your ability to hear through the stethoscope and take accurate readings.

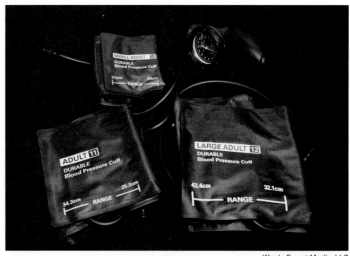

Figure 11.27   When taking an adult blood pressure, three cuff sizes are available—small adult, adult, and large adult.

Procedure 11.9   Taking a Patient's Blood Pressure—Manual and Electronic

Rationale

Blood pressure is a measure of the force of the blood pushing against the body's arterial walls. A blood pressure reading that is outside the normal range may indicate a disease or health issue.

Preparation: Manual Device

1. Assemble the following equipment:
   - a sphygmomanometer—aneroid or mercury
   - an appropriately-sized cuff—pediatric, small adult, adult, or large adult
   - a stethoscope
   - antiseptic wipe(s)
   - a pen and pad, or a form for recording the blood pressure

2. Wash your hands to ensure infection control.

3. Explain in simple terms what you are going to do, even if the patient is not able to talk or is disoriented.

The Procedure: Manual Device

4. Provide privacy. Screen around the patient, close the curtains, or close the door to the room, if appropriate.

5. Have the patient rest quietly, either lying comfortably on the bed or sitting in a chair.

6. When appropriate, give the patient a choice as to which arm they want you to use for a blood pressure and whether they want to sit up or lie down.

7. If the patient is in bed, lock the wheels and raise the bed to a comfortable working level. If the patient is on an examining table, stand next to the patient, or sit in a chair in front of the patient so you can get a clear view of the dial.

8. Remember, when using the mercury or aneroid sphygmomanometer, the measuring scale should always be level with your eyes (Figure 11.28).

9. Clean the earpieces and the diaphragm of the stethoscope with antiseptic wipes.

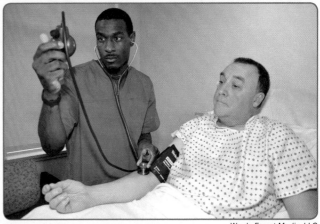

Figure 11.28   *Wards Forest Media, LLC*

10. Place the patient's arm so that it is resting at the level of the heart with the palm turned upward. Provide support, if needed (Figure 11.29).

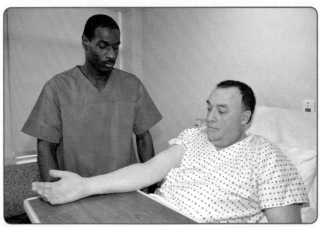

Figure 11.29   *Wards Forest Media, LLC*

11. Expose the upper arm so that you are placing the cuff on bare skin.

12. Unroll the blood pressure cuff and loosen the valve on the bulb of the sphygmomanometer by turning it counterclockwise (Figure 11.30).

13. Squeeze the cuff to expel any remaining air.

14. With your fingertips, locate the brachial artery at the inner aspect of the elbow (Figure 11.31).

15. Wrap the cuff smoothly and snugly around the arm about one inch above the elbow.

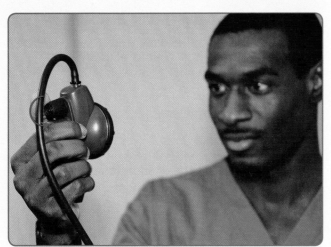

Figure 11.30   Wards Forest Media, LLC

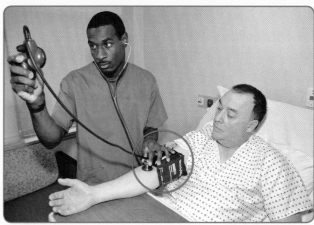

Figure 11.32   Wards Forest Media, LLC

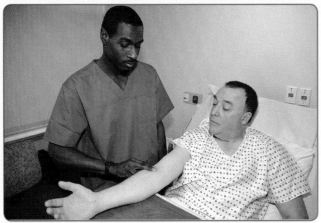

Figure 11.31   Wards Forest Media, LLC

16. Place the center of the cuff, usually marked with an arrow, above the brachial artery.

17. Close the valve on the bulb by turning it clockwise. Be careful not to turn it too tightly.

18. Place the earpieces of the stethoscope in your ears.

19. Find the brachial pulse.

20. Place the warmed diaphragm of the stethoscope over the brachial artery.

21. Inflate the cuff to 180 mmHg. You should not be able to hear the pulse. If you do, inflate to 200 mmHg.

22. The stethoscope diaphragm should be held firmly against the skin, close to the cuff, but not placed under the cuff (Figure 11.32).

23. Deflate the cuff by slowly turning the valve on the bulb counterclockwise at an even rate of two to four millimeters per second.

24. Listen carefully while the cuff is deflating. Note the dial reading when you hear the first sound (beat). This is the systolic pressure.

25. Continue deflating the cuff slowly and evenly. Note the dial reading when the sound (beat) disappears. This is the diastolic pressure.

26. Completely deflate the cuff and remove it from the arm. Remove the stethoscope earpieces from your ears.

27. Write the results on a pad or form for recording the blood pressure. Report abnormal results to the appropriate provider immediately.

28. Return the cuff to its case or wall mount.

29. Clean the earpieces and diaphragm of the stethoscope with antiseptic wipes.

30. Return the stethoscope and cuff case (if appropriate) to their storage location.

Preparation: Electronic Device

31. Assemble the following equipment:
   - an electronic blood pressure device
   - the appropriately-sized cuff, disposable cuff, or tubes needed
   - antiseptic wipes
   - a pen and pad, or a form for recording the blood pressure

Procedure 11.9   Taking a Patient's Blood Pressure—Manual and Electronic (continued)

32. Wash your hands to ensure infection control.

33. Explain in simple terms what you are going to do, even if the patient is not able to talk or is disoriented.

The Procedure: Electronic Device

34. Provide privacy. Screen around the patient, close the curtains, or close the door to the room, if appropriate.

35. Bring the electronic blood pressure unit near the patient and plug it into a source of electricity.

36. Clean the cuff with an antiseptic wipe or cover with a disposable paper cover.

37. Have the patient rest quietly, either lying comfortably on the bed or sitting in a chair.

38. If the patient is in bed, lock the wheels of the bed. Raise the bed to a comfortable working level. If the patient is on an examining table, stand next to the patient, or sit in a chair in front of the patient so you can get a clear view of the digital display.

39. Remove any restrictive clothing from the patient's arm. Again, you can ask the patient which arm they would prefer, if appropriate.

40. Locate the *Power* switch and turn the machine on.

41. Squeeze any excess air out of the cuff.

42. Connect the cuff to the connector hose.

43. Wrap the cuff smoothly and snugly around the patient's arm. Check to make sure that only one finger can fit between the cuff and the skin.

44. Make sure the artery arrow marked on the outside of the cuff is correctly placed over the brachial artery.

45. Check to make sure the connector hose between the cuff and the machine is not kinked.

46. Press the *Start* button. The cuff should begin to inflate and then deflate as the reading is being taken.

47. You will see and/or hear the signal when the reading is completed.

48. Note that if you will be taking periodic, automatic measurements, you should set the machine for the designated frequency of blood pressure measurements. Set the upper and lower alarm limits for systolic, diastolic, and mean blood pressure readings, according to facility policy.

49. Record the results on a pad or form for recording the blood pressure. Report abnormal results to the appropriate provider immediately.

50. Clean the tubing and cuff with an antiseptic wipe. Discard the disposable sleeve, if used.

51. Remove the machine and place it in its appropriate storage location.

52. If the cuff is to remain on the arm between blood pressure readings, loosen it. Remove the cuff at least every two hours and rotate the site to the other arm, if possible. Evaluate the skin for redness and/or irritation. Report any abnormal observations to the appropriate provider.

Follow-up: Manual or Electronic Readings

53. Make sure the patient is safe and comfortable.

54. Wash your hands to ensure infection control.

Reporting and Documentation

55. Communicate any specific observations, complications, or unusual responses to the appropriate provider. Also record this information in the patient's chart or EMR.

56. Use your facility's standard policy and forms to record the blood pressure.

Real Life Scenario — Checking Blood Pressure

Jane has been asked to perform a blood pressure check on a patient who has been complaining of a headache this morning. She checks the last blood pressure reading taken and finds that it was 124/78 yesterday morning. She uses an electronic device to measure the patient's blood pressure and finds that it is now 162/98.

Apply It

1. Should Jane take the blood pressure again? Why or why not?
2. Should Jane use different equipment to take the blood pressure? Why or why not?
3. What might be causing the high blood pressure reading?
4. This patient's high blood pressure could be a symptom of what problems or diseases?

Height and Weight

Height and weight are usually measured upon admission to a healthcare facility and may be done during a patient's stay. These measurements are also taken during a patient visit to a doctor's office. How often (daily, weekly, or monthly) these measurements are taken depends on the doctor's orders for a health condition or disease. For example, a patient with kidney disease or a heart condition may need daily weights to help determine if they have **edema**. If the patient is admitted to a healthcare facility, the facility's policy may also dictate how often these measurements are taken.

The purpose of keeping track of height and weight is to determine nutritional status and medication dosage, and to monitor health. The relationship between height and weight is also important because it can provide an indication of a patient's overall health status. Height and weight are used to calculate **ideal body weight (IBW)** and body mass index (BMI). These calculations help determine whether a patient is overweight so a doctor can plan calorie intake, protein, and fluid needs.

edema
excess build-up or retention of fluid in the bodily tissues that causes swelling, usually in the legs and feet

ideal body weight (IBW)
the healthiest weight for an individual; determined primarily by height, but also takes gender, age, build, and muscular development into account, using adjusted statistical tables

Extend Your Knowledge ▶ Body Mass Index

The Centers for Disease Control and Prevention (CDC) uses body mass index (BMI) to define when a person is overweight or obese. BMI is the measurement of body fat based on height and weight that applies to both men and women between the ages of 18 and 65 years.

BMI is generally a good indicator of body fat for most adults. It is not so reliable for athletes or the elderly. A BMI between 18.5 and 24.9 is considered normal weight. You can determine your BMI by going to the CDC website and finding the BMI Calculator.

Apply It

1. Visit the CDC's website and calculate your BMI using either the adult calculator (if you are over the age of 18) or the child and teen calculator (if you are younger than 18).
2. Review your results. Is your BMI within the healthy range? If not, what could you do to adjust your BMI?

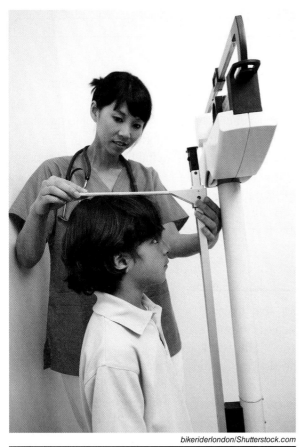

Figure 11.33 When using an upright, balance scale to measure height, lower the bar until it rests on the top of the patient's head.

Think It Through

How often do you weigh yourself and keep track of your height? Are you happy with how much you weigh and how tall or short you are? If you could, what changes would you make to your weight and height?

Measuring Height

Height can be measured one of two ways. When a patient is able to walk, you can use an upright, balance scale to measure his height (Figure 11.33). If the patient is bedridden, you will need to use a tape measure. Height should be measured in feet (') and inches (") or in centimeters (cm), depending on facility policy.

If the patient is able to walk, have him stand very straight on the center of the scale with his arms and hands down at his sides. Lower the rod until it rests on the top of the head. The height is read at the movable part of the ruler.

If the patient is bedridden, use a tape measure. If allowed, have the patient lie on his back, as straight as possible with his arms straight at his sides and legs extended. Straighten and tighten the bed sheet. With the help of another healthcare worker, extend the tape measure along the patient's side from the top of the head to the bottom of the heel. Measure the distance between the two points.

Measuring Weight

A patient's weight is often used to calculate medication dosage, so accurate measurement is essential. Weight can also be an indicator of certain conditions, such as malnutrition (poor nourishment) or edema. There are different ways of measuring weight. This measurement can be taken using a balance or digital scale or by using a lift or bed scales, if the patient is bedridden.

Weight should be measured at the same time each day in the same or similar clothing and using the same scale, if possible. Be sure the patient has urinated before measurement. Always calculate additional items that may add weight such as shoes, casts, catheters, colostomy bags, or other bodily devices. Weight can be measured standing, sitting, or in bed. Weight should be measured in pounds (lbs) or in kilograms (kg), depending on facility policy.

If standing and using a balance or digital scale, have the patient stand straight on the center of the scale with her arms and hands down at her sides. If you are using a balance scale, move the weights on the balanced scale bar to zero. Move the lower and upper weights until the balance pointer is in the middle (Figure 11.34). Add the amounts of the two bars together to determine the weight.

If using a lift or bed scale, be sure to follow the facility policy and instructions for the equipment. You will need another healthcare worker to assist in this procedure.

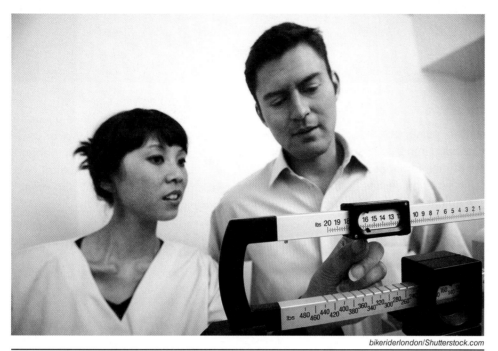

bikeriderlondon/Shutterstock.com

Figure 11.34 Once the scale has been balanced, add the numbers on the top and bottom bar to determine the patient's weight.

Safety Concerns When Measuring Height and Weight

Always be aware of safety issues when measuring a patient's height and weight, particularly if he or she is frail or has problems with fainting or dizziness. Pay attention to infection control by washing your hands before and after these procedures and document them accurately and in a timely fashion. Notify the appropriate provider if there are any irregularities with your measurements.

Check Your Understanding ✓

1. If a doctor tells his patient that the patient has hypertension, should the patient try to raise or lower his blood pressure?

2. For a healthy, normal patient, which number will be higher, her diastolic pressure or her systolic pressure?

3. A patient's blood pressure is 118/77. Which number represents his diastolic pressure? Which number represents his systolic pressure?

4. What are the average ranges for both diastolic and systolic blood pressure for teenagers?

5. Describe two important reasons to measure height and weight.

6. What equipment should you assemble to measure the height and weight of a bedridden patient?

7. How do you determine weight using an upright balanced scale?

8. What units of measurement can you use to record height and weight?

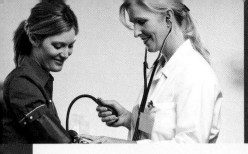

Chapter 11
Review and Assessment

Summary

Vital signs, including temperature, pulse, rate of respirations, and blood pressure, provide important information needed to determine whether someone is well or ill. Vital signs have well-established guidelines for adults and children that provide guidance to identify whether a measurement is in the normal range or not. Vital signs are recorded in the patient's chart or electronic medical record (EMR) and usually on a form provided by your facility.

Body temperature measures a patient's body heat in degrees. Body temperature should be monitored frequently as it can change over the course of a day. Oral, rectal, axillary, tympanic, or temporal artery temperatures can be taken using thermometers designed for each location.

Pulse measures the pressure of the blood against the wall of an artery as the heart beats. It is an important indicator of how well the cardiovascular system is working. The two common pulse locations are radial (located on the thumb side of the wrist) and apical (found at the bottom left portion of the heart). When appropriate, a carotid pulse can also be used. Pulse is taken by counting the number of beats for a set period of time and is reported per minute.

The rate of respiration is a measurement of breathing and how well oxygen is being supplied to the body cells. Rate of respiration can be determined by counting full breaths. Oxygen saturation in the blood is measured by using a pulse oximeter. Respiration rate provides information regarding potential conditions such as asthma, heart disease, and even infections.

Blood pressure is the force of blood pushing against the body's arterial walls. Blood pressure measurements can indicate if there is too much pressure on the walls of the arteries or the possibility of a specific disease. Two pressure levels are measured—systolic pressure and diastolic pressure.

Height and weight are often measured with vital signs. The relationship between height and weight can provide an indication of a patient's overall health status, can help determine nutritional status and medication dosage, and be used to monitor health.

When taking and recording vital signs and measuring height and weight, be sure to take accurate measurements and ask for help if needed. *Never* make up a reading. Be familiar with the normal range for each vital sign and understand the factors that may influence a reading. Always report any abnormal readings to the appropriate provider.

Review Questions

Answer the following questions using what you have learned in this chapter.

True or False 📲 Assess

1. *True or False?* The most accurate way to measure body temperature is using an oral thermometer.

2. *True or False?* Hypoxia means not having enough oxygen.

3. *True or False?* An aneroid sphygmomanometer is a device used to measure blood pressure.

4. *True or False?* Normal ranges for vital signs are the same for adults and children.

5. *True or False?* Blood pressure is measured in degrees.

6. *True or False?* An axillary temperature is taken in the armpit.

7. *True or False?* Dyspnea is the absence of breathing.

8. *True or False?* The normal adult range for respirations is 18 to 30 breaths per minute.

Multiple Choice 📲 Assess

9. Mrs. Garrett had her blood pressure taken this morning and it was 160/110. This reading is much higher than when it was taken yesterday. Which reading below was yesterday's?

    A. 165/112

    B. 155/105

    C. 100/70

    D. None of the above.

10. When taking an apical pulse, the stethoscope should be placed _____.

   A. above the sternum

   B. above the right nipple on the chest

   C. below the sternum

   D. below the left nipple on the chest

11. When is the best time to count respirations?

   A. right before taking the temperature

   B. right after taking the blood pressure

   C. right after taking the pulse

   D. right before taking the pulse

12. Which of the following resting pulse rates is *not* considered normal for an adult?

   A. 90

   B. 70

   C. 85

   D. 101

13. Mr. Laila has a rectal temperature of 100.6°F. What does this mean?

   A. His body temperature is low, indicating hypothermia. He should have his temperature taken again in the next few hours.

   B. His body temperature is in the normal range and all is okay. No action needs to be taken.

   C. His body temperature is high, indicating his body is building defenses. He should have his temperature taken again in the next few hours.

   D. His body temperature is high, indicating his body is building defenses. He should have his temperature taken again tomorrow.

14. Mrs. Tong had an early breakfast before vital signs were taken. How long should you wait before taking her oral temperature?

   A. 1 to 3 minutes

   B. 5 to 10 minutes

   C. 10 to 15 minutes

   D. 15 to 30 minutes

15. When a blood pressure is taken, there is a phase in the reading where the heart beat is no longer heard because the heart relaxes. This is called _____.

   A. dyspnea

   B. diastole

   C. systole

   D. sclerosis

16. A _____ is used to measure the oxygen's saturation in the blood.

   A. pulse oximeter

   B. sphygmomanometer

   C. stethoscope

   D. probe

17. Which position is preferred when measuring height using an upright, balance scale?

   A. standing on the center of the scale with arms and hands on their sides

   B. standing facing the healthcare worker

   C. standing on the center of the scale with arms and hands raised

   D. standing at the back of the scale looking forward

Short Answer

18. What are vital signs? Why are they important?

19. What device is used to measure two different vital signs?

20. Name the different types of thermometers that can be used to measure a patient's temperature. Which ones are the most effective?

21. Identify the two primary locations where you can take a patient's pulse. What is the reason for selecting one location over another?

22. How long should you count a pulse?

23. Describe the process for measuring respiration rate. What can you do to be sure you are observing the normal rate for the patient you are measuring?

24. What does blood pressure measure?

25. What is the difference between hypotension and hypertension?

26. Identify three guidelines you need to be aware of when taking a patient's blood pressure.

27. When is height and weight usually measured?

Critical Thinking Exercises

28. Vital sign measures must always be as accurate as possible. What specific guidelines or steps can be followed to ensure vital signs are accurate?

29. When taking vital signs, infection control must be maintained. Explain how this can be accomplished for each of the vital signs.

30. Research and then describe the ethical practices that must be used when taking vital signs and measuring height and weight.

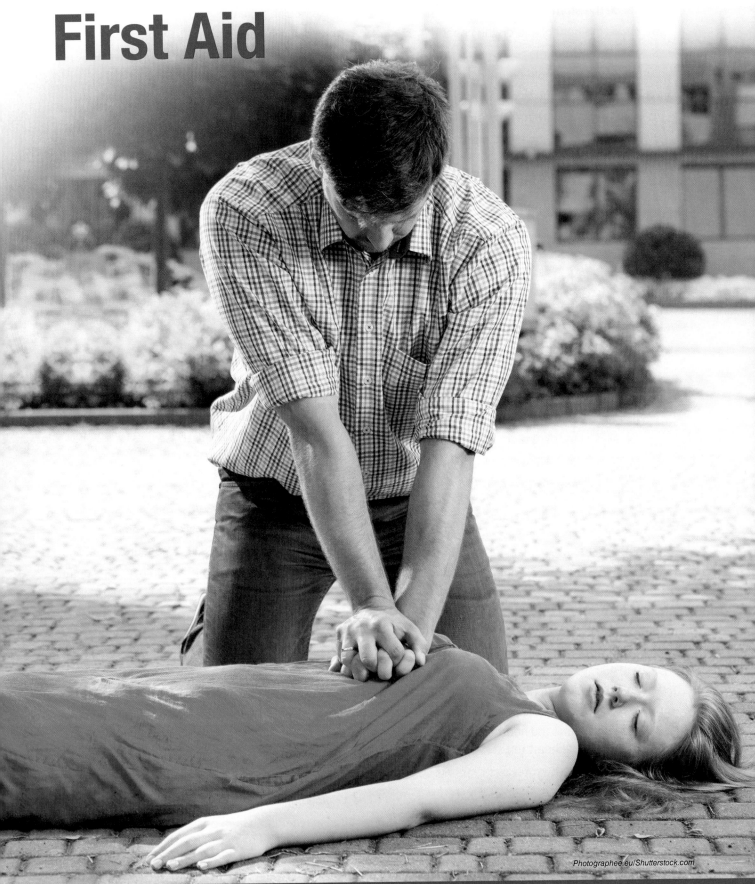

Chapter 12
First Aid

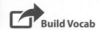
allergen

anaphylaxis

antihistamine

asphyxia

automated external defibrillator (AED)

cardiopulmonary resuscitation (CPR)

cyanotic

fibrillation

grand mal seizure

hands-only CPR

Heimlich maneuver

hemorrhage

petit mal seizure

rule of nines

shock

syncope

Chapter Objectives

- Describe the healthcare worker's role during medical emergencies.
- Explain first aid guidelines.
- Describe the steps necessary to perform hands-only CPR.
- Recognize the differences between hands-only and conventional CPR, and when each should be used.
- Explain the proper use and application of an AED.
- Explain how the body reacts to anaphylaxis, poisoning, hemorrhage, choking, burns, fainting, and seizures.
- Demonstrate emergency procedures for anaphylaxis, poisoning, hemorrhage, choking, burns, fainting, and seizures.

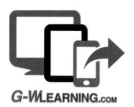

While studying, look for the activity icon to:

- **Build** vocabulary with e-flash cards and interactive games.
- **Assess** progress with chapter and unit review questions.
- **Expand** learning with animations and illustration labeling activities.
- **Simulate** EHR entry with healthcare documents.

www.g-wlearning.com/healthsciences/

First aid is the process of observing and responding to a medical emergency such as an injury, poisoning, or burns, or a medical issue such as a heart attack or stroke. First aid is performed at the onset of, and during, an emergency. It begins with determining the extent of an emergency and includes taking the correct and best course of action and treatment based on standards of care.

Every emergency situation is different, but in all instances timing is crucial. Professional help should always be sought immediately; however, there are general first aid guidelines you can follow that can make the difference between a person's life and death.

First Aid Guidelines

If you witness an emergency situation and are not yet a trained healthcare worker, first and foremost, do not panic. Call for help (9-1-1) immediately (Figure 12.1). Once you are speaking with a 911 dispatcher, remember the following guidelines:

1. Provide as much factual information as possible.
2. Give the dispatcher the person's name (if you know it), gender, and approximate age.
3. Describe the symptoms, but only what you see or are told. This might include bleeding and location, site of burns, or complaint of chest pain.
4. Describe your exact location and how trained medical professionals can get there.
5. Answer any questions you are asked to the best of your ability.

Pay attention to your own safety. Notice your surroundings and evaluate the situation. For example, never jump into a pool to save a drowning person if you are not a good, strong swimmer.

Always consider infection control. If you suspect the person may have a contagious disease, wear gloves and a mask, if possible. Avoid direct contact with the person's blood. If contact does occur, be sure to clean the blood off you as soon as possible.

Do not move the person unless it is for safety reasons, such as fire. Moving the person may increase the chance of paralysis or death due to spinal cord damage.

If the person's condition or situation is *not* getting worse, always wait for trained medical professionals to arrive. Remember: *do no harm*. You can further injure a person who is stable by performing a procedure for which you have no training. Be honest with yourself about what you are able to do.

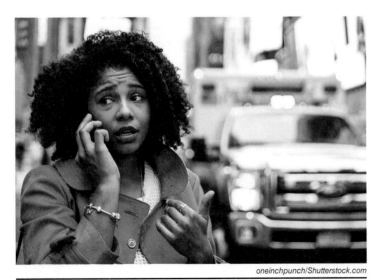

oneinchpunch/Shutterstock.com

Figure 12.1   If you witness an emergency situation, call for help as soon as possible. Give the 9-1-1 dispatcher as much factual information as possible and stay with the victim until help arrives.

Reassure the person that trained medical professionals have been called, and that you will stay with them until they arrive (Figure 12.2). This support can help him or her to remain calm and not feel alone.

Cardiopulmonary Resuscitation (CPR)

In many of the emergencies you may encounter, one of the first actions you can take to help someone is performing cardiopulmonary resuscitation (CPR).

Cardiopulmonary resuscitation (CPR) is an emergency lifesaving procedure for a person whose breathing or heartbeat has stopped. The term *cardiopulmonary* means "pertaining to the heart and lungs," while

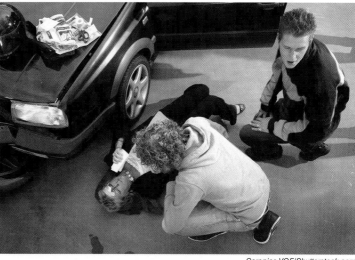

Corepics VOF/Shutterstock.com

Figure 12.2 If you encounter a medical emergency, do not perform any procedure you are not trained to execute. You may, instead, provide comfort by reassuring the victim that help is on the way and you will stay with her until trained medical professionals arrive.

resuscitation means "to revive." CPR supports blood circulation and breathing. It can include manual external chest compressions (to make the heart pump) and rescue breaths (to restore breathing until trained medical professionals arrive). CPR may be necessary after a person suffers an electric shock; drowning; or cardiac arrest (when the heart stops beating), which can occur as a result of a heart attack.

According to the American Heart Association, nearly 383,000 sudden cardiac arrests occur in the United States each year. Of those cardiac arrests, 88 percent happen at home.

When a person is experiencing cardiac arrest, the heart stops suddenly, without warning. The person will become unconscious, stop breathing, and have no pulse. The skin will be cool, pale, and gray. The person often appears healthy right before a cardiac arrest.

Acting quickly during a cardiac arrest can help prevent death. The chance for survival drops 7 to 10 percent for every minute a normal heartbeat is not restored. Therefore, CPR performed immediately can double or triple a person's chance of survival.

cardiopulmonary resuscitation (CPR) *an emergency lifesaving procedure in which a series of chest compressions and rescue breaths are given to a person whose breathing or heartbeat has stopped; supports blood circulation and breathing*

Did You Know?   **Maintaining a Calm Demeanor**

Medical emergencies are frightening for those involved. Whether the emergency is happening to you or someone else, keep centered and calm. If you are the one aiding another person, focus on what you know how to do. Do not try to be a hero. Rather, be helpful. Remember that the person can "feel" your emotional state. A calm demeanor during an emergency can make a positive difference in recovery.

The American Heart Association offers guidelines on the best approach for CPR based on the amount of training a person has received:

hands-only CPR
uninterrupted chest compressions given to restore heartbeat and promote blood circulation; an alternative procedure for those not trained in conventional CPR

- For those *not* trained in CPR, provide **hands-only CPR**. This means performing uninterrupted chest compressions at a rate of around 100 compressions per minute until trained medical professionals arrive. The chest compressions force the blood through the cardiovascular system.

- For those trained in CPR and confident in their ability, conduct conventional CPR. Conventional CPR begins with chest compressions, but also includes clearing the airway and performing rescue breathing. The acronym *CAB* will help you remember these steps: Compressions, Airway, and Breathing.

Hands-Only CPR

Hands-only CPR is CPR *without* rescue, or mouth-to-mouth, breathing. Hands-only CPR can be used for teens or adults who suddenly collapse and are not breathing. Conventional CPR with compressions and rescue breathing is recommended for infants and children.

The steps to follow for hands-only CPR include the following:

- Call 9-1-1 (or send someone to do so) and follow the first aid guidelines discussed earlier in the chapter.

- Before starting hands-only CPR, check to see if the person is conscious. You can tap or shake the shoulder and ask, "Are you okay?" (Figure 12.3). Also look at the person's chest to see if she is breathing (the chest is rising and falling). If the person is unconscious and not breathing, proceed. You can also check the carotid pulse located on the side of the person's neck (Figure 12.4). Place your index and middle fingers on the neck to the side of the windpipe to feel the pulse. Check for a pulse for no more than 10 seconds. If there is no pulse, proceed.

- Be sure the person is lying on her back (in supine position) and, if possible, on a hard surface. Get on your knees and bend over one side of the person.

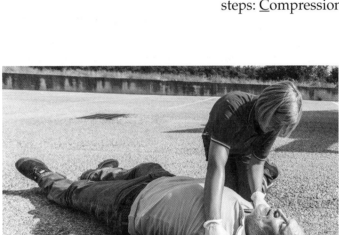

William Perungi/Shutterstock.com

Figure 12.3 Before beginning hands-only CPR, determine the person's level of consciousness by gently shaking him and asking if he is okay.

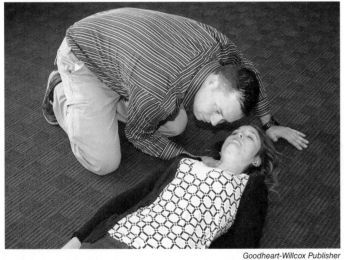

Goodheart-Willcox Publisher

Figure 12.4 Check for a carotid pulse by placing your index and middle fingers on the person's neck, to the side of the windpipe.

- Use the heels of your hands, placing one hand on top of the other (Figure 12.5). Interlock your fingers. Your dominant hand should be the one on the person's chest. With your arms straight and your shoulders directly over your hands, use your body weight to push hard and fast in the center of the chest, on the sternum. Time your compressions to the beat of the disco song "Stayin' Alive," or use some familiar method so you are providing 100 chest compressions per minute with no interruptions. For teens and adults, the chest should be compressed to a depth of two inches. It is helpful to count out loud while allowing the chest to move back to its normal position between compressions. Continue chest compressions until the person starts to move, or until trained medical professionals arrive.

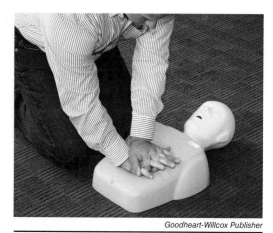

Figure 12.5 When you are performing chest compressions, it is important to properly place your hands on the person's sternum, or *breastbone*. Place your dominant hand on the chest and interlock your fingers.

Hands-only CPR improves a person's chance of survival and it should not be feared.

Conventional CPR

When conventional CPR is performed, it includes chest compressions, clearing of the airway, and rescue breathing (CAB). Remember that clearing the airway and performing rescue breathing should never be attempted without formal training.

To best understand the differences between conventional CPR and hands-only CPR, review the following guidelines.

Chest Compressions—C

- Check the carotid pulse located on the side of the person's neck. Place your index and middle fingers on the neck to the side of the windpipe to feel the pulse. Check for a pulse for no more than 10 seconds.

- If there is no pulse, start chest compressions (Figure 12.6). Be sure the person is lying on her back (in supine position) and, if possible, on a hard surface. Get on your knees and bend over one side of the person.

- Use the heels of your hands, placing one hand on top of the other. Interlock your fingers. Your dominant hand should be the one on the person's chest. With your arms straight and your shoulders directly over your hands, use your body weight to push hard and fast in the center of the chest, on the sternum. Perform 30 chest compressions with no interruptions. For teens and adults, the chest should be compressed to a depth of two inches. It is helpful to count out loud while allowing the chest to move back to its normal position between compressions.

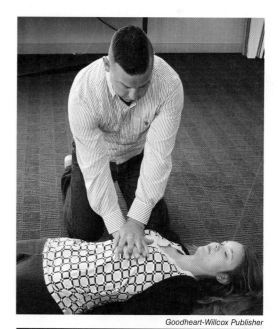

Figure 12.6 Lean over the person, straighten your arms, and use your body weight to give hard, fast chest compressions. Why do you think it is helpful to use your body weight when giving chest compressions?

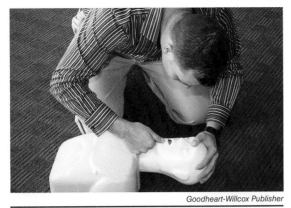

Goodheart-Willcox Publisher

Figure 12.7 The head-tilt, chin-lift maneuver can be used to check and clear the person's airway.

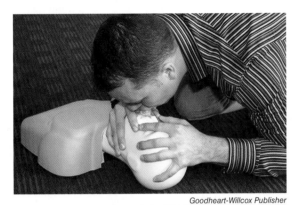

Goodheart-Willcox Publisher

Figure 12.8 Rescue breathing may be performed with direct mouth-to-mouth contact, or a CPR mask may be used to form a barrier between the two mouths. A CPR mask could be classified as what type of equipment?

automated external defibrillator (AED)
a medical device that delivers an electric shock through the chest to the heart to stop an irregular heart rhythm and allow a normal heart rhythm to resume

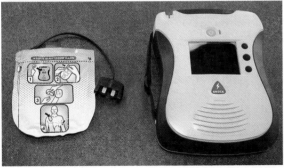

Goodheart-Willcox Publisher

Figure 12.9 An AED machine comes with disposable pads, which must be connected to the unit before use.

Airway—A

- After 30 chest compressions, clear the airway by using the head-tilt, chin-lift maneuver (Figure 12.7). Put your palm on the person's forehead and gently tilt the head back. With your other hand, gently lift the chin forward to open the airway.

Rescue Breathing—B

- After clearing the airway, quickly check for normal breathing, taking no more than 10 seconds. Determine breathing by looking for chest motion, listening for normal breath sounds, and feeling the person's breath on your cheek and ear. If the person is gasping, this is not considered normal breathing. If the person isn't breathing or gasping, then begin rescue breathing.

- Rescue breathing can be mouth-to-mouth breathing or mouth-to-nose if the mouth is injured or can't be opened. After ensuring an open airway and covering the mouth to form a seal, give two rescue breaths—each lasting one second (Figure 12.8). After the first breath, quickly watch to see if the chest rises. Then give the second breath. Then resume chest compressions. The cycle is 30 chest compressions, followed by two rescue breaths.

- Five cycles are usually performed (taking two minutes) prior to using an automated external defibrillator (AED), if available. An AED is used if the person is still not responding to CPR. It can be used twice between the five CPR cycles. If an AED is not available, continue CPR until the person starts to move, or until trained medical professionals arrive.

Using an Automated External Defibrillator (AED)

The rate and rhythm of the heartbeat is controlled by an internal electrical system in the heart. Some people have problems with their heart rhythm. The heart can beat too fast or too slow, beat irregularly, or stop due to a cardiac arrest.

An **automated external defibrillator (AED)** is a medical device that delivers an electric shock through the chest to the heart (Figure 12.9). This shock to the heart can stop an irregular heart rhythm such as

fibrillation, allowing a normal heart rhythm to resume. Along with calling 9-1-1 and performing CPR (compressions first), using the AED is an important part of responding to a medical emergency.

fibrillation
an irregular heart rhythm

AEDs are located in a variety of places such as ambulances and police cars, and in public and private locations such as doctors' offices, airports, and sports arenas. They are lightweight, battery operated, and easy to use. Voice prompts are provided to inform you if and when a shock should be sent to the heart. Visual and vocal prompts from an AED provide step-by-step instructions based on its reading of the person's heart rhythm.

To use an AED, follow these guidelines:

- Provide two minutes of CPR at your level of training. After the two minutes of CPR, use the AED.

- Always practice safety with an AED. Since an AED emits an electrical shock, check for any water near the unconscious person. Make sure you are not near water either. Water conducts electricity, so using an AED in or near water poses a risk that the rescuer will be shocked as well. If there is water, only move the person if you have to.

- Turn on the AED's power.

- Expose the person's chest if it is not already exposed. Remove any metal necklaces or underwire bras, and check for body piercings that may be in the way. Metal can conduct electricity and cause burns. You can cut the center of a bra and pull it away from the skin. If the person has a lot of chest hair, use the tools provided with the AED to trim or shave it.

- AEDs have sticky pads with sensors called *electrodes*. Apply the pads to the person's chest (Figure 12.10). Be sure the chest is dry. As you lean over the person, place one pad on the right center of the person's chest, above the nipple. Place the other pad slightly below the other nipple and to the left of the ribcage. Make sure the sticky pads make a good connection with the skin. If the connection is not good, a *check electrodes* message will appear on the AED's screen.

- Check for a medical alert bracelet to see if there may be implanted devices, such as a pacemaker. These are visible under the skin on the chest or abdomen. Move the defibrillator pads at least one inch away from any implanted devices or piercings so the electric current can flow freely between the pads. Also remove any medicine patches that are on the chest and wipe the skin.

- Check that the wires from the electrodes are connected to the AED. Make sure no one is touching the person, and then press the AED's *Analyze* button. Stay clear while the machine checks the person's heart rhythm. The AED will determine if a shock is needed to help resume the heart rhythm. If a shock is needed, the AED will prompt you. The shock may be delivered automatically by the AED, or you may be prompted to press the *Shock* button.

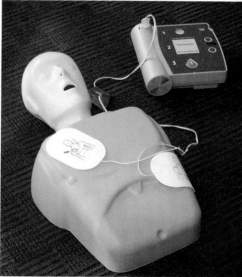
Goodheart-Willcox Publisher

Figure 12.10 AED machines are easy to use, even if you have not had formal training. The pads will often come with drawings to indicate the proper placement on the person's chest.

- Stand clear of the person and make sure others are clear before you push the AED's *Shock* button.
- After the shock, resume CPR.
- The AED will automatically reanalyze the person's heart rhythm to determine if another shock is needed.
- If a shockable heart rhythm is not detected, the AED will prompt you to check the person's pulse and continue to perform CPR.
- If the person is still not responding, continue CPR until the person moves, or until trained medical professionals arrive. Stay with the person until help arrives. Report all the information that you know.

Check Your Understanding ✔

1. When is it appropriate for someone to perform conventional CPR?
2. How many compressions should be done in hands-only CPR and how many should be done in conventional CPR?
3. What is the appropriate depth of chest compressions in CPR?
4. Describe the differences between hands-only CPR and conventional CPR.
5. Explain how an AED works and when it should be used.

Anaphylaxis

anaphylaxis
a severe allergic reaction that can affect the whole body

allergen
any substance that causes an allergy

Many people have allergies to medications such as aspirin or antibiotics; foods such as nuts, fish, and shellfish; and insect stings. Some respond with mild to moderate allergic reactions and others experience **anaphylaxis**, a severe allergic reaction that can affect the whole body. An allergic reaction usually occurs within minutes of exposure to an **allergen**. An allergen is any substance (often a protein) that causes an allergy (Figure 12.11). However, anaphylaxis can occur a half hour or longer after exposure to an allergen.

Not everyone has the same allergic reactions. Symptoms of an allergic reaction may include

- skin reactions such as hives and itching, as well as flushed or pale skin;
- swelling of the face, eyes, lips, or throat;
- a feeling of warmth throughout the body;
- the sensation of a lump in the throat;
- constriction of airways, which can cause wheezing and troubled breathing;
- a weak, rapid pulse;
- nausea, vomiting, or diarrhea; and
- dizziness, fainting, or unconsciousness.

Common Allergens

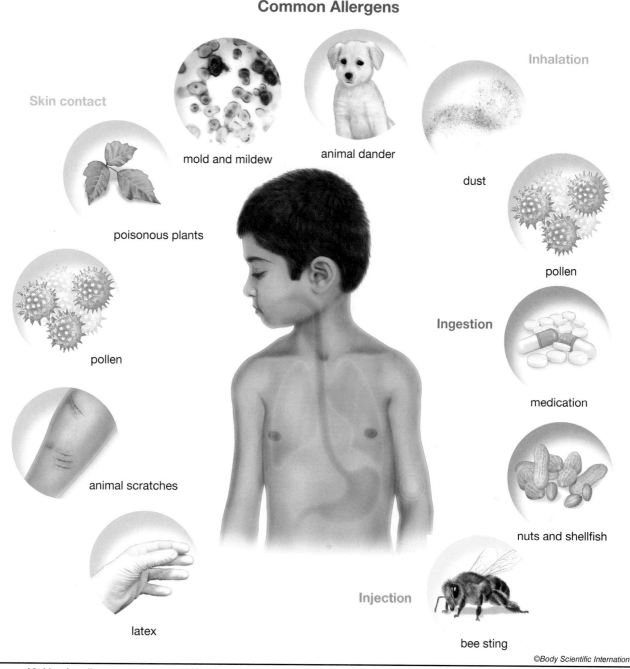

Skin contact

mold and mildew

animal dander

Inhalation

dust

poisonous plants

pollen

pollen

Ingestion

medication

animal scratches

nuts and shellfish

latex

Injection

bee sting

©*Body Scientific International*

Figure 12.11 An allergen may present itself in the form of an injection, through contact with the skin, or it may be ingested or inhaled.

If you are with someone experiencing moderate to severe symptoms of an allergic reaction or anaphylaxis, do not wait to see if they get better. Seek emergency treatment right away. In severe cases, untreated anaphylaxis can lead to death within 30 minutes. Be aware that only taking an oral **antihistamine** will not work fast enough if someone is in anaphylaxis. These symptoms must be acted on immediately. Get emergency treatment even if symptoms start to improve.

antihistamine
a drug that slows down or stops the actions of histamine, the substance that causes an allergic reaction

Take the following actions if you are with someone who experiences an allergic reaction:

1. • Call 9-1-1 immediately and follow the first aid guidelines discussed earlier in the chapter.

2. • Determine if the person has an epinephrine auto-injector to treat the allergic reaction. If so, ask if the person needs help with the injection. If help is needed, press the auto-injector against the person's thigh (Figure 12.12).

3. • Have the person lie still on his or her back and loosen tight clothing. Cover the person with a blanket, if available.

4. • Do not give the person anything to drink. If there is vomiting or bleeding from the mouth, turn the person to the side to prevent choking.

5. • If there are no signs of breathing, coughing, or movement, begin hands-only or conventional CPR (depending on your level of training) until the person starts moving or until trained medical professionals arrive.

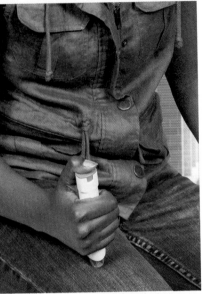

Rob Byron/Shutterstock.com

Figure 12.12 People with a known, severe allergy may carry epinephrine pens, which can be quickly administered during a severe allergic reaction or anaphylaxis.

Poison

People are injured by or die as a result of poisons every day. Most poisons—such as cyanide, paint thinners, or household cleaning products—are ingested, or swallowed, but poisons can also enter the body through the skin, by breathing them in, intravenously (by injection), through radiation exposure, or by eating spoiled food.

Poisoning is categorized as

• unintentional or accidental (such as a child ingesting a cleaning product); or

• intentional (deliberate self-poisoning).

A person can be poisoned and not show symptoms for hours, days, or even months. For example, a person may be taking a large dose of aspirin for extreme pain, which seems harmless, but over a long period of time the prolonged effects of the aspirin cause an overdose as it slowly poisons the person. This is dangerous because the delay in seeking medical help can result in long-term or permanent damage.

Did You Know?   **People are Poisoned Every Day**

According to the American Association of Poison Control Centers, the US Poison Control Center manages approximately 5,995 poisoning cases each day and receives a call about a poisoning every 14.4 seconds. The CDC estimates about 48 million Americans get food poisoning each year. They also report that about 9,500 children under the age of six are hospitalized each year in the US after taking a family member's prescription medication. About 25 percent of children who are exposed to a toxic substance are poisoned again within a year.

It can also be difficult to determine what type of poisoning has occurred. Some signs and symptoms of poisoning can be similar to those of common illnesses such as strokes, seizures, head injuries, and others. Typical signs and symptoms of poisoning can include

- abnormal skin color;
- burns or redness around the mouth and lips;
- breath that smells like chemicals, such as gasoline or paint thinner;
- nausea and vomiting;
- difficulty breathing;
- restlessness and agitation;
- seizure; and
- confusion or disorientation.

If poisoning is suspected, look for clues such as empty pill bottles; scattered pills; and burns, stains, or odors on the person or nearby objects. Children may have applied medicated patches to their skin or swallowed a small battery. If the person has no symptoms, but it appears they may have taken a potentially dangerous poison, call the US National Poison Control Center at 1-800-222-1222 or the Regional Poison Control Center to ask questions about possible poisoning. Have the pill bottle, medication, cleaning product, or other suspected container or material available so you can talk about it when speaking with the poison control center.

Call 9-1-1 or go to the local emergency department if the person is displaying active signs of poisoning, if it is an infant or toddler suspected of being poisoned, or if something has been taken to intentionally cause harm, even if the substance itself may not be harmful. After calling 9-1-1, you may take the following actions until trained medical professionals arrive:

- If poison has been swallowed, check the person's mouth and remove anything that remains. If they ingested household cleaner or another chemical, read the container's label and follow instructions for accidental poisoning.

- If poison is on the skin, remove any contaminated clothing using gloves. Rinse the skin for 15 to 20 minutes in a shower or with a hose.

- If poison is in the eye, gently flush the eye with cool or lukewarm water for 20 minutes or until help arrives (Figure 12.13).

- If poison has been inhaled, move the person into fresh air as soon as possible.

- If the person is vomiting, turn the head to the side to prevent choking.

- If the person shows no signs of life, begin and continue hands-only CPR until trained medical professionals arrive.

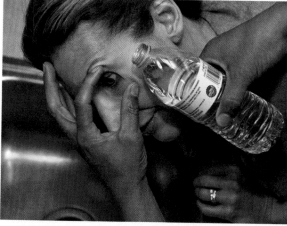

Wards Forest Media, LLC

Figure 12.13   If a poisonous substance enters the eye, gently flush the eye with cool or lukewarm water. A water bottle may be useful to help direct and control the stream of water.

Be sure to gather pill or vitamin bottles, packages or containers with labels, plants, and any other information about the suspected poison. Be ready to describe the symptoms; the age and weight of the person; other medications being taken; and any information about the suspected poisoning, such as the amount ingested and how long it has been since the poisoning occurred.

Real Life Scenario   Is It Poison?

Imagine you arrive home from grocery shopping and you find your young niece, who is visiting, playing with the cat. You notice an empty container of plant fertilizer next to her, and a small amount of fertilizer that has been spilled on the floor. Since the fertilizer was recently purchased, you wonder where the rest of it has gone.

While your niece looks okay, you do see something white and frothy near her lips.

Apply It

1. How would you react to this scenario? What is the first action you should take?
2. What steps should you take next?

Hemorrhages

hemorrhage
excessive blood loss over a short period of time due to an internal or external injury

A **hemorrhage**, which is excessive blood loss over a short period of time, is a medical emergency. You must act quickly if this occurs.

There are two types of hemorrhages—internal, which you cannot see, and external, which you can see. Internal hemorrhages occur inside the body's tissues and cavities. The signs of an internal hemorrhage are pain, shock, vomiting, coughing up blood, and loss of consciousness. In external hemorrhage, blood may be spurting, which indicates it is coming from an artery. If the blood has a steady flow, the hemorrhage is coming from a vein.

shock
a condition in which the body experiences a lack of sufficient oxygen available to the organs and tissues

When a person loses a large amount of blood, he or she may go into **shock**. This is because there is not enough oxygen available to the organs and tissues. When a person is in shock, the blood pressure drops; the pulse is rapid and weak; the skin is cool, clammy, and pale; and the person may lose consciousness. To prevent death, immediate treatment by trained medical professionals who can replace needed fluids is essential.

The signs and symptoms of an external hemorrhage include

cyanotic
blue discoloration of the skin

- a pale or **cyanotic** (blue discoloration) face;
- low blood pressure;
- increased, but weak heart rate;
- rapid, shallow respirations;
- feeling weak and helpless;
- restlessness;
- complaints of thirst; and
- feeling cold, shaking, or trembling.

To control bleeding, you can use direct or indirect pressure. Direct pressure is applied to the bleeding wound. Indirect pressure is achieved by applying pressure to a pressure point nearest to the wound. Pressure points are places on the body where blood vessels are located close to the surface (Figure 12.14).

Pressure Points

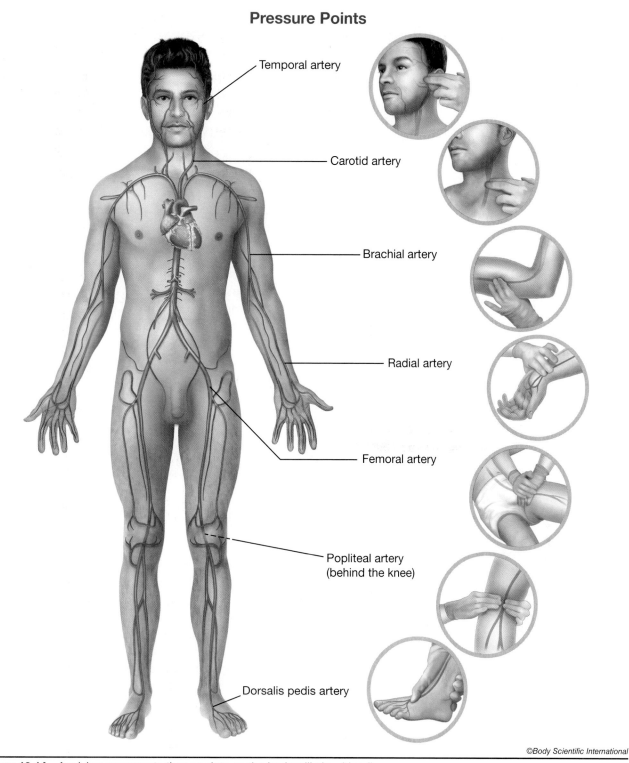

©Body Scientific International

Figure 12.14 Applying pressure to these points on the body will slow bleeding.

When these points are pressed, blood flow to the wound is slowed. When combined with direct pressure, this will help stop the bleeding. Pressure can be applied with the fingers, thumb, or heel of the hand.

Pressure points, especially the carotid artery, should be used with extreme caution. Indirect pressure can cause tissue damage.

The following is a first aid procedure that can be performed to control bleeding.

Procedure 12.1 | Responding to and Controlling Bleeding

Rationale

A hemorrhage can be life threatening if not stopped. Hemorrhages can occur internally or externally, and they are often caused by an injury.

Preparation

1. Follow the first aid guidelines and remain calm.

The Procedure: Internal Hemorrhage

2. Call for help or have someone else call for help. If you are in a healthcare facility, press the emergency call light, otherwise, call 9-1-1.
3. Reassure the person who is experiencing a hemorrhage that you are there to help.
4. Keep the person flat, warm, and quiet.
5. Do not give the person any fluids.
6. Do not remove any objects that may have caused the hemorrhage.
7. Wait calmly with the person for trained medical professionals to arrive.

The Procedure: External Hemorrhage

8. If you are in a healthcare facility, press the emergency call light; otherwise, call 9-1-1.
9. Reassure the person who is experiencing the hemorrhage that you are there to help.
10. Do not remove any objects that may have caused the hemorrhage.
11. Use standard precautions by wearing gloves, if possible.
12. Apply direct pressure to the bleeding site with the palm of your hand (Figure 12.15). Do not stop applying pressure until the bleeding stops.

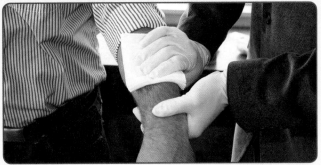

Figure 12.15   *Goodheart-Willcox Publisher*

13. Apply a sterile dressing, if available. If a sterile dressing is not available, use a clean material such as a towel or cloth and secure it with a bandage or tape.
14. If possible, elevate the affected area of the body—hand, arm, foot, or leg. This will help to minimize blood flow to the area. Bind the wound when the bleeding stops.
15. Watch for bleeding through the bandage. With knowledge, you may apply indirect pressure on a pressure point to try to slow the bleeding.
16. Keep the person warm by covering him or her with a blanket.
17. Do not give the person anything to eat or drink.

Follow-up

18. Make sure the person is comfortable.
19. Wash your hands to ensure infection control.

Reporting and Documentation

20. Communicate any specific observations, complications, or unusual responses to the appropriate provider. Also record this information in the patient's chart or EMR, if appropriate.

Check Your Understanding ✔

1. What is anaphylaxis?
2. What should you do if you are with someone who is experiencing a moderate to severe allergic reaction?
3. What are three signs or symptoms to look for if you think someone has been poisoned?
4. Describe the two types of hemorrhages.
5. What are pressure points and why are they important when controlling bleeding?
6. Identify the signs and symptoms of shock.

Choking

Choking is considered a medical emergency because it cuts off oxygen to the brain and blocks the flow of oxygen to the lungs. The lack of oxygen leads to **asphyxia**, a condition in which the body is deprived of oxygen, leading to loss of consciousness or death. Therefore, you must act quickly when you witness someone who is choking. For adults, a piece of food usually causes choking. For children, swallowing a small object usually causes choking.

There are two types of blockage that can cause choking—partial and complete:

1. **Partial blockage**. The person is coughing vigorously, can speak, and can breathe. Encourage the person to continue to cough. Stay with the person and call 9-1-1 for help. Do not strike the person on the back.

2. **Complete blockage**. The person cannot speak and makes high-pitched sounds or clutches at his throat with his hands (Figure 12.16). These are universal signs of distress. Take quick action using the **Heimlich maneuver**.

The Heimlich maneuver may be combined with a series of back blows. When giving a back blow, lean the person forward and strike his back between the shoulder blades five times using the heel of your hand (Figure 12.17). The American Red Cross suggests using the five-and-five method, in which five back blows are followed by five abdominal thrusts using the Heimlich maneuver. The American Heart Association's recommended response to choking does not include back blows, but focuses solely on the use of abdominal thrusts when responding to conscious choking. Procedure 12.2 describes those guidelines.

asphyxia
a lack of oxygen that causes breathing to stop; may be caused by an obstruction or swelling of the trachea

Heimlich maneuver
a series of abdominal thrusts performed to remove an object that is lodged in a person's airway, preventing the person from breathing

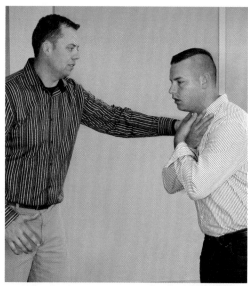

Goodheart-Willcox Publisher

Figure 12.16 A person who is clutching at his throat is exhibiting the universal sign of choking.

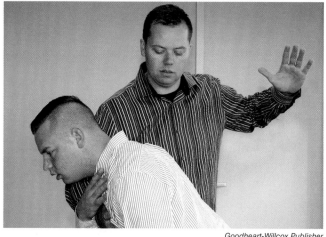

Goodheart-Willcox Publisher

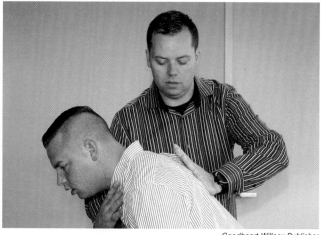

Goodheart-Willcox Publisher

Figure 12.17 When performing a back blow, strike the victim's back between the shoulder blades using the heel of your hand.

Procedure 12.2   Responding to Choking Using the Heimlich Maneuver

Rationale

Foreign bodies can obstruct a person's airway, which causes choking. Relieving choking prevents injury or death. The following procedure should be used with adults and children over one year of age.

Preparation

1. Follow the first aid guidelines and remain calm.

The Procedure: Choking—A Conscious Adult or Child (Over One Year of Age)

2. Call for help or have someone else call for help. If you are in a healthcare facility, press the emergency call light; otherwise, call 9-1-1.

3. Reassure the person that you are there to help.

4. If the person is standing or sitting, use an abdominal thrust (the Heimlich maneuver).

5. Stand or kneel behind the person. Wrap your arms around his waist and have his arms hang free (Figure 12.18).

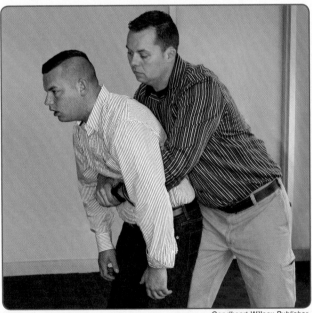

Figure 12.18   *Goodheart-Willcox Publisher*

6. Make a fist with one hand.

7. Place the thumb side of your clenched fist against the person's abdomen, slightly above the navel and well below the sternum, or *breastbone*.

8. Grasp your clenched fist with the other hand. Do not tuck your thumb inside the fist and avoid pressing on the ribs with your forearms.

9. Press forcefully into the abdomen with the thumb side of your fist, using quick inward and upward thrusts (Figure 12.19).

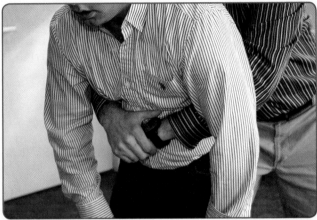

Figure 12.19   *Goodheart-Willcox Publisher*

10. Repeat the thrusts five times and check to see if the object is visible or expelled.

    Remove the foreign object, if you see it. To open the person's airway, use the head-tilt, chin-lift method (Figure 12.7). Look into the person's mouth for the object. Grasp and remove the object, if it is within reach.

    If the object is not visible or has not been expelled, keep doing thrusts until the object is expelled or the person loses consciousness (is not responding).

11. If the person loses consciousness, lower him to the floor or ground and proceed to step 12.

The Procedure: Choking—An Unconscious Adult or Child (Over One Year of Age)

12. If you are in a healthcare facility, press the emergency call light; otherwise, call 9-1-1. Put on gloves, if available.

13. Turn the person so that he is lying in supine position.

Procedure 12.2	**Responding to Choking Using the Heimlich Maneuver (continued)**

14. Begin conventional CPR if trained, or use the guidelines for hands-only CPR until trained medical professionals arrive.
15. Each time the person's airway is open, look for the foreign object in his mouth.
16. If the foreign object is seen, remove it, but avoid pushing it farther down into the throat.
17. Continue CPR until the object is expelled or help arrives.

Follow-up

18. Make sure the person is comfortable.
19. Wash your hands to ensure infection control.

Reporting and Documentation

20. Communicate any specific observations, complications, or unusual responses to the appropriate provider. Also record this information in the patient's chart or EMR, if appropriate.

Burns

Burns pose a serious threat to a person's health. Remember, the skin is the body's first line of defense against infection. A burn is a break in the skin, so there is a risk of infection at the burn site and potentially throughout the body.

The amount of damage a burn can cause depends on its location, depth, and the body surface it covers. The **rule of nines** provides a guide to assess the percentage of the body that has been burned (Figure 12.20). It is used to help determine treatment including fluid replacement. This rule is applied only to second- and third-degree burns. It is done by estimating the body surface area (BSA) using multiples of nine. For example, using the rule of nines, a burn to the head and neck would be reported as nine percent. This rule works better for adults who have been burned than children.

Burns are also classified based on their depth. There are three classifications—first degree, second degree, and third degree. It is important to note that the degree of a burn can change over time. For example, sunburn that was originally considered a first-degree burn can blister and become a second-degree burn over a few hours.

First-Degree Burns

First-degree burns are superficial, meaning they exist only on the surface or outer layer of the skin. They are the least serious of all burns and usually take a few days to a week to heal. Briefly touching a hot pan is an example of a first-degree burn. First-degree burns can be characterized by symptoms such as redness, mild swelling, skin that is tender to touch, and pain.

rule of nines
a method of calculating the surface area of the body that has been affected by burns

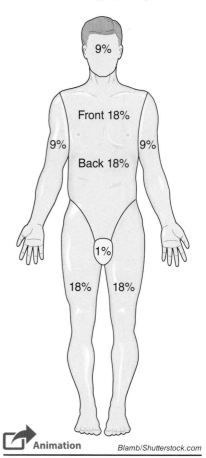

Animation *Blamb/Shutterstock.com*

Figure 12.20 The rule of nines assigns a percentage, in multiples of nine, to each region of the body, accounting for 100 percent of the body's total surface area.

Did You Know? **Burn Statistics**

According to the American Burn Association, approximately 450,000 patients receive hospital and emergency room treatment for burns each year. More men than women are burned. Of these burn injuries, about 3,400 result in deaths. The CDC states that burns and fires are the third leading cause of death in the home.

Considered a minor burn, most first-degree burns are easily treated by following these guidelines:

- Hold the burned area under cool (not cold) running water for 10 to 15 minutes or until the pain eases. You can also apply a clean towel dampened with cool tap water to the burned area.
- Remove any jewelry or tight items in the burned area. Do this quickly and gently before swelling occurs.
- Apply moisturizer, aloe vera lotion or gel, or low-dose hydrocortisone cream to the burned area. These products may provide relief.
- Over-the-counter pain relievers may also help.

If the burn involves a large portion of the hands, feet, face, groin, buttocks, or a major joint, emergency medical attention should be sought.

Second-Degree Burns

Second-degree burns are more serious than first-degree burns because they are deeper. These burns may cause permanent injury and scarring. If they are not too deep, second-degree burns will usually take two to three weeks to heal. Signs of a second-degree burn include red, white, or splotchy skin; swelling; pain; and blistering of the skin.

If a second-degree burn is no larger than three inches (7.6 centimeters) in diameter, treat it the same way you would a first-degree burn. If the burned area is larger or covers the hands, feet, face, groin, buttocks or a major joint, treat it as you would a third-degree burn. Do not break small blisters (those that are no bigger than a small fingernail). However, if blisters break on their own, gently clean the area with mild soap and water, apply an antibiotic ointment, and cover it with a nonstick gauze bandage.

Seek medical help if large blisters develop, as these are best removed, but only by a medical professional. Do not attempt to remove these blisters on your own. Also seek medical help if there are signs of infection, such as oozing from burned areas, increased pain, redness, and swelling.

Third-Degree Burns

The most serious burn, a third-degree burn, involves all layers of the skin and underlying fat. Nerves, blood vessels, muscle, and bone can be affected. Third-degree burns will likely result in permanent injury and scarring, and usually take more than three weeks to heal.

Burned areas may be charred black or white and become leathery, and the person may experience difficulty breathing. If smoke inhalation also occurred, the person may experience other toxic effects as well.

Because third-degree burns are considered major burns, the affected person must receive medical attention as soon as possible. Call 9-1-1 immediately and use the guidelines provided in the earlier part of this section. Stay with the person.

Until help arrives, you may also take these actions:

- Protect the burned person by safely checking that there is no further contact with smoldering materials or exposure to smoke or heat.

- Check for signs of breathing, coughing, or movement. If the person is unconscious, perform CPR (using hands-only CPR if you are not certified in conventional CPR) until trained medical professionals arrive.

- If possible, remove jewelry, belts, and other restrictive items (especially from around burned areas and the neck), as swelling will occur rapidly. But do *not* remove burned clothing that is stuck to the skin.

- Elevate burned areas above the heart, if possible.

- Do not use cold water for large severe burns. This may cause a serious loss of body heat (known as *hypothermia*) or a drop in blood pressure and decreased blood flow (shock). Rather, cover the burned area with a cool moist bandage or clean cloth.

Fainting

Fainting is a brief loss of consciousness, and it is considered a medical emergency. It is also called **syncope** (SING-kuh-pee) or *passing out*. Fainting is caused by a drop in the blood flow to the brain. There are many reasons for someone to faint, including fatigue, hunger, certain medications, dehydration, heart conditions, age, or even the temperature or ventilation in a room. Signs that a person may faint include

syncope
fainting

- a face that is pale in color;
- skin that feels cold and clammy (moist);
- perspiration;
- a weak pulse;
- shallow breathing;
- trembling and shaking; and
- complaints of dizziness or blurred vision.

Consider any or all signs of fainting a medical emergency even if the person only says they feel like they might faint. This prevents possible injury.

Procedure 12.3   **Responding to Fainting**

Rationale

Fainting is a sudden loss of consciousness due to an inadequate supply of blood to the brain. When consciousness is lost, the person is likely to fall, and injuries can occur.

Preparation

1. Follow the first aid guidelines and remain calm.

The Procedure

2. Call for help or have someone else call for help. If you are in a healthcare facility, press the emergency call light; otherwise, call 9-1-1.

3. Reassure the person that you are there to help.

4. If you have observed signs that a person is about to faint, assist her to a safe position using proper body mechanics. Help her to sit or lie down before fainting occurs.

5. If the person is sitting, have her bend forward and place her head between her knees (Figure 12.21). If lying down, place the person on her back and raise or elevate her legs.

6. Check the clothing around the person's neck, chest, and abdomen. Loosen any tight clothing that may restrict breathing.

7. If fainting has occurred, raise or elevate the legs approximately 12 inches so that they are above the heart. Check breathing and pulse.

8. Do not let the person get up for at least five minutes after fainting.

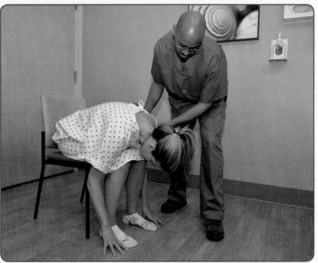

Figure 12.21   *Wards Forest Media, LLC*

9. Do not give the person anything to eat or drink unless directed to do so by a trained medical professional.

10. Do not leave the person alone.

Follow-up

11. Make sure the person is comfortable.

12. Wash your hands to ensure infection control.

Reporting and Documentation

13. Communicate any specific observations, complications, or unusual responses to the appropriate provider. Also record this information in the patient's chart or EMR, if appropriate.

Seizures

Seizures are a sudden change in the brain's normal electrical activity that causes an altered or loss of consciousness. A seizure may be the result of a disease such as epilepsy, tumors, or nervous system disorders. Seizures can also be the result of a head injury, so you must act quickly if you witness someone experiencing a seizure. Seizures can occur at any age and generally last from a few seconds to several minutes.

There are two different types of seizures—partial and generalized. Partial seizures can include motor seizures, sensory seizures, and autonomic seizures. Motor seizures occur in the muscles and are observed as jerking of hands and fingers. Sensory seizures are reported as tingling sensations. Autonomic seizures cause changes in the rate of respirations, sweating, or an increase in the heart rate.

Generalized seizures can be of two types—petit mal seizures and grand mal seizures. A person experiencing a **petit mal seizure** will have impaired awareness and responsiveness, may stare, and may have facial or body twitches.

A person having a **grand mal seizure** will experience a combination of tonic and clonic phases. In the tonic phase, muscles stiffen and air is forced out of the lungs. The person usually groans, and then loses consciousness. The person may also fall to the floor, turn blue, and bite his tongue. In the clonic phase, muscles contract and relax, which causes jerking and rhythmic movements of the arms and legs. Bowel and bladder control may be lost. Consciousness returns slowly and gradually after a grand mal seizure.

petit mal seizure
a generalized seizure in which the person has impaired awareness and responsiveness, and may lose consciousness

grand mal seizure
a generalized seizure in which a person may experience a loss of consciousness and violent muscle contractions

Procedure 12.4   Responding to Seizures

Rationale

Preventing injury and maintaining an open airway are primary goals when responding to a person experiencing a seizure.

Preparation

1. Follow the first aid guidelines and remain calm.

The Procedure

2. If you are in a healthcare facility, press the emergency call light; otherwise, call 9-1-1.
3. Reassure the person that you are there to help.
4. Never try to stop a seizure.
5. Note the time the seizure started.
6. Lower the person to the floor (if not already there) to protect the person from falling.
7. Maintain an open airway. Turn the person on her side and make sure her head is also turned to promote drainage of any saliva or vomit.
8. Protect the person's head by placing something soft under her head. This will help to prevent the head from striking the floor during the seizure. Use a pillow, chair cushion, folded jacket, blanket, or towel, or cradle the person's head in your lap.
9. Loosen tight clothing and jewelry around the person's neck. Clear the area of equipment or sharp objects. The person may strike these objects during the seizure.

10. Do not force the mouth open. Do not put any objects or your fingers between the teeth. Do not try to restrain or control movements.
11. Note the time the seizure ends and place the person in a recovery position (lying on her side), with the head turned to the side to allow saliva to drain from the mouth (Figure 12.22).

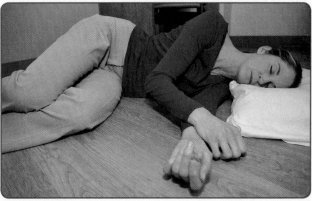

Figure 12.22   *Wards Forest Media, LLC*

Follow-up

12. After the seizure is over, make sure the person is comfortable.
13. Wash your hands to ensure infection control.

Reporting and Documentation

14. Communicate any specific observations, complications, or unusual responses to the appropriate provider. Also record this information in the patient's chart or EMR, if appropriate.

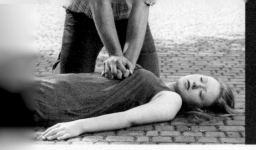

Chapter 12
Review and Assessment

Summary

Medical emergencies can range from trauma such as severe cuts, burns, and broken bones to life-threatening medical conditions such as strokes and heart attacks. No matter what the origin or cause of a medical emergency, response and care must be immediate. First aid is the initial process of observing and responding to a medical emergency. It is at this time that a person's condition is determined to be an emergency and the correct and best course of action or treatment is taken. Every emergency situation is different, but timing is always crucial.

When you encounter a medical emergency, you must remain calm and focus on what you can do to help. If you are not in a healthcare facility, call 9-1-1 and provide basic first aid. When responding to an emergency in a healthcare facility, turn on the emergency call light immediately.

Cardiopulmonary resuscitation (CPR) is an emergency lifesaving procedure for a person whose breathing or heartbeat has stopped. CPR supports circulation and breathing. It can include manual external chest compressions (to make the heart pump) and manual ventilation to restore breathing until trained medical professionals arrive. Those not certified in CPR should perform hands-only CPR (uninterrupted chest compressions only, of about 100 a minute) until trained medical professionals arrive. Those trained in CPR and confident in their abilities may perform conventional CPR, which begins with 30 chest compressions and continues with checking the airway and performing rescue breathing. The acronym *CAB* will help you remember the steps of conventional CPR—compressions, airway, and breathing.

Using an automated external defibrillator (AED) can also be an important part of this medical emergency when it occurs outside of a healthcare facility. AEDs are typically located in public places.

Other medical emergencies you may encounter can include allergic reactions and anaphylaxis, accidental and intentional poisoning, hemorrhages, choking, burns, fainting, and seizures. Understanding how to properly respond to each of these emergencies improves your ability to help.

Review and practice each of the procedures in this chapter with the assistance and supervision of your teacher. Learning how to administer first aid is important, particularly if you intend to pursue a career in healthcare.

Review Questions

Answer the following questions using what you have learned in this chapter.

True or False Assess

1. *True or False?* All people have the same reaction to allergens.
2. *True or False?* The cycle for conventional CPR is 30 chest compressions to two rescue breaths.
3. *True or False?* When someone is cyanotic, the skin is pale and gray.
4. *True or False?* The most serious burn is a second-degree burn.
5. *True or False?* In the tonic phase of a seizure, muscles stiffen, air is forced out of the lungs, there is a groan, the person loses consciousness, and he or she may fall to the floor.
6. *True or False?* When dealing with a person whom you suspect has been poisoned, you should look for clues.
7. *True or False?* If a person is sitting and feels like he is about to faint, have him lie down and elevate his legs.
8. *True or False?* Always remove the object that causes a hemorrhage immediately after encountering the person.
9. *True or False?* You should not consider it a medical emergency if someone says she feels like she might faint.
10. *True or False?* It is best to try to stop a seizure to keep the person from being injured.

Multiple Choice Assess

11. A second-degree burn is best characterized by which of the following?
    A. redness
    B. white leathery skin
    C. blisters
    D. chalky-looking skin
12. Hands-only CPR means that you _____.
    A. perform chest compressions with your hands
    B. give rescue breaths without using your hands
    C. perform breathing and chest compressions
    D. do nothing at all but call for help

13. Mrs. Garcia is clutching at her throat with her hands. What is she trying to communicate?
    A. She is having a seizure.
    B. She is having a stroke.
    C. She is choking.
    D. She is having a heart attack.

14. When performing the Heimlich maneuver, _____ are used to stop choking and clear the victim's airway.
    A. rhythmic breathing
    B. abdominal thrusts
    C. chest compressions
    D. firm back slaps

15. Which of the following degrees of burn would you *not* treat using cool water to alleviate the pain?
    A. second degree
    B. first degree
    C. tenth degree
    D. third degree

16. An AED is used to help during which emergency medical procedure?
    A. control of bleeding
    B. CPR
    C. Heimlich maneuver
    D. seizure

17. When arriving at a medical emergency, what is the first thing you should do?
    A. check for consciousness
    B. take vital signs
    C. reassure the person
    D. call for help

18. Ms. Cho is eating lunch and appears to have the signs of fainting. What should you do after calling for help?
    A. continue to talk with her to divert her attention
    B. have her bend forward and place her head between the knees
    C. offer her a glass of water and some crackers
    D. move her to her bed so she is lying flat

19. Jody has a severe allergic reaction that affects her whole body when she eats nuts. This is called _____.
    A. anaphylaxis
    B. aphagia
    C. asphyxia
    D. angina

20. Along with always calling for help, what is another important guideline in first aid?
    A. stand back and let others help
    B. take control and tell others what to do
    C. do as much as you can do to help
    D. know your limits when helping

Short Answer

21. What is one important guideline of first aid?
22. How do most poisons enter the body?
23. Where should the AED's electrodes be placed?
24. What should you do if someone is choking do to a partial blockage?
25. What does *CAB* mean?
26. How would someone check an airway?
27. What is an AED used for?
28. In what ways might an allergen present itself?
29. Discuss the body's reaction to a hemorrhage.
30. Describe the procedure used when someone has a seizure.

Critical Thinking Exercises

31. Describe a situation in which you had to perform first aid or respond to a medical emergency. How did you feel about it? What did you do? Were you scared? Did someone help you during or after the emergency? If they did, what did they do? Did it make you feel better?

32. Review the first aid guidelines at the beginning of the chapter. Which one(s) do you feel you could perform appropriately? Are there any you feel unqualified to perform? Select the guideline that you are least comfortable performing and describe two actions you can take to improve your skills.

33. Go to a website such as the American Heart Association (AHA), or the American Red Cross, or one of your choosing, and describe two new facts or guidelines about first aid you did not know. Brainstorm ways you can apply this information when responding to an emergency.

34. How can infection control be maintained when performing first aid procedures?

35. Research, list, and describe any of your state's laws that you need to know when performing first aid and CPR. Does your state have a Good Samaritan law, for example?

Chapter 13
Assisting with Mobility

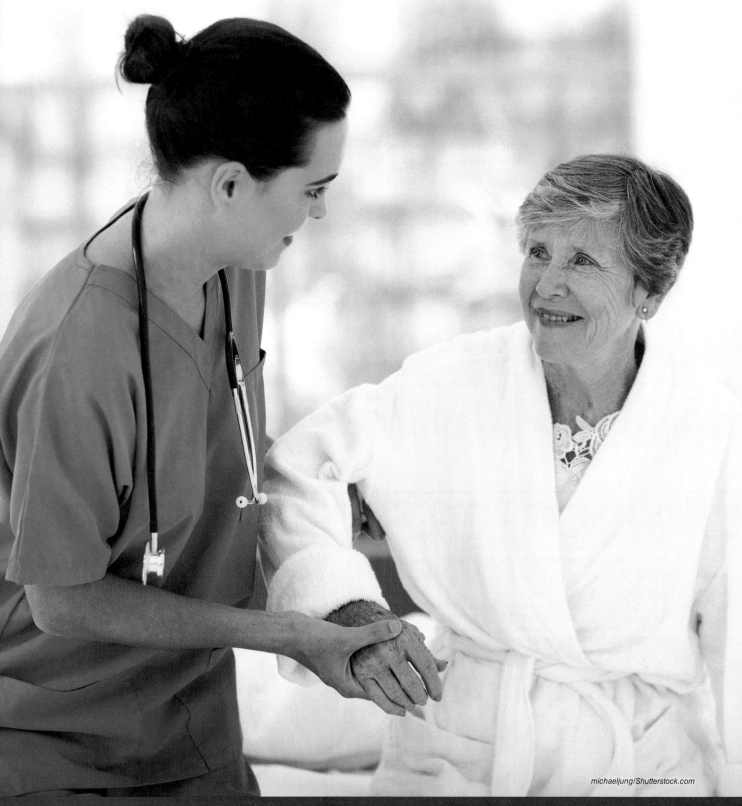

michaeljung/Shutterstock.com

Terms to Know

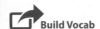 **Build Vocab**

activity of daily living (ADL)	contracture	immobility
ambulation	contraindicated	necrotic
ankylosis	decubitus ulcer	posture
atony	embolus	thrombus
atrophy	foot drop	traction
body alignment	gait belt	trochanter roll

Chapter Objectives

- Explain why exercise and ambulation are important.
- Identify the benefits of proper posture and good body alignment.
- Display correct body mechanics.
- Perform the procedures to assist with ambulation and the use of canes, crutches, and walkers.
- Demonstrate the procedures for positioning, turning, lifting, and transferring patients.
- Perform passive range-of-motion exercises.

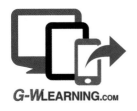

While studying, look for the activity icon to:

- **Build** vocabulary with e-flash cards and interactive games.
- **Assess** progress with chapter and unit review questions.
- **Expand** learning with animations and illustration labeling activities.
- **Simulate** EHR entry with healthcare documents.

www.g-wlearning.com/healthsciences/

contracture
a condition characterized by the tightening or shortening of a body part, such as muscle, tendon, or skin, due to lack of movement

atony
lack of sufficient muscular tone

atrophy
a decrease in size or wasting away of a body part or tissue

thrombus
a blood clot that forms in a blood vessel and remains at the site of formation

embolus
a mass, most commonly a blood clot, that becomes lodged in a blood vessel and obstructs the flow of blood

activity of daily living (ADL)
any basic self-care task, including grooming, bathing, and eating

posture
position of the body when sitting or standing

body alignment
the optimal placement of body parts so that bones are used efficiently and muscles have to do less work to get the same effect

The human body is designed for motion and activity. Regular exercise contributes to a healthy body and well-being, while immobility has a negative effect. A joint that has not moved sufficiently can begin to stiffen within 24 hours and will eventually become inflexible. Long periods of joint immobility may also negatively affect tendons and muscles. Therefore, exercise is very important, particularly for someone who is immobile.

Exercise has many benefits, including

- maintaining joint mobility;
- preventing **contractures**, **atony**, and **atrophy** of muscles;
- promoting circulation to prevent **thrombus** and **embolus** formation;
- improving coordination; and
- building and maintaining muscle strength.

Most people move and exercise their joints and muscles when they perform **activities of daily living (ADL)**. Some have regular exercise plans. Maintaining proper **posture** and body alignment also plays an important role in achieving proper mobility.

Figure 13.1 provides the meaning of several abbreviations and acronyms commonly used in healthcare to describe mobility. You will see how these terms are used while reading this chapter.

Body Alignment, Posture, and Body Mechanics

Body alignment is the optimal placement of body parts so that bones and muscles are used efficiently. To obtain correct posture, you must have good body alignment. Therefore, it is critical that patients maintain proper body alignment at

Mobility Abbreviations and Acronyms	
Abbreviation or Acronym	*Meaning*
AAROM	active assistive range of motion
ABD	abduction
ADL	activities of daily living
Amb	ambulation
BR	bedrest
BRP	bathroom privileges
CPM	continuous passive motion
HOB	head of bed
OOB	out of bed
ROM	range of motion
Up ad lib	up as desired
W/C	wheelchair

Goodheart-Willcox Publisher

Figure 13.1   These common abbreviations and acronyms are often used when discussing patient mobility in healthcare.

all times. This includes any time healthcare workers position, turn, lift, or transfer a patient. The goal is to reduce the amount of stress on joints and skin. If body parts are in correct alignment they remain functional, healthy, and stress free.

Good posture and body alignment are also important for healthcare workers. Many people who work in healthcare can run the risk of developing musculoskeletal disorders (MSDs) because of the physically demanding nature of their jobs. MSDs common among healthcare workers often occur while moving and repositioning patients, resulting in high rates of back and shoulder injuries. These injuries can be prevented if proper body mechanics are used. Body mechanics were discussed in more detail in chapter 4.

Your mobility—when you walk, climb stairs, or drive a car—happens through constriction of muscles. These muscles move bones with the help of the connective tissue that joins the two together. For example, there are two muscle groups that constrict to move your upper arm: the biceps brachii located on the front of your upper arm, and the triceps brachii on the back of your upper arm. Their constriction is aided by connective tissue. This represents the *mechanics* in the term *body mechanics*.

Using good body mechanics, such as properly picking up and lifting items during your everyday life, leads to good posture, which

- aligns bones and joints, reducing any stress that may occur;
- reduces wear and tear on joints;
- strengthens the spine and muscles; and
- conserves energy.

> ### Think It Through
>
> What is your posture like? Have you been told that you stand up straight or that you slump? When standing, are your feet apart, tailbone tucked in and pelvis tilted, shoulder blades back, chest lifted and forward, and knees straight? Is your head erect and your face forward? Is your chin lifted and jaw and mouth relaxed?

Did You Know?   How We Move

The brain is more efficient at recognizing movement than it is at isolating a particular muscle. This means that body mechanics training involves practicing movement patterns similar to the intended activity, and then correcting the muscles needed to do that activity. To hit a ball, golfers and tennis players must use their abdominal muscles. Ice skaters mainly use their hips and lower body, but they must also depend on their abdominal and back muscles to lean forward to skate—but not too far, or they may lose their balance.

Some healthcare facilities ask that healthcare workers wear specially designed back belts to help protect against back injuries they may suffer when giving patient care (Figure 13.2). Unless required, wearing a back belt is a matter of choice, as research has not shown that they will actually prevent back injuries. If a back belt is used, it should be worn properly and should never be a substitute for correct body mechanics and good lifting skills.

There are several types of back belts. The ones typically used in the workplace are lightweight and designed as an elastic belt worn around the lower back. Some back belts also have suspenders to hold them in place.

Healthcare workers are essential to promoting and maintaining the mobility of their patients. They provide the encouragement, support, and assistance needed to ensure that patients remain mobile, feel comfortable using assistive

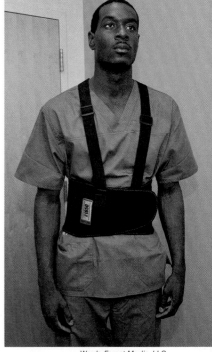

Wards Forest Media, LLC

Figure 13.2 When worn properly, a back belt may help prevent back strain and injury.

devices (such as canes, crutches, and walkers), and receive proper positioning and range-of-motion exercises when needed. Proper body mechanics are also an important part of ensuring safety for yourself and your patients.

Ambulation

ambulation
the ability to walk from one place to another

Ambulation, or the ability to walk around, is key to performing activities of daily living. It improves circulation and muscle tone, preserves lung tissue and airway function, and helps promote muscle and joint mobility. Ambulation is essential for optimal well-being. When hospital patients are able to ambulate early in their stay, their lung function has been found to improve greatly. In a recent study, patients who increased their walking by at least 600 steps between the first and second 24-hour days in the hospital were discharged approximately two days earlier than those who did not.

Ambulation requires an action called *double pendulum*. When people walk, their leg leaves the ground, swinging forward from the hip. This is the first pendulum. When that leg strikes the ground, with the heel touching first and rolling through to the toe, this motion is the second pendulum. When walking, the movement of the two legs is coordinated so that one foot is always in contact with the ground.

Walking differs from running. When walking, one leg is always in contact with the ground, while the other is swinging. When running, there is a ballistic phase that occurs when both feet are off the ground at the same time.

> ### Think It Through
>
> How are your body mechanics? Think about how you lift something or bend down to pick up an object from the floor. Do you bend your knees to a full squat position, bring the object close to you, and then hold it close to your body as you pick it up? Do you tighten your abdominal muscles to support your movements so you can lift from your legs to a standing position? Do you avoid twisting and making quick, jerky actions? Ask a friend to watch you and give you feedback.

> ### Did You Know? Average Walking Speed
>
> On average, children first walk independently at approximately 11 months old. By adulthood, the average walking speed is about 3.1 miles per hour (mph), though walking speed for older adults is slower.
>
> Walking speed varies depending on a person's height, weight, age, fitness level, effort, and culture. The ground, surface, and how much a person is carrying also influence walking speed.

The Stages of Patient Ambulation

There are usually three stages needed to assist a patient in moving from a bed to being able to ambulate. Healthcare workers have an important role to play in each of these stages. They are also responsible for making sure these stages occur safely and appropriately.

The three stages of assisting a patient to ambulate follow:

1. Assist the patient to lift his body from lying in bed to sitting on the side of the bed. This is called *dangling* because the patient's legs and feet are hanging off the side of the bed (Figure 13.3). Having patients dangle after lying in bed avoids a drop in blood pressure, helping prevent potential dizziness and possibly fainting when standing. This is called *orthostatic hypotension*, a condition you learned about in chapter 11.

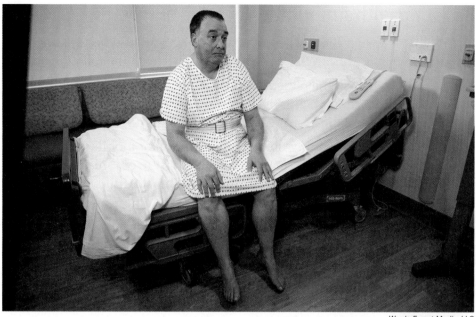

Wards Forest Media, LLC

Figure 13.3 During the first stage of ambulation, the patient is assisted into a dangling position, where he is seated at the edge of the bed with his feet dangling off the side.

gait belt
a device made of canvas, nylon, or leather that is used by healthcare workers to safely move (transfer) patients to a standing position or to assist them during walking

2. Assist the patient to stand. A **gait belt** (or *transfer belt*) is a safety device that can be used by healthcare workers to move patients, both when standing and ambulating. The gait belt is worn by the patient, who may be too weak to support himself. This helps prevent falls. It also decreases the risk of healthcare workers sustaining back injuries. Gait belts come in a variety of sizes and material, such as canvas, nylon, or leather (Figure 13.4).

3. In this stage, the patient begins ambulating. Sometimes it is helpful to assist the patient to a chair so that he may rest prior to ambulating.

There are extra safety precautions if you are helping someone ambulate in his or her home:

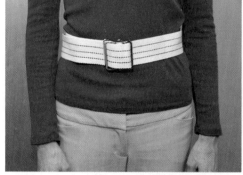

Wards Forest Media, LLC

Figure 13.4 A gait belt may be worn by a patient during ambulation, allowing the healthcare worker to help move the individual.

- Remove any small rugs or electrical cords, clean up any spills on the floor, and move anything else that may cause a fall.

- Place nonslip bath mats in the bathroom. It is helpful if there are grab bars installed, a raised toilet seat, and a shower tub seat (Figure 13.5).

- Make sure everyday household items are easily accessible.

- Encourage the use of a backpack, fanny pack, apron, or briefcase to enable the person to carry things during ambulation.

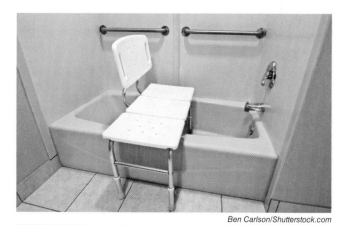

Ben Carlson/Shutterstock.com

Figure 13.5 Grab bars and a tub seat have been installed in this bathroom to ensure the elderly homeowner's safety while bathing.

Assisting with Ambulation

When preparing for any procedure in which you will be assisting with ambulation in a healthcare facility, you should perform the following steps:

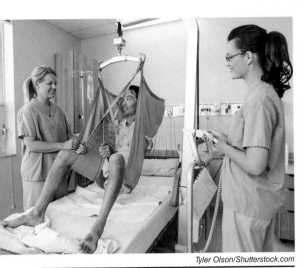

Figure 13.6 Electronic patient lifts may be mounted to the ceiling or mobile, as shown here.

Tyler Olson/Shutterstock.com

1. Ask the patient if she is feeling any pain. If she is, consult with the appropriate provider about her pain medication schedule before beginning the ambulation.

2. Depending on the patient's level of mobility, various equipment may be used to assist in ambulation. This equipment may include mechanical, full-body lifts (Figure 13.6); mobile, sit-to-stand lifts; or gait belts. These help reduce the load of the patient's body weight on the healthcare workers who are assisting. Know how the equipment works and understand the procedure being implemented.

3. Gather the appropriate supplies, equipment, and other staff members, if needed.

4. Organize the physical environment and the equipment to ensure safe completion of the procedure. This includes locking the wheels of the bed or chair, putting the bed or stretcher at the correct height, and making sure any mobile equipment is charged. Identify and remove any tripping hazards such as electrical cords, throw rugs, and clutter.

5. If other healthcare workers are needed to conduct a procedure, make sure they know what they need to do.

6. Tell the patient what actions you expect from her.

7. Show the patient what to do and help her during the procedure.

8. When assisting patients, be sure you have good posture and are using proper body mechanics.

9. If the patient you are assisting begins to collapse during ambulation, do not try to carry, hold up, or catch her. Rather, assume a broad stance with your preferred foot slightly ahead of the other and between the patient's legs. Grasp the patient's body firmly at the waist or under the axilla (armpit), and allow her to slide down against your leg (Figure 13.7). Ease the patient slowly to the floor, using your body as an incline. If necessary, lower your body along with hers. Remember to always use proper body mechanics.

10. If there are family members or friends available who would like to assist, they may do so as long as the appropriate provider has given permission and each person understands and is comfortable with the procedure. Family members and friends must know how to avoid any risks or harm to themselves and the patient as described here. This may require you to provide instructions and assistance the first few times they assist with ambulation. Also, be sure to show them what to do if the patient collapses or begins to fall.

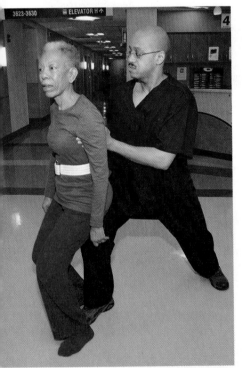

Wards Forest Media, LLC

Figure 13.7 Do not try to catch or carry a collapsing patient. Instead, assume a wide stance and slowly ease her to the floor, using your body as an incline.

When people do not feel well, they often want to stay in bed. Therefore, assisting with mobility is one of the most important responsibilities of healthcare workers. Maintaining mobility is essential for patient well-being. The following procedure provides information about how to encourage and help patients move out of their beds and ambulate.

Procedure 13.1 | Assisting with Ambulation

Rationale

Assisting a patient with ambulation can improve mental and physical health.

Preparation

1. Make sure you have a written doctor's order for ambulation.
2. Assemble the following equipment:
   - a robe, if needed to ensure the patient is not exposed
   - nonslip, properly fitting, low-heeled footwear
   - a gait belt (check that it is in good condition and is functional)
3. Wash your hands to ensure infection control.
4. Explain in simple terms what you are going to do before assisting with ambulation.

The Procedure

5. Provide privacy. You can draw the bed curtain or put a screen around the bed, if needed.
6. If the patient is in bed, lower the bed to its lowest position and lock the wheels.
7. If the patient is in bed, assist her to a dangling (sitting) position on the side of the bed. The patient may be seated in a chair.
8. Help the patient put on the nonslip, properly fitting shoes and robe, if needed.
9. Apply the gait belt by putting the belt around the patient's waist, over her clothing. The buckle should be in the front. Thread the belt through the teeth of the buckle and through the other two loops to lock it.
10. Check that the belt is snug but that there is still enough room to place your fingers under the belt.
11. Whether in a bed or sitting in a chair, face the patient and use an underhand grasp on the gait belt for greater safety (Figure 13.8).

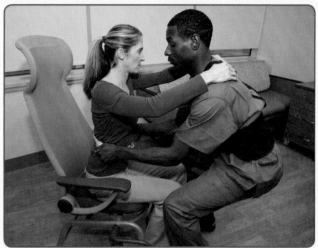

Figure 13.8   *Wards Forest Media, LLC*

12. Using the gait belt, assist the patient to a standing position (Figure 13.9). Lift the patient using your arm and leg muscles. Bend your knees and keep your back straight. Do not twist your body.

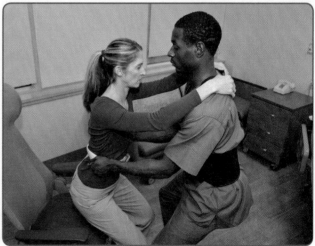

Figure 13.9   *Wards Forest Media, LLC*

13. Continue to hold on to the gait belt while the patient gains her balance. Have her stand erect with her head up and back straight.

Procedure 13.1   Assisting with Ambulation (continued)

14. Walk behind the patient and to one side during ambulation.

15. Hold on to the belt directly from behind. Watch for signs of a possible patient collapse. *Do not attempt to catch a patient who begins to collapse during ambulation. Instead, slowly ease the patient to the floor, using your body as an incline.*

16. Determine if the patient has a weak side. If so, position yourself accordingly:
    - weak right side: stand between the 4 and 5 o'clock positions (Figure 13.10A)
    - weak left side: stand between the 7 and 8 o'clock positions (Figure 13.10B)

17. Let the patient set the pace while keeping a firm grasp on the gait belt, if used.

18. Encourage the patient to achieve the ordered distance, but be observant. Watch for signs of patient fatigue. If collapse occurs, follow the steps discussed earlier.

19. When the ambulation is completed, help the patient return to her room (or bed). Remove and put away the gait belt, robe, and shoes.

Follow-up

20. Make sure the patient is safe and comfortable. Place the call light and personal items within easy reach.

21. Wash your hands to ensure infection control.

Reporting and Documentation

22. Communicate any specific observations, complications, or unusual responses to the appropriate provider. Also record this information in the patient's chart or EMR.

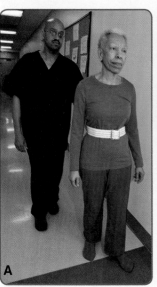 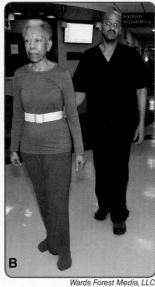

Figure 13.10   *Wards Forest Media, LLC*

Check Your Understanding ✓

1. Name at least three benefits of exercise.

2. What is the goal of proper body alignment?

3. Do bones move muscles, or do muscles move bones?

4. Are healthcare workers required to wear back belts when assisting patients, or is each healthcare worker allowed to decide for himself or herself?

5. Why is it important to anticipate the needs of patients during ambulation?

6. What possible safety risks and hazards might occur when assisting with ambulation?

7. How can family members assist patients with ambulation?

Ambulating with Assistive Devices

Some people require assistive devices to ambulate. These usually include canes, crutches, and walkers. The decision as to which device is used typically depends on how much support is needed.

Canes are particularly useful for those people who may have had surgery and are not yet able to maintain balance or need extra stability. The elderly may use a cane if they have recovered from a stroke and are not yet able to fully ambulate, or if they have arthritis that has resulted in restricted movement.

Crutches are often used for short-term conditions such as a sprained ankle or broken leg. Though in some cases, when a patient has had an amputation or a disability, crutches may be the assistive device of choice because they provide better support over time. Canes and crutches do require upper body strength.

Walkers are helpful for people who may have had surgery on their lower limbs, such as a hip or knee replacement. The walker is used during rehabilitation with the goal of reaching full ambulation. Walkers are also used by the elderly when they begin to lose their balance and stability and need extra assistance. Walkers are often selected over canes or crutches because walkers allow the patient's weight to be more evenly distributed, and upper body strength is not as critical (although the patient using a walker must be able to pick it up).

Ambulating with a Cane

There are several different types of canes that can be used (Figure 13.11). The type of cane a patient chooses often depends on their preferred grip, balancing ability, and need.

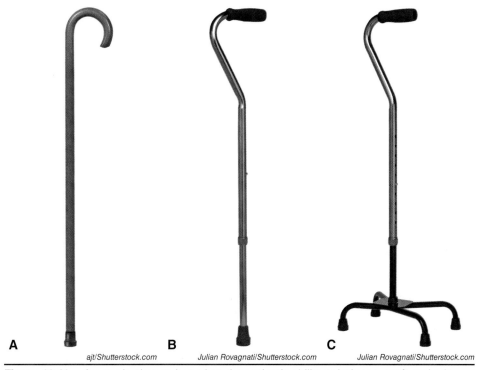

Figure 13.11 A cane is chosen based on the patient's ability to balance, preferred grip, and personal need. Three types of canes are shown here—a C cane (A), a functional grip cane (B), and a quad cane (C).

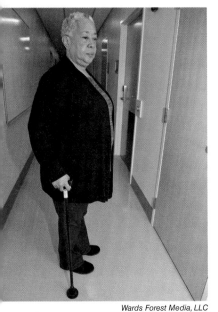

Figure 13.12 Check the cane's fit before the patient begins using it during ambulation.

Wards Forest Media, LLC

Canes with a single shaft are known as *C canes*. The C shape resembles a candy cane. These are used for temporary walking impairment and are available at local pharmacies. This type of cane usually has a slip-resistant tip.

A functional grip cane is another type of single-shaft cane. This type has a straight handle for a steadier grip. While the C and functional grip canes provide support, they do not assist with balance.

The quad cane has a base with four prongs, each with a skid-resistant tip. It offers more stability than a single-shaft cane. This cane offers support, provides a functional grip, and assists with balance.

To successfully ambulate with a cane, a patient's cane must be fit and used properly (Figure 13.12). The top of the cane should be in line with the patient's wrist crease (the wrinkle that separates the arm from the hand) when she stands up straight and her arms are hanging loosely at her sides. The patient should be able to slightly bend her elbow (approximately 15–20 degrees) while using the cane. The cane should always be held in the hand on the stronger side of the body (opposite the side that needs support).

Procedure 13.2   Assisting with Ambulation Using a Cane

Rationale

Assisting a patient who is ambulating with a cane reduces the chance of injury and promotes safe ambulation by helping achieve balance and giving support.

Preparation

1. Make sure you have a written doctor's order for ambulation with a cane.
2. Assemble the following equipment:
   - a robe, if needed to ensure the patient is not exposed
   - nonslip, properly fitting, low-heeled footwear
   - a cane with one, two, three, or four tips for added support (check the cane for flaws, cracks, bends, or missing parts)
   - a gait belt (check that it is in good condition and is functional)
3. Wash your hands to ensure infection control.
4. Explain in simple terms what you are going to do before assisting with ambulation with a cane.

The Procedure

5. Provide privacy. You can draw the bed curtain or put a screen around the bed, if needed.
6. If the patient is in bed, lower the bed to its lowest position and lock the wheels.
7. If the patient is in bed, assist him or her to a dangling (sitting) position on the side of the bed. The patient may be seated in a chair.
8. Help the patient put on the nonslip, properly fitting shoes and robe, if needed.
9. Apply the gait belt, if needed. Put the belt around the patient's waist, over her clothing, with the buckle in the front. Thread the belt through the teeth of the buckle and through the other two loops to lock it. Make it snug, but leave enough room to place your fingers under the belt.
10. The patient should hold the cane on her stronger side.
11. While facing the patient, use an underhand grasp on the gait belt for greater safety.

Procedure 13.2   Assisting with Ambulation Using a Cane (continued)

12. Using the gait belt, assist the patient to a standing position. Lift her using your arm and leg muscles. Bend your knees and keep your back straight. Do not twist your body.

13. Continue to hold on to the gait belt while the patient gains her balance. Have her stand erect with her head up and back straight.

14. The cane should be positioned and the patient stabilized with the cane before ambulation begins.

15. When ambulation begins, the cane should be moved forward about 6 to 10 inches (Figure 13.13).

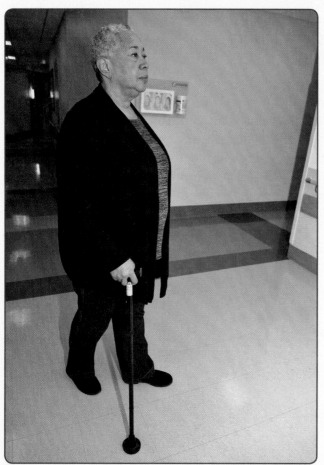

Figure 13.13   *Wards Forest Media, LLC*

16. The patient should follow, first with the weak leg and then with the strong leg.

17. If using a gait belt, stand slightly behind the patient on her weaker side to provide additional support as needed.

18. Grasp the gait belt with an underhand grip from the back, if needed.

19. Encourage the patient to use handrails, if available.

20. Let the patient set the pace while keeping a firm grasp on the gait belt, if used. Encourage the patient to achieve the ordered distance, but be observant. Watch for signs of patient fatigue or possible collapse. *Do not attempt to catch a patient who begins to collapse during ambulation. Instead, slowly ease the patient to the floor, using your body as an incline.*

21. If permissible, and the patient is strong enough, she may be assisted with climbing stairs with a cane. Before beginning, check to be sure that she is able to safely walk on flat surfaces.

22. Have the patient grasp the handrail (if possible) with the hand on her weak side. Ask her to hold the cane in her opposite, strong hand.

23. The patient should step up the stair using her strong leg first. Once balanced, the cane should then be moved up the stair, followed by the weak leg. This is repeated to move up the stairs.

24. To come down stairs, the cane should be placed on the step first, followed by the weaker leg and then the stronger leg.

    Remember to have the patient face forward and "go up with the good, down with the bad." When going up, lead with the strongest leg. When going down, lead with the weaker one.

25. When the ambulation is completed, help the patient return to her room (or bed). Remove and put away the gait belt, robe, cane, and shoes.

Follow-up

26. Make sure the patient is safe and comfortable. Place the call light and personal items within easy reach.

27. Wash your hands to ensure infection control.

Reporting and Documentation

28. Communicate any specific observations, complications, or unusual responses to the appropriate provider. Also record this information in the patient's chart or EMR.

Ambulating with Crutches

There are times when patients need to keep weight off their legs or feet. Normally this is due to an injury or surgical procedure. In these cases, the patient may have to use crutches. Crutches are seldom recommended for older adults because they require upper body strength.

Types of Crutches. There are several different types of crutches (Figure 13.14):

- *Standard underarm* or *axillary crutches* are generally made of wood or aluminum and can be adjusted for height. They have padding on the underarms and also have hand holds. These crutches are usually for short-term use.

- *Strutter crutches* are similar to standard crutches but have a u-shaped underarm support that distributes weight over a larger area of the skin surface and also has a larger base. This provides better balance and helps alleviate any possible injury of nerves and blood vessels in the axilla.

- *Platform crutches* use the same base as standard crutches but feature a horizontal, padded armrest. The patient using these crutches straps his arms onto each armrest and is then able to maneuver the crutches.

- *Forearm crutches* are typically used for patients with disabilities. While these crutches can be used temporarily, they are often selected for long-term use. These crutches are designed so they can be slipped on and off through a forearm cuff that provides stabilization and allows for a tighter grip on the handholds. The cuff is usually aluminum or plastic and is shaped like a half-circle (open cuff) or complete circle (closed cuff).

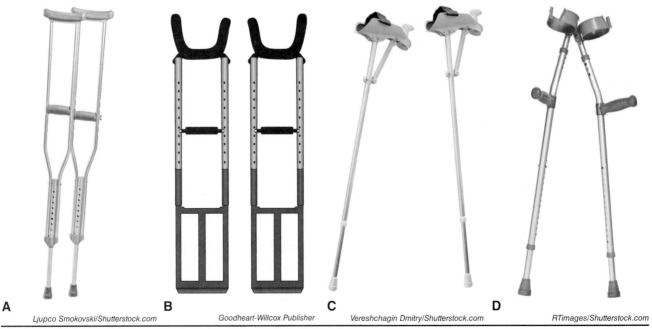

A *Ljupco Smokovski/Shutterstock.com*   B *Goodheart-Willcox Publisher*   C *Vereshchagin Dmitry/Shutterstock.com*   D *RTimages/Shutterstock.com*

Figure 13.14   Four types of crutches include the standard underarm crutches (A), strutter crutches (B), platform crutches (C), and forearm crutches (D).

In addition to these, there are newer, hands-free crutches. A knee walker or knee scooter is a wheeled device that supports the injured leg. The knee of the injured leg is placed in a padded seat while the good leg pushes the scooter. The patient uses the scooter handles to maneuver and make turns.

Guidelines for Using Crutches. Some healthcare facilities may have special procedures or training for healthcare workers who will be assisting patients to ambulate with crutches.

The fit and size of standard crutches is important. Before allowing a patient to ambulate with crutches, the fit and size of the crutches must be deemed appropriate for that patient (Figure 13.15). The tops of the crutches (crutch pad) should be about one and a half inches below the axilla, while the patient is standing up straight and shoulders are relaxed. The handgrips of the crutches should be even with the hips. The elbows should be able to bend slightly when the handgrips are used. The crutch length should equal the distance between the axilla and about six inches in front of the patient's shoe. The tops of the crutches should be held tightly to one's sides, but never pressing into the axilla, which can damage the nerves. The bottoms of the crutches should always have rubber tips.

Before helping the patient to ambulate with crutches, check for flaws (cracks in wooden crutches and bends in metal crutches) and tighten all the bolts on the crutches, if appropriate.

Using the Appropriate Gait. Equally important to properly sizing crutches is knowing which crutch walking gait is ordered by the doctor so proper instructions can be given. Each gait starts in a tripod position (Figure 13.16). The crutch tips are placed about four to six inches to the side and slightly in front of each foot. The strong foot bears the weight of the body.

A four-point gait is used when there is some weight-bearing ability on both legs. Start with the tripod position. Then follow the sequence for the four-point gait (Figure 13.17 on the next page).

A three-point gait is used when there should be no weight bearing on the affected, or injured leg. Start with the tripod position and follow the sequence for the three-point gait (Figure 13.18 on the next page). When using the three-point gait, the non-weight-bearing leg should move forward along with the crutches.

A two-point gait is used when both legs can bear some weight. This is an alternative to the four-point gait, which also allows for some weight to be placed on each foot. Start with the tripod position and follow the sequence for the two-point gait (Figure 13.19 on the next page).

A swing-through gait is used when the legs are paralyzed and in braces. Start with the tripod position and follow the sequence for the swing-through gait (Figure 13.20 on the next page).

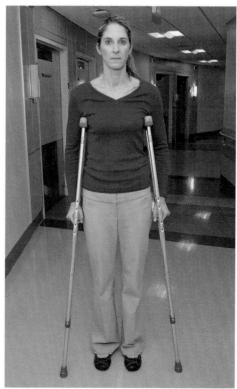

Wards Forest Media, LLC

Figure 13.15   Before a patient uses crutches to ambulate, check that they properly fit the patient and are in good condition.

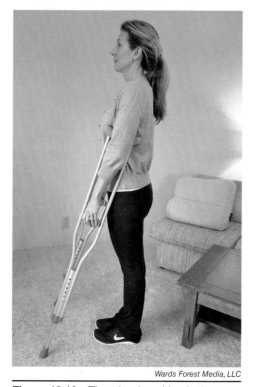

Wards Forest Media, LLC

Figure 13.16   The tripod position is the neutral starting position for ambulating with crutches.

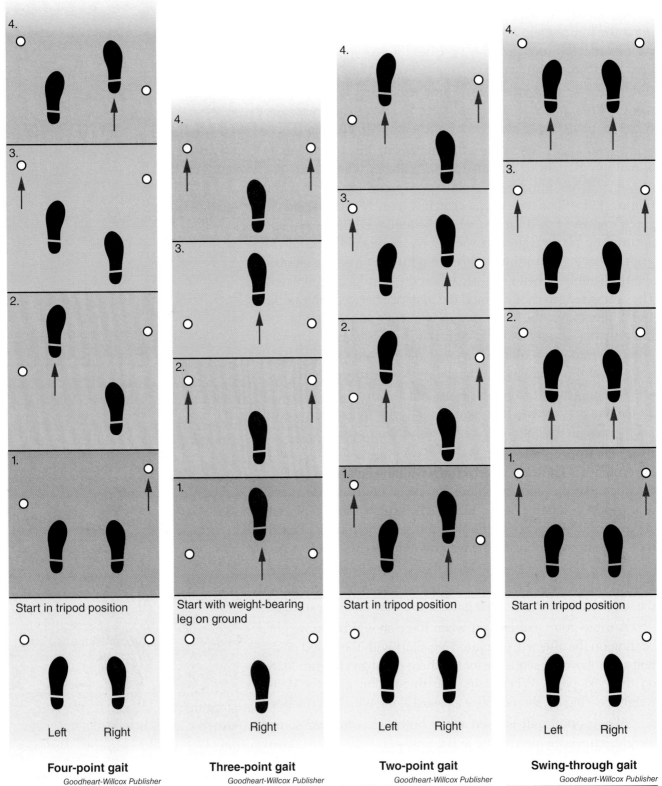

Four-point gait
Goodheart-Willcox Publisher

Three-point gait
Goodheart-Willcox Publisher

Two-point gait
Goodheart-Willcox Publisher

Swing-through gait
Goodheart-Willcox Publisher

Figure 13.17 Four-point gait using crutches. In step 1, the right crutch moves forward.

Figure 13.18 Three-point gait using crutches. In step 1, the weight-bearing leg moves forward.

Figure 13.19 Two-point gait using crutches. In step 1, the left crutch and the right leg move forward together.

Figure 13.20 Swing-through gait using crutches. In step 1, the two crutches move forward together.

Procedure 13.3   Assisting with Ambulation Using Crutches

Rationale

Assisting patients ambulating with crutches reduces the chance of injury and helps promote safe ambulation.

Preparation

1. Make sure you have a written doctor's order for ambulation with crutches.

2. If the facility has a specific policy and procedure for ambulating with crutches, be sure to follow it.

3. Assemble the following equipment:
   - a robe or well-fitting clothing
   - nonslip, properly fitting, low-heeled footwear
   - gait belt (check that it is in good condition and is functional)
   - a pair of crutches that have been properly sized and are in working condition

4. Wash your hands to ensure infection control.

5. Explain in simple terms what you are going to do before assisting the patient to ambulate with crutches.

The Procedure

6. Provide privacy. You can draw the bed curtain or put a screen around the bed, if needed.

7. If the patient is in bed, lower the bed to its lowest position and lock the wheels.

8. If the patient is in bed, assist him or her to a dangling (sitting) position on the side of the bed. The patient may be seated in a chair.

9. Help the patient as she puts on the nonslip, properly fitting shoes and a robe, if needed.

10. Apply the gait belt, if needed. Put the belt around the patient's waist, over her clothing, with the buckle in the front. Thread the belt through the teeth of the buckle and through the other two loops to lock it. Make it snug, but leave enough room to place your fingers under the belt.

11. Ensure the crutches fit properly. Discuss any concerns with the appropriate provider.

12. The crutches should be in the tripod position. Hands should be on the hand grips to absorb the patient's weight. There should not be any weight placed on the axilla.

13. Determine the gait that has been ordered by the patient's doctor and have the patient follow the sequence.

14. Remind the patient to maintain an erect posture and keep focused on where she is ambulating to by looking straight ahead and not at her feet.

15. Stay safely to the side of the patient. Watch for signs of a possible patient collapse. *Do not attempt to catch a patient who begins to collapse during ambulation. Instead, slowly ease the patient to the floor, using your body as an incline.*

16. Let the patient set the pace while keeping a firm grasp on the gait belt, if used.

17. Encourage the patient to achieve the ordered distance, but be observant. Watch for signs of patient fatigue. If the patient collapses, follow the steps discussed earlier.

18. If permissible, the patient may climb stairs with her crutches. She must have the strength and flexibility needed. One approach is to hold the handrail with one hand, tucking both crutches under the opposite axilla. When going up stairs, have the patient lead with the strong foot, keeping the weak foot raised behind. When going down stairs, the patient should hold the weak foot up and in front of the body, hopping down each stair on the strong foot, taking it one step at a time (Figure 13.21 on the next page). Place yourself in back of the patient when she is going up the stairs and in front when going down, to assist if needed.

Procedure 13.3   Assisting with Ambulation Using Crutches (continued)

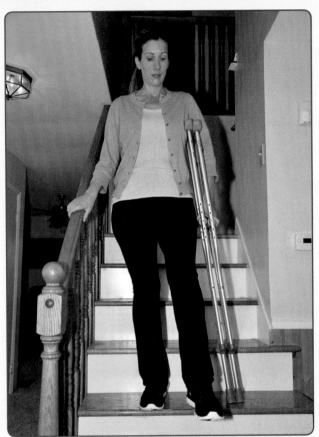

Figure 13.21   *Wards Forest Media, LLC*

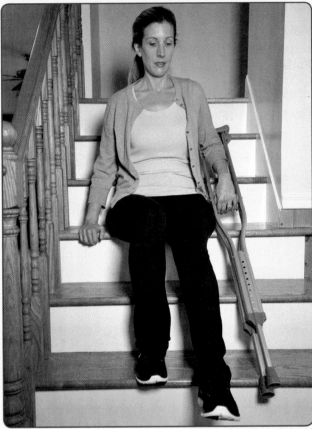

Figure 13.22   *Wards Forest Media, LLC*

Another approach is for the patient to sit on the stairs and inch up or down each step (Figure 13.22). The patient should hold the weak leg out in front of her body, and carry both crutches flat against the stairs in the hand opposite the railing. She should scoot her bottom up or down to the next step, using the free hand and strong leg for support.

19. When ambulation is complete, help the patient return to her room (or bed). Remove and put away the gait belt, robe, crutches, and shoes.

Follow-up

20. Make sure the patient is safe and comfortable. Place the call light and personal items within easy reach.

21. Wash your hands to ensure infection control.

Reporting and Documentation

22. Communicate any specific observations, complications, or unusual responses to the appropriate provider. Also record this information in the patient's chart or EMR.

Ambulating with a Walker

Some patients need more support with ambulation than a cane or crutches can provide. In such cases, a walker is often a better option. The walker lets patients take all or some of their weight off their lower body by using their arms as they ambulate. A patient should never try to climb stairs or use an escalator with a walker.

There are different types of walkers (Figure 13.23). A standard, pickup walker is made of lightweight metal and has four solid legs with rubber

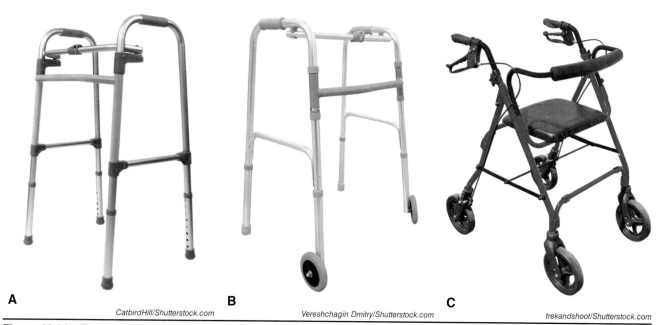

A

CatbirdHill/Shutterstock.com

B

Vereshchagin Dmitry/Shutterstock.com

C

trekandshoot/Shutterstock.com

Figure 13.23 The three types of walkers include the pickup walker (A), the rolling walker (B), and a rolling walker with hand brakes and a platform (C).

tips on the bottoms of the legs, which provide a wider base of support. This type of walker is used when the patient is able to pick up the walker while ambulating.

A rolling walker, or *rollator*, has wheels or casters on the end of each of the four legs so the walker rolls during ambulation. To provide stability, some rolling walkers have two wheels on the front two legs and no wheels on the back two legs. Some also have four wheels and hand brakes, along with platforms and pouches to carry personal items. Rolling walkers let the patient push the walker rather than lift it while ambulating. The patient will still need enough strength to lift the walker when needed.

Once a walker that best suits the patient's needs has been selected, it must be properly fitted (Figure 13.24). The handles or top of the walker should be at a height even with the patient's wrist when she is standing in an upright position with arms relaxed at her sides. When holding on to the walker, the patient's elbows should be bent in a comfortable and natural position. The patient should never be stooped over while using the walker.

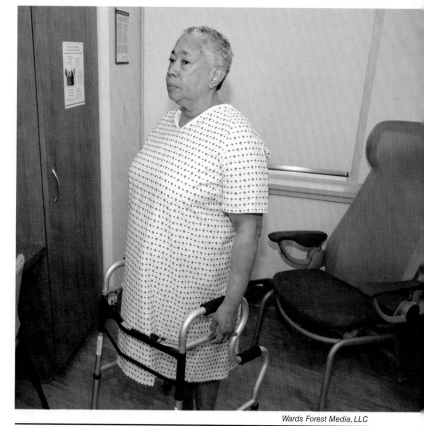

Wards Forest Media, LLC

Figure 13.24 Ensure the walker fits the patient appropriately before she uses it to ambulate.

Procedure 13.4   Assisting with Ambulation Using a Walker

Rationale

Assisting a patient to ensure a walker is used correctly reduces the chance of injury and promotes safe ambulation.

Preparation

1. Make sure you have a written doctor's order for ambulation with a walker.

2. Assemble the following equipment:
   - a robe or well-fitting clothing
   - nonslip, properly fitting, low-heeled footwear
   - a standard or rolling walker
   - gait belt (check that it is in good condition and functional)

3. Wash your hands to ensure infection control.

4. Explain in simple terms what you are going to do before assisting the patient to ambulate with a walker.

The Procedure

5. Provide privacy. You can draw the bed curtain or put a screen around the bed.

6. If the patient is in bed, lower the bed to its lowest position and lock the wheels.

7. If the patient is in bed, assist him or her to a dangling (sitting) position on the side of the bed.

8. Help the patient as she puts on the nonslip, properly fitting shoes and robe, if needed.

9. Apply the gait belt, if needed. Put the belt around the patient's waist, over her clothing, with the buckle in the front. Thread the belt through the teeth of the buckle and through the other two loops to lock it. Make it snug, but leave enough room to place your fingers under the belt.

10. While the patient is sitting on the bed, position her so she is centered in front of and inside the frame of the walker.

11. The walker should be placed about one step ahead of the seated patient, making sure the legs of the walker are level on the ground and stable.

12. Using both hands, have the patient grip the top of the walker for support, stand, and walk into it. Then have her take the first step with her weakest leg. The heel of the foot should touch the ground first and the foot should flatten.

13. As the step is completed, the next step should be taken with the patient's strong leg. As the patient ambulates, position yourself behind her and slightly to the side.

14. The first step is repeated with the weak leg and then followed by the strong leg. This sequence is repeated. Do not hurry the patient.

15. Make sure the patient does not step all the way to the front bar of the walker. Have her take small steps when she turns.

16. Let the patient set the pace while keeping a firm grasp on the gait belt, if used.

17. Encourage the patient to achieve the ordered distance, but be observant. Watch for signs of patient fatigue or a possible collapse. If this occurs, follow the steps discussed earlier.

18. To move the patient to a sitting position, have her begin by standing so her back is to the chair (Figure 13.25A). Make sure the patient is close enough to sit down on the chair. The patient should slide her weaker leg forward and shift her weight to the stronger leg. Have her switch hands from the walker to the arms of the chair and sit down slowly (Figure 13.25B).

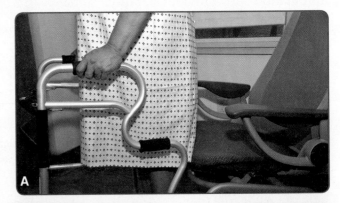

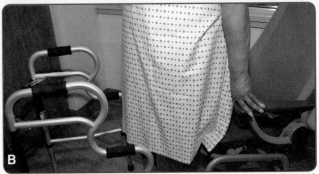

Figure 13.25   *Wards Forest Media, LLC*

19. To have the patient get up from a chair, put the walker in front of the chair. Have the patient move forward in the chair, placing her hands on the arms of the chair and pushing up. She should then move her hands to the grips of the walker. The patient should stand for enough time to be sure she has stability and balance before beginning to ambulate.

20. When ambulation is complete, help the patient return to her room (or bed). Remove and put away the gait belt, robe, walker, and shoes.

Follow-up

21. Make sure the patient is safe and comfortable. Place the call light and personal items within easy reach.

22. Wash your hands to ensure infection control.

Reporting and Documentation

23. Communicate any specific observations, complications, or unusual responses to the appropriate provider. Also record this information in the patient's chart or EMR.

Check Your Understanding ✓

1. Describe the types of assistive devices that can be used to help someone ambulate, and explain under what conditions each type should be selected.

2. Describe the proper fit of a cane.

3. Identify four types of crutches.

4. Describe the procedure you should use if a patient starts to collapse when he or she is walking with a cane, crutches, or a walker.

Positioning, Turning, Lifting, and Transferring Patients

Some healthcare workers, particularly those working in a hospital or long-term care facility, have the responsibility of monitoring and changing patient or resident positions. This may include positioning a patient in bed, lifting the patient, or helping (transferring) the patient into a wheelchair. Patient positions must be changed because being in any position, even one that feels comfortable, can become unbearable after a long period of time. It can also be helpful to reposition patients who are restless, uncomfortable, or having trouble sleeping. An immobile patient should be repositioned at least every two hours, whether he is in a bed or seated in a chair. Some patients may need to be repositioned more often.

Benefits of Positioning

There are many reasons why it is important that a patient's position is changed periodically and that she is positioned correctly:

1. to increase comfort and to help the patient relax

2. to restore body function—changing positions can improve respiratory and gastrointestinal function and stimulate circulation

ankylosis
the stiffening or immobility of a joint resulting from disease, trauma, surgery, or bone fusion

foot drop
a condition characterized by the inability to lift the front part of one or both feet due to weakness or paralysis of the muscles in the foot; causes the toes to drag on the ground while walking

3. to prevent deformities—muscles can atrophy (waste away) and cause contractures (shortening) and **ankylosis** (stiffening) when they are not actively moving

   If the patient has **foot drop** due to illness or injury, she will be unable to lift the front part of one or both feet due to muscle weakness or paralysis. This can cause the toes to drag on the ground while walking. When in bed, proper positioning and support will be especially important for this condition.

4. to relieve pressure and strain on the skin and to prevent the formation of a decubitus ulcer

Preventing Decubitus Ulcers

Many patients require assistance when moving and turning due to **immobility**. Certain conditions may also make it impossible for a patient to turn on his own, such as when he has serious fractures that require **traction** appliances (Figure 13.26). These appliances may be a supporting brace or suspended weights used to help injuries heal. It is especially important that immobile patients are turned regularly to prevent skin breakdown and the formation of a **decubitus ulcer** (also known as a *bedsore* or *pressure sore*).

A decubitus ulcer is caused by pressure that restricts blood circulation to the skin. This pressure can be the result of immobility, but also the rubbing of a cover or clothing on the skin, wrinkled or wadded up sheets, irritation

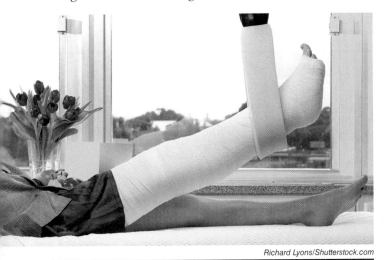
Richard Lyons/Shutterstock.com

Figure 13.26 Traction appliances help support injured limbs such as a broken leg.

immobility
a condition characterized by a limited, or complete lack of, ability to move

traction
the use of a pulling force to treat muscle and skeletal disorders

decubitus ulcer
a skin sore that is a result of lying in one position too long; caused by pressure that interferes with blood circulation to the skin

from tubing on or around the body, or even food crumbs among the bedding. Fragile skin is particularly susceptible to decubitus ulcers.

Stages of Decubitus Ulcers

The appearance of a decubitus ulcer can range from very mild, pink coloration of the skin to a severe wound that extends to the bone and sometimes into internal organs. The severity of decubitus ulcers is identified using four stages (Figure 13.27):

- **Stage 1:** the skin is not open but is discolored, turning red on people with light complexions and blue or purple on those who have a darker complexion. If the skin does not turn to white when pressed, this is a sign that a decubitus ulcer has already started to form.

- **Stage 2:** the decubitus ulcer is still considered superficial (or shallow) but the skin is now open. A blister filled with fluid, an abrasion, or a shallow sore that looks like a crater can be seen, and the surrounding area may be irritated and red in color.

Stages of Decubitus Ulcers

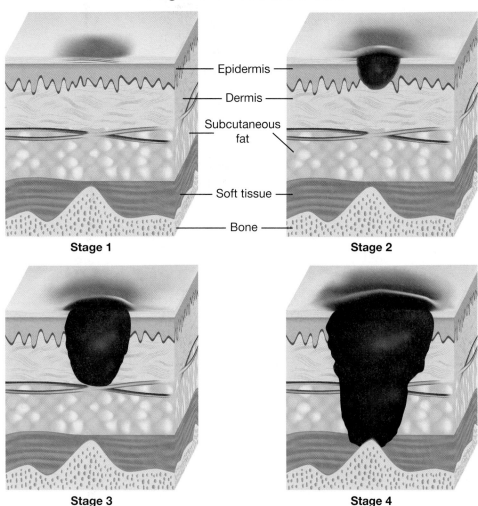

Figure 13.27 Decubitus ulcers have four stages of severity.

- **Stage 3:** the ulcer is much deeper than in stage 2 and may affect the underlying connective tissue. The sore looks more like a crater and may ooze, bleed, or contain pus.

- **Stage 4:** the damage is deep and may reach the muscle, tendons, ligaments, joints, and bone. The ulcer will bleed and the skin and tissue become **necrotic**.

Decubitus Ulcer Pressure Points

Certain areas of the body are more likely to develop decubitus ulcers than others. These are known as *pressure points* (Figure 13.28). Pressure points can be found where the skin covers bony areas of the body.

Positioning is important to avoid decubitus ulcers, but so is providing good skin care each time you change a patient's position. This means keeping pressure points dry and clean, changing any wet or creased dressings and bandages, and making sure bed linens are smooth and free from crumbs. Continuous observation is critical, as is noting any existing ulcers prior to admitting the patient to your healthcare facility.

necrotic
term that describes dead cells or tissues

Pressure Points for Decubitus Ulcers

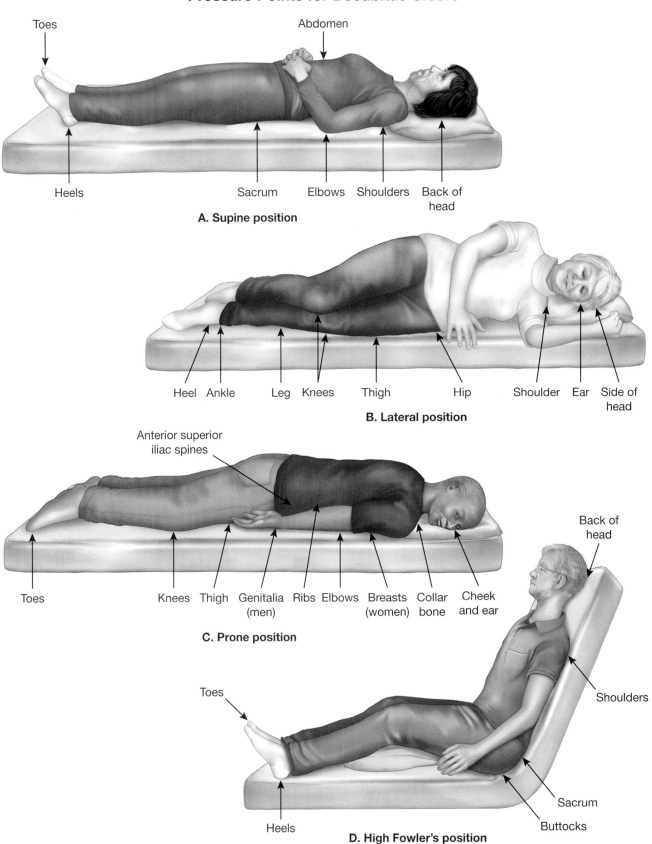

A. Supine position

Toes · Abdomen · Heels · Sacrum · Elbows · Shoulders · Back of head

B. Lateral position

Heel · Ankle · Leg · Knees · Thigh · Hip · Shoulder · Ear · Side of head

C. Prone position

Anterior superior iliac spines · Toes · Knees · Thigh · Genitalia (men) · Ribs · Elbows · Breasts (women) · Collar bone · Cheek and ear

D. High Fowler's position

Back of head · Shoulders · Sacrum · Buttocks · Toes · Heels

©Body Scientific International

Figure 13.28   The weight of a body in bed or the pressure of a sheet or blanket covering a bedridden patient may cause decubitus ulcers to form at specific pressure points.

Safe Patient-Handling Techniques

It is vital that you follow safe patient-handling techniques at all times when positioning or moving patients. Some general safety guidelines include the following:

- Maintain a wide, stable base with your feet.
- Position the bed at the correct height (waist level when you provide care, hip level when moving a patient).
- Try to keep the work directly in front of you to avoid rotating your spine.
- Keep the patient as close to your body as possible to minimize reaching.
- Give skin care to pressure points before and after a change in position. Protect the patient from tubing that may rub his or her skin, if possible.
- Provide the most support to the heaviest part of the patient's body and avoid placing one body part directly on top of another.
- Move the patient smoothly.
- Always check the bed linens to be sure they are clean, dry, and smooth so that folds in the sheets or food crumbs do not rub the skin and increase the risk of decubitus ulcers.

Positioning Guidelines

Properly positioning and repositioning patients requires knowledge of the different types of available positions, familiarity with the equipment, and attention to the condition of the patient and the patient's skin. Always practice safety by using proper body mechanics and asking for assistance from others if the patient is frail, is overweight, or has equipment or devices attached to his body, such as tubes or an intravenous (IV) catheter.

Different types of equipment and devices are used for positioning. If you are uncertain about the type of positioning equipment or devices to use, or how to use them, check with the appropriate provider. (Note: some devices can be interpreted as a type of restraint, which is contraindicated.)

Examples of positioning equipment and devices you may use include

- pillows of various sizes to help protect the skin; prop up a limb; or support the head, a limb, or the back for comfort;
- folded or rolled towels and blankets to prop up and support the patient and maintain proper body alignment;
- **trochanter rolls** made from rolled towels or blankets placed from the top of the pelvic bone to mid-thigh to prevent external rotation of the hip (Figure 13.29);
- a turning sheet, also called a *pull sheet*, *draw sheet*, or *lift sheet*, is used by the healthcare worker to turn the patient;
- cotton padding to protect skin and bony areas;
- a foot board, which is a flat panel used at the end of the bed to prevent foot drop; and
- a hip abduction wedge, which is usually made of a stiff foam rubber material cut in a wedge to prop up the hip (Figure 13.30).

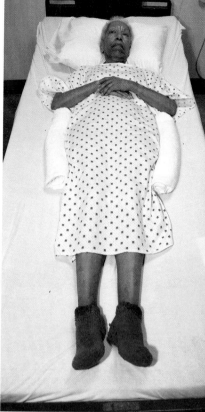

Wards Forest Media, LLC

Figure 13.29   Trochanter rolls prevent the patient's hips from externally rotating.

trochanter roll
a rolled towel or blanket placed along the hip that prevents the hips from rotating externally

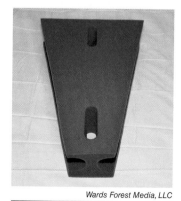

Wards Forest Media, LLC

Figure 13.30   Hip abduction wedge

Positioning a Patient in Bed

Some doctors may prescribe a specific schedule to make sure patients are placed in different positions, particularly when they are confined to a bed, or *bedridden*. Whether or not there is a doctor's order, patients should be moved every two hours. At minimum, they should be rotated through at least four body positions, unless a particular position is **contraindicated**, or harmful. Position changes and the types used should be recorded to make sure the schedule is maintained.

contraindicated
term that describes any situation or condition that causes a particular type of treatment to be improper or undesirable

Fowler's Position

- The patient is seated in bed and the head of the bed is raised to a 45° angle (Figure 13.31).
- The patient's knees may be elevated by placing a pillow under the knees.

Semi-Fowler's Position

- The patient is seated in bed and the head of the bed is raised to a 30° angle (Figure 13.32).
- Support the patient's head with a pillow.
- The patient's knees may be elevated by placing a pillow under the knees.
- Use a foot support such as a foot board to prevent foot drop, if prescribed by the appropriate provider.

Supine Position

- The patient is lying face up, flat on her back (Figure 13.33).
- The bed is flat and both of the patient's arms and legs are extended.
- Support the patient's head with a pillow.
- Support the patient's arms and hands with pillows, if necessary.
- Support the small of the patient's back with a small rolled towel or blanket. You may also place a small folded towel under the knees to relieve strain on the back.

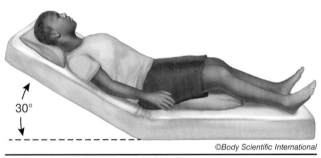

45°

©Body Scientific International

Figure 13.31   Fowler's position

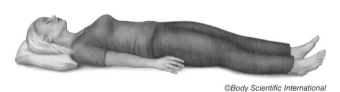

30°

©Body Scientific International

Figure 13.32   Semi-Fowler's position

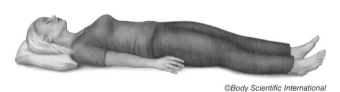

©Body Scientific International

Figure 13.33   Supine position

- If prescribed by the appropriate provider, a foot board may be used to prevent foot drop.
- A trochanter roll may be used to prevent the patient's hips from rotating outward.
- Use padding to protect pressure points on the patient's elbows, knees, and the tailbone.

Prone Position

- The patient is lying face down, flat on the abdomen (Figure 13.34).

- The patient's legs are extended and his head is to one side.

- The patient's arms are bent upward at the elbows or extended down at the sides.

- The patient's head and abdomen may be supported with pillows, if preferred.

- A pillow may also be placed under the patient's lower legs to reduce pressure on the toes, if necessary. The patient's feet may also hang off the bed to relieve pressure on the toes.

Lateral Position

- The patient is lying on her left side, called *left lateral*, or right side, called *right lateral* (Figure 13.35).

- Support the patient's head with a pillow and place a pillow against her back to maintain the position.

- To relieve pressure on the back, the patient's upper leg and hip is bent at the knee.

- You may place a pillow between the patient's knees for protection and alignment.

- The patient's lower arm should be flexed. You may place a small pillow under the arm.

Sims' Position

- Sims' position is a partly left-side lying and partly prone-lying position (Figure 13.36).

- Support the patient's head and shoulder with a pillow.

- The patient's left leg and arm are extended and the right leg and arm are flexed.

- The patient's left arm rests behind him.

- The flexed right leg is supported with a pillow.

- The flexed right hand and arm are supported with a pillow.

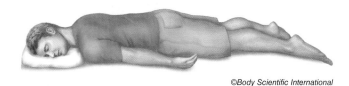
©Body Scientific International
Figure 13.34   Prone position

Think It Through

Positioning patients helps them relax and promotes sleep. Think about what position helps you relax and sleep. You may also find that certain bedding or special pillows help you feel comfortable. In addition, you may reduce light, turn off the radio or television, or play soothing music. What more could you do to help a patient feel more comfortable?

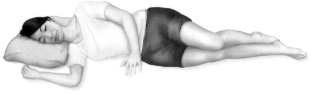
©Body Scientific International
Figure 13.35   Lateral position

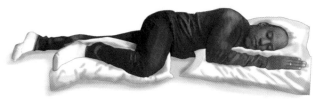
©Body Scientific International
Figure 13.36   Sims' position

Procedure 13.5   Positioning a Patient in Bed

Rationale

Proper positioning and repositioning provides good body alignment, helps to prevent decubitus ulcer formation, and promotes comfort.

Preparation

1. Assemble the necessary equipment based on how the patient will be positioned.
2. Be aware of all pressure points and natural curves of the body that may need care and support.
3. Wash your hands to ensure infection control.
4. Explain in simple terms what you are going to do before positioning. Do this even if the patient is unable to communicate or is disoriented.

The Procedure

5. Provide privacy by drawing the bed curtains or putting a screen around the bed.
6. Ask the patient how he would be most comfortable, if there are any pressure concerns, and about personal preferences.
7. Use proper body mechanics when positioning the patient. Raise or lower the bed to a comfortable level for working and lower the bed rails. Lock the wheels of the bed, if needed.
8. Depending on the position desired, place pillows, soft rolled towels, or blankets under various body areas, such as
    - the head, shoulders, and small of the back;
    - the arms and elbows;
    - the thighs (tucking under to prevent external hip rotation); and
    - the ankles, calves, and knees (to raise the heels off the bed). Be sure to support the knees and calves when raising the ankles.
9. The knees may be flexed and supported with a small pillow or blanket roll.
10. A small pillow or blanket roll may be added at the feet to prevent foot drop. (Use a foot board only if approved by the appropriate provider.)
11. Position or reposition the patient so the body is properly aligned. Then straighten the bed linens.
12. Raise the head of the bed to a level that is appropriate for the position. Lower the bed and raise the bed rails, if needed.
13. Ensure that any tubing the patient may have is carefully handled and reattached, if needed. If there is an IV catheter, be sure it remains intact during the positioning. If there is any concern, ask the appropriate provider to assist by checking that the IV or other tubing is functioning properly after the positioning is completed. If the patient has a foley catheter, which is used to drain urine from the bladder, be sure it is secured below the bladder.

Follow-up

14. Make sure the patient is safe and comfortable. Place the call light and personal items within easy reach.
15. Wash your hands to ensure infection control.

Reporting and Documentation

16. Communicate any specific observations, complications, or unusual responses to the appropriate provider. Also record this information in the patient's chart or EMR.

Turning a Patient

You may be asked to help turn patients for a variety of reasons such as to position the patient, to prepare the patient for transfer to a stretcher, or to provide hygiene care such as washing the patient's back. Always practice safety by asking for assistance from others if the patient is frail, overweight, or has equipment or devices attached to his body, such as tubes or an IV catheter.

Procedure 13.6 Turning a Patient in Bed

Rationale

Turning helps to prevent skin breakdown, promote comfort, and prepare patients for actions such as transfer.

Preparation

1. Assemble the following equipment, as needed:
   - pillows of various sizes, if available and needed for support
   - turning sheet
2. Wash your hands to ensure infection control.
3. Explain in simple terms what you are going to do before turning in bed. Do this even if the patient is unable to communicate or is disoriented.

The Procedure

4. Provide privacy by drawing the bed curtains or putting a screen around the bed.
5. Use proper body mechanics when turning the patient in bed. Raise or lower the bed to a comfortable level for working and lower the bed rails. Lock the wheels of the bed, if needed.
6. To turn a patient, adjust the bed to waist height. The head of the bed should be flat. Follow the doctor's order for turning, if specified.
7. Move any tubes, IVs, or medical devices carefully out of the way before turning the patient.
8. Stand at the side of the bed, lower the bed rail, and face the patient. Put a pillow between the patient's knees (Figure 13.37).
9. If possible, ask the patient to grab the opposite bed rail with her hand on the opposite side (Figure 13.38).
10. Roll the edge of the turning sheet on your side and grab it. Pull the turning sheet up so the patient slowly rolls from her back to her side.
11. Keep the head, torso, and legs in line. The body should stay straight during the turn.
12. Cross the patient's arms over her chest so they are not trapped under the body during the turn (Figure 13.39).

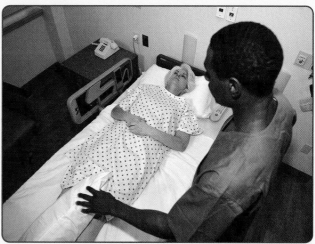

Figure 13.37   *Wards Forest Media, LLC*

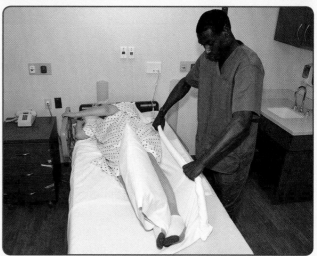

Figure 13.38   *Wards Forest Media, LLC*

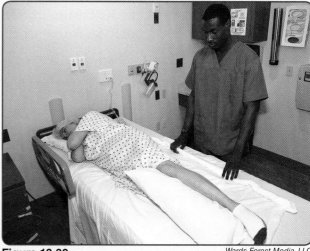

Figure 13.39   *Wards Forest Media, LLC*

Procedure 13.6   Turning a Patient in Bed (continued)

13. Once the patient is turned, place pillows behind the back and buttocks to help keep her on her side comfortably (Figure 13.40).

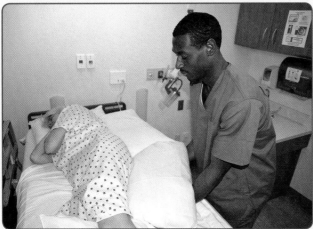

Figure 13.40   Wards Forest Media, LLC

14. Do not drag or pull the patient because doing so can tear or break skin.

15. Turn the patient so her body is properly aligned and then straighten the bed linens. Lower the bed, if needed, and raise the bed rails.

Follow-up

16. Make sure the patient is safe and comfortable. Place the call light and personal items within easy reach.

17. Wash your hands to ensure infection control.

Reporting and Documentation

18. Communicate any specific observations, complications, or unusual responses to the appropriate provider. Also record this information in the patient's chart or EMR.

Transferring a Patient

Transferring patients from their bed to a chair, wheelchair, or stretcher (and back again) is another procedure that requires concentration and safety awareness. Transfer sheets, slides, or roll boards, as well as wood or plastic slide or transfer boards are typically used for bed and stretcher transfers. Gait belts can be useful during transfers to chairs or wheelchairs. For patients who are extremely overweight or cannot bend their bodies, mechanical or electronic lifts may be used.

There are several steps in the transfer procedure. Remember the steps that need to be done prior to the transfer such as washing your hands; greeting the patient; and explaining, in simple terms, what you are planning to do. Ensure that any tubes, medical devices, or IVs are secure enough to transfer with the patient.

Real Life Scenario   What's in a Position?

Mrs. Gallagher, an elderly widow, has suffered a severe stroke. She has been in the hospital for several days and is unable to get out of bed. You have been asked to care for her today and one of your responsibilities is to position and turn her to prevent her from getting a decubitus ulcer. She has had no visitors. Her children live in Europe and her sister, who lives locally, is much older and cannot visit. As a result of her stroke, Mrs. Gallagher cannot speak and is paralyzed on her left side. When you enter her room, she is restless and looks very depressed.

Apply It

1. What actions should you take to be sure you are positioning and turning Mrs. Gallagher correctly?

2. What can you say and do for Mrs. Gallagher to help her feel more comfortable?

The following guidelines should be followed when transferring a patient to a chair or wheelchair:

- Position the chair or wheelchair close to the bed. Be sure the chair is stabilized or the wheelchair wheels are locked. If you are using a wheelchair, also remove the armrest nearest to the bed and swing both leg rests out of the way.

- Help the patient turn over in the bed toward you. Put an arm under the patient's neck with your hand supporting the shoulder blade. Put your other hand under the patient's knees (Figure 13.41).

- Swing the patient's legs over the edge of the bed. Help her to sit up, and then have her move to the edge of the bed. Wait a few minutes before the next step to give the patient time to adjust to the sitting position.

- Put your arms around the patient's chest and clasp your hands behind the patient's back (Figure 13.42). Alternatively, you may use a gait belt.

- Support the patient's leg farthest from the wheelchair between your legs, lean back, shift your weight, and lift (Figure 13.43). Avoid injuring your back by bending your knees and keeping your back straight.

- Pivot toward the chair as you continue to clasp your hands around the patient. You may want to have someone assist by supporting the wheelchair or patient from behind.

- As the patient moves toward you, bend your knees and lower the patient into the chair or wheelchair.

The following are guidelines for transferring a patient from a bed to a stretcher or stretcher to bed. This transfer requires two healthcare workers.

- Lower the side rails of the bed and position the stretcher as close as possible to the bed.

- Adjust the stretcher so it is at a working height and adjust the bed to the same level as the stretcher. Ensure the stability of the bed and stretcher by locking the brakes on each.

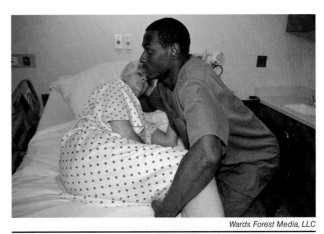
Wards Forest Media, LLC

Figure 13.41   Support the patient's head and neck as you begin moving her into a seated position.

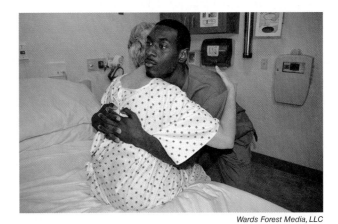
Wards Forest Media, LLC

Figure 13.42   Wrap your arms around the patient to ensure you have a strong grasp as you continue the transfer.

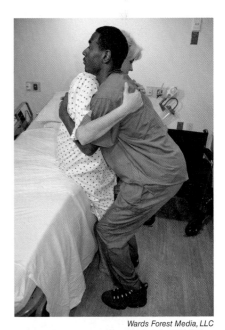
Wards Forest Media, LLC

Figure 13.43   Observe proper body mechanics as you begin lifting the patient from bed.

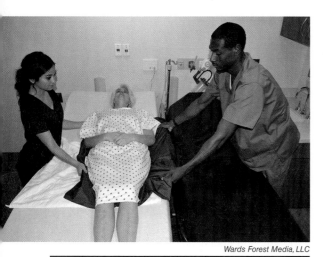

Wards Forest Media, LLC

Figure 13.44 With the transfer sheet beneath her, the patient is prepared for healthcare workers to begin moving her from the bed to the stretcher.

- With the bed and stretcher close together, stand on the side where the patient will be moving (Figure 13.44). The stretcher will be positioned between your body and the patient's bed. The other healthcare worker should be standing on the other side of the patient's bed.

- If there is a gap between the bed and the stretcher, use a plastic or wood slide board (also called a *transfer board*) to fill the open space.

- Lay the transfer sheet or slide at the back of the patient from the shoulder down to the hips. If the patient is too weak to move his head, adjust the sheet so it will also support the head.

- Ask the patient to move closer to the edge of the stretcher or bed he is on, so that he is closer to the surface to which he'll be transferred.

- Ask the patient to do as much of the transfer as possible. If the patient is too weak, grasp the transfer sheet firmly and instruct the patient to tuck his chin to his chest to avoid hyper-extending his neck as he is lifted from the bed. Also be aware of arm placement. If the patient is unable to assist in the transfer, have him place his arms across his chest.

- Prepare the patient and other healthcare worker for the lift and transfer. Count to three and then begin the transfer. You will usually transfer the lower body of the patient first and then move the upper body second. Some patients require the lift to occur in one motion to prevent any further injury.

- Cover the patient with a sheet or blanket. Elevate the side rails of the stretcher or bed and release the brake. Make sure the patient's body is in alignment and that she is comfortable. Wash your hands to ensure infection control.

Lifting a Patient

Lifting patients from their bed to a chair, wheelchair, or stretcher is a procedure that requires concentration and safety awareness. It also requires special training. General lifting, as described in positioning and transferring, usually requires manual equipment and good body mechanics.

Lifting those who are overweight or frail may require a device that uses slings and mechanical or electronic equipment. In some states and facilities, only healthcare workers over the age of 18, or those who have had special training, may operate mechanical or electronic lifting devices.

Remember the tasks that need to be done prior to lifting, such as washing your hands; greeting the patient; and explaining, in simple terms, what you are planning to do. Ensure that any tubes, medical devices, or IV catheters are secure enough to remain intact during the lift.

Next, determine any possible limitations on your involvement with the procedure if it involves the use of mechanical or electronic lifts. Are you old enough?

Have you received the proper training? Healthcare workers who are able to use mechanical or electronic lifts should pay attention to the following guidelines:

- Follow all directions given by the appropriate provider and the equipment instructions.

- Be sure the equipment is in working order and that the type of the sling being used is appropriate and the right size for the patient.

- This procedure requires assistance. At least two healthcare workers will be needed.

- Always ensure the bed, stretcher, or wheelchair (depending on the required lift), and the lifting equipment have locked wheels.

- Carefully place the sling, making sure the lower part is behind the patient's knees, with the upper part beneath the patient's upper shoulder.

- The lift frame must be in an open position and any open hooks should be turned away from the patient.

- Be sure all attachments between the sling and the device are secure.

- Ask the patient to fold his arms across his chest. Lift the patient away as the other healthcare worker supports his legs.

- Position the patient above the chair, wheelchair, or stretcher and gently lower him as he is being guided by the other healthcare worker.

- Make sure the patient's feet and hands are in a comfortable position, and then lower the lift's bar so that you can easily unhook the sling. The sling is usually left beneath the patient if another lift is anticipated.

- Position the patient's feet and hands and cover them with a blanket, if needed. Be sure he is positioned appropriately and safely. Wash your hands to ensure infection control.

Check Your Understanding ✓

1. How often should a bedridden patient's position be changed?
2. Describe the stages of decubitus ulcers.
3. How can you prevent decubitus ulcers?
4. Describe the lateral position.
5. *True or False?* Any healthcare worker can operate a mechanical lift, regardless of his or her age.

Range-of-Motion Exercises

When a patient is immobile or on long periods of bed rest, there are several exercises that can be used to promote circulation and increased flexibility. These are called *range-of-motion (ROM) exercises*. ROM exercises are standardized, structured movements that help people move each joint through as full a range as possible without causing pain. The goal is for patients to do these exercises themselves; however, patients who experience pain and have diseases or conditions in which they are immobile or injured will need healthcare workers to provide support and assistance.

Types of ROM Exercises

There are three types of range-of-motion exercises. Depending on the patient's abilities, one type or a combination of exercises may be used. The patient's doctor determines which range-of-motion exercises are appropriate.

1. **Active range of motion:** used when there is a full range of motion of one or more parts of the body and the patient does not require physical help to perform exercises. Healthcare workers may need to remind or observe the patient to make sure exercises are being done correctly.

2. **Active-assistive range of motion:** used when the patient needs help with a full range of motion for one or more body parts because the muscles are too weak or stiff. Healthcare workers help with range of motion by encouraging normal muscle function.

3. **Passive range of motion:** used when a patient cannot move one or more body parts. Healthcare workers perform the full range of motion without any help from the patient. Passive exercises will not preserve muscle mass, but they will keep joints flexible.

Active-assistive and passive range-of-motion exercises are done in a slow, gentle manner to avoid hurting the patient or harming joints and bones. If there is pain, the exercises must be stopped and the appropriate provider notified. Sometimes weights are used with active range of motion and active-assistive range of motion. Some patients may also need to wear a splint or brace to support their limbs during their exercises. Parallel bars and gait belts help to provide stability and balance and also assist movement.

Range-of-motion exercises require people to use a variety of body movements. Some of these body movements are described in Figure 13.45.

Contraindications for ROM Exercises

It is important to remember that there may be contraindications for range-of-motion exercises. Range-of-motion exercises may be contraindicated for people with heart and respiratory diseases and conditions, as they may make the heart beat too fast and cause shortness of breath, chest pain, and fatigue. Range-of-motion exercises can also put stress on the soft tissues of joints and on bony structures. Therefore, range-of-motion exercises should not be performed if joints are swollen or inflamed, or if there has been injury to the muscles or bones near the joint.

General Guidelines for ROM Exercises

Before you conduct range-of-motion exercises with a patient, it is important to familiarize yourself with the following general guidelines as well as your facility's policies.

Body Movements		
Movement	**Description**	**Example**
Flexion	the act of bending a joint	bending the arm at the elbow
Extension	the act of straightening a joint	lowering the arm back down at the elbow
Hyperextension	an exaggerated, or extreme, extension	moving the arm from the side so that it extends behind the body
Abduction	lateral (sideways) movement away from the midline (an invisible line running vertically through the body)	moving the leg away from the body
Adduction	lateral movement toward the midline of the body	moving the leg toward the body
Rotation	turning of a body part around an axis, or fixed point	rotating the ankle outward so that the foot moves away from the body
Circumduction	rotating a body part in a complete circle	moving the pointer finger in a circular motion
Supination	rotating a body part from the body	rotating the forearm so that the palm faces upward
Pronation	rotating a body part toward the body	rotating the forearm so that the palm faces downward

Goodheart-Willcox Publisher

Figure 13.45 Body movements can be described using these directional terms.

Create a Schedule

Create a schedule for when range-of-motion exercises should be done. Consulting patients as you plan may make them more willing to participate voluntarily. Always explain what you are going to do before beginning any exercise. Remember to maintain proper body mechanics as you carry out these exercises to avoid hurting or straining yourself.

Range-of-motion exercises should be performed at least twice daily. Doing these exercises as the patient bathes is beneficial because the warm water relaxes the muscles and can reduce muscle spasms. Exercising before bedtime may be another option. Immobile patients must have their joints exercised once every eight hours to prevent contractures. Begin each exercise slowly, using smooth and rhythmic movements appropriate for the patient's condition.

Use the Best Approach

Begin the exercises with the neck and work your way down the body. Put each joint that requires exercise through the range of motion a minimum of three times (five times is preferable). Do not do the exercises to the point of patient fatigue. When passively exercising the joints of the arm or leg, make sure you support that extremity. Never force a joint to the point of pain. Instead, move each joint until you feel slight resistance. Always return the joint to a neutral position when you have completed the exercise.

Pay Attention

You can cause serious injury if you do not perform ROM exercises properly. Check with the appropriate provider for specific instructions or limitations. For example, some facilities do *not* allow healthcare workers to exercise the neck. Remember, only exercise the joints that require exercise, and always stop and notify the appropriate provider if the patient complains of pain.

Think It Through

Think about your own range of motion. Do your joints get enough exercise? Try to flex and extend your head, arms, wrists, fingers, legs, knees, feet, and toes. Were you able to do this easily? If not, which joints were more difficult to move or caused pain? What can you do to make sure your joints are getting enough exercise?

Procedure 13.7 | Range-of-Motion Exercises

Rationale

Range-of-motion exercises are critical to maintain flexibility, preserve movement, and prevent skin inflammation or injury, such as a decubitus ulcer.

Preparation

1. Make sure you have a written doctor's order and instructions from the appropriate provider to perform range-of-motion exercises.
2. Assemble the following equipment:
   - towels and/or bath blankets

   Note: When exercising limbs, perform all of the steps listed here on one side of the body, and then move to the other side.

The Procedure

3. Lower the bed rail near you, if it is up.
4. Position the patient supine (flat on the back).
5. Fanfold the top linens to the foot of the bed. Expose only the body part being exercised.
6. Exercising the neck
   - Exercise the neck *only* if it is allowed by your facility and/or if you have been instructed to do so.
   - Support the patient's head and jaw with both hands (Figure 13.46). The head should be in a neutral position to start.

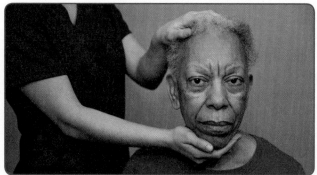

Figure 13.46   *Wards Forest Media, LLC*

- Flexion—bring the head forward (Figure 13.47A). Unless contraindicated, the chin should touch the chest.
- Extension—bring the head back (Figure 13.47B). Avoid hyperextension, or extending the neck beyond its normal limits.

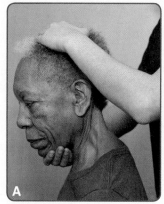
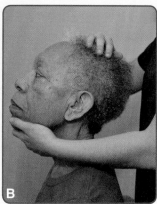

Figure 13.47   *Wards Forest Media, LLC*

- Rotation—turn the head from side to side (Figure 13.48).

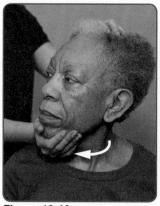
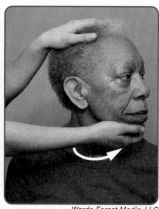

Figure 13.48   *Wards Forest Media, LLC*

- Lateral flexion—move the head to the right and to the left (Figure 13.49).

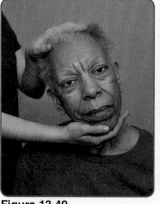
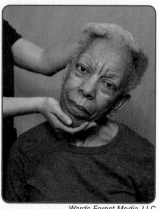

Figure 13.49   *Wards Forest Media, LLC*

7. Exercising the shoulder
   - Grasp and support the patient's wrist with one hand and the elbow with your other hand.
   - Flexion—raise the arm straight out in front of the patient and over the head (Figure 13.50A).
   - Extension—bring the arm down to the side (Figure 13.50B).

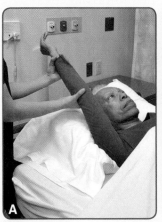
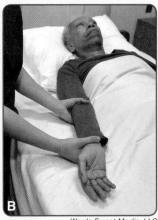

Figure 13.50

Wards Forest Media, LLC

   - Abduction—move the straight arm away from the side of the body (Figure 13.51A).
   - Adduction—move the straight arm to the side of the body (Figure 13.51B).

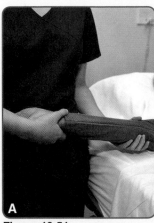
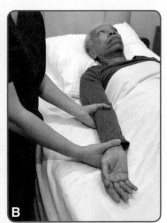

Figure 13.51

Wards Forest Media, LLC

   - Internal rotation—bend the elbow (Figure 13.52A). Unless contraindicated, place the elbow at the same level as the shoulder. Move the forearm down toward the body.
   - External rotation—move the forearm toward the head (Figure 13.52B).

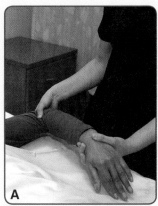
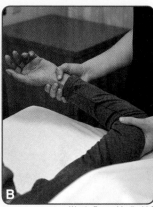

Figure 13.52

Wards Forest Media, LLC

8. Exercising the elbow
   - Grasp and support the patient's wrist with one hand and the elbow with your other hand.
   - Flexion—bend the arm so the same-side shoulder is touched, if possible (Figure 13.53A).
   - Extension—straighten the arm (Figure 13.53B).

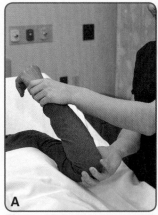
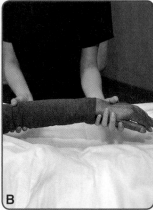

Figure 13.53

Wards Forest Media, LLC

Procedure 13.7   Range-of-Motion Exercises (continued)

9. Exercising the forearm
   - Grasp and support the patient's wrist with one hand and the elbow with your other hand.
   - Pronation—turn the hand so the palm is facing down.
   - Supination—turn the hand so the palm is facing up (Figure 13.54)

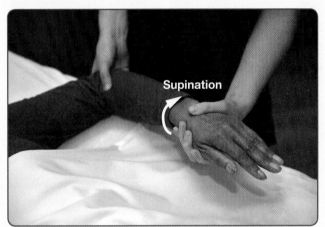

Figure 13.54   *Wards Forest Media, LLC*

10. Exercising the wrist
    - Hold the wrist with both of your hands.
    - Flexion—bend the hand down.
    - Extension—straighten the hand (Figure 13.55).

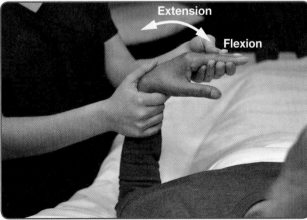

Figure 13.55   *Wards Forest Media, LLC*

   - Radial flexion—with the hand straight up, turn the hand toward the thumb approximately 20°, as if the patient is waving.
   - Ulnar flexion—with the hand straight up, turn the hand toward the little finger approximately 30°.

11. Exercising the thumb
    - Hold the patient's hand with one hand and grasp the patient's thumb with your other hand.
    - Abduction—move the thumb out, away from the index finger (Figure 13.56A).
    - Adduction—move the thumb in, toward the index finger (Figure 13.56B).

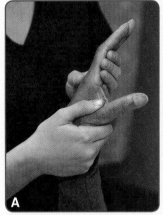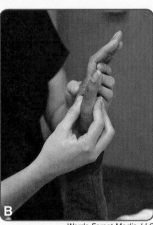

Figure 13.56   *Wards Forest Media, LLC*

   - Opposition—touch each fingertip with the thumb (Figure 13.57).

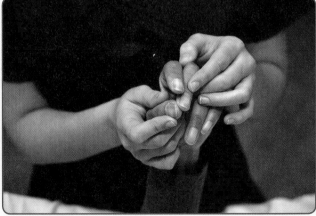

Figure 13.57   *Wards Forest Media, LLC*

- Flexion—bend the thumb into the hand (Figure 13.58A).
- Extension—move the thumb out to the side of the fingers (Figure 13.58B).

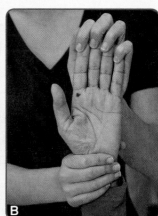
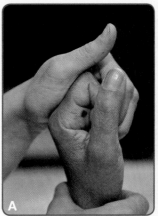

Figure 13.60   *Wards Forest Media, LLC*

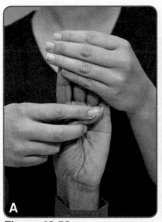
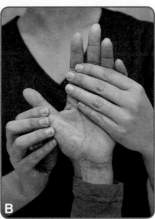

Figure 13.58   *Wards Forest Media, LLC*

12. Exercising the fingers

- Abduction—spread the fingers and the thumb apart (Figure 13.59A).
- Adduction—bring the fingers and thumb together (Figure 13.59B).

13. Exercising the hip

- Support the leg by placing one hand under the patient's leg and your other hand under the patient's knee.
- Flexion—raise the leg and bend the knee (Figure 13.61A).
- Extension—straighten the leg (Figure 13.61B).

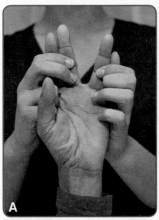
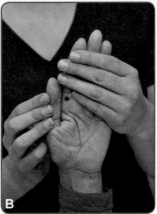

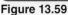
Figure 13.59   *Wards Forest Media, LLC*

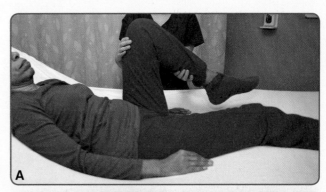

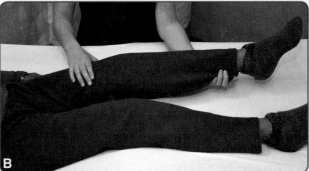

- Flexion—curl the fingers up to make a fist (Figure 13.60A).
- Extension—open the hand so the fingers, hand, and arm are straight (Figure 13.60B).

Figure 13.61   *Wards Forest Media, LLC*

Procedure 13.7   Range-of-Motion Exercises (continued)

- Abduction—move the leg away from the body (Figure 13.62A).
- Adduction—move the leg toward the other leg (Figure 13.62B).

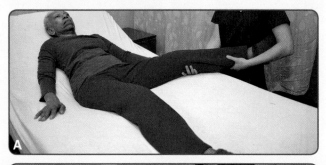

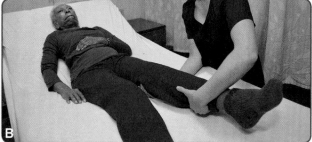

Figure 13.62   *Wards Forest Media, LLC*

- Internal rotation—turn the leg inward (Figure 13.63A).
- External rotation—turn the leg outward (Figure 13.63B).

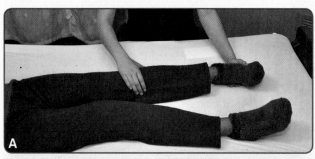

Figure 13.63   *Wards Forest Media, LLC*

14. Exercising the knee
- Support the knee by placing one hand under the patient's knee and your other hand under the patient's ankle.
- Flexion—bend the knee (Figure 13.64A).
- Extension—straighten the knee (Figure 13.64B).

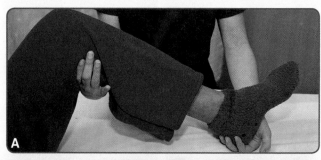

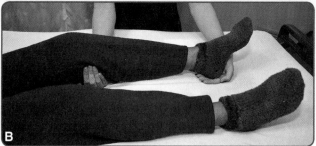

Figure 13.64   *Wards Forest Media, LLC*

15. Exercising the ankle
- Support the foot and ankle by placing one hand under the patient's foot and your other hand under the patient's ankle.
- Dorsal flexion—pull the foot forward; push down on the heel at the same time (Figure 13.65A).
- Plantar flexion—turn the foot down or point the toes (Figure 13.65B).

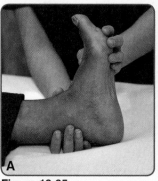
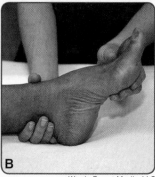

Figure 13.65   *Wards Forest Media, LLC*

16. Exercising the foot
    - Support the foot and ankle by placing one hand under the patient's foot and your other hand under the patient's ankle.
    - Pronation—turn the outside of the foot up and the inside down (Figure 13.66A).
    - Supination—turn the inside of the foot up and the outside down (Figure 13.66B).

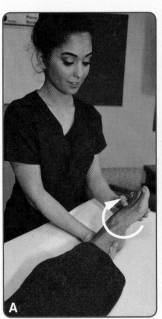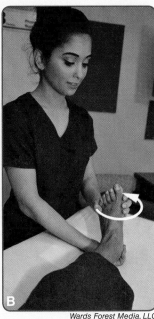

Figure 13.66   *Wards Forest Media, LLC*

17. Exercising the toes
    - Flexion—curl the toes (Figure 13.67A).
    - Extension—straighten the toes (Figure 13.67B).

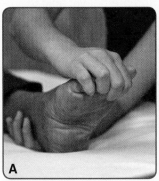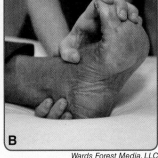

Figure 13.67   *Wards Forest Media, LLC*

- Abduction—spread the toes apart (Figure 13.68).
- Adduction—pull the toes together.

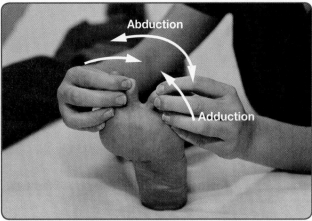

Figure 13.68   *Wards Forest Media, LLC*

18. Cover the patient's leg and raise the bed rail, if used.
19. Go to the other side of the bed and lower the bed rail, if it is up.
20. Repeat these exercises for the other side of the body from the shoulder down.

Follow-up

21 Make sure the patient is safe and comfortable. Place the call light and personal items within easy reach. Lower the bed and raise the bed rails, if needed.
22. Wash your hands to ensure infection control.

Reporting and Documentation

23. Communicate any specific observations, complications, or unusual responses to the appropriate provider. Also record this information in the patient's chart or EMR.

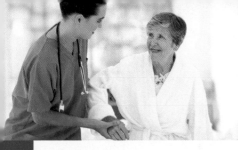

Chapter 13
Review and Assessment

Summary

Regular exercise and movement has many benefits, including contributing to a healthy body and well-being. A joint that has not moved sufficiently can begin to stiffen within 24 hours and will eventually become inflexible and cause immobility. Long periods of joint immobility may also negatively affect tendons and muscles, making it particularly important for healthcare workers to regularly assist patients with ambulation and range of motion.

Body alignment is the optimal placement of body parts so that bones and muscles are used efficiently and remain functional, healthy, and stress free. Body alignment is needed for correct posture. This is true for both patients and healthcare workers who, if not using proper body mechanics, may develop musculoskeletal disorders.

Helping patients ambulate is an important part of a healthcare worker's daily responsibilities. Ambulation improves circulation and muscle tone, preserves lung tissue and airway function, and helps promote muscle and joint mobility.

Before assisting a patient with ambulation, check if he or she needs medication for pain; assemble appropriate equipment and supplies; solicit the help of a coworker, if needed; be sure you understand the procedures fully; create a safe environment; show patients what to do; and help him or her during the procedure. Remember safety precautions in case a patient begins to collapse.

Some people require assistive devices to ambulate, which can include canes, crutches, and walkers. Which device is used typically depends on how much support is needed.

Another responsibility of healthcare workers is monitoring and changing patient or resident positions. This may include positioning a patient in bed, lifting the patient, or helping a patient into a wheelchair. Some patients may need to be repositioned more often. Changing positions increases patient comfort; helps them relax; improves body functions; corrects deformities such as atrophy; and relieves pressure and strain on the skin, preventing the formation of decubitus ulcers.

When a patient is immobile or on long periods of bed rest, range-of-motion exercises (ROM) are used to promote circulation, prevent decubitus ulcers, and increase flexibility. ROM exercises are standardized, structured body part movements. The goal is for patients to do ROM themselves; however, some patients need support and assistance. There are three types of ROM depending on a patient's abilities: active, active-assistive, and passive.

Review Questions

Answer the following questions using what you have learned in this chapter.

True or False Assess

1. *True or False?* A joint can be exercised as many times as a healthcare worker decides will be helpful for better mobility.

2. *True or False?* One way to prevent a decubitus ulcer is to keep the skin clean and dry.

3. *True or False?* During the ballistic phase of walking, both feet are off the ground.

4. *True or False?* When getting a patient ready to use a walker, the walker should be placed about one step ahead of the seated patient.

5. *True or False?* To turn a patient, adjust the bed to waist height. The head of the bed should be flat.

6. *True or False?* A transfer sheet stretches from the patient's waist down to his hips.

7. *True or False?* When a treatment is contraindicated, it means it is one that is desirable.

8. *True or False?* The tripod position means that crutch tips are placed two to three inches in front of the patient's feet.

9. *True or False?* A cane is most useful for patients who have had surgery and are not yet able to maintain balance or need extra stability.

Multiple Choice Assess

10. The main purpose of positioning and turning is to _____.

    A. avoid low blood pressure

    B. provide daily exercise

    C. decrease pressure on body parts

    D. create stimulation

11. Mr. Deng's doctor has written an order that states he can use a walker. You have been assigned to help him walk his first time. First, he should _____.

   A. touch the heel of his foot to the ground

   B. put the walker one step ahead

   C. step all the way to the front of the walker

   D. lift his toes off the ground on the first step

12. Healthcare workers can help patients perform active ROM exercises by _____.

   A. instructing how to perform the range of motion

   B. informing the patient that he should be mobile when home

   C. taking the patient outdoors so he can have fresh air

   D. moving the patient in his wheelchair to the dining room

13. Which device is used to maintain proper foot alignment when in bed?

   A. headboard

   B. backboard

   C. transfer board

   D. foot board

14. Healthcare workers should always lift and move patients on the count of _____.

   A. five

   B. two

   C. three

   D. four

15. When Linda, a healthcare worker, was asked to lift the patient in Room 525, she knew she would need to use good body mechanics. Which of the following should she *not* do?

   A. bend over the patient

   B. push, not pull

   C. stay close to the patient

   D. take small breaks

16. Which of the following statements about range-of-motion (ROM) exercises is *true*?

   A. ROM exercises should be done once a day.

   B. ROM exercises help prevent strokes and paralysis.

   C. ROM exercises are often performed during ADLs such as bathing or dressing.

   D. ROM exercises require at least 10 repetitions of each exercise.

17. When ambulating, a gait belt is often _____.

   A. worn around the nurse assistant's waist for back support

   B. used to keep the patient positioned properly

   C. used to help stand the patient, and then removed before walking

   D. put around the patient's waist to provide a way to hold onto the patient

Short Answer

18. What are two benefits of having a proper posture?

19. What types of disorders are healthcare workers at risk of developing? When do these injuries typically occur?

20. What is good body alignment?

21. Describe the three stages of patient ambulation.

22. List three actions that help you prepare to assist with ambulation.

23. Why is it important for patients to change positions?

24. What are three safety guidelines to follow when positioning or moving a patient?

25. What areas of the body are more likely to develop decubitus ulcers?

26. Explain the guidelines for transferring a patient.

27. Identify the difference between flexion and extension.

Critical Thinking Exercises

28. Find and read one article that discusses current research on two best safety practices for healthcare workers to use when assisting patients with ambulation and discuss how this information can be used in a healthcare facility.

29. Answer the following question by doing research. "Do people who run regularly have good body alignment, mechanics, and posture?" Give the rationale for your findings.

30. Describe words of encouragement and support you can use when helping patients with their ambulation or when conducting range-of-motion exercises. Discuss why this type of communication is helpful.

31. You are caring for Mrs. Garrett, who recently had a stroke. She does not speak well and has paralysis on her left side. She has a large family and they want to be as helpful as possible. What can you do and say to them to include them in Mrs. Garrett's care?

Chapter 14
Working in Healthcare

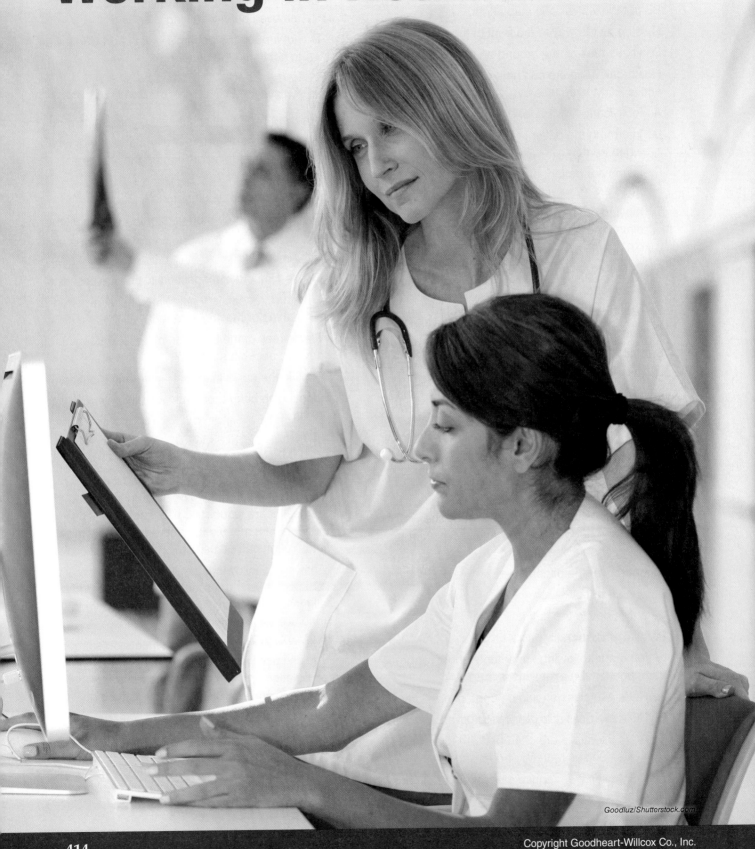

Goodluz/Shutterstock.com

Terms to Know

 Build Vocab

delegate	ophthalmoscope	plaque
discharge plan	oral prophylaxis	speculum
laryngeal mirror	otoscope	

Chapter Objectives

- Examine the roles, responsibilities, and required education and training of selected healthcare careers.
- Compare and contrast procedures performed by various healthcare workers who provide direct care.
- Discuss the differences between healthcare facility admission, transfer, and discharge.
- Demonstrate the admission, transfer, and discharge procedures.
- Gather the equipment and perform the steps needed to prepare for a physical examination.
- Perform the actions necessary to safely fill a prescription.
- Use the teaching guidelines to instruct patients on proper oral care.
- Demonstrate positioning a person who is unconscious.

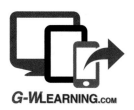

While studying, look for the activity icon to:

- **Build** vocabulary with e-flash cards and interactive games.
- **Assess** progress with chapter and unit review questions.
- **Expand** learning with animations and illustration labeling activities.
- **Simulate** EHR entry with healthcare documents.

www.g-wlearning.com/healthsciences/

There are many career opportunities in healthcare that allow you to provide direct care to patients in a variety of healthcare facilities. Chapter 1 provided an overview and description of these different healthcare facilities. In chapter 2, you began exploring various healthcare career pathways that may interest you. These include the therapeutic, diagnostic, health informatics, support services, and biotechnology research and development pathways. You learned about career possibilities in each of these pathways.

This chapter examines, in more detail, careers that emphasize the therapeutic services pathway. Procedures in which you will have direct, hands-on experiences with patients are also introduced. The focus of these careers is to deliver direct care to patients to help them improve their health and well-being.

The career paths examined more closely in this chapter are nursing assistant, patient care technician, health unit coordinator (HUC), medical assistant, dental assistant, pharmacy technician, physical therapy assistant, and emergency medical technician (EMT). Each of these healthcare workers uses unique knowledge, skills, and abilities to deliver safe and competent care. Each career path has a specific education and training program. For some, there is a requirement for licensure or certification.

While each of these healthcare workers offers a unique contribution to care, some learn and perform several of the same procedures. For example, all direct healthcare workers are expected to be able to perform cardiopulmonary resuscitation (CPR) and first aid. Nursing assistants, medical assistants, and EMTs all learn how to take vital signs (temperature, pulse, respiration, and blood pressure). Nursing assistants, medical assistants, and physical therapy assistants help patients exercise and ambulate. Nursing assistants, patient care technicians, and HUCs can admit, transfer, and discharge patients.

No matter what their roles and responsibilities are, all healthcare workers must have passion for and the desire to help others. It is essential to always maintain infection control. You must properly wash your hands to help prevent the spread of infection and wear personal protective equipment (PPE) such as masks, gloves, and a gown when necessary. Maintaining a safe environment free from potential safety hazards is also important.

To learn how these selected healthcare workers can provide their own unique care while also sharing the same procedures, a brief review of their roles and responsibilities, as well as the education, training, and certification they require follows.

Nursing Assistant

Nursing assistants care for patients under the supervision of licensed nurses, registered nurses (RNs), or licensed practical/vocational nurses (LPNs or LVNs). Nursing assistants work in healthcare facilities such as hospitals, long-term care facilities, hospices, or specialty clinics.

Providing direct patient care is a nursing assistant's number one responsibility. This includes activities of daily living (ADL) such as bathing, grooming, dressing, eating, toileting, lifting, moving, positioning, ambulating (walking), and exercising (Figure 14.1). These workers may assist in dressing and undressing those who are unable to do this for themselves. Other important responsibilities include setting up meals, feeding patients and residents, documenting what and how much is eaten, and recording the level of fluid intake.

Another important responsibility is measuring, recording, and reporting vital signs and height and weight. Nursing assistants also apply non-sterile dressings; provide skin and oral care; and admit, transfer, and discharge patients. Nursing assistants collect specimens from patients to assist in diagnosing their illnesses or evaluating how well they are progressing. Specimen samples collected may include feces (stool), urine, hair, and swabs from wounds or infection sites on the body.

Nursing assistants are often the first to communicate with those they care for and their families. This is because nursing assistants spend most of their work time at a patient's bedside, making sure all daily needs are met. Nursing assistants are also responsible for recording necessary information in electronic or paper charts, answering the telephone, and taking messages.

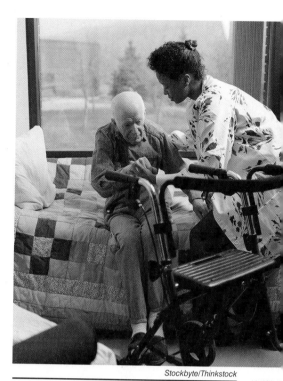

Stockbyte/Thinkstock

Figure 14.1 Nursing assistants work closely with patients.

In 1987, Congress passed the Omnibus Budget Reconciliation Act (OBRA), standardizing the minimum requirements for certified nursing assistant training programs and evaluation. OBRA regulations are specific to nursing assistants working in nursing homes that receive federal funding. Today, nursing assistant education and training courses that lead to certification must continue to meet OBRA standards. Since OBRA was passed, states have taken the responsibility of making sure education and training programs meet these standards and also provide the process for obtaining certification.

Requirements for education, training, and certification may vary from state to state, as will scope of practice. Some nursing assistant programs are located in high schools where students may take the training program during their senior year. Other programs are located in private and community colleges where a high school diploma or GED may be required. Classroom instruction ranges from a minimum of 75 hours to over 150 hours. Supervised clinical training may be 24 hours or more in long-term care facilities. In addition, some programs include hospital and other related clinical experiences.

Upon completion of a state-approved education and training program, the graduate is expected to take a certification examination offered by the state. The examination consists of a written portion and a hands-on clinical skill demonstration. After successfully passing this examination, the nursing assistant becomes certified and is usually called a *certified nursing assistant* (CNA).

Patient Care Technician

Like nursing assistants, patient care technicians also work under the supervision of licensed nurses. They work in healthcare facilities such as hospitals, long-term care facilities, hospices, and clinics.

Patient care technicians perform some of the same tasks as a nursing assistant, such as ADLs and vital signs. In addition to the nursing assistant responsibilities, a patient care technician may also draw blood (phlebotomy) or help perform EKGs or ECGs after receiving specialized training (Figure 14.2). They may also assist other healthcare providers, such as helping a doctor with a physical examination. Patient care technicians may perform administrative tasks such as answering telephones; processing orders for admission, discharge, or transfer; and scheduling diagnostic tests.

Many healthcare facilities require that patient care technicians first become nursing assistants and earn their certification (CNA). Additional training such as drawing blood and performing ECGs are often learned at the healthcare facility through on-the-job training programs. Other healthcare facilities require only the completion of a formal patient care training program available through the state or on-the-job training. This career path does not require certification or licensure unless the person must be a CNA before becoming a patient care technician.

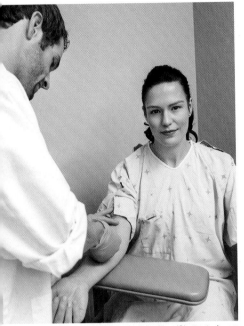

Tyler Olson/Shutterstock.com

Figure 14.2 A patient care technician may be asked to draw a patient's blood, which is a skill that can be learned through on-the-job training.

Health Unit Coordinator (HUC)

The health unit coordinator (HUC), sometimes known as a *unit secretary* or *unit clerk*, is trained to "run the desk." This means the HUC is responsible for overseeing the administrative and support functions of a healthcare facility, usually a hospital or long-term care facility. The responsibilities of a health unit coordinator may include processing doctors' orders; ordering dietary trays; scheduling X-rays; and processing orders for admission, discharge, or transfer within the facility or to other healthcare facilities (Figure 14.3).

HUCs often receive training at a technical school or community college. Some have a high school diploma and are trained on the job. HUCs work closely with nursing assistants and patient care technicians.

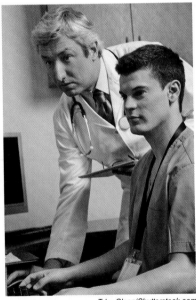

Tyler Olson/Shutterstock.com

Figure 14.3 Health unit coordinators work closely with healthcare providers to ensure the unit's administrative tasks are completed accurately and efficiently.

Admission, Transfer, and Discharge

The various people responsible for admission, transfer, and discharge include doctors, who write the orders; licensed nurses, who are responsible for carrying out the doctor's orders; and healthcare workers, to whom licensed nurses **delegate** the actual procedure. These workers may be nursing assistants, patient care technicians, or health unit coordinators (HUC).

delegate
to assign the accountability and responsibility of one's task to another worker

When people are admitted to hospitals, they are called *patients*. When they are admitted to long-term care facilities, they are called *residents* because their stay is typically much longer. For some, this stay lasts until the end of their lives. In other settings, such as in community or public health, and also in therapeutic relationships, people might be called *clients*.

Healthcare facilities usually follow similar procedures for admission, transfer, and discharge. However, some have procedures specific to the facility, such as rehabilitation or outpatient surgery. Other facilities may include special forms or have additional steps unique to their policies. As a result, you will need to learn the general procedures, as well as any specific procedures observed at your facility.

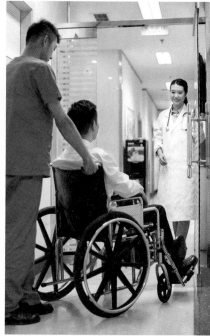

XiXinXing/Shutterstock.com

Figure 14.4 Hospital admissions may be completed by a single healthcare worker, but sometimes the responsibility is shared among a health unit coordinator, patient care technician, and nursing assistant.

> ## Did You Know? Admissions to US Healthcare Facilities
>
> Each year, there are an estimated 35 million admissions in US Registered Hospitals (American Hospital Association). A recent estimate by the CDC revealed that there are also 1.4 million residents in long-term care facilities.

Admission

Admission occurs when people have serious illnesses or conditions, or if they can no longer take care of themselves. They are usually admitted into (enter) a hospital or long-term care facility. In hospitals, there are two major types of admissions: emergency and elective. Emergency admission occurs when someone goes to the emergency room. From there, the person may be admitted to the hospital. Elective admission usually occurs if a person has a scheduled procedure or surgery (Figure 14.4). Sometimes people are admitted to a hospital because they need to be observed for a short period of time until a decision is made about their condition or illness.

Specific policies and procedures are used to collect needed information and prepare for admission. Sometimes one healthcare worker completes the entire admission process. Other times, it is a shared responsibility in which the paperwork is completed by a HUC and the room is prepared by a nursing assistant or patient care technician.

The information needed for admission usually includes personal information, employment, closest relative, insurance carriers, reason for admission, allergies, and medications the person may be taking. There are also other forms for signature, such as privacy practices and treatment agreements. This procedure also focuses on making sure people are oriented to, and made comfortable in, the facility and their room; that they are aware of their rights; and that the room is prepared with needed supplies and equipment.

Expand

Hospitals usually have an admissions kit that includes a water pitcher, cup, basin, and other hygiene items such as toothpaste and brush, soap, and lotion (Figure 14.5). In long-term care facilities, the admissions kit might not include hygiene items such as a toothbrush or paste, as residents often bring their own. Once patients or residents are settled into their room, treatments ordered by their doctors are started. Admissions documents are used to aid in collecting necessary information. A clothing and personal belongings list is also a part of the admissions process and is completed to safeguard items that remain in the facility.

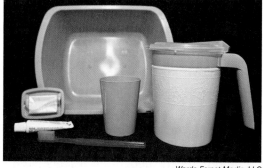

Wards Forest Media, LLC

Figure 14.5   A basic hospital admissions kit

Procedure 14.1   Admission to a Healthcare Facility

Rationale

The admission process allows healthcare workers to gather necessary information about patients or residents and orient them to the healthcare facility and their room.

Preparation

1. Obtain the admission forms for the patient or resident. You may have to ask the appropriate provider for these forms. In some facilities, admissions forms are filled out electronically using a tablet, laptop, or computer on wheels.

2. Wash your hands to ensure infection control.

3. Assemble the following equipment:
   - admissions kit, including a wash basin, water pitcher and cup, toothbrush, toothpaste, soap, and other items
   - a bed pan and urinal (for men)
   - instruments for measuring vital signs, such as a thermometer, sphygmomanometer, and stethoscope
   - towels and washcloths
   - an IV pole, if needed
   - any other items requested by the licensed nurse

4. Place the thermometer, sphygmomanometer, and stethoscope at the bedside, and place admission forms on the over-bed table.

5. Place the water pitcher and cup within reach of the bed.

6. Leave an empty urine specimen container for collection of a sample, if ordered by the doctor. Unless otherwise directed, the container can be left by the sink in the bathroom for later collection of the specimen.

7. Place the following items in the bedside stand:
   - an admissions kit
   - a bedpan and urinal
   - a gown or pajamas
   - towels and washcloths

8. Prepare the bed by pulling back the bed covers and adjusting the bed position to a level that is easy for the patient to sit down and enter the bed.

9. Attach the call light to the bed linens and place it within the patient's reach (Figure 14.6).

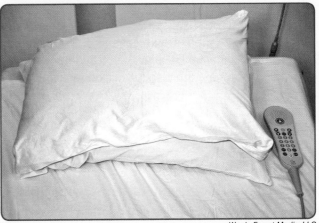

Figure 14.6   *Wards Forest Media, LLC*

The Procedure

10. When the patient arrives at the room, check the patient's name with the admission forms.

11. Place an identification band on the patient's wrist if she is not already wearing one.

12. Explain the admission process in simple terms before and during the procedure. It is important to provide privacy. If family members or friends are present, determine whether they will stay during the admission process.

13. Ask the patient the questions on the admissions forms if they have not already been completed. If the patient is disoriented or unable to answer your questions, you may ask an accompanying family member your questions.

14. If the patient will have a roommate, make introductions.

15 Let the patient stay dressed, if approved, or help her change into a gown or pajamas.

16. Help the patient into bed or a chair, as directed by the appropriate provider.

17. The licensed nurse will usually be doing a patient assessment. Assist with the assessment by taking vital signs and measuring height and weight.

18. Complete the clothing and personal belongings list (per facility policy). Along with the appropriate provider, sign the list to verify which belongings have been left in the room, or if any valuables have been put into the facility's safe. If you are in a long-term care facility, label the resident's belongings.

19. Unless a family member or friend wishes to assist, put away the clothes and personal items.

20. Explain any ordered activity limits such as bed rest or ambulation restrictions.

21. Explain when meals are served and how to request snacks.

22. If oral fluids are allowed per doctor's orders, fill the water pitcher and cup.

23. Provide a denture cup, if needed, and label it with the patient's name, room number, and bed number. If handling dentures, wash your hands before and after to ensure infection control.

Follow-up

24. Make sure the patient is safe and comfortable. Place the bed in its lowest position and be sure the wheels are locked. Place the call light and personal items within easy reach.

25. Wash your hands to ensure infection control.

Reporting and Documentation

26. Communicate any specific observations, complications, or unusual responses to the appropriate provider. Also record this information in the patient's chart or EMR.

Transfer

When a patient's condition changes, he may be transferred to a different location in the same healthcare facility or to another facility entirely. For example, if a patient had a serious car accident, the hospital stay may end when his condition is stabilized but he is not ready to go home. The patient may lack mobility due to broken bones and a head injury, and he may not be able to fully dress or bathe without help. As a result, the patient would likely be transferred to a rehabilitation center for physical or occupational therapy to help him regain limited or lost function.

Transfer is voluntary. Prior to a transfer, patients are provided the opportunity to accept or refuse the transfer. If a transfer is refused, the patient is usually discharged with documentation stating that they refused the transfer against the recommendation of the healthcare provider.

Forms are also used for this procedure. Like admission, transfers are conducted based on the doctor's written orders. Licensed nurses may delegate transfer responsibilities to nursing assistants, patient care technicians, or health unit coordinators. A staff member from social services often assists patients and their families in locating a facility that will meet their treatment needs and is covered by their insurance. Transfer forms usually request information about the facility that has been selected for transfer, patient diagnosis, medications being taken, treatments being provided, allergies, physical and mental assessments, level of independence, safety concerns, and a list of valuables.

Expand

As a healthcare worker, you may find that some patients become frightened during a transfer procedure, such as the elderly who may not understand the reasons for the transfer. It is essential that you stay calm and reassure and reorient the patient as necessary. Seek assistance from a coworker to help with a transfer, if needed.

If the transfer occurs between units in a facility, the patient is accompanied by a healthcare worker to the new unit. The healthcare worker checks in with the licensed nurse on the new unit and transfers the patient's paper chart, if it has not already been sent electronically.

If the transfer is to another facility, a licensed nurse will contact the new facility about the patient's arrival. A healthcare worker accompanies the patient to the transport vehicle, where transport workers then take the responsibility for the patient; the patient's documents, such as the chart; and any belongings and valuables not taken by the family.

Procedure 14.2   Transfer within a Healthcare Facility or to Another Facility

Rationale

Following this procedure will ensure smooth and safe care when it is necessary for a patient or resident to be moved to another location in the healthcare facility or to a different healthcare facility.

Preparation

1. Check to be sure there are written doctor's orders for transfer to another unit or facility.

2. Prepare the patient for the transfer by explaining what is about to happen. This can help to decrease any anxiety and stress they may be feeling.

3. Healthcare workers must provide patients with information about the transfer and give them the right to refuse it. If the transfer is refused, discharge from the healthcare facility is discussed.

The Procedure

4. Assist in moving or packing the patient's belongings and any needed equipment.

5. Manually transport the patient's paper chart to the new unit, enter the information about the transfer into the EMR, or prepare needed documentation for transfer to the new facility, depending on the situation.

6. Monitor vital signs during the transfer per the facility's policy and instructions given by the appropriate provider.

7. If you are transferring the patient to a unit within the same facility, alert the appropriate provider that the patient has arrived.

Follow-up

8. Make sure the patient is safe and comfortable. If transferring within the same facility, make sure the bed in the new unit is in its lowest position. Place the call light and personal items within easy reach. If not in the same facility, make sure the patient is moved safely into the transport vehicle.

9. Wash your hands to ensure infection control.

Reporting and Documentation

10. Communicate any specific observations, complications, or unusual responses to the appropriate provider. Also record this information in the patient's chart or EMR.

Discharge

Patients are discharged from (leave) a healthcare facility to go home when their health has improved and they have the ability and resources to take care of themselves. A nursing assistant, patient care technician, or health unit coordinator may conduct the discharge based on orders from a doctor and delegation by the licensed nurse. Sometimes a transportation aide or volunteer will take the patient to the waiting vehicle once the discharge is completed in the room.

Expand A discharge form must be completed before a patient can leave. Discharge forms are used to ensure all of the necessary information is retrieved, which usually includes patient personal information, medical diagnoses, insurance carrier, and a clothing and personal belongings list. This form is signed by the doctor in charge.

Expand In addition to the discharge forms, there is also a **discharge plan**, which provides instructions for medications, activity levels, treatments to continue at home, and when to next visit the doctor.

Practice safety during the discharge process, such as making sure the patient does not trip or fall while getting ready to leave and safely moving the patient from the discharge wheelchair to the patient's transport vehicle (Figure 14.7). Get assistance from a coworker, if needed.

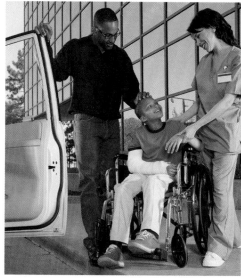

Blend Images/Shutterstock.com

Figure 14.7   Once discharged from a healthcare facility, the patient should be escorted to his vehicle by a healthcare worker.

discharge plan
a set of instructions regarding the patient's treatment and medications for use after leaving a healthcare facility

---

Procedure 14.3   Discharge from a Healthcare Facility

Rationale

The discharge procedure allows healthcare workers to help patients safely and efficiently leave a healthcare facility.

Preparation

1. Check to be sure there are written doctor's orders for discharge.
2. Prepare for the discharge by explaining what is about to happen to the patient. This can help to decrease any anxiety and stress the patient may be feeling.

Procedure

3. Provide privacy by closing the bedside curtains or hospital room door, or by putting up a screen.
4. Help the patient get dressed. Then collect and pack their belongings.

5. Return any valuables that have been kept in the facility's safe. Check the belongings against the list created during admission.
6. During discharge, observe and report issues regarding the patient's ability to complete activities of daily living (ADLs), as well as any concerns or fears, to the appropriate provider.
7. Notify the licensed nurse when the patient is ready for final discharge instructions. The licensed nurse will
   - provide prescriptions written by the doctor;
   - communicate the discharge instructions; and
   - have the patient sign the clothing and personal belongings forms.
8. Help escort the patient in a wheelchair from the facility to the transport vehicle.
9. Lock the wheelchair and assist the patient into the transport vehicle.

(continued)

Procedure 14.3   Discharge from a Healthcare Facility (continued)

10. Help put the belongings into the transport vehicle.

Follow-up

11. Return the wheelchair and cart (if used) to the storage area for cleaning.

12. Hospital housekeepers may share some of the following duties:
    - Strip the bed and clean the room.
    - Clean the wheelchair and cart.
    - Dispose of dirty linen.
    - Make the bed using clean linen.

13. Wash your hands to ensure infection control.

Reporting and Documentation

14. Communicate any specific observations, complications, or unusual responses to the appropriate provider. Also record this information in the patient's chart or EMR.

It is important to learn about and understand the admission, transfer, and discharge procedures so safe, quality, and competent care is given.

Check Your Understanding ✓

1. How are the procedures for admission, transfer, and discharge different?
2. List two examples each of information collected upon admission, transfer, and discharge?
3. What do you need to do to prepare a room for a patient admission?
4. What actions should you take to ensure safety during admission, transfer, and discharge?
5. What can you do to provide support for the patient and family during admission, transfer, and discharge?

Medical Assistant

Medical assistants (MAs) work with doctors and other healthcare workers in doctor's offices and clinics. An important role for MAs is helping patients feel at ease during their office visit. As you learned in chapter 2, front office medical assistants are usually cross-trained to perform administrative and clinical responsibilities. Requirements for education, training, and certification may vary from state to state, as will scope of practice. Medical assistants usually attend a formal training program or complete an educational program that offers an associate's degree, diploma, or certificate of completion. Many states and employers require national certification.

With the emphasis on helping patients to realize their most optimal levels of health and well-being, medical assistants are being trained to help support wellness treatment regimens prescribed by doctors. This has led to many medical assistants expanding their responsibilities to the role of "coach." Under the doctor's supervision, MAs may provide information about treatments and education regarding nutrition and exercise.

Some daily responsibilities typically include

- answering telephones and greeting patients;
- scheduling appointments;
- maintaining medical records;
- coding and filling out insurance forms;
- handling correspondence, billing, and bookkeeping;
- arranging for hospital admissions, laboratory services, and referrals;
- taking brief medical histories;
- explaining basic treatments, medications, and special diets when directed and instructed to by the doctor;
- preparing for physical examinations;
- assisting the doctor during exams (Figure 14.8);
- collecting and preparing laboratory specimens and communicating the results as directed;
- performing basic laboratory tests;
- preparing and administering medications as directed;
- drawing blood;
- performing electrocardiograms;
- removing sutures and changing dressings; and
- authorizing prescription refills as directed.

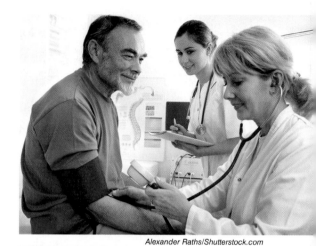

Alexander Raths/Shutterstock.com

Figure 14.8   Assisting a doctor with a physical examination is among the many responsibilities of a medical assistant.

Physical Examination

Physical examinations (sometimes abbreviated PEs) usually take place in medical offices, doctor's offices, or clinics. When performed in a hospital or long-term care facility, a physical examination may occur in a patient's room or an examining room. Medical assistants are usually responsible for preparing a room and the patient for a physical examination; however, nursing assistants or patient care technicians may also be asked to perform this procedure if it is done in a hospital or long-term care facility.

There are several types of physical examinations. These include routine healthcare screening, comprehensive annual exams, pre-employment physicals, travel physicals (may include specific immunizations), well-women and well-baby exams, and physical exams for special diagnostic procedures and examination of specific body parts.

Physical exams are performed to determine the status of a patient's bodily systems and functions. During the physical examination, the doctor, nurse practitioner, or physician assistant will typically take a medical history to determine past and current issues or complaints, and to identify related family conditions, past surgeries and hospitalizations, and current use of medications. Depending on the type of physical, a head-to-toe examination of the body systems is then performed.

Examination Equipment

Different types of equipment are used to conduct a physical examination in addition to tests and screening tools (Figure 14.9). This equipment includes

- a sphygmomanometer, to measure blood pressure;
- a stethoscope, to measure blood pressure, heart and lung sounds, and pulse;
- a flashlight, to examine pupils for dilation;
- a thermometer;
- a tongue depressor, to examine the throat;
- an **otoscope**, to examine the ears;
- an **ophthalmoscope**, to examine the eyes;
- a **laryngeal mirror**, to examine the mouth, tongue, and teeth;
- a tuning fork, to test hearing;
- a percussion or reflex hammer, to tap body parts to test reflexes;
- a vaginal **speculum**, to examine the vagina and other parts of the female reproductive system;
- an eye chart, for vision screening;
- sheets or drapes, to cover the patient;
- a disposable covering for the examination table;
- a container for soiled instruments;
- disposable gloves;
- lubricant; and
- tissues.

Once the physical examination is completed, normal and abnormal results are reviewed by the doctor, nurse practitioner, or physician assistant, and recommendations are given for treatments and follow-up visits.

otoscope
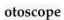
a lighted medical device used to examine the ear and eardrum

ophthalmoscope
a lighted medical device used to examine the interior of the eyes

laryngeal mirror
a device used to examine the mouth, tongue, and teeth

speculum
a medical device designed to enter a body opening such as the vagina, rectum, or nose, making those areas visible for an examination

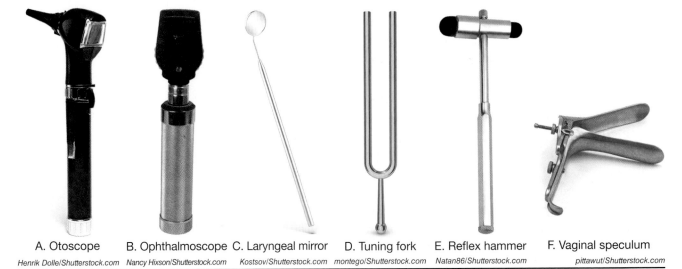

| A. Otoscope | B. Ophthalmoscope | C. Laryngeal mirror | D. Tuning fork | E. Reflex hammer | F. Vaginal speculum |

Henrik Dolle/Shutterstock.com Nancy Hixson/Shutterstock.com   Kostsov/Shutterstock.com   montego/Shutterstock.com   Natan86/Shutterstock.com   pittawut/Shutterstock.com

Figure 14.9   Various equipment may be required during a physical exam.

Extend Your Knowledge ▶ **Finding "Clues" during Physical Examinations**

During the head-to-toe physical examination, the doctor or appropriate healthcare provider may use the following actions. These actions can lead to clues that help determine the outcome of the physical examination.

1. **Inspection:** examining a body part using one's eyes, such as looking at the color of the skin or determining if there is any bruising or discoloration on the body

2. **Palpation:** using the hands to feel an object, such as a lump on the body or a mass in the body, to determine its location, size, shape, and hardness

3. **Percussion:** placing one hand on the surface of the body and then striking or tapping a finger on that hand with the index finger of the other hand to determine underlying body structure issues such as fluid in the abdominal or chest cavities

4. **Auscultation:** listening to the internal sounds of the body, such as the heartbeat, using a stethoscope

Apply It

1. Inspect another person's skin on their arms. Describe what you see. What clues might you discover? For example, if the person's arms have many brown marks, that might mean they have been out in the sun a lot. This clue would likely prompt a question about tanning habits.

2. What body sounds have you heard using a stethoscope? If it was a heartbeat, were you able to hear it clearly? Describe the sound and the rate of the heartbeats. The sound and the rate of heartbeats are clues about possible diseases and conditions that may be found during a physical examination.

Draping and Positioning for Physical Exams

There are a variety of positions and draping used for physical examinations. The type of examination being performed determines which positions and draping are used. In some examinations, the patient stands on the floor or sits on the examining table. In other examinations, the following positions are used (Figure 14.10 on the next page):

- **Dorsal recumbent position** is used to examine the vagina or rectum. The patient lies flat on the back with the knees bent and feet flat on the table. The drape is placed in a diamond shape, covering the chest and perineal area (between the anus and the scrotum on the male, and between the anus and the opening to the vagina on the female).

- **Fowler's position** is often used to examine the legs and feet. The patient is seated on the table with the backrest at a 45° angle. The legs are extended flat on the table. The drape should cover the legs.

- **Knee-chest position** is used to examine the rectum. The patient kneels on the table with buttocks raised. The head and chest remain on the table. Arms are extended above the head, and the elbows are bent. The head is turned to one side. A pillow under the chest may provide comfort. The drape covers the back and legs.

- **Lithotomy position** is used to examine the vagina. The patient lies on her back, and her hips and buttocks are brought to the corners of the table. Her legs are bent and her feet are placed in padded stirrups. The drape is placed in a diamond shape, and it covers the body but not the head.

- **Prone position** is used to examine the spine and legs. The patient lies on the abdomen with arms and hands to each side. The head is turned to the side. The drape extends from the shoulders to the legs and may cover the feet.

Think It Through

Think about the last time you had a physical examination. What would you have liked to know before, during, and after the examination? What would have made you feel more comfortable during and after the examination?

- **Sims' position** is sometimes used to examine the rectum or vagina. It is a left-side lying position. The lower arm is bent and behind the back. The upper knee is bent and raised toward the chest and supported by a pillow. There should be a pillow under the bottom of the foot so that the toes do not touch the table. The drape extends from shoulders to toes. When being examined, to expose the rectum or vagina, the drape is folded back to the near corner.

- **Supine position** is used for examination of the front of the body and breasts. The patient lies flat on the back with the arms at each side. The drape extends from under the armpits to the toes.

It is very important to maintain a calm, friendly attitude while preparing the patient for the examination. The patient may need assistance in dressing, undressing, or being positioned on the examination table. Provide that assistance when needed.

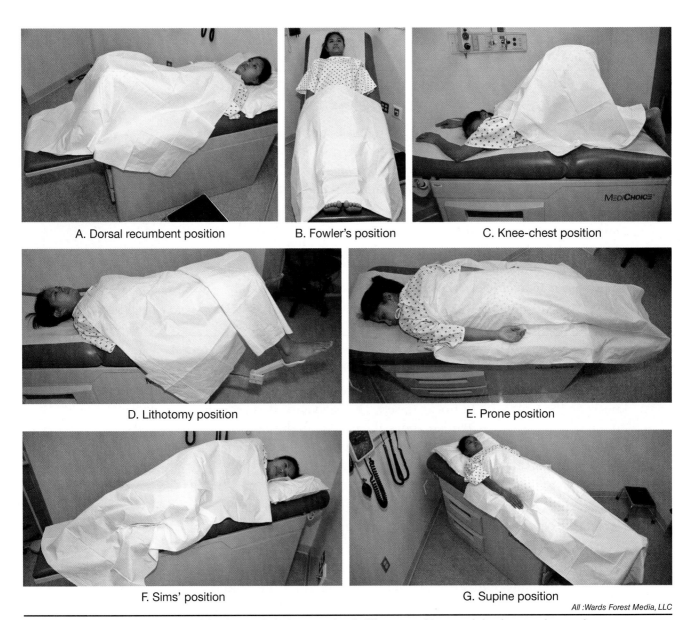

A. Dorsal recumbent position

B. Fowler's position

C. Knee-chest position

D. Lithotomy position

E. Prone position

F. Sims' position

G. Supine position

All :Wards Forest Media, LLC

Figure 14.10   Depending on which body area is being examined, different positions and draping may be used.

Procedure 14.4 | **Preparing for a Physical Examination**

Rationale

Appropriate positioning and draping for an examination provides comfort and promotes a safe and accurate examination. Proper draping helps limit exposure to only the body part(s) being examined.

Preparation

1. Assemble the equipment needed for the prescribed type of examination. If electronic health records are used, prepare the appropriate screen.
2. Cover the examining table with a disposable table sheet.
3. Prepare the equipment and instruments needed for the specific exam. Lay out the equipment and instruments for easy access during the examination. Make sure you understand any specific approaches the healthcare provider likes to use during the examination, such as the location of certain equipment. Make sure there are adequate supplies, including lubricant and tissues.
4. Prepare the needed drapes.
5. Explain, using simple terms, what you are going to do to prepare for the examination. Do this even if the patient is unable to communicate or is disoriented.
6. Encourage the patient to use the bathroom before the examination. Also measure height and weight if the scale is outside of the examining room.

Procedure

7. Provide privacy and safety. Screen the patient or close the door to the room.
8. Have the patient remove only the clothes required for the examination.
9. Have the patient put on a gown. Explain whether the gown should be tied in the front or the back of the body and where clothes may be stored, if appropriate. Provide assistance if needed. If not, step out of the room until the patient has indicated he is ready.

10. Be sure there is adequate lighting.
11. Measure the patient's vital signs, as instructed. Measure the patient's height and weight if the scales are in the examining room.
12. Help the patient onto the examining table, if appropriate.
13. Sometimes a special position is needed for an examination. Prepare the patient for the needed position and explain why the position is required.
14. Make sure the patient is safe and comfortable. Do not leave the patient alone in the room once he is positioned.
15. Drape the patient for the examination during and after positioning. Ensure warmth and show respect for privacy.

Follow-up

16. Provide assistance during the examination as requested.
17. After an examination of the vagina or rectum, provide the patient with tissues to wipe or clean off the lubricant used during the examination.
18. Assist with dressing or returning to bed, if appropriate.
19. Respond to any questions the patient may have.
20. Discard disposable items. Clean and store reusable items according to the facility's policy. Send the speculum or other equipment to the supply area for sterilization.
21. Wash your hands to ensure infection control.

Reporting and Documentation

22. Communicate any specific observations, complications, or unusual responses to the appropriate provider. Also record this information in the patient's chart or EMR, as appropriate.

Dental Assistant

Dental assistants work in dentists' offices, dental clinics, and in dental specialty practices. Dental assistants are one of three healthcare workers who work in dental offices. These include the dentist, who supervises other workers and provides professional dental services; the dental hygienist, who may remove stains and **plaque** from teeth surfaces, apply preventive tooth decay treatments, make molds of patient's teeth, and remove sutures and dressings; and the dental assistant.

plaque
a sticky substance found on teeth

Typical responsibilities for a dental assistant include clerical and administrative duties such as scheduling appointments, answering patient questions, maintaining patient records, and assisting with billing and payments. These workers also prepare the room and patients for dental examinations, help the dentist with dental procedures (Figure 14.11), assist with dental X-rays and dental laboratory work, instruct patients on proper oral care and hygiene, sterilize dental instruments and equipment, and ensure that supplies and equipment are available and in working order. The procedures dental assistants are allowed to perform vary from state to state.

There are four procedures that dental assistants may perform, if within state regulations:

1. coronal (crown) polishing: removing soft deposits such as plaque from the surfaces of the teeth

2. sealant application: painting a thin, plastic substance over teeth to keep food particles and acid-producing bacteria from causing cavities

3. fluoride application: applying fluoride directly on the teeth to prevent cavities

4. topical anesthetics application: applying a topical anesthetic that temporarily numbs an area in the patient's mouth

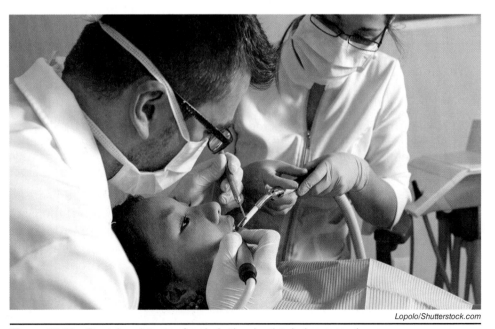

Lopolo/Shutterstock.com

Figure 14.11   Dental assistants often help the dentist during procedures.

While dental assistants may be trained on the job, some states require that they complete an accredited, one-year training program. Upon successful completion of their program, they must also pursue certification.

Providing Oral Care

Dental hygienists are primarily responsible for cleaning teeth in the dental office. Dental assistants are responsible for teaching people how to perform oral care properly at home. Nursing assistants and patient care technicians also have a responsibility to ensure their patients receive proper oral care in healthcare facilities.

Humans have 20 deciduous teeth (commonly called *baby teeth*), which are eventually replaced by 32 permanent (*adult*) teeth. Teeth cleaning is a critical part of daily oral care to ensure that teeth remain healthy. Routine teeth cleaning consists of daily brushing and flossing and a visit to the dentist twice a year.

Oral prophylaxis is a procedure performed in the dentist's office to thoroughly clean the teeth. Prophylaxis is an important dental treatment for dealing with inflammation and gum disease. Some benefits of prophylaxis include tartar and plaque removal, both above and below the gum line. It also helps remove stains on the teeth, leads to fresher breath, and identifies any potential health problems.

oral prophylaxis
term for actions taken to maintain oral health and prevent the spread of disease

Between prophylaxis teeth cleanings, you should properly brush and floss your teeth. Follow these guidelines when doing so:

- Brush your teeth twice a day for two minutes with a soft-bristled brush. The toothbrush should be a size and shape that fits your mouth, allowing you to easily reach all areas in your mouth (Figure 14.12).

- Replace your toothbrush every three to four months. Do this sooner if the bristles are frayed to prevent using a worn toothbrush.

- Use a toothpaste that has an American Dental Association (ADA) seal.

Brushing your teeth is only part of a complete teeth cleaning. Daily flossing of the teeth is also important. Flossing removes up to 80 percent of the film that hardens to plaque.

Procedure 14.5 provides the steps necessary for dental assistants to instruct patients on how to achieve proper oral care. This procedure is also helpful for nursing assistants and patient care technicians who assist in oral care in healthcare facilities.

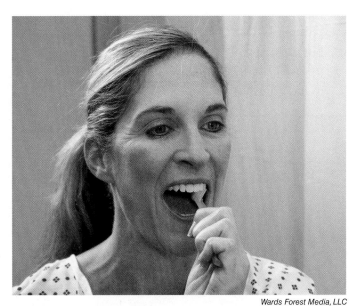

Wards Forest Media, LLC

Figure 14.12   To properly clean your teeth, a toothbrush must be the appropriate size for your mouth, allowing it to easily reach all surfaces of the teeth.

Procedure 14.5 | Providing Oral Care

Rationale

Oral care is an essential part of a person's daily activities. Oral care freshens the mouth, cleans the teeth, provides moisture, and reduces bacteria in the mouth.

Preparation

1. Assemble the following equipment:
   - soft-bristled toothbrush
   - toothpaste
   - disposable gloves
   - facecloth
   - paper towels
   - towels
   - face mask
   - dental floss
   - mouthwash

2. Wash your hands to ensure infection control. Put on disposable gloves if you are giving care or touching the patient's mouth.

3. Explain in simple terms what you are going to do or show the patient.

4. Be prepared to brush a patient's teeth yourself if you are in a healthcare facility and the patient is unable to brush his own teeth.

Procedure

5. The patient should be in a sitting position. If you are in a healthcare facility, raise the bed to a comfortable level for working and lock the wheels. Also spread a towel across the patient's chest.

6. Put toothpaste on a wet, soft-bristled toothbrush.

7. Place the toothbrush on the teeth at a 45° angle to the gums (Figure 14.13).

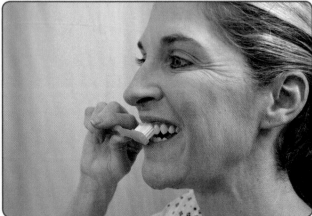

Figure 14.13   Wards Forest Media, LLC

8. Gently move the brush back and forth in short (tooth-wide) strokes.

9. Brush the outer surfaces, inner surfaces, and chewing surfaces of the teeth (Figure 14.14).

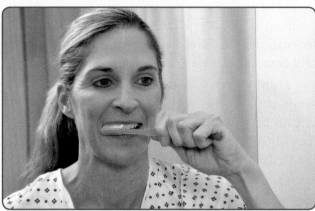

Outer Surface

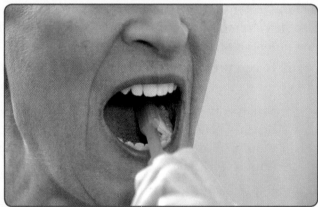

Inner Surface

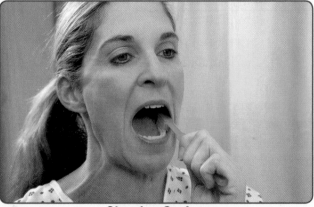

Chewing Surface

Figure 14.14   All: Wards Forest Media, LLC

10. To clean the inside surfaces of the front teeth, tilt the brush vertically and make several up-and-down strokes.

11. Brush the tongue to remove bacteria and keep the breath fresh, but take care not to brush so far back that gagging occurs.

12. To floss teeth:
    - Cut a piece of floss 18 inches long.
    - Wrap the ends of the floss around the middle finger on each hand with the other fingers placed out of the way (Figure 14.15).
    - Hold the dental floss stretched tight between the middle fingers.

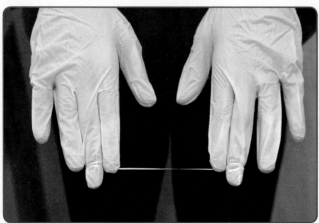

Figure 14.15 *Wards Forest Media, LLC*

- Gently insert the floss between each pair of teeth and slide the strand around both sides of each tooth.
- Do not press the floss into the gum.

13. When finished, offer the patient mouthwash solution or fresh water to rinse the mouth. Remove and discard your gloves. Clean and store equipment according to the facility's policy. Discard disposable equipment.

Follow-up

14. If you are in a healthcare facility, make sure the patient is safe and comfortable, and that the bed is in its lowest position. Place the call light and personal items within easy reach.

15. If instructing a patient in the dentist's office, ask if there are any further questions.

16. Wash your hands to ensure infection control.

Reporting and Documentation

17. Communicate any specific observations, complications, or unusual responses to the appropriate provider. Also record this information in the patient's chart or EMR.

Check Your Understanding ✓

1. How often should someone brush their teeth and for how long each time?
2. What type of toothbrush should be used and at what angle should it be held when brushing?
3. Describe the process of tooth brushing.
4. What are the reasons for flossing your teeth?
5. How often should someone floss their teeth?
6. What is the best way to floss?

Pharmacy Technician

Pharmacy technicians work in hospitals, long-term care facilities, assisted-living facilities, retail or mail-order pharmacies, or health and personal-care stores. These technicians are supervised by licensed pharmacists.

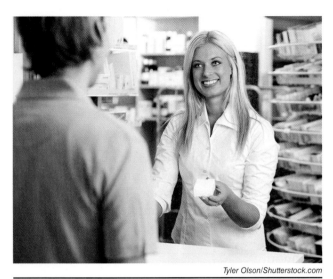

Tyler Olson/Shutterstock.com

Figure 14.16   Pharmacy technicians work closely with customers.

A pharmacy technician's primary responsibility is to receive and fill medication prescriptions. Prescription requests can come from hospitals, doctor's offices, or patients who receive them from their doctors. When a prescription is filled or refilled, a licensed pharmacist must check the completed prescription before it is given to the patient. Prescription filling or refilling usually includes tasks such as

- counting, pouring, measuring, mixing, and weighing medications;
- selecting the appropriate medication container;
- creating prescription labels;
- determining the cost of medications; and
- maintaining patient prescription files.

Pharmacy technicians also interact with patients by answering phones, completing cash register transactions, and responding to questions (Figure 14.16). They may also prepare insurance claim forms and take inventory.

Pharmacy technicians attend formal training programs or complete their education at community colleges, where they earn an associate's degree. Many states and employers require that pharmacy technicians become certified.

Filling a Prescription

Medications are most often prescribed by doctors. In some states, nurse practitioners and physician assistants also have this responsibility included in their legal scope of practice. Prescriptions can be written for patients who are in healthcare facilities or at home. Under the supervision of a licensed pharmacist, pharmacy technicians are able to fill prescription medications.

Did You Know?   **Prescriptions in the United States**

Many people in the United States, particularly the elderly, take more than one prescribed medication. It was reported by the CDC that nearly 48 percent of people use at least one prescription drug, 22 percent use three or more prescription drugs, and nearly 11 percent use five or more.

The Mayo Clinic reported that seven out of ten Americans take at least one prescription drug. The most commonly prescribed drug is antibiotics—taken by 17 percent of Americans—followed by antidepressants and opioids, which are each taken by 13 percent of Americans.

Getting medication prescriptions filled or refilled requires one of the following:

- an order for the medication sent to a healthcare facility pharmacy

- a written paper prescription taken to a local pharmacy

- a call or an e-mail to a pharmacy from the doctor's office

- a prescription sent to the pharmacy via a computer linked to the electronic health record (EHR)

Prescriptions must include the patient's full name, the medication name, the dosage, directions for taking the medication, the doctor's signature, the Drug Enforcement Administration (DEA) registration number (if it is a controlled substance, such as a narcotic), and refill information (Figure 14.17).

Prescriptions can be filled and refilled by a healthcare facility's in-house pharmacy, a local retail pharmacy, a mail-order pharmacy, or an online pharmacy.

Medication prescription fills and refills can be paid for in a variety of ways. Insurance policies may completely cover the cost of a medication prescription, or they may cover only a portion of the cost. If insurance pays for only a portion of the prescription, the patient will be required to pay for the remainder. The portion the patient must pay for is called a *copayment*, or *copay*. Some prescriptions may not be covered at all and must be paid for in cash. If a patient is unable to afford a prescription as written, he may ask that his doctor be called. The doctor can determine if there are any substitutions for the medication, or if there is another medication that will be as effective at a lower cost.

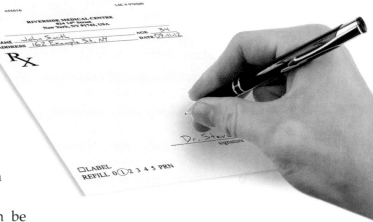

piotr_pabijan/Shutterstock.com

Figure 14.17 Before filling a medication, a pharmacy technician must check that the doctor has included all of the necessary information on the prescription.

Procedure 14.6 describes the steps pharmacy technicians must follow to fill a prescription. Attention to detail is very important. A major focus during this procedure is ensuring that no errors are made. One strategy to achieve this is to reduce any distractions when possible—both internally and environmentally. Lessen stress and balance workloads so there is sufficient time to perform the procedure. Always check the bottle's label and confirm the national drug code (NDC) number in the computer. The NDC is a unique, three-segment number that is a universal product identifier for drugs. Also, be sure to store drugs properly so there are no mix-ups or the possibility of using look-alike drugs. Remove expired medications from the shelves. Finally, always thoroughly check and double-check all prescription fills and refills.

Procedure 14.6 | Filling a Prescription

Rationale

Information provided in a prescription must be accurate, and care must be taken during the filling of a prescription so that it is performed correctly.

Preparation

1. Make sure all necessary information is listed on the prescription.

2. Consult with the pharmacist to interpret any prescriptions that are difficult to read.

3. Enter the prescription into the pharmacy's computer program. The computer prints a prescription label, which the pharmacist checks for accuracy. The pharmacist also checks which other medications the patient is taking. If drug interactions are possible, the pharmacist contacts the doctor.

4. Wash your hands to ensure infection control.

The Procedure

5. Select the correct medication from the stock shelf area.

6. Check the bottle's label and confirm the national drug code number in the computer to make sure it matches the prescription.

7. Count out the necessary amount of the medication and fill the container, taking care not to touch the medication (Figure 14.18).

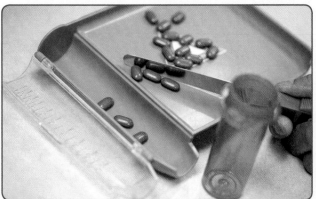

Figure 14.18   Volt Collection/Shutterstock.com

8. Select and attach the correct lid based on container size and the patient's preference for a childproof or easy-open lid.

9. Attach the label to the container and initial the bottom right-hand corner of the printed label.

10. Attach auxiliary labels (Figure 14.19). These give additional information, such as whether the medication is to be taken with water or on an empty stomach.

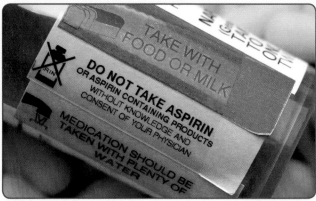

Figure 14.19   Steve Cukrov/Shutterstock.com

11. Place the medication on top of the original prescription.

12. Present the medication and prescription to the pharmacist for final approval.

Follow-up

13. If you work in a retail pharmacy, the insurance company will let you know how much, if any, of the prescription cost will be paid for by the company. The copayment will be paid by the patient. If you work in a healthcare facility's pharmacy, the cost of the medication will be included in patient billing.

14. Package and store the medication per facility policy.

15. Wash your hands to ensure infection control.

16. Advise the patient the order has been filled via phone, e-mail, or text message.

17. When the patient picks up the prescription, process the sale.

18. Ask patients if they have any questions about the medication. If it is a first-time medication, ask if they want to talk with the pharmacist. This is called *patient counseling*.

Recording and Documentation

19. Enter needed information about the medication fill or refill into the computer to maintain a patient history.

Physical Therapy Assistant (PTA)

The physical therapy assistant (PTA) works under the supervision of a physical therapist in hospitals, long-term care facilities, home health agencies, physical therapy offices, clinics, rehabilitation hospitals or clinics, or fitness centers. Physical therapy assistants help physical therapists by providing rehabilitation services to people who have diseases or conditions that limit their mobility and daily functioning. Responsibilities of a PTA include

- teaching exercises, as directed (Figure 14.20);
- assisting patients in performing physical activities and using assistive devices such as crutches and canes (as you learned in chapter 13);
- performing treatments using massage, heat and cold, and traction;
- monitoring progress through patient management plans;
- maintaining treatment records; and
- possibly administering ultrasound and electric current treatments.

The goal of physical therapy is to reduce pain, prevent further injuries, promote wellness, and practice health maintenance.

PTAs graduate from an accredited program from which they earn an associate's degree. Licensure or certification is required in most states.

Emergency Medical Technician (EMT)

Emergency medical technicians (EMTs) work for ambulance companies (land and air), in emergency rooms, with fire services, with search and rescue, and in some clinic and community settings. There are usually three levels of EMTs: EMT-basic, EMT-intermediate, and EMT-paramedic.

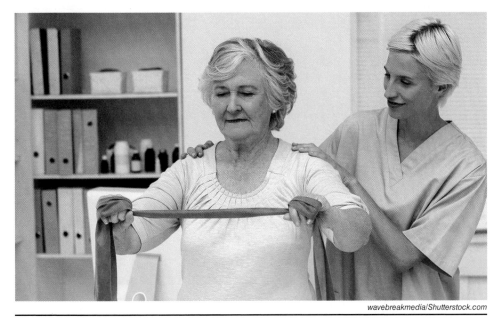

wavebreakmedia/Shutterstock.com

Figure 14.20 Physical therapy assistants work under the supervision of physical therapists to instruct and guide patients through rehabilitative exercises.

The differences among these levels are in each one's scope of practice, which is based on training and education. For example, state regulations do not allow basic EMTs to give shots or start an IV. Usually, basic EMTs can only use oxygen, glucose, asthma inhalers, and epinephrine auto-injectors to treat patients. Intermediate EMTs have additional training and can perform intravenous (IV) therapy. EMT-paramedics, usually called *paramedics*, can do everything basic and intermediate EMTs can do, as well as give shots and provide more advanced airway management. Paramedics may also be trained in the use of several medications, depending on the state.

Licensure for EMTs is required everywhere in the United States. EMT training programs are often offered at basic, intermediate, and paramedic levels. The length of a program depends on the level of licensure desired. A basic EMT program may take six months, but a paramedic program may be an associate's degree program that takes two years to complete.

As you learned in chapter 2, the most critical responsibility of any EMT is determining the extent of emergency through observation. EMTs must respond quickly and efficiently to the medical needs of those who are sick or injured. EMTs must also determine a patient's level of consciousness (LOC) and take vital signs (Figure 14.21).

If needed, and depending on level, EMTs maintain airways; provide ventilation; administer CPR; use AEDs; control hemorrhages; treat shock; bandage wounds; immobilize painful or swollen body parts; assist in emergency childbirth; deal with altered mental and physical states; and respond to allergic reactions, seizures, poisoning, and environmental emergencies. If working in ambulance services, EMTs provide en route care and transfer patients to the emergency room. EMTs are also responsible for inventory, restocking, replacing, disinfecting, and checking all equipment and supplies in the ambulance.

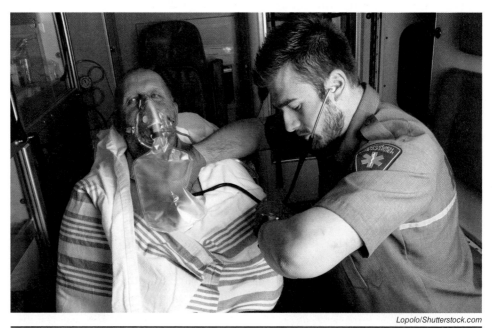

Lopolo/Shutterstock.com

Figure 14.21   One way an EMT assesses a patient's medical condition is by monitoring vital signs.

Properly positioning and moving patients are some of an EMT's most important responsibilities. EMTs must always position, lift, and carry patients in a manner that ensures the safety of the patients and themselves.

Positioning an Unconscious Person

EMTs and paramedics are often the healthcare workers responsible for positioning an unconscious patient during an emergency. Loss of consciousness may be the result of a head injury or trauma from an accident, a heart attack, or a stroke.

When people are conscious, they are awake, aware, and alert, or they are in an accepted state of normal sleep from which the person can easily awaken. When someone is injured; loses a lot of blood; or experiences a heart attack, stroke, or other serious condition, loss of consciousness may occur. Abnormal states of consciousness are not simply or easily defined, but the following classifications may be used to identify a patient's level of consciousness:

- **Clouding of consciousness** is a very mild form of altered mental status. The person is inattentive and sleeps more than usual.

- **Confusion** is a more profound lack of awareness in which the person may be disoriented and bewildered and have difficulty following commands.

- **Lethargy** is a severe drowsiness. The person can be aroused but will then drift back to sleep.

- **Obtundation** is similar to lethargy. The person has a lessened interest in the environment, has slowed responses to stimulation, and sleeps more than normal with drowsiness in between.

- **Stupor** is a state in which only vigorous and repeated stimuli will arouse the person. When left undisturbed, the person will immediately become unresponsive.

- **Coma** is described as unarousable unresponsiveness.

Real Life Scenario   Responding to an Unconscious Patient

Imagine you are an EMT and the ambulance company you work for is called to Mrs. Gonzales's house at 1:00 a.m. She called 9-1-1 to say that she tripped on an area rug and hit her head on one of her tables. She said that this happened about an hour ago and she was able to stop the bleeding on her arm and forehead. Now she feels very dizzy and is not sure she should be alone.

When the ambulance arrives at her house, you find Mrs. Gonzales lying on the floor with one arm under her head and one leg bent. She looks like she is in her 60s and she lives alone. You call her name and she does not respond. You then put pressure on

one of her nail beds and she moans. You repeat the pressure and again she moans.

Apply It
(Read the next page and Procedure 14.7 before answering.)

1. What should you have done before the AVPU assessment?

2. Using the AVPU assessment, what do you think her level of consciousness might be?

3. Should you leave Mrs. Gonzales in the position you found her or should you move her? Explain your answer.

One accepted tool used to determine consciousness is the AVPU scale, which is an acronym that stands for *alert, voice, pain,* and *unresponsive.* It is a quick assessment, particularly during an emergency, to determine the following levels of consciousness:

1. **Alert:** The person is awake and alert. This does not necessarily mean the person is orientated to time and place or responding normally.

2. **Voice:** The person is not fully awake but does respond to verbal commands.

3. **Pain:** The person is difficult to rouse and only responds to painful stimuli, such as putting pressure on a person's nail bed.

4. **Unresponsive:** The person is completely unconscious and cannot be roused.

Procedure 14.7   Positioning an Unconscious Person

Rationale

It is important to maintain proper body alignment for an unconscious patient. The unconscious patient is unable to communicate discomfort and/or maintain normal bodily function.

Preparation

1. Even though the patient appears unconscious, reassure her that you are there to help.

2. Determine level of consciousness using the AVPU assessment.

3. Put on disposable gloves.

4. Remain calm.

Procedure

5. Check the patient to see if she is breathing (and continue to do this while positioning).

6. Check the pulse (do this before, once during, and again after positioning).

7. If at any time the breathing or pulse has stopped, position the patient onto her back and begin cardiopulmonary resuscitation (CPR).

8. If you think there is a spinal injury, leave the patient in the position you found her (as long as she is breathing).

9. If the patient is breathing and lying on her back, and you do not think there is a spinal injury, carefully roll the patient toward you onto her side. Do not allow the patient's arms to be caught under her body. Maintain the patient's body alignment and support her neck and back (Figure 14.22).

10. Bend the patient's legs so both the hips and knees are at right angles (Figure 14.23).

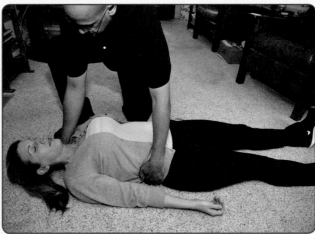

Figure 14.22   *Wards Forest Media, LLC*

(continued)

Procedure 14.7   Positioning an Unconscious Person (continued)

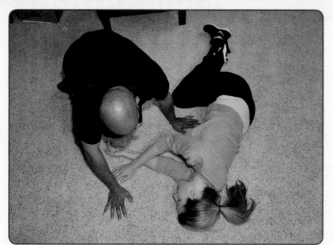

Figure 14.23   *Wards Forest Media, LLC*

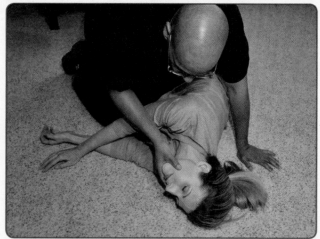

Figure 14.24   *Wards Forest Media, LLC*

11. Gently tilt the patient's head back to keep the airway open (Figure 14.24).
12. If the patient vomits, roll her entire body onto her side at one time. Support her neck and back to keep her head and body in the same position.
13. Keep the person warm while preparing for transport.

Follow-up

14. When appropriate, prepare and move the patient for transport according to guidelines and policy.

15. Discard gloves when appropriate.
16. Wash your hands to ensure infection control.

Reporting and Documentation

17. Communicate any specific observations, complications, or unusual responses to the appropriate provider. Also record this information in the patient's chart or EMR, if appropriate.

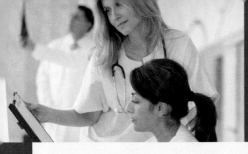

Summary

Several healthcare careers are discussed in this chapter, including nursing assistant (NA), patient care technician (PCT), health unit coordinator (HUC), medical assistant (MA), dental assistant (DA), pharmacy technician, physical therapy assistant (PTA), and emergency medical technician (EMT). Those working in these professions are expected to provide safe and competent hands-on patient care. These healthcare workers must complete specific education and training and programs and, for some, there is a requirement of licensure or certification.

When people have serious illnesses or conditions, they may be admitted into a hospital or long-term care facility. When a patient's condition changes, she may be transferred to a different location in the same healthcare facility or to another facility entirely. Patients are discharged from a healthcare facility to go home when their health is improved.

Typically, medical assistants help prepare for physical examinations by assembling equipment and supplies, positioning and draping the patients, and assisting when appropriate. Physical exams are performed to determine the status of a patient's bodily systems and functions, and they often require different types of equipment, positioning, and draping.

Teeth cleaning is a critical part of daily oral care to ensure teeth remain healthy. Routine teeth cleaning consists of daily brushing and flossing, and a visit to the dentist twice a year. Oral prophylaxis is performed in a dentist's office to thoroughly clean the teeth and prevent inflammation and gum disease. Dental assistants educate patients on proper brushing and flossing techniques.

Pharmacy technicians can fill and refill medication prescriptions under the supervision of a pharmacist. To do this, they must follow strict procedures. This procedure requires close attention to detail to ensure that no errors are made.

EMTs and paramedics are responsible for positioning an unconscious patient during an emergency. Loss of consciousness may occur when someone is injured; loses a lot of blood; or experiences a heart attack, stroke, or other serious condition. EMTs can determine a patient's level of consciousness (LOC) using the AVPU scale. It is a quick assessment that determines the patient's level of consciousness. Breathing is also assessed before proper positioning can take place.

Review Questions

Answer the following questions using what you have learned in this chapter.

True or False Assess

1. *True or False?* In the Fowler's position, the patient is seated on the examining table with the backrest at a 90° angle.

2. *True or False?* Healthcare workers need to bring patients to their transport vehicles upon transfer or discharge.

3. *True or False?* Pharmacy technicians are able to fill prescriptions without asking a pharmacist to check their work.

4. *True or False?* An otoscope is a medical device used to inspect the throat.

5. *True or False?* A medical assistant is the only healthcare worker whose education is determined by federal law.

6. *True or False?* EMTs must check an unconscious person's breathing before positioning.

7. *True or False?* When a patient is in the prone position, the drape extends from shoulders to knees.

8. *True or False?* A patient's call light can be placed anywhere as long as the patient can see it.

Multiple Choice Assess

9. Which of the following statements about flossing your teeth is *true*?

   A. The floss should be 12″ long and should slide between each pair of teeth with focus on the molars.

   B. The floss should be 6″ long and should slide between the teeth using a back-and-forth method.

   C. The floss should be 18″ long and should slide between each pair of teeth.

   D. The floss should be 20″ long and should be used only for the front teeth.

10. Imagine you are a medical assistant helping with an examination and the doctor asks you for an ophthalmoscope. What is this?

   A. a lighted medical device used to examine the interior of the eyes

   B. a lighted medical device used to examine the interior of the ears

   C. a lighted medical device used to examine the vagina

   D. a lighted medical device used to examine the throat

11. Before a prescription can be filled, the pharmacy technician needs to look for the _____ on the written or electronic prescription.

   A. patient's birth date

   B. patient's driver's license number

   C. medication's side effects

   D. medication name and dosage

12. James, an EMT, is first on the scene of a traffic accident. He sees a woman on the ground next to her car. The first action he should take is _____.

   A. move her out of the way of oncoming cars

   B. make sure her purse is safe

   C. check for consciousness and breathing

   D. look for her children to be sure they are okay

13. The medical assistant positions the patient so she is lying on her back and her hips and buttocks are brought to the corners of the table. Her legs are bent and her feet are in padded stirrups. Which position is the patient in?

   A. lithotomy

   B. Sims'

   C. semi-Fowler's

   D. supine

14. How can an EMT determine if painful stimuli arouse a patient when assessing LOC?

   A. Loudly ask the patient if he is in pain.

   B. Shake the patient's shoulders and check for a response.

   C. Gently pinch the patient's ears.

   D. Put pressure on the patient's nail beds.

Short Answer

15. Identify one position used for a physical examination and explain how the patient should be draped in that position.

16. Explain two differences between an EMT-basic and a paramedic.

17. If a patient is not fully awake, but groans when you call her name, what is her level of consciousness on the AVPU scale?

18. List three pieces of information that need to be on a prescription.

19. Which healthcare workers can admit, transfer, and discharge patients?

20. How can EMTs determine level of consciousness (LOC)?

21. What is one difference between a dental assistant and dental hygienist?

22. Describe three safety precautions that must be undertaken during admission, transfer, or discharge.

23. Which of the healthcare workers discussed in this chapter require professional certification?

24. Identify and describe the use of five pieces of equipment that can be used for a physical examination.

Critical Thinking Exercises

25. Talk to a healthcare worker who provides care in a hospital and a healthcare worker who provides care in a long-term care setting. Ask these workers about their daily responsibilities. What do they like the best about their jobs, and what they do not like as much? Describe the differences between the workers' jobs and the care each one gives. Identify which position you might like to pursue and why.

26. Find and read one article about helping patients follow hospital discharge instructions. Discuss the findings and explain how healthcare workers can help patients adhere to these instructions.

27. Imagine you are an EMT called to the home of a person who does not speak English. You are unable to communicate with the person in his native language. Describe how you would use verbal and nonverbal communication in this scenario.

28. In the chapter, you learned that drugs must be stored properly so there are no mix-ups between look-alike and sound-alike drugs. Explain look-alike and sound-alike drugs. Give two examples and explain how pharmacy technicians can increase safety awareness by being alert to these.

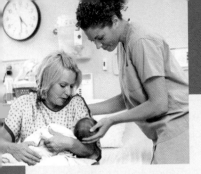

Review Questions

Answer the following questions using what you have learned in this unit.

True or False

1. *True or False?* Apnea is difficult and labored breathing.

2. *True or False?* Emergency situations differ, but timing is crucial in all emergencies.

3. *True or False?* It does not matter if the earpieces of a stethoscope fit in your ears as long as they are warm to the touch.

4. *True or False?* When a person loses a large amount of blood, he or she can go into shock.

5. *True or False?* When draping for the supine position, the patient lies on his stomach with his arms at each side. The drape extends from under the armpits to the toes.

6. *True or False?* When taking a patient's blood pressure, the cuff size is as important as the placement on the patient's arm.

7. *True or False?* You should always ask a person who is having an allergic reaction if he has an epinephrine auto-injector.

8. *True or False?* When a doctor orders that a patient be transferred, this should occur even if the patient refuses.

9. *True or False?* One important benefit of regular oral prophylaxis is to identify any potential health problems.

Multiple Choice

10. The doctor has ordered that Mr. Young start ambulating. He has not been out of bed since his surgery. You know that he might feel faint, so you decide to first have him _____.
    A. dangle at the side of the bed
    B. sit in the chair at the side of the bed
    C. wear a back belt for stabilization
    D. put on a pair of slippers to prevent a fall

11. Two parts of a stethoscope are the _____ and the _____.
    A. lens, bulb
    B. diaphragm, bell
    C. bulb, bell
    D. diaphragm, lens

12. Mr. Garcia has just eaten some food when he starts choking and cannot breathe. He has a(n) _____.
    A. partial blockage
    B. mid-airway blockage
    C. incomplete blockage
    D. complete blockage

13. Which of the following describes tachycardia?
    A. a slow pulse of less than 60 beats per minute
    B. a thready, weak, and slow pulse
    C. a fast pulse of over 100 beats per minute
    D. None of the above.

14. Mrs. Grant has pyrexia, which is a condition characterized by _____.
    A. fast pulse
    B. fever
    C. low blood pressure
    D. slow pulse

15. Janet has just gotten a poisonous substance in her eye. Which of the following first aid guidelines should she follow first?
    A. Put a cold compress on the eye for 10 minutes.
    B. Flush the eye with warm water for 5 to 10 minutes.
    C. Flush the eye with cool water for 20 minutes.
    D. Flush the eye with saline eye drops for 5 minutes.

16. What might you take into a patient's room if you want to correctly position her?
    A. trochanter roll
    B. towels
    C. foot board
    D. All of the above.

17. If a patient is beginning to fall, which of the following procedures should you follow?

   A. Ease the patient slowly to the floor, using your body as an incline.

   B. Grab the gait belt and lift the patient up slowly.

   C. Lift the patient up by putting your arms under his or her axilla.

   D. Call for help immediately.

Short Answer

18. List the information you should give a 9-1-1 dispatcher during an emergency.

19. Describe three daily responsibilities of a medical assistant or physical therapy assistant.

20. Explain the procedure for measuring the weight of a bedridden patient.

21. Name three pieces of equipment that might be used during a physical exam and explain how each one is used.

22. List the contents of an admissions kit.

Critical Thinking Exercises

23. Measure the vital signs of five of your classmates. Record your findings. List the differences you found and explain two possible reasons for these differences.

24. Select one emergency situation discussed in the chapter that you still don't know much about or feel uncomfortable treating. Conduct research to increase your knowledge of this situation. Describe what about the situation makes you uncomfortable and develop a plan of action to improve your confidence regarding this emergency.

25. You have just completed passive range-of-motion exercises with your patient, Mrs. Lord. What types of information should you report about how she did with the exercises? What information should be documented?

Career Exploration

Biomedical Engineer

Biomedical engineering has become an important part of healthcare. People are living longer and staying active, so they often need biomedical devices and procedures, such as hip and knee replacements.

Biomedical engineers (BMEs) combine medical and biological sciences with engineering principles to support and enhance healthcare. They design and build equipment, medical devices, computer systems, and software, and improve processes for important work such as genomic testing.

BMEs work in hospitals, medical and educational research facilities, and government regulatory agencies. To become a BME, a degree in biomedical engineering or bioengineering from an accredited program is necessary.

It is expected that the need for BMEs will grow up to 23 percent in the next 10 years. The median annual income for a BME is $86,950.

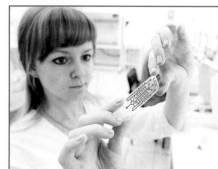

science photo/Shutterstock.com

Further Research

1. Research one of the related careers using the *Occupational Outlook Handbook* and other reliable Internet resources. What is the outlook for this career?

2. Review the educational requirements for this career. What level of education is necessary? What classes would you need to take to pursue a related degree?

3. What is the salary range for this job?

4. What do you think you would like about this career? What might you dislike? Compare the job you have researched to the description of a biomedical engineer. Which job appeals to you more? Why?

> **Related Careers**
> Biochemist
> Biophysicist
> Chemical engineer
> Mechanical engineer
> Surgeon

Unit 5

College and Career Readiness

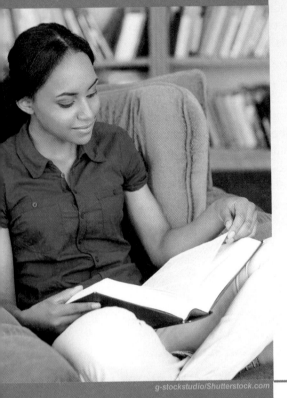

g-stockstudio/Shutterstock.com

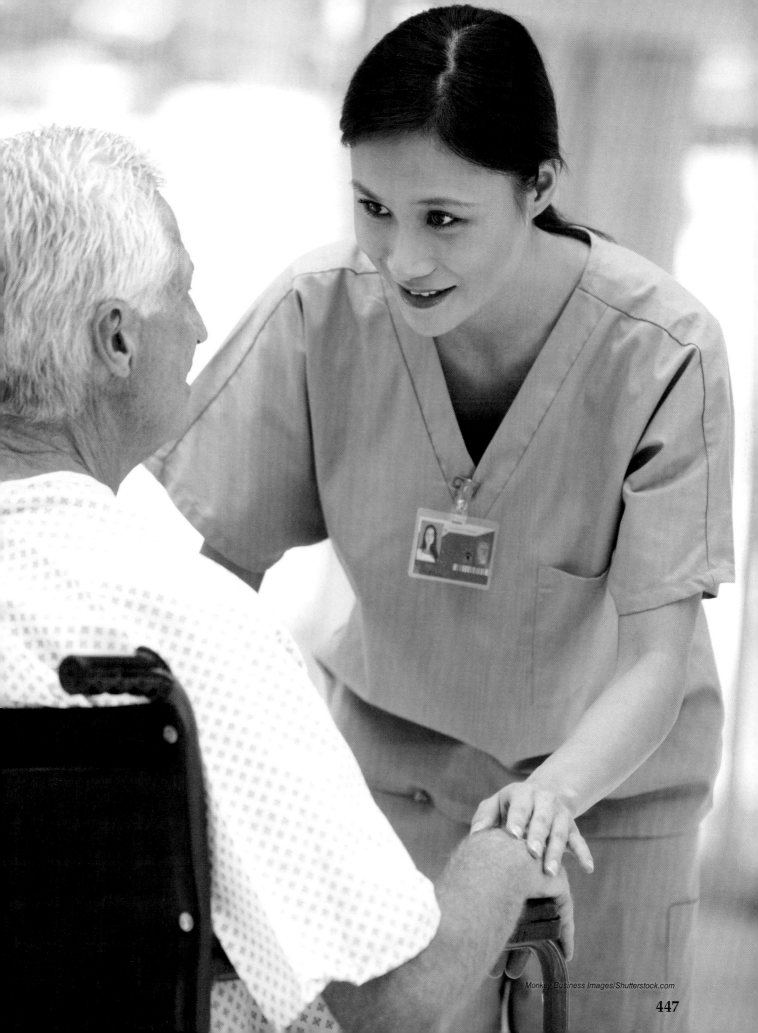

447

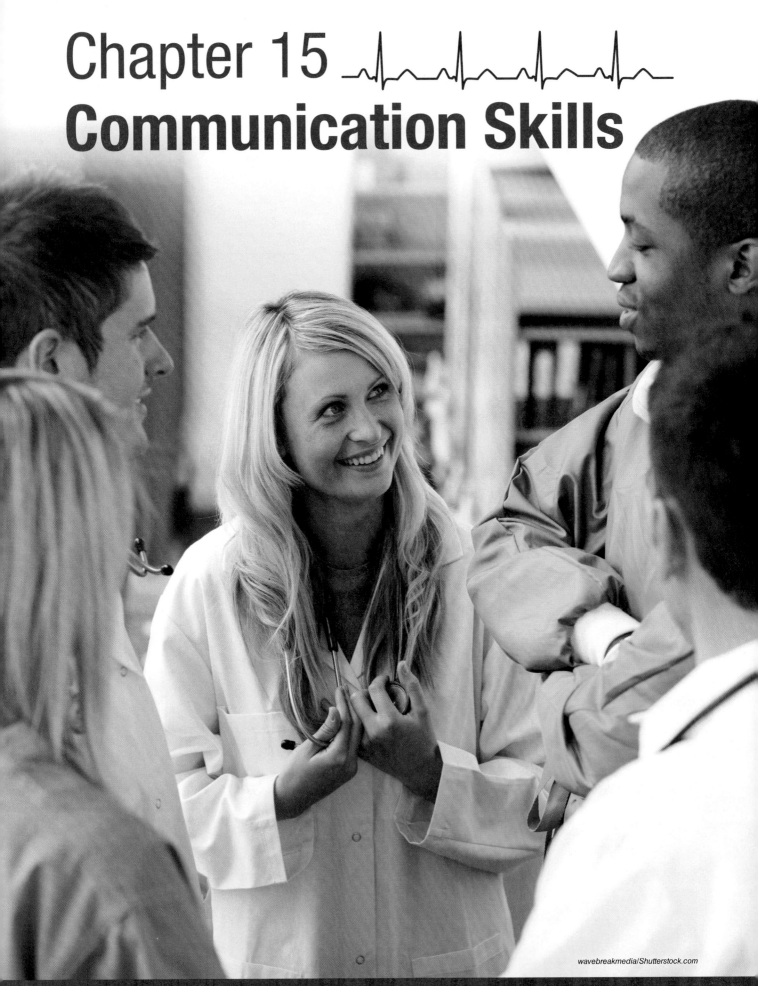

Chapter 15
Communication Skills

wavebreakmedia/Shutterstock.com

Terms to Know Build Vocab

active listening

aphasia

nonverbal communication

objective writing

proxemics

sender-receiver communication
  model

stereotype

subjective writing

verbal communication

Chapter Objectives

- Describe the role that verbal communication skills play in the workplace.
- Identify potential communication barriers and challenges when interacting with patients.
- Discuss the sender-receiver communication model.
- Describe how to take a complete telephone message.
- Describe strategies for giving a successful presentation.
- Discuss the general rules for attending and holding a meeting.
- Discuss the significance of nonverbal communication in healthcare.
- Define *proxemics* and discuss the types and significance of personal territory.
- Identify steps that can be taken to actively listen.
- Explain the importance of active listening and the barriers that can occur.
- Identify different types of writing.
- Describe how to format and send e-mails, texts, and faxes in a professional setting.

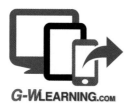

While studying, look for the activity icon to:

- **Build** vocabulary with e-flash cards and interactive games.
- **Assess** progress with chapter and unit review questions.
- **Expand** learning with animations and illustration labeling activities.
- **Simulate** EHR entry with healthcare documents.

G-WLEARNING.com

www.g-wlearning.com/healthsciences/

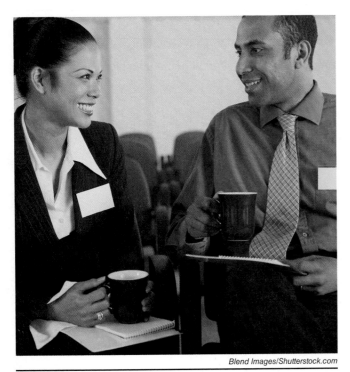

Blend Images/Shutterstock.com

Figure 15.1   A smile enhances communication.

If you list your daily activities, you will find that much of your time is spent communicating in some way—be it verbal, nonverbal, or written communication. Communication skills affect your ability to be understood and to understand others, to establish positive relationships, and to perform your job well. For some people, communicating with others is one of the biggest challenges they face in their jobs. This chapter will provide you with tips and tools for improving your communication skills.

Being a good communicator is important in both personal and professional aspects of life. Being able to communicate clearly with patients and coworkers is vital in the healthcare industry. Miscommunication can lead to serious physical, and even legal, consequences. When you become a healthcare worker, you *must* be able to communicate precisely and effectively. Effective communication skills are essential to working with your healthcare team to provide quality care.

One tip to remember is that a simple smile can improve your ability to communicate. A smile can reassure an anxious patient or welcome a new coworker on her first day (Figure 15.1).

Verbal Communication

verbal communication
expressing your thoughts out loud; also known as speaking

Verbal communication, or *speaking*, is an important form of communication in a healthcare facility. During the course of a work day most healthcare workers spend time talking with coworkers, supervisors, managers, and patients. Planning and organizing your thoughts is a critical part of verbal communication. This involves thinking about who will receive the message and what you want to convey. Making notes before a phone call, having an agenda for a meeting, or researching information you wish to give to someone in advance are all methods you can use to ensure clear communication.

According to motivational speaker and entrepreneur Pat Croce, effective communication involves much more than choosing the right words. Croce recommends five rules to incorporate while conveying a message. These are known as the *5 Cs of Communication*:

1. **Clear.** Speak in black-and-white terms to clearly state your message. Allow questions from the recipient of your communication to ensure you are understood.

2. **Concise.** Do not ramble. Your important message can be lost in the nonessential information you include—get to the point.

3. **Consistent.** Make your message consistent at all times. If you are telling your supervisor about an incident that you have observed, do not change your story to make it more dramatic. Report your findings in a consistent, accurate manner. Do not tell one person what you saw and later change your observations as you retell the story to another person.

4. **Credible.** People can tell if your words are insincere—make sure your message is real. Do not heap praise on someone just because you want to win his or her favor. It is important that you mean what you say.

5. **Courteous.** Words and phrases such as "hello," "thank you," "please," "excuse me," and "I'm sorry" are easy, effective ways to demonstrate respect. Being courteous when you communicate sets the right tone and attitude. Courtesy is mandatory in the workplace, even if you are interacting with someone you dislike. Keep your personal feelings out of your work interactions.

Having an open mind during verbal communication is also very important. Making assumptions about what someone is going to say before he or she speaks might cause you to miss the essence of the message. If you have had disagreements with the speaker, you might negatively translate a message into your assumption about what you are hearing. Keeping an open mind and listening respectfully without emotion is critical to open, clear communication.

Engagement

To provide the best possible patient care, be aware of ways to fully engage patients in your care. Patients enter healthcare facilities because they are ill or injured, or because they can no longer care for themselves. Most often, they feel stress and anxiety. Some are lonely and depressed. Others are feeling hopeless, and some are going through withdrawal. Those healthcare workers who are dealing closely with patients (admitting personnel, nurses, transporters, doctors, and so on) can make a huge difference in a patient's mental and emotional well-being.

Did You Know?   Listening and Attention

Several studies have shown that 20 minutes is about the maximum amount of time listeners can stay attentive (Figure 15.2). After 20 minutes, listeners' attention levels begin to drop. Speaking is more stimulating than listening, so although it may be exciting to talk for long periods of time, chances are your listeners may be having a hard time staying focused.

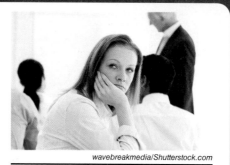

wavebreakmedia/Shutterstock.com

Figure 15.2   When a speaker sees that the audience is being inattentive, he may call for a break.

Engagement means that you are able to focus your attention completely on the patient. Take time to address needs and desires of the patient, ignoring your own. It has been found that satisfaction and even pain reduction increase when a healthcare worker takes notice of and responds to the needs of the patient. This satisfaction can decrease stress and anxiety, leading patients to heal more rapidly, be more willing to follow treatment plans, and cooperate more readily.

Asking Open-Ended Questions

One way to encourage patient engagement and communication is by asking open-ended questions. For example, asking, "Did you sleep well last night?" may receive a one-word answer of "yes" or "no." If you ask instead, "How many hours did you sleep?," the patient may respond with a more detailed answer, such as "Although I slept about six hours, I had a hard time falling asleep and had strange dreams." Asking open-ended questions allows you to get more information you will need to provide safe care for your patient.

Forming Positive, Professional Relationships

The most successful communicators in healthcare form positive relationships with coworkers and patients through mutual respect and professionalism (Figure 15.3). Having a bad day is no excuse for using an irritated tone when speaking with a patient or coworker. Personal problems should not be brought into the workplace.

It is also important to be aware of how patients wish to be addressed. Some patients, especially the elderly, may feel disrespected if you call them by their first names. To be safe, use the titles Mrs., Mr., or Ms. and their last name when speaking to adult patients. They may ask you to call them by their first names, which is acceptable with permission. Pet names like *Honey* or *Sweetie* could offend patients, who may feel you are talking down to them.

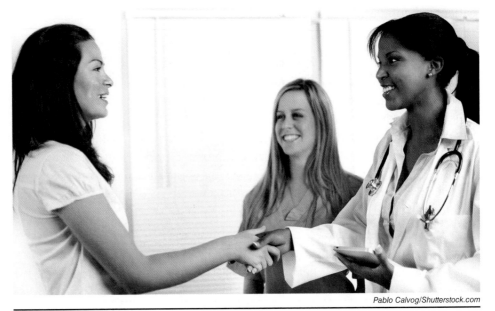

Pablo Calvog/Shutterstock.com

Figure 15.3   A healthcare worker can put a patient at ease with a warm greeting.

When addressing your patient, speak clearly and use a tone that can be easily heard. Shouting or mumbling will not help get your point across. Careless slang expressions, especially vulgarities, are also unacceptable when dealing with patients.

Any communication with patients must be appropriate for the therapeutic setting. Sharing personal information with patients is not appropriate. Keep your conversation focused on medical information.

Did You Know? **Addressing Patients**

To comply with HIPAA regulations, you should not call patients by their full names in the reception area. In the interest of confidentiality, use their first or last name only. For example, when addressing a patient in front of other patients, use Mr. Mercer rather than John Mercer.

Communicating Needs, Wants, and Emotions

As a healthcare worker interacting with your healthcare team, how do you communicate your needs, wants, and emotions effectively in the workplace? How do you control your anger and stress? How do you let your team know that you need something you are not getting from them? Answering these questions can be challenging, but developing strategies to effectively communicate needs, wants, and emotions will help you be successful in your healthcare career.

Expressing Wants and Needs

Being assertive means expressing your wants and needs in an open and honest way, while standing up for yourself and respecting others. You do not want to be hostile, aggressive, or demanding. Being an effective communicator is always about understanding the other person, not about winning an argument or forcing your needs on others.

You also have to learn to say "no." Do not let others take advantage of you, but look for alternatives that allow everyone to feel good about the outcome of the conversation.

Emotions

When you are emotionally overwhelmed or stressed, you may misread other people, sending confusing signals to your coworkers and patients. You need to pause to collect your thoughts and recognize when you are getting emotional. Your body will tell you. Are your muscles getting tight? Are your hands clenched? Is your breathing getting shallow?

Take some deep breaths. Recall a soothing image. Postpone a conversation if you can and gather your thoughts. Be willing to compromise to reduce the stress of the moment. If you are interacting with a coworker, you may want to agree to disagree and take time away from a stressful situation so everyone involved can calm down. Take a quick break and possibly take a walk outside.

Verbal Communication Challenges

Anything that interferes with communication can lead to a misinterpretation of your message. However, various factors can interfere specifically with your ability to communicate verbally with your patients. Do you have a tendency to be sarcastic? If so, this could affect your ability to communicate effectively with patients. Stereotyping patients may also impact your communication. Patients such as the hearing impaired, some intellectually disabled individuals, or those who do not speak your language pose challenges to verbal communication, possibly requiring the use of a translator. Speaking may be difficult for a patient who has suffered a stroke or stutters badly.

In addition to these considerations, communication often must be geared toward a patient's ability to understand. This often means substituting basic terms for challenging medical terms that could confuse some people. Even if a coworker is translating for you, you can't assume that a fellow employee unfamiliar with your specific field will understand your use of technical terms. You may want to simplify your language for both the translator and the patient.

Sarcasm

Some people have a tendency to be sarcastic, or use words that mean the opposite of what they feel, to express frustration or in an attempt to be funny. Sarcasm must be avoided with patients and coworkers. Sarcasm adds a biting edge to words and can be hurtful or misunderstood.

Stereotypes and Communication

We all have a tendency to see what we want to see, forming an impression from a small amount of information or one experience, and assuming that to be highly representative of the whole person or situation. **Stereotypes** form when you judge all people with a similar trait to be the same. For example, it is not fair to assume that all elderly patients are senile, or losing their memory.

Treat each patient as an individual and approach each interaction with an open mind. Stereotypes may affect how you communicate with a person, if you let them. All patients deserve the best care available.

stereotype
an impression that is formed from a small amount of information or one example, assuming that the information or example represents a whole person, group of people, or situation

aphasia
a collection of language disorders caused by brain damage

Patients with Aphasia

Aphasia, a collection of language disorders caused by brain damage, is most commonly caused by a stroke. Other causes can be epilepsy, Alzheimer's disease, brain tumor, or a head injury. The symptoms differ from patient to patient and can range from having trouble finding the right word to use to losing the ability to read, write, and speak altogether. Aphasia does not affect a person's intelligence.

Hearing-Impaired Patients

Communicating with someone who is hearing impaired presents special challenges. If you have the opportunity, learning American Sign Language (ASL) would be valuable to your healthcare career (Figure 15.4).

However, many deaf people can read lips. If this is the case with your hearing-impaired patient, speak slowly and face the patient in a well-lighted area.

When a hearing-impaired patient is accompanied by an ASL interpreter, your conversation is still with the patient, not the interpreter. Face your patient and speak directly with her. Speak in a normal tone of voice, slowly, and clearly. People often speak loudly when talking to a deaf person, but this is unhelpful and should be avoided.

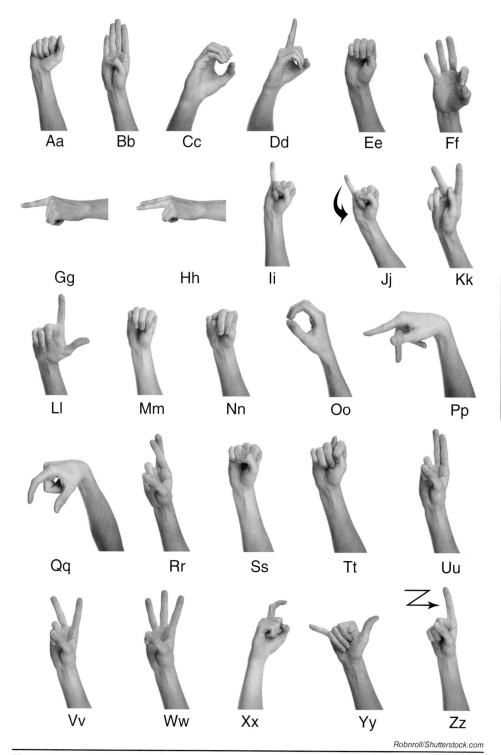

Think It Through

Have you had an experience communicating with a hearing-impaired individual? If so, what methods did you use to ensure you understood one another?

Robnroll/Shutterstock.com

Figure 15.4 The ASL alphabet

Visually-Impaired Patients

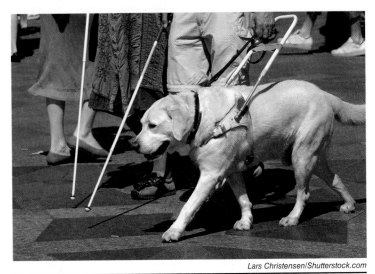

Lars Christensen/Shutterstock.com

Figure 15.5   Do not distract a service dog who is accompanying a visually-impaired person.

Patients with visual impairments present unique communication challenges. Verbal communication is one of the main ways a visually challenged person communicates with the outside world. When working with a visually-impaired patient, you must hone your verbal skills so you are able to communicate successfully with your patient.

Many blind patients will be accompanied by someone who will help them adjust to the environment. However, the patient may be left alone with you temporarily, perhaps in a treatment room. Introduce yourself and address the patient by name, so he knows you are addressing him and not another person in the room. If the patient is standing, guide the patient to a chair by placing his hand on the chair. Remember to ask the patient what assistance is needed instead of making assumptions.

Ensure that the patient is included in discussions about procedures and medical plans. Visually-impaired individuals can still hear and understand what is being said. Be sure to inform the patient what you are doing throughout each step of the procedure. For instance, you do not want the patient to be startled when you apply a blood pressure cuff. Let him know what you are about to do by saying, "Now I'm going to place the cuff around your arm."

Visually-impaired patients may have a service animal (Figure 15.5). The animal must stay with the patient throughout the entire visit, including when the patient visits other facilities. Remember that the service animal is working and should not be petted or otherwise distracted.

Patients with Severe Mental Illness

Severe mental illness may affect patients' judgment, making them incompetent, or unqualified to make decisions on their own. Most patients who have a mental illness that interferes with their judgment will be accompanied by a legal guardian. When communicating with someone who is seriously mentally ill or incompetent, you should speak to the patient first and then to the guardian. Repeat any instructions you may give the patient, making sure that the guardian understands as well. You might also want to demonstrate to the guardian any task that the patient has been shown.

Distressed Patients

Patients can become nervous, confused, scared, sick, and angry when they enter the unfamiliar environment of a healthcare facility. Becoming angry or frustrated with an unsettled patient will only make the situation worse. Remain calm and speak in a steady, confident voice.

Be sympathetic when you see the patient's distress. Sentiments such as "I am so sorry you are upset" and "Let's see if we can make things easier for you" can be very helpful and calming to the patient. Put yourself in the patient's place and respond with compassion. Hopefully, the distressed patient has brought someone to help her understand what you are trying to communicate. If not, proceed slowly and carefully as you work with distressed, unaccompanied patients.

Communicating with Young Patients

When treating children, you must remember that the child is the patient, but the parent is also important in such interactions. Serious illness in children is overwhelming for all parents, but even minor illness can be frightening. The following points are important to remember when you work with children in a healthcare facility:

- Find out where the child is most comfortable—on a parent's lap or on the floor playing with toys.
- Pay attention to the distance between you and the child— many children like you to physically be at their level.
- Work with the child using an unstructured, open approach, perhaps even incorporating play during your time with a small child.
- Take the child seriously and do not talk down to him or her.
- Offer the child support and praise.
- A child may be more relaxed during a procedure if you first demonstrate the procedure on a stuffed animal so the child will know what to expect (Figure 15.6).

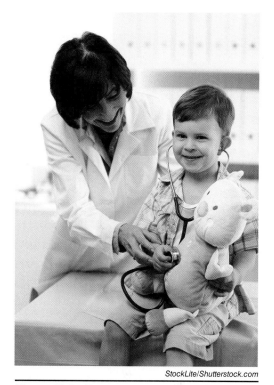

StockLite/Shutterstock.com

Figure 15.6 Toys can make a child more comfortable during a medical examination.

Did You Know? **Children and the Truth**

Part of treating a child with respect is being honest with him or her. Telling a child that a shot or a blood test is not going to hurt may cause lasting distrust of healthcare workers. Telling a child, "you may feel a little pinch" may be more appropriate.

Language Barriers to Communication

Some patients will not be able to communicate with you because they speak another language. Most hospitals have a policy in place to deal with this situation. Additionally, many facilities have a list of employees who speak languages other than English. Be particularly careful to avoid slang expressions, as these can be especially confusing to non-English speakers.

Most importantly, make sure that the patient can understand the information being communicated. You should also make sure you understand any questions that the patient wants to communicate.

The Sender-Receiver Communication Model

sender-receiver communication model
a model designed to describe communication between two people

Most everything that has been and will be accomplished by humans involves communication. An unsatisfactory relationship between two people is often caused by inadequate communication. The **sender-receiver communication model** attempts to describe communication between two people (Figure 15.7).

In this model, the sender encodes, or translates her thoughts or ideas into a message that can be understood by the receiver. The sender's thoughts can be sent using either verbal or written communication. The message is sent to the receiver, but encounters noise on its way. This noise may affect the receiver's ability to decode, or understand the message. Examples of noise include language differences, cultural barriers, the distance between the sender and receiver, or any of the other communication challenges you have learned about in this chapter.

Once the receiver has decoded the message, he must prepare his response and encode his thoughts into a feedback message. The message is sent, and once again encounters noise along the way. When it arrives, the message is decoded and the exchange is complete.

Effective communication includes one's ability to transfer information and express ideas to others. When done well, this can result in successful, meaningful relationships. Successful communication with coworkers and patients helps you provide excellent care.

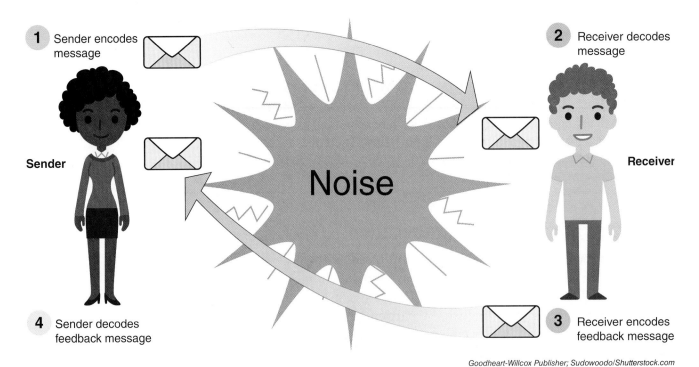

Goodheart-Willcox Publisher; Sudowoodo/Shutterstock.com

Figure 15.7 Communication between two people may be complicated by the influence of noise as messages travel between the sender and the receiver.

Telephone Etiquette

Expand

Regardless of where you work in a healthcare facility, sooner or later you will be answering the telephone. The following steps are an introduction to proper telephone etiquette:

- Answer a ringing phone promptly! If you need to put someone on hold, get his or her permission before doing so. For example, you might say, "May I put you on hold, please?" Do not leave the caller on hold for more than a minute or two without returning to see if he or she wishes to continue to hold. Your healthcare facility may have different guidelines for this.

- When answering the phone, identify the facility or department in which you work, and give your name and title. For example, "Laboratory, this is Jean Smith, laboratory assistant. May I help you?"

- Before making a call, plan what you are going to say.

- When you leave a telephone number, speak slowly and repeat the number twice.

- Speak clearly with a pleasant, professional tone (Figure 15.8).

- Take a clear, concise message. Ask the caller to repeat the message if you are not sure whether you have heard or recorded it properly.

- A proper message must include the date and time of the call, the caller's name spelled correctly, and the telephone number (including the area code). You should also include your name as the person who took the call. Always repeat all numbers, including telephone numbers, addresses, numerical results, and times. Be sure to double-check that you have taken the message down correctly.

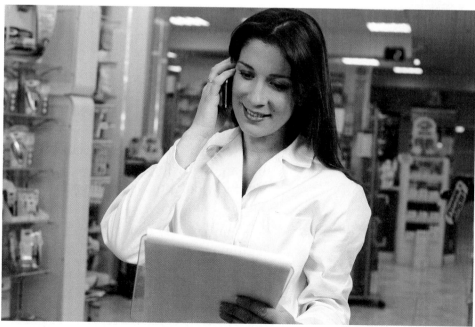

Federico Marsicano/Shutterstock.com

Figure 15.8 You sound friendlier on the telephone when smiling.

- If the message is for someone else, be sure you deliver the message to the correct person. If you are the recipient of a message, return the call as soon as possible.

- Pay special attention to the spelling of the caller's name. Ask for a full name in case the caller has a common name.

- Use "please" and "thank you," and avoid using slang expressions.

- Hold the receiver an inch or an inch and a half from your mouth and speak directly into the receiver.

- Make sure you have confirmed all aspects of the message before you hang up.

- When a doctor calls, answer questions promptly, or transfer the call as soon as possible.

- Remember that you are not authorized to give medical information to a family member or friend of a patient unless the patient has given written permission to do so. Usually, your immediate supervisor should also give permission.

- Do not allow any conversation that identifies a patient or contains personal information to be overheard by other patients or visitors.

Public Speaking

You may be called on to give a presentation in class or in your role as a healthcare worker. Whether you are giving a short talk to fellow classmates or explaining a procedure to fellow workers, there are several public speaking strategies to keep in mind.

- Be prepared. Practice your presentation several times. Know more about your material than you include in your speech. Use humor, personal stories, and conversational language if relevant.

- Look at the audience and establish direct eye contact. Smile, develop rapport, and notice if your audience looks like they are following what you are saying or if they look puzzled or confused (Figure 15.9).

- Relax and slowly count to three before beginning to allow yourself time to calm down. Don't apologize for being nervous. Realize that people want you to succeed.

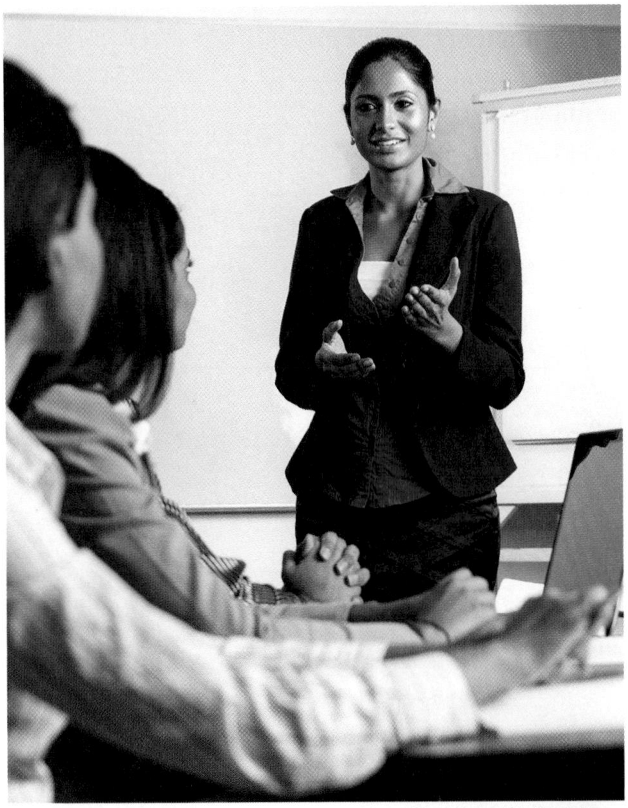

Stuart Jenner/Shutterstock.com

Figure 15.9 Direct eye contact is critical when giving a presentation.

- Know your room. Arrive early to the venue and walk around the speaking area. Practice using the microphone if possible, and make sure any visual aids you may have are present and in working order.

- Remember to be concise and avoid a long, repetitive presentation. Be aware of signs of lagging attention in your audience.

- Develop visuals if appropriate. You may use projected visuals, handouts, PowerPoint® presentations, or demonstrations. Visuals can effectively reinforce your speech. Make sure any technology you might need to use for your visuals is working before the presentation begins.

- Be well-acquainted with your topic. Reading continually from note cards loses your audience's attention. Write down key phrases, quotes, and stories in large letters on note cards to jog your memory as you are talking. Show enthusiasm for your topic.

- Practice, practice, practice! Speak slowly and calmly, but louder than your usual speaking voice (unless you are using a microphone).

Did You Know? | **Overcoming a Fear of Public Speaking**

If you find yourself having to give presentations in your job, and you feel inadequate to do so, you might want to consider joining an organization like *Toastmasters*. This is a nonprofit organization that helps people develop public speaking skills through practice and feedback. There may be many opportunities for you to speak in front of people, such as accepting an award, delivering a eulogy, providing technical information, giving a sales pitch, introducing speakers, and so on.

Meetings

When you become a healthcare worker, you will be asked to attend many meetings. As you take on more responsibility in your job, you may be asked to hold meetings as well.

Attending a Meeting

Meetings vary in importance. Some will be brief, and others will be lengthy. Whatever type of meeting you are asked to attend, there are some general rules that need to be followed:

- **Know the details of the meeting.** Where will it be? What time does it start? What topics will be discussed? Reconfirm these details before the meeting starts to make sure the location and time have not changed.

- **Be on time!** Arrive a few minutes early so that you can get organized before the meeting begins.

- **Come prepared.** You may need paper and pen to take notes. What you will need to bring with you will depend on the type of meeting you're attending.

- **Dress respectfully, yet comfortably.** Your appearance will vary depending on what type of meeting you're attending. If you wear a uniform, make sure it is clean and free from stains. If the meeting is more formal, make sure you wear nicer clothing. Check ahead of time to make sure you won't be underdressed or overdressed.

- **Pay close attention and listen carefully.** Turn your cell phone off and resist the temptation to bring other electronic devices that could divert your attention. The organizer of the meeting will expect you to understand what is being said. If you do not understand, ask questions at an appropriate time to clarify. Try not to yawn.

- **If your participation is needed or expected, make sure you take part in the meeting.** Participation shows that you are listening and are engaged in the conversation. Make sure you show respect for everyone attending.

Holding a Meeting

Meetings can be very productive, but they can also be a waste of time. Ineffective meetings not only stop normal workflow with little gain, they can also be frustrating and lower employee morale. You need to know how to run a meeting that will generate productive results. Here are some techniques to follow:

1. **Send out a meeting request.** Make sure key players can attend at the requested time. Set up another time if the people you want to attend cannot come due to scheduling conflicts. In your request, state the purpose of the meeting. Also, create an agenda after thinking through and preparing each topic of discussion. Your meeting request should be sent with meeting material, such as an agenda, at least two days before the meeting.

2. **Make copies of relevant materials for everyone attending the meeting.** It is important to supply each attendee with the documents to be discussed during the meeting.

3. **Start the meeting on time.** Wait no more than five minutes for latecomers.

4. **Set up ground rules for the meeting.** Make it clear that you will need attendees' full attention, and ask them to turn off all electronic devices.

5. **Get to the point!** Allow a minute or two of pleasantries; make it clear when it is time to get down to business.

6. **Prioritize meeting subjects.** If you have ten topics to discuss, start with the most important items.

7. **Follow your agenda.** Do not allow anyone to get off topic. Be firm when it is time to move on.

8. **Take notes.** This will assure participants that you are listening to their points. If the meeting is complex with many topics, try to have someone else take minutes, or notes, for you.

9. **Know when to end the meeting.** If you have set a time to end the meeting, do not go over your time limit. If topics are not discussed, you may have to hold a follow-up meeting. Watch for signs from your audience that you have talked long enough. If the group starts to fidget, look at their watches, or seem inattentive, it is time to stop. Go over action items that may have been discussed during the meeting and ask for questions.

10. **Send out an overview after the meeting.** The overview should contain a record of who attended, what was discussed, any agreements that were reached, and action items that were assigned. The overview should be completed soon after the meeting is over.

When done correctly, meetings are a good way to make employees feel valued and knowledgeable or informed.

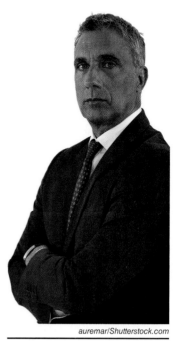

auremar/Shutterstock.com

Figure 15.10 What does this man's body language suggest? Does he seem welcoming?

Check Your Understanding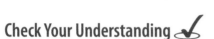

1. What are the 5 Cs of Communication?
2. What communication challenge does aphasia present?
3. Name three techniques for communicating with young patients.
4. What is the sender-receiver communication model?
5. Name three points to remember when holding a meeting.

Nonverbal Communication

Nonverbal communication, or *body language*, is a critical form of communication. This natural, unconscious language reveals your true feelings and intentions in any given moment.

When you interact with others, you continuously give and receive wordless signals. All of your nonverbal behaviors—the gestures you make, the way you sit, how fast or loud you talk, how close you stand to others, whether or not you make eye contact—send strong messages. These messages do not stop when you stop speaking. Even when you are quiet, you're still communicating your thoughts and feelings (Figure 15.10).

nonverbal communication *any form of communication that does not involve speech, including gestures, the way one sits, eye contact (or lack of), and facial expressions; also known as* body language

Real Life Scenario **Inattention**

Rusty is quite anxious to discuss an upcoming exam, so he makes an appointment with his instructor. The instructor greets Rusty and asks him to sit down. However, as Rusty begins to ask questions, the instructor continues to look at his e-mail.

Apply It

1. What message does the instructor's inattention send to Rusty?
2. What are some possible consequences of the instructor's inattention?

Some nonverbal messages are subtle, such as posture. What message does the posture of the students in Figure 15.11 give to their instructor during a lecture?

Frequently, what we say and what we communicate through body language are two different things. When faced with these mixed signals, the listener has to choose whether to believe your verbal or nonverbal message. Often, a listener will be more influenced by nonverbal signals because these tend to be more reliable than words.

Gender Differences in Nonverbal Communication

Studies have shown that men and women differ in their use of nonverbal communication. Women use facial expressions to express emotion more often than men. Women are also more likely to smile and use facial and body expressions to show friendliness. Men do not smile as much. Women may demonstrate more friendly nonverbal cues, but their posture tends to be tenser than men's. Men seem more relaxed and will use more gestures, whereas women tend to rely more on verbal communication.

Women tend not to stare, while men use staring to challenge a powerful person. Men will often wait for the other person to turn away from an initial gaze, whereas women are more likely to avert their eyes. The differences in nonverbal signals between men and women further add to the complexity of communication.

Cultural Differences in Nonverbal Communication

Hand and arm gestures, touch, and eye contact (or lack of eye contact) are some aspects of nonverbal communication that can vary significantly depending on a person's cultural background. Of course, it is important to remember that, within cultures, there is great variation in communication. This discussion can be used to guide your communication so that you do not needlessly offend someone.

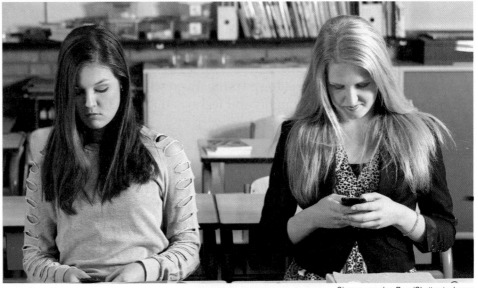

Simone van den Berg/Shutterstock.com

Figure 15.11   Do these students look like they are listening to the instructor?

Gestures

Some gestures commonly used in the United States may be offensive to someone from another culture. An example of this is the use of a finger or hand to indicate for someone to "come here." In some cultures, this gesture may be used to call dogs. Pointing with one finger is not done in some Asian cultures and may be considered rude. Some cultures use the entire hand to point to something.

Touch

In the United States, it is common for someone to pat a child's head as an affectionate gesture. However, in some Asian cultures, this might be considered inappropriate because they believe the head to be a sacred part of the body. In many Muslim cultures, touch between people of the opposite sex who are not related is considered inappropriate.

Eye Contact

In Western culture, direct eye contact is understood to convey attentiveness and honesty. In many cultures (Hispanic, Asian, and Middle Eastern, for example), eye contact may be seen as disrespectful and rude. Women in some cultures may especially avoid eye contact with men as it could be taken as a sign of sexual interest.

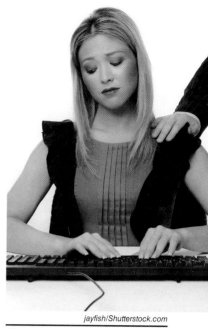

jayfish/Shutterstock.com

Figure 15.12   Has this woman's personal space been violated? Does she seem comfortable with his touch?

Proxemics

Proxemics is the study of our use of space. Proxemics can be divided into two categories: physical territory (rooms and furniture arrangements) and personal territory (the distance you keep between yourself and others).

Personal territory is the area surrounding a person that they psychologically regard as their own. Most people value their personal territory and feel uncomfortable, angry, or anxious when another person enters, or "invades," their personal territory (Figure 15.12). How much you permit another person to enter into your personal territory, or to what degree you enter somebody else's personal territory, can reveal your relationship with that person. Understanding the concept of personal territory when working with patients, coworkers, and visitors increases your ability to provide the best possible care.

There are four types of personal territory. These include intimate space, personal space, social space, and public space (Figure 15.13).

proxemics
the study of humans' use of space; includes physical territory and personal territory

Proxemics		
Personal Territory	*Reserved For*	*Distance*
intimate space	significant others, children, close family	18 inches or less
personal space	friends, coworkers	1.5–4 feet
social space	new acquaintances, strangers	4–12 feet
public space	speeches, lectures, and theater	Greater than12 feet

Goodheart-Willcox Publisher

Figure 15.13   Distances of personal territory can vary among cultures as well as individuals.

The size of an individual's personal territory can vary by locale. People living in a densely populated area tend to have a smaller personal territory, whereas people living in less crowded areas may have a much larger personal territory. What is considered intimate space in one culture may fit another culture's description of social space.

Men and women may also differ in their personal territory requirements. Women tend to stand close to others, while men seek more personal territory. However, men may be more likely to invade someone else's personal territory, if necessary, when asserting themselves during disagreements or emergencies.

Personal Territory and Touch

There are various types of touch, and each type can be received in many ways. Touch can be comforting—such as a pat on the back—or it can be offensive, possibly leading to a sexual harassment lawsuit. People who have experienced sexual abuse or other traumatic experiences may not want to be touched at all. You must be extremely careful when using touch as a communication tool.

In today's society, lawsuits are plentiful, and any touching without a person's consent could be mistaken for something unwanted. Touch should be used with great caution. While providing care, many healthcare workers have to enter a patient's intimate space and should be sensitive to the patient's reaction.

Although a common method of greeting is the handshake, it is not appropriate in many situations in the healthcare facility. Handshakes are typically avoided to help reduce the spread of infection among the patients and healthcare workers.

The type and amount of touching that is appropriate varies with culture, age, gender, and family background. Some families hug every time they part, while others rarely hug. In some cultures and in many of the healing arts, touch is used to promote healing.

If you want to communicate more successfully in all areas of your life, you should strive to become more sensitive to body language and other nonverbal cues. This sensitivity will help you be more in tune with the thoughts and feelings of others. You also need to be aware of the signals you are conveying to ensure that the messages these signals send match what you really want to communicate.

Active Listening Skills

When you think of communication, listening skills may not immediately come to mind. However, listening is a key element in all communication. If you do not receive the message that is being sent, communication has not taken place. If you understand how to be a good listener, you will be a far better healthcare worker, spouse, friend, and communicator.

Active listening is not the same as simply hearing what has been said. Active listening is the decision to be fully attentive and to understand the intent of the speaker. It requires physical and mental attention, energy, concentration, and discipline. As part of your career in healthcare, you will be attending meetings, following directions, working with patients, and giving and receiving feedback. All of these activities require active listening.

active listening
the act of listening intently to not only hear the words being spoken, but to understand the complete message being sent

Strategies for Active Listening

Applying the following active listening strategies can help you build effective relationships in school, in the healthcare environment, and in life.

- **Desire to be a good listener.** You must want to be a better listener. Is your intention to learn about and understand the other person? Or do you feel restless until the speaker stops talking because you want to prove your intelligence and have a chance to shine?

- **Be open and willing to learn.** When listening to someone giving you instruction, are you resistant to learning new information? Be open to different points of view, different styles of lecturing, and new ideas.

- **Show interest.** When you are speaking one-on-one with a patient, it is important to show interest in the other person. Good eye contact, a gentle touch if appropriate, and other body language shows that you are interested in what the patient has to say. If you tune out the message due to disinterest, communication will not take place. Pay attention to the speaker.

- **Resist judgment.** If the speaker is wearing strange clothing, has a reputation for being troublesome, speaks in an annoying voice, or displays other distracting features, focus on the message the person is conveying. Try not to be distracted by these less important aspects of the person.

- **Do not interrupt.** Have you ever been continually interrupted when trying to get a point across to a friend? Recall how frustrating you found the interruptions. Allow the speaker to give you his entire message without interrupting him. If you need to ask a question, wait until the speaker finishes his general message.

- **Show empathy and respect.** Focus on understanding the message and viewpoint of the speaker. Look for common views and ways in which you are alike. Listen with the intent to understand.

- **Look as if you are listening.** Active listening requires high energy—sit up and uncross your legs. Maintain eye contact with the speaker and lean slightly forward.

- **Give feedback.** Repeat what you think the speaker meant. For example: "If I understand you correctly…," "Please correct me if my understanding is wrong…," "What I believe you are saying is…"

Barriers to Active Listening

There are many situations in which active listening is challenging. It is important to listen closely to your patients and coworkers, particularly in a healthcare facility where the well-being of your patients is concerned. People often fail to listen when they face the following situations:

- You are interrupted by someone coming into the room, a telephone ringing, or other people talking loudly nearby.

- You move ahead in the listening process when you think you have heard what the person is saying, thinking to yourself, "I've heard all this before."

- You do not agree with what is being said and, therefore, refuse to listen (Figure 15.14).

- You cannot hear what the patient is saying because of his or her soft voice.

- You do not understand what the patient is saying because he or she has a speech problem, uses challenging vocabulary, or has a thick accent.

- Your mind starts wandering, interfering with your concentration.

To be a good listener, you must concentrate on what is being said, showing a sincere interest in what the speaker is saying. To avoid being distracted, block out everything except the speaker's voice. Do not interrupt the speaker unless you cannot understand what is being said. Ask the speaker to explain what he or she is saying in greater detail. Remember that active listening can be improved with practice. Being a good listener makes you a much better employee and improves the quality of care you deliver as a healthcare worker.

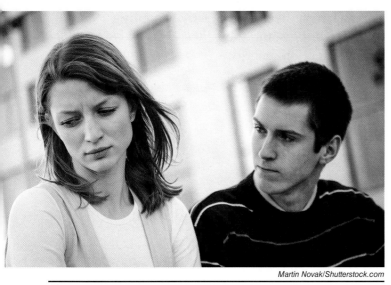

Martin Novak/Shutterstock.com

Figure 15.14   Are these two people demonstrating active listening?

> **Think It Through**
>
> Can you remember times when you have felt that someone was not listening to you? How did it make you feel? How did you make yourself heard, if at all? How can you be a better listener?

Check Your Understanding ✓

1. What is meant by *proxemics*?
2. In regard to nonverbal communication, what are two general differences that may occur between men and women?
3. Explain active listening.
4. Name the four types of personal territory.

Written Communication Skills

Many employers consider written communication to be one of the most important job skills an employee can have. Studies have indicated that the ability to write well seems to be diminishing among students. Therefore, if you can write a message clearly and accurately, that skill will benefit you in the working world. As you study to become a healthcare worker, you must practice using clear, concise writing in your assignments.

Composing written communications can be done effectively if you possess good writing skills. Written communication requires the presentation of clear, logical thoughts. Grammar, an important component of good writing, is covered in Background Lesson 1. Today, few written communications are actually written by hand, except quick notes like telephone messages. The vast majority of written communications are prepared electronically (Figure 15.15). As a result, keyboard skills are essential in today's healthcare world.

Patients entering a healthcare facility may find the experience complicated, and many people struggle with understanding medications, instructions, and follow-up plans. A healthcare worker who communicates with patients through written instructions helps to minimize confusion and provides better patient care.

Written communications offer an excellent opportunity to make a good impression on others, but developing these skills takes time and effort. Throughout your healthcare career, you might be asked to write a variety of communications such as original letters, memos, responses to information requests, telephone messages, e-mails, patient instructions, and supply orders. You will also fill out a variety of forms on a regular basis.

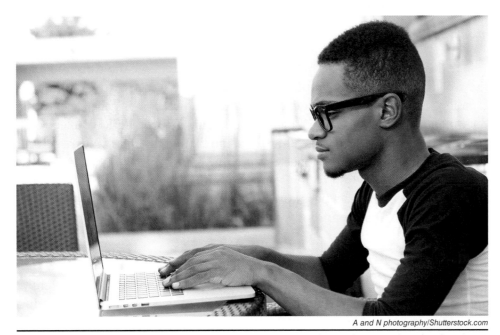

A and N photography/Shutterstock.com

Figure 15.15 Technological advances have made it easy for students and professionals to send written communications electronically.

Of course, to obtain a job you may be asked to present a cover message, job application, and résumé—all of which will require strong writing skills. Job seeking information is covered in-depth in Chapter 18, *Employability Skills*.

Strong writing uses several key elements to get the point across. These elements include using grammar correctly; recognizing and correctly using the parts of speech; spelling and punctuating properly; and using clear, concise words.

Objective Versus Subjective Writing

objective writing
writing based on evidence you can see and evaluate

Most of the writing that you will be doing in healthcare will be **objective writing**. Objective writing is based on evidence you can see and evaluate. Objective writing uses facts and figures. The purpose of this type of writing is to inform the reader.

subjective writing
writing based on evidence you cannot evaluate

Subjective writing is based on evidence you cannot evaluate. You have to accept or reject what the person says. This type of writing emphasizes personal feelings, judgments, opinions, or thoughts.

Consider the case of a medical assistant whose patient reports that his leg hurts a lot. The medical assistant would not write that the patient says that his leg hurt when she sees a gaping wound on his shin. When written objectively, the report would state *patient has a 12-inch gash on his left shin*, rather than a report written subjectively, which would state *patient has leg pain that hurts a lot*.

Some healthcare reports may have both objective and subjective writing. A doctor may share subjective information in the electronic medical record by quoting a patient. For example, the doctor may state that the "patient indicates his leg hurts a lot."

Technical Writing

Technical writing is often used in healthcare. Technical writing is objective, so subjective details should be avoided, unless you are directly quoting a patient in his chart. Documentation is done using physical or electronic documents such as a patient's electronic health record (EHR) or electronic medical record (EMR). Technical writing can be used in a healthcare setting when, for instance, an employee is asked to record *exactly* what happened when a patient fell while trying to get out of her hospital bed. This type of writing requires an exact description of what happened, including the time, place, who was present, and other details.

Writing an Effective E-mail

When you are writing a business e-mail—to an instructor, a fellow employee, or supervisor about a work-related subject—keep the following guidelines in mind:

- **Include a specific subject line.** If you do not put anything in the subject line, chances are your e-mail will not be a top priority. Instead of a subject line that says *Quiz*, a better effort would be *Question concerning 12/8 quiz for Anatomy Class, Section 4*.

- **Keep your message focused.** E-mails are meant to be short and to the point. Long, rambling messages may be only partially read or ignored.

- **Identify yourself.** When e-mailing an instructor, be sure to include the following: your name; the course name and its section number (if it has one); the days on which the course is offered; and your brief, focused message. Do not assume that the instructor knows immediately who you are by your name.

- **Do not e-mail an angry message.** If you find yourself e-mailing in anger, resist the urge. Instead, politely ask the intended recipient (maybe it is your instructor or supervisor) if you may have a meeting with them concerning the topic you wish to discuss. By the time you have the meeting, you may have calmed down and will be able to speak rationally.

- **Proofread your e-mail.** Your point will be taken more seriously if you express yourself intelligently with excellent spelling and grammar.

- **Be courteous.** When asking for assistance and requesting a response, thank the sender by saying something like, "thank you for your quick response," or "I appreciate your assistance in this matter."

- **Do not assume that your e-mail is private.** Your message can be easily intercepted. Do not include any private information about a patient. Be professional in your communications and refrain from gossiping.

- **Avoid any fancy fonts.** Keep your message clear by using a standard font such as Times New Roman or Helvetica.

Sending a Fax

Expand

Even though sending a fax may seem outdated, many offices and facilities still use the fax machine. You may need to know how to write a message for the fax machine and observe certain rules to protect the confidential information you are sending.

When sending a fax, always include a cover page. Your cover page should be simple, free of unnecessary information or artwork. Include your name and contact information, the number of pages you are sending (including the cover sheet), the recipient's name, and any other pertinent information. Keep the page professional, as people other than its intended recipient may look at it.

Use discretion when faxing personal or confidential information. You might want to call ahead to the recipient telling him that the fax is arriving. You can avoid this problem by using an online faxing service, which sends faxes directly to a personal computer.

After sending the fax, make a follow-up call to the recipient to confirm it was received and ask him if he has any questions about the content of the fax.

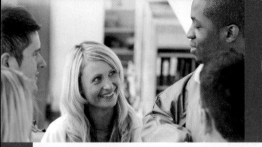
Summary

To be a competent communicator, you must understand and practice English language usage rules. Your ability to communicate successfully is dependent upon your understanding of language. This is true in speaking and listening, as well as written communication such as letters, reports, essays, e-mails, and faxes. Communicating clearly while giving a presentation and holding a meeting is critical for succeeding in both endeavors. If you use incorrect English in your written and verbal communications, you may be misunderstood.

Another way to communicate is through the use of body language. Reading others' body language and being aware of your own body language does much to enhance your communication skills. If you are unaware of the message your body language is sending, you may be sending a message to a patient, a coworker, supervisor, or visitors that is not what you intended at all. You must also be aware of cultural differences regarding gestures, touch, and proxemics.

There are many different types of writing. When writing a report as a healthcare worker, technical writing, devoid of opinion or emotion, is most often used, particularly when documenting patient care and incidents that occurred in the healthcare facility.

Review Questions

Answer the following questions using what you have learned in this chapter.

True or False

1. *True or False?* Meetings should start and end promptly.
2. *True or False?* It is important to read your presentation to the audience.
3. *True or False?* A healthcare worker must be respectful of a patient's personal territory.
4. *True or False?* If you are a new employee, you should not speak up in meetings.
5. *True or False?* It is permissible to leave a caller on hold for up to five minutes.
6. *True or False?* Meetings can sometimes be a waste of time.

7. *True or False?* You should use pet names for patients to make them feel welcome.
8. *True or False?* You should never tell a child that a procedure could be painful.
9. *True or False?* Personal space requirements are universal in all cultures.
10. *True or False?* In general, men seek more personal space than women.

Multiple Choice

11. Which guideline would *not* be appropriate when sending a professional e-mail?
    A. Include a subject in the subject line.
    B. Being honest, even angry, is permissible when sending a professional e-mail.
    C. Be focused with your message.
    D. Proofread your e-mail.
12. Which of the following are barriers to active listening?
    A. people speaking loudly in a nearby room
    B. an inability to understand a patient who has a speech problem
    C. disagreeing with the speaker and not listening
    D. All of the above.
13. Aphasia is _____.
    A. another word for stereotyping
    B. a language disorder caused by brain damage
    C. a disorder that affects intelligence
    D. a form of cancer
14. According to Pat Croce, which of the following are *not* considered part of the 5 Cs of Communication?
    A. confident, casual
    B. consistent, credible
    C. courteous
    D. clear, concise
15. The maximum amount of time listeners can stay attentive to a speaker is _____.
    A. 15 minutes
    B. 20 minutes
    C. 30 minutes
    D. 50 minutes

16. You are stressed and feeling emotional. You are about to have a difficult conversation with a coworker. Which of the following should you *not* do?

    A. Take deep breaths.

    B. Take a walk outside in the fresh air before the conversation.

    C. Take this opportunity to tell your coworker how you really feel.

    D. Recall a soothing image.

17. Which of the following statements about objective writing is *false*?

    A. Objective writing is based on judgments.

    B. Objective writing is based on evidence you can see.

    C. Objective writing uses facts and figures.

    D. Objective writing informs the reader.

18. Nonverbal communication _____.

    A. is also called *body language*

    B. should be used unconsciously

    C. is when you are quiet but still can communicate your thoughts

    D. Both A and C are correct.

19. Which term is *not* associated with personal territory?

    A. intimate space

    B. private space

    C. social space

    D. public space

20. Which statement about sarcasm is true when used in a healthcare setting?

    A. Sarcasm always cheers patients up.

    B. Sarcasm is universally understood by most patients.

    C. Sarcasm can be misunderstood and hurtful.

    D. You should only use sarcasm with coworkers.

Short Answer

21. List three barriers to communication that you might encounter while working in healthcare.

22. Explain the term *proxemics*.

23. Describe three errors you could make while holding a meeting.

24. Briefly explain the sender-receiver communication model.

25. Discuss three responsibilities as a good employee when attending a meeting.

Critical Thinking Exercises

26. On a scale of one to ten, one being a poor communicator and ten being a successful communicator, how would you rate your communication skills? If you did not give yourself a 10 in communication skills, what can you do to improve your verbal, nonverbal, and written communication skills?

27. Public speaking is the number one fear reported by people in the United States. Do you fear getting up in front of people to deliver a speech or presentation? Think about the public speakers you have heard—for example, your instructor might speak in front of many people in a lecture hall. When were you excited about a lecture or presentation you observed? What was it about the speaker that interested you? When were you bored and restless during a presentation? Why?

28. With a partner, role play the following scenarios, both partners taking turns being the healthcare worker and being the patient:

    A. Explain to a child that you are going to take some blood.

    B. Reassure a frightened elderly patient that she will be well taken care of in the hospital.

    C. You are admitting a blind patient with a guide dog into the hospital. Do you interact with the guide dog?

    D. As a nurse, you are assigned to a profoundly deaf patient. How will you communicate?

    E. You are a medical assistant. Your patient cannot speak a word of English. How will you communicate?

29. Have you ever had the experience of calling a business or a healthcare facility and being treated rudely by the person who takes your call? Have you been put on hold for a long time? If you were answering the phone at that business or facility, how would your telephone etiquette differ from the person who took your call?

30. Role play a meeting situation in which you express your needs, wants, and emotions and practice saying "No." Change roles, then evaluate communication and conflict resolution strategies.

31. Are you bothered when someone approaches you and stands too close? Do you prefer to keep a large distance between yourself and others? How might these preferences affect your future healthcare career?

Chapter 16
Medical Math Skills

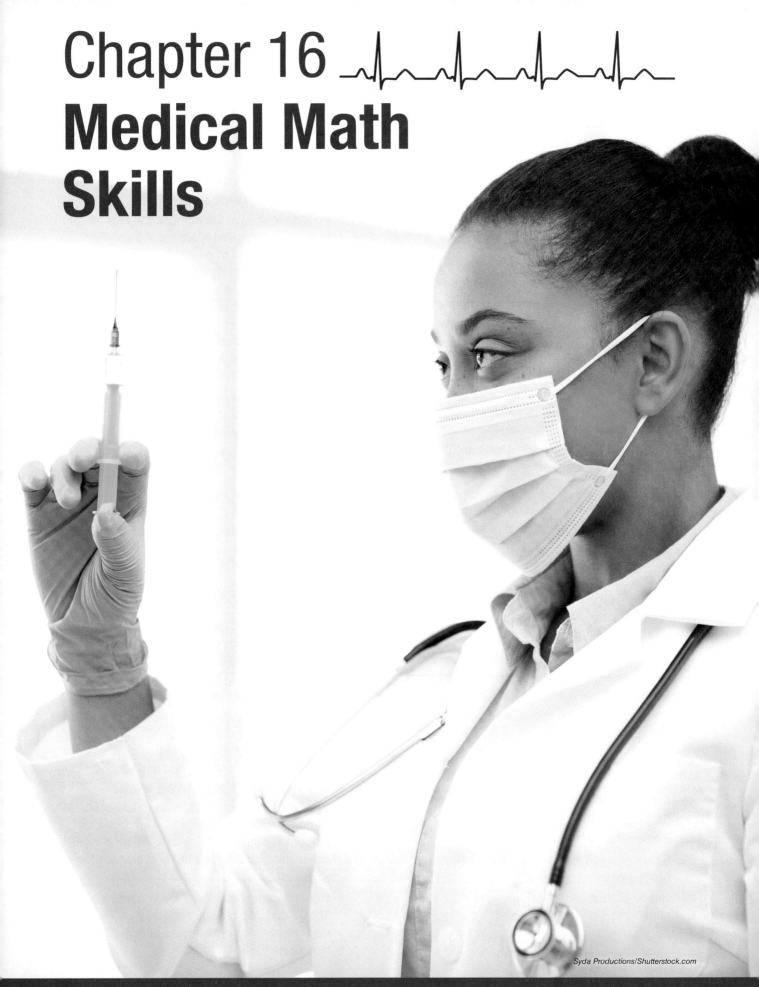

Terms to Know

 Build Vocab

12-hour clock	English system of measurement	on-hand dose
24-hour clock	equations	percentage
administration unit	expiration date	proportion
algebra	generic name	ratio
concentration	mean	Roman numerals
database	median	spreadsheet
decimals	metric system of measurement	trade name
dosage unit	mode	

Chapter Objectives

- Describe the uses of decimal fractions, percentages, and ratios in healthcare settings.
- Perform computations using decimal fractions, percentages, and ratios.
- Explain how algebra can be applied to problem solving in healthcare.
- Identify uses of Roman numerals in healthcare.
- Explain the possible functions of graphs and charts when displaying healthcare information.
- Discuss the importance of the metric system in healthcare and recognize key terms and prefixes used in the metric system.
- Demonstrate how to convert Fahrenheit temperatures to Celsius temperatures.
- Explain how the 24-hour clock works and why it is used in healthcare facilities.

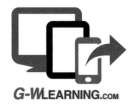

While studying, look for the activity icon **to:**

- **Build** vocabulary with e-flash cards and interactive games.
- **Assess** progress with chapter and unit review questions.
- **Expand** learning with animations and illustration labeling activities.
- **Simulate** EHR entry with healthcare documents.

G-WLEARNING.com

www.g-wlearning.com/healthsciences/

Math is an important skill for anyone seeking to become an effective healthcare worker. No matter which healthcare field you choose for your career, you will be required to perform some math calculations. It is important that you become skilled at performing these calculations because they can contribute to the delivery of quality care and prevent potential tragedies.

You might be wondering, "Why do I need to learn math to be a nurse, medical assistant, or dental hygienist?" Perhaps math has been a challenging subject for you, and you have been hoping that a healthcare career would not require you to do or know much math. If you have thought this or have ever felt overwhelmed by math problems or math classes, you are not alone. Math is difficult for many students.

The good news is, however, that math becomes easier for many people when they see how it used in the real world. In fact, learning some real world healthcare-related math may help you improve your grades in standard math classes.

 Pretest

Throughout this chapter, you will review basic math and make connections to your career goal in healthcare. If you need to brush up on the most basic math operations, refer to Background Lesson 2 at the back of this book. You may want to take the math pretest on the companion website first.

Decimal Fractions

decimals
fractions that are expressed in the base 10 system;
also known as decimal
fractions

If you are considering a healthcare career as a nurse, doctor, or pharmacist, it is vital that you have a strong understanding of calculations involving decimal fractions. Decimal fractions are often called **decimals**, and they are fractions expressed in the base 10 system. Decimals are used when writing prescriptions, administering medications, and providing other types of treatments.

Decimals are special types of fractions that most people find easier to work with than traditional fractions. Like traditional fractions, decimals represent parts of the whole. For example, 0.5 is 1/2 of 1 and 0.75 is 3/4 of 1.

Decimal fractions are always expressed in multiples of ten. Each numeral in a decimal number has a value based on its location in relation to the decimal point. Figure 16.1 shows the place values for the whole numbers and decimal numbers typically used in the healthcare field.

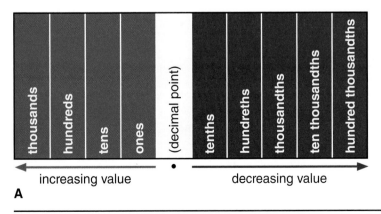

A

Expressing Parts of a Whole		
Decimal	**Fraction**	**Written-Out**
.1	1/10	One-tenth
.01	1/100	One-hundredth
.001	1/1,000	One-thousandth
.0001	1/10,000	One ten-thousandth

B

Goodheart-Willcox Publisher

Figure 16.1   A above shows the place values for the whole numbers to the left of the decimal point and the decimal fractions to the right of the decimal point. B shows the three different ways to express decimals.

Example: 28.74 is a decimal fraction. 28 is the whole number, the (.) is a decimal point, and the numbers to the right of the decimal point represent the decimal itself. This number is read as twenty-eight and seventy-four one hundredths, or as twenty-eight point seventy-four.

In the healthcare field, it is standard to always place a zero to the left of the decimal point when there is not a digit in that value (for example, 0.95). Putting a zero before the decimal point prevents misinterpretation, such as reading .95 as the number 95. This will help you avoid potential life-threatening errors when you are calculating drug dosages, for example.

When writing an equation that features a decimal fraction, you must remember to properly align all of the numbers. Make sure that when you add or subtract decimal fractions, you line up the decimal points from each number.

Example:

```
     23.45
      1.40
+   451.23
   _____
    476.08
```

Converting a Fraction to a Decimal

You will sometimes need to convert fractions to decimals. Converting a fraction to a decimal is done through a division problem. The first step is to divide the numerator (top or first number) of the fraction by the denominator (bottom or second number). If your fraction is 2/3, you should divide 3 into 2.

Example: Change the fraction 7/8 to a decimal number.

```
        0.875
   8 )7.000
      64
      __
      60
      56
      __
       40
       40
       __
        0
```

Check Your Understanding ✓

Convert the following fractions to decimals. Round to the thousandth, if necessary.

1. $\dfrac{3}{4}$ = _____

2. $\dfrac{2}{5}$ = _____

3. $\dfrac{7}{10}$ = _____

4. $\dfrac{5}{6}$ = _____

5. $\dfrac{5}{20}$ = _____

6. $\dfrac{5}{12}$ = _____

7. $\dfrac{3}{12}$ = _____

8. $\dfrac{5}{9}$ = _____

9. $\dfrac{2}{7}$ = _____

10. $\dfrac{2}{3}$ = _____

Real Life Scenario   Working with Decimal Fractions

Suzanne is a part-time occupational therapist. Her schedule for next week has her working some partial shifts as well as a full shift. Suzanne's schedule looks like this:

Monday: 5-1/2 hours
Tuesday: 5-1/4 hours
Wednesday: 6-1/2 hours
Thursday: 3-1/4 hours
Friday: 8 hours

Apply It

1. Convert the mixed numbers shown here into decimal fractions. See the explanation of mixed numbers in Background Lesson 2 if you need help.

2. Add the decimal fractions together to find out how many total hours Suzanne will be working next week.

3. Suzanne wakes up on Thursday with a sore throat. She calls her supervisor to tell him she will not be working Thursday, but will be in on Friday. Now how many hours will Suzanne work for the week?

Rounding Decimal Fractions

Decimal fractions can be rounded up or down for the specific degree of accuracy required. The rounding off rule states that if the digit to the right of the number you are rounding is 5 or greater, round the number *up* to the next highest number. If the digit is less than 5, round the number *down*, which means leaving the original number unchanged and deleting the digits that follow it.

Example:
Round 3.99 to the nearest tenth.
Identify the number to the right of the tenths place: 3.99
Is that number greater than or less than 5? (greater than)
Since the second 9 in 3.99 is greater than 5, add 0.1.
3.9 + 0.1 = 4.0 or 4

In the example above, the number was rounded to the nearest tenth. Now suppose that a decimal must be accurate to the nearest hundredth, or two place values to the right of the decimal point. To round a number such as 17.363 up or down to two decimal places, first locate the digit two places to the right of the decimal point. In this case, that number is 6. Next, look at the number to the right of that digit, which is 3. Since that number is less than 5, round the number off to 17.36. In the case of the number 17.367, the number 7 is greater than 5, so you would have rounded the 6 up to a 7, making the number 17.37.

Let's look at a couple examples. A hospital administrator wants to know how many females are having surgery compared to males. In her calculations she found that, for every male having surgery, there were 3.2 females having surgery. To best present this data to the nursing staff, the administrator must round off this number. She knows that a fraction of a person cannot have surgery, so she rounds *down* to the nearest whole number, 3, because 2 tenths is less than 5.

In some cases, you will need to round to the nearest tenth. Assume that you are going to start your new healthcare position next week, and you need to buy a set of blue scrubs. You find just the right set for $55.30. Sales tax is 3 percent, so you should calculate $55.30 \times 0.03 = \$1.659$. You will need to pay $1.66 in tax because the 9 in the hundredths place is more than 5.

Rounding decimals is an important skill to learn, and you will use it often in your healthcare profession. Rounding decimals is especially important when administering medications. Healthcare workers such as nurses and pharmacists require this foundational knowledge to ensure that their patients are safe. Incorrect rounding can lead to an inaccurate medication amount, which could result in injury, harm, and possible death.

Medications are administered in several different forms, including liquid, powder, tablets, capsules, injections, and infusions. The most common forms of medication that you may prepare and administer are liquid and tablets. More often than not, when you prepare and administer a liquid or injectable medication, you will need to round to the nearest tenth. This is a common situation in which you will need to use your knowledge of rounding decimal fractions.

Extend Your Knowledge ▶ To Divide or Not Divide a Medication

When your calculated dose is not a whole number, you must determine if the dosage form can be safely divided. Certain types of medications, such as the following, cannot or should not be divided:

- unscored tablets
- extended-release medications (designated with *XL*, *XR*, or *ER*)
- enteric coated tablets (designated with *EC*), which don't dissolve until exposed to fluids in the intestines
- capsules

These types of medications cannot be broken or divided safely. Trying to do so would cause the drug to be improperly absorbed and utilized by the body. Some tablets are scored with one or two dividing lines. These tablets can be broken safely in half or in fourths.

Apply It

Assuming tablets are scored only in halves, which of the following medication amounts can be given safely?

1. 2.0 extended release capsules
2. 1.5 enteric coated tablets
3. 0.75 scored tablets
4. 0.75 unscored tablets
5. 1.5 scored tablets

Check Your Understanding ✓

Round the following numbers to the nearest tenth.

1. 26.73 = _____
2. 5679.76 = _____
3. 0.88 = _____
4. 32.562 = _____
5. 215.08 = _____
6. 804.99 = _____
7. 0.0783 = _____
8. 609.37 = _____
9. 69.89 = _____
10. 0.088 = _____

Round the following numbers to the nearest hundredth.

11. 57.337 = _____
12. 0.785 = _____
13. 42.5676 = _____
14. 0.2390 = _____
15. 0.0068 = _____
16. 7,704.129 = _____
17. 672.981 = _____
18. 90.2456 = _____
19. 426.078 = _____
20. 42.735 = _____

Percentages

percentage

an amount per one hundred

A term used to describe part of a whole number is **percentage**. Percent means "per one hundred." Thirty percent, written as 30%, means 30 parts out of 100 parts. Written as a fraction, it would be expressed as 30/100. A number can be written as a fraction, a decimal, or a percentage (Figure 16.2). To solve mathematical problems, you may need to convert a percentage to a fraction or decimal fraction.

Percentages are very important in healthcare. From the infection control nurse, to the radiologist and the healthcare administrator, healthcare workers of all types use percentages to calculate and document information. When documenting meal intake, for example, the nursing assistant might use percentages to document how much of the meal the patient ate.

When we work with percentages, we must remember that the percentage reflects a portion of the whole. For example, if the patient ate the whole plate of food, he would have eaten 100%. If the patient ate half of the food on the plate, the assistant would document that he ate 50% of the total meal.

Calculating Percentages

To calculate a percentage, you must divide the part by the whole. Then convert the resulting decimal to a percentage by moving the decimal point two places to the right and adding a percent sign (%). This will tell you what percentage represents the specified part of the whole.

Example: Grace is in a health occupations class. There are 35 students in the class. A high percentage of the students are interested in a nursing career. The total number of students interested in a nursing career is 28, representing 80% of the students. The calculation to establish this percentage is: 28 ÷ 35 = .80, or 80%.

Converting a Percentage to a Decimal Fraction

To convert a percentage into a decimal fraction, you must divide by 100 or move the decimal point two places to the left and drop the percent sign.

Examples: 14% = 14.0 = 0.14
29.9% = 0.299

Fractions, Decimals, and Percentages		
Fraction	**Decimal**	**Percentages**
3/20	0.15	15%
1/5	0.20	20%
5¼	5.25	525%

Goodheart-Willcox Publisher

Figure 16.2 This table shows three different ways to express the same value. Do you feel more comfortable with one of these methods as compared to the other two?

In the same manner, a decimal fraction can be converted to a percentage by multiplying by 100, or by moving the decimal point two places to the right and adding a percent sign.

Examples: 0.41 = 41%
0.042 = 4.2%

Percentages are often used in your daily life. For example, you are charged a sales tax on every purchase you make. The sales tax is always a percentage of the total bill. You will also see percentages used during department store sales. The sale price represents a percentage of the original price (Figure 16.3).

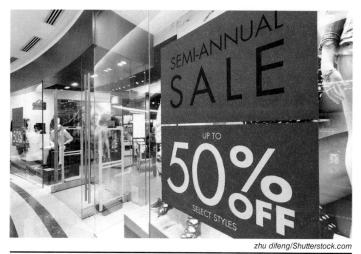

zhu difeng/Shutterstock.com

Figure 16.3 Percentages are often used to broadcast discounts in department store sales.

Check Your Understanding ✓

Answer the following. If necessary, round to the correct whole number using the rounding rules you learned earlier in this chapter.

1. 84 is what percentage of 200?
   A. 25%
   B. 5%
   C. 42%
   D. 75%

2. 30 is what percentage of 40?
   A. 5%
   B. 45%
   C. 75%
   D. 15%

3. Of the 40 RNs on staff at Jacksonville Hospital, only 6 are male. What percentage of the nursing staff is male?
   A. 25%
   B. 15%
   C. 5%
   D. 75%

4. Of the 1,200 active patients at Rosa Villa Medical Center, 60 have accounts that are past due. What percentage of the patients are past due?
   A. 15%
   B. 5%
   C. 25%
   D. 75%

5. There are 15 CNAs available to work nights in the Sunnyvale Long-Term Care Center. This represents only 20% of the CNAs on staff. How many CNAs are on staff?
   A. 35
   B. 75
   C. 15
   D. 42

6. A box of table salt (sodium chloride) contains 40% sodium. If a box of salt weighs 26 ounces, how many ounces of sodium are in the box of salt?

7. 30 people at Eastridge Hospital had surgery on May 21st—4 were children, 12 were men, and 14 were women. What percentage of the people who received surgery on May 21st were children?

8. Dr. Levin, an orthopedist, has 36 patients who suffer from osteoporosis. This condition causes the bones to become brittle and break more easily than healthy bones. This year, 15 patients had broken hips, 11 had collapsing vertebrae, and 10 had broken wrists. What percentage of Dr. Levin's osteoporosis patients had broken hips this year?

Ratios and Proportions

ratio
a mathematical expression that compares one quantity with another, similar quantity

A **ratio** expresses the relationship between two numbers. Ratios can be used to show how many times one number can be found within another number. Healthcare professionals use ratios and proportions in a variety of ways. For example, nurses, doctors, veterinarians, and pharmacists use their knowledge of ratios when administering medications.

The quantities that are compared in a ratio are called the *terms,* or components, of the ratio. The components are written with a colon (:) or the word *to* between them. A ratio can also be expressed as a fraction.

> Example: In Eastridge High School's medical terminology class, there are 15 girls and 10 boys. What is the ratio of girls to boys?
> 15:10, or 15 to 10, or 15/10

Ratios, like fractions, can be reduced, or simplified. Because both 15 and 10 can be divided by 5, you can use that number to reduce the ratio.

> 15 ÷ 5 = 3
> 10 ÷ 5 = 2
> The ratio expressed in its lowest terms would be: 3:2, or 3 to 2, or 3/2

A ratio is written in the same order as the words describing it are written. For instance, the newborn nursery in Eastridge Hospital has one nurse for every four newborns, so the ratio of nurses to newborns would be expressed as 1:4. However, if you wish to express that there are four newborns in the nursery for every one nurse, you would write the ratio 4:1.

If a ratio is known, you can determine what percentage one of the components is of the whole. To do so, first add the components together to get the total. Then, divide the component for which you want to find the percentage by the total. Your answer will be a decimal fraction and you can determine the percentage by multiplying the decimal by 100.

> Example: In Eastridge Extended Care Hospital, the ratio of male patients to female patients is 1:4. What is the percentage of male patients at the hospital?
> The ratio is 1:4, males to females.
> The total number of patients is 1 male + 4 females = 5
> The percentage of males in the hospital is 1/5 or 0.2
> Multiply 0.2 by 100 to get the percentage. 0.2 × 100 = 20%

Supervisors use ratios in many different scenarios. One example is in determining how many nursing assistants will be required to care for the patients in a facility. Suppose that a facility's standard rule is that one nursing assistant can care for eight residents, which is a ratio of 1:8. If, at a particular time, that facility has 160 residents, how many nursing assistants will be needed? Since each nursing assistant can care for 8 residents, you can divide 160 by 8, which equals 20 nursing assistants. Do you see that 1:8 is the same ratio as 20 to 160?

Dietary services workers use ratios in the preparation of recipes. For example, suppose that a dietary services worker knows that he must mix four ounces of milk powder with one quart (32 ounces) of water to produce one quart of liquid milk. In other words, he knows that the ratio of powder to water is 4:32, or 1:8 in lowest terms. So if the dietary services worker needed to prepare a gallon (128 ounces) of milk, how much powder would he need? You can divide 128 by 8, which equals 16 ounces of milk powder.

Check Your Understanding ✓

1. Last month at Eastridge Hospital, 32 infants were born. Of these 32 deliveries, doctors performed 8 Caesarean sections (surgical removal of a baby). What is the ratio of Caesarean sections to normal deliveries expressed in lowest terms?

2. On his flight last week, Jamal sat next to a woman who was coughing and sneezing throughout the entire trip. There were 8 people seated in direct contact with the sick woman. Jamal and two other people became sick a few days later. Of the people exposed to the germs, what was the ratio of those who became sick to those who did not? What percentage of people exposed became sick?

A **proportion** is an equation with a ratio on each side. To use a proportion, the ratios must be equal to each other.

proportion
a statement of the equality of two ratios

Example: 8:4 = 2:1

Another way of expressing this is 8/4 = 2/1 or: $\dfrac{8}{4} = \dfrac{2}{1}$

One way proportions are used by healthcare professionals is in determining dosages of medicine.

Example: John is a 150-pound man. The dosage directions for one of John's medications say to give a 150-pound man 10 milliliters (mL) of the liquid medicine. What if John weighed 300 pounds (lb)? What dosage would he be given then? A proportion can be used to find the answer.

$$\dfrac{150}{10} = \dfrac{300}{x \text{ (or unknown)}}$$

Cross multiply to begin solving for x. Multiply the numerator of the first fraction by the denominator of the second. Repeat this step with the numerator of the second fraction and the denominator of the first. In this case, you end up with:

150x = 3,000

To find the value of x, divide 3,000 by 150. This will isolate x on the left side of the equation.

3,000 ÷ 150 = x
x = 20
A 300-pound man would need 20 mL of the medication to receive the proper dose.

Check Your Understanding ✓

1. The Eastridge Hospital Emergency Department reported that 1 out of 6 patients arriving on the second Saturday in December had the flu. If 78 people were admitted, how many of these patients had the flu?

2. If the ratio of patients on a hospital floor needing special meals is 1:15, and there are 64 patients on the floor, how many special meals are needed?

Introduction to Algebra

Suppose that you are the only nurse on a healthcare unit, and the doctor writes orders for intravenous (IV) fluids for a patient. As you may know, IV fluids can be infused with a manual control or an infusion pump. Regardless of the method, you will be responsible for calculating the correct IV flow rate. How will you accurately calculate the flow rate? A foundational knowledge of algebra can help you with situations such as this one.

Basic Algebra

algebra
the branch of mathematics that substitutes letters for numbers; involves solving for the unknown

Algebra is the branch of mathematics that substitutes letters for numbers to solve for unknown quantities. The term *algebra* comes from the Arabic *al-jebr*, meaning "reunion of broken parts." Algebra problems are designed to find an unknown quantity with the answer represented by a letter—typically x or y. When you learned how to solve for x in this chapter's section on proportions, you were using algebra. This section will briefly explain how algebra can be used while treating patients.

The mathematics involved in an algebraic equation can be described as balancing a scale (recall the scale used to illustrate the scale of justice). What is done on one side must be done to the other side to balance the scale. In the case of an algebra problem, what is done to one side of the problem must be done to the other. Moving from arithmetic (simple math including addition, subtraction, multiplication, and division) to algebra will look something like this:

Arithmetic: $3 + 4 = 4 + 3$
Algebra: $x + y = y + x$

equations
mathematical statements containing expressions composed of numbers and/or letters; two sides of an equation are separated by an equal sign and must be equal to one another

The examples above are **equations**. An equation consists of expressions (collections of numbers and letters) separated by an equal sign. The two sides of the equation must be equal, like a scale that has equal weights on both sides.

When solving an algebra problem, you must first write out the equation and identify the unknown quantity you plan to solve for. Then, use your basic arithmetic skills—addition, subtraction, multiplication, and division—to isolate the unknown on one side of the equation. This will help you determine the value of the unknown.

Example: $3x - 5 = 10$

Add 5 to both sides of the equation to isolate the $3x$ on the left.

$3x - 5 + 5 = 10 + 5$
$3x + 0 = 15$
$3x = 15$

Now, divide each side by 3, so that only the x remains on the left-hand side of the equation.

$3x \div 3 = 15 \div 3$
$x = 5$

To check your answer, insert 5 into the equation where *x* appears.

3(5) − 5 = 10
15 − 5 = 10
10 = 10

Because the two sides of the equation are equal, you know that 5 is the correct answer.

Check Your Understanding ✓

Solve for *x*.

1. 5*x* − 5 = 20   3. 5*x* = 100   5. 20*x* − 20 = 400
2. *x* + 30 = 50   4. 400 × 5 = 2*x*

Using Algebra to Calculate Dosages

A common use of algebra in healthcare is for calculating medicine dosages. Licensed nurses, in particular, are responsible for performing these calculations and administering the proper amount of medicine to a patient. Before learning how to solve algebraic equations involving dosages, you should learn some basic information about medicines and medication packaging. Figure 16.4 is a sample of a typical medication label.

Names that appear on medication labels are of two basic types. **Trade names** are assigned to drugs by their manufacturers. These names vary from one company to another. For example, you may be familiar with the over-the-counter pain relievers Advil and Motrin. These are two

trade name
the name assigned to a drug by its manufacturer

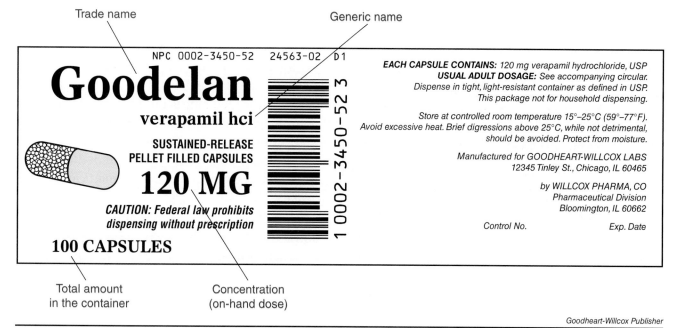

Trade name   Generic name

NPC 0002-3450-52   24563-02 D1

Goodelan
verapamil hci

**SUSTAINED-RELEASE
PELLET FILLED CAPSULES**

120 MG

*CAUTION: Federal law prohibits
dispensing without prescription*

100 CAPSULES

EACH CAPSULE CONTAINS: *120 mg verapamil hydrochloride, USP*
USUAL ADULT DOSAGE: *See accompanying circular.*
Dispense in tight, light-resistant container as defined in USP.
This package not for household dispensing.

*Store at controlled room temperature 15°–25°C (59°–77°F).
Avoid excessive heat. Brief digressions above 25°C, while not detrimental,
should be avoided. Protect from moisture.*

*Manufactured for GOODHEART-WILLCOX LABS
12345 Tinley St., Chicago, IL 60465*

*by WILLCOX PHARMA, CO
Pharmaceutical Division
Bloomington, IL 60662*

Control No.   *Exp. Date*

Total amount   Concentration
in the container   (on-hand dose)

Goodheart-Willcox Publisher

Figure 16.4   Drug labels contain much valuable information for the healthcare worker calculating proper doses to administer to patients.

generic name
the official name assigned to a drug in the United States

different trade names, manufactured by two different companies, for the same drug. In this case, that drug is ibuprofen, which is the **generic name** for this medication.

The generic name for a drug is assigned to the drug officially in the United States. There is only one generic name for each drug, and all drug labels must list the drug's generic name in addition to any trade names so that the drug can be identified by its official name. The generic name of a drug is generally written in lowercase letters. If you look closely at a bottle of Advil or Motrin, you will see that the each bottle's label states that it contains ibuprofen, which is the drug's official or generic name.

dosage unit
the unit of measurement that indicates a drug's weight or action

Dosage units are the units of measurement that indicate a drug's weight or action. These units are used whenever a doctor writes an order for a drug. The most common dosage units are *milligrams, grams, micrograms, grains, units,* and *mil-equivalents.*

administration unit
the unit of measurement used when giving a patient a drug

Administration units refer to the methods in which the medicine is actually measured and given to the patient. Healthcare workers usually measure drugs to be administered by their volume or by counting the number of units. The most common administration units are tablets, capsules, teaspoons, tablespoons, ounces, drops, liters, and milliliters. The total amount is simply the total number of administration units contained in a particular package of the drug.

concentration
the dosage strength of a drug; describes the amount of medication per administration unit

Concentration, or dosage strength, describes the amount of medication per administration unit. For example, drug manufacturers produce tablets and capsules of different strengths. Some capsules might have 120 milligrams of a particular medicine, while others have 80 milligrams. The amount of medication per capsule is its concentration, or strength. This amount is also referred to as **on-hand dose**.

on-hand dose
the amount of medication per capsule or other delivery method

expiration date
the date on which a medication is no longer fit for use

All drugs have an **expiration date**, which is usually preceded by the abbreviation *EXP*. Before giving a drug to a patient, you should always check that the current date, the date on which you are administering the drug, occurs before the drug's expiration date.

When a doctor writes an order for a particular drug, the order almost always requests the drug in dosage units, such as milligrams. However, the medicine is rarely available in a form (administration units) that matches exactly the amount needed by the patient. This means that healthcare workers must calculate how many administration units will be needed to deliver the proper dosage before giving a patient any medication.

Suppose that you have a doctor's order to administer 600 mg of pentoxifylline. The pentoxifylline you have on hand is in a bottle that has a label like the one in Figure 16.5. Looking at the label, you see that the bottle has 100 tabs of pentoxifylolline and that one tablet of pentoxifylline has a strength of 400 mg. How many tablets of this 400 mg strength pentoxifylline should you give to the patient, who is supposed to get a 600 mg dosage? You can use algebra to solve this problem.

Willcal
(pentoxifylline)*
400 MG
CAUTION: Federal law prohibits dispensing without prescription. Do not use of bottle closure seal is broken.

100 TABLETS

Goodheart-Willcox Publisher

Figure 16.5 If the prescribed dose was 600 mg, how many tablets of this medication should the healthcare worker administer?

Several different methods can be used to calculate dosages. The following examples use one common formula. The formula works with all types and strengths of medication, including tablets, capsules, and liquids.

$$\frac{D \text{ (prescribed dose)}}{H \text{ (dose on hand)}} \times Q \text{ (quantity of on-hand dose)} = x \text{ (amount to be administered)}$$

Example 1: A vial of medication states that there are 300 mg (dose on hand) of the medicine per 0.5 mL (quantity of on-hand dose). The doctor orders 600 mg (prescribed dose) of medication to be administered to the patient. How many mL of the medication should the nurse inject?

$$\frac{600 \text{ mg}}{300 \text{ mg}} \times 0.5 = x$$

$600 \div 300 = 2$

$2 \times 0.5 = x$

$x = 1 \text{ mL}$

You should administer 1 mL of the medicine to achieve the desired dose of 600 mg.

Example 2: A doctor orders 500 mg (prescribed dose) of amoxicillin for a patient. You have access to amoxicillin tablets (1 tablet will be your quantity on hand). The tablets are each 250 mg (on-hand dose).

$$\frac{500 \text{ mg}}{250 \text{ mg}} \times 1 = x$$

$500 \div 250 = 2$

$2 \times 1 \text{ tablet} = x$

$x = 2 \text{ tablets}$

You should administer 2 tablets of the medicine to achieve the desired dose of 500 mg. But what if the doctor order looked like this:

Example 3: A pulmonologist orders 125 mg (prescribed dose) of amoxicillin for a patient. You have access to 250 mg (on-hand dose) amoxicillin tablets (1 tablet is the quantity). The same formula is used to make the proper dosage calculation.

$$\frac{125 \text{ mg}}{250 \text{ mg}} \times 1 = x$$

$125 \div 250 = 0.5$

$0.5 \times 1 \text{ tablet} = x$

$x = 0.5 \text{ tablets}$

You should administer half of a tablet to deliver the prescribed amount.

Real Life Scenario — Using Algebra to Calculate Vacation Days

Judy works in the human resources department of Eastridge Hospital. She is told to calculate how many vacation days will be given to new, full-time employees in one year if the employee earns one-and-a-half vacation days every two months.

Apply It

1. How would you set up an algebraic equation for this calculation?

2. How many vacation days would an employee earn per year?

The same formula can also be used to solve the problem at the bottom of page 486 regarding the doctor's order for pentoxifylline. In this case, be careful in choosing what should serve as the quantity in your equation. According to the information, it may seem like your quantity should be 100, as there are 100 tables in the bottle of medication. However, the quantity should be 1 because that is the quantity you're working with for each individual patient.

$$\frac{600 \text{ mg}}{400 \text{ mg}} \times 1 = x$$

$$600 \div 400 = 1.5$$

$$1.5 \times 1 \text{ tablet} = x$$

$$x = 1.5 \text{ tablets}$$

You should administer one and a half tablets to the patient.

Check Your Understanding ✔

For the following problems, use the formula $D \div H \times Q = x$, in which D represents the prescribed dose, H is the on-hand dose (strength or concentration), and Q is quantity, to tell how much of the medication you should give the patient.

1. A medicine vial states that there are 200 mg of medicine per 0.5 mL. The doctor orders 400 mg of medication to be given to the patient. How many mL of the medication should the nurse administer?

2. When working with a patient, a nurse is instructed to give an injection of 75 mg of liquid medication. The medication bottle reads 125 mg/mL. How many mL of the medicine should be administered to achieve the desired dosage of 75 mg?

3. The doctor's order reads: Give the patient 0.4 mg by mouth. The bottle of tablets is labeled 0.2 mg.

4. The doctor's order reads: Give the patient 0.75 g by mouth. The bottle of capsules is labeled 250 mg.

5. The doctor's order reads: Give the patient 90 mg by mouth. The bottle of tablets is labeled 60 mg.

6. A patient needs 600,000 units of a medication. The medicine bottle states that there are 400,000 units per mL. Identify the proper dosage in milliliters to be given to the patient.

Roman Numerals

Roman numerals
letters used by the ancient Romans to represent numbers

You may be surprised to see **Roman numerals** in a textbook about healthcare careers, but this information is important for certain healthcare workers to learn. If you are considering a career as a pharmacist or a pharmacy technician, you will need to review your Roman numerals. These ancient symbols are still used on prescription drug orders and on packaging to designate Drug Enforcement Administration (DEA) schedules for controlled substances. For example, can you interpret a doctor's order that calls for "aspirin gr X"? If you know that the abbreviation *gr* means grains, and that the Roman numeral X means 10, you know that the order calls for 10 grains of aspirin.

Roman numerals originated in Rome, and they were used by the ancient Romans almost 2,000 years ago. The numerals were originally independent symbols. In this system, seven symbols are used: I, V, X, L, C, D, and M. The following Arabic numerals are assigned to each symbol:

- I = 1
- V = 5
- X = 10
- L = 50
- C = 100
- D = 500
- M = 1,000

The numbers represented are 1, 5, and multiples of 5 and 10. There is no zero in this system. Other numerals, such as 2, 3, and 6, are represented with these symbols by placing them in a row and adding or subtracting. It is important to memorize which Arabic numerals each symbol represents.

Did You Know? Counting Sheep

Some historians trace Roman numerals back to shepherds counting their flocks by marking notches on their staffs. When they reached four notches, the fifth sheep would be represented by a "V." Every tenth notch looked like an "X."

Roman numerals were used by bankers and bookkeepers until the eighteenth century because they did not trust symbols like 6, 8, or 9, which could easily be changed into other numbers. The chart in Figure 16.6 shows Arabic to Roman numeral conversions.

Arabic	Roman	Arabic	Roman
1	I	23	XXIII
2	II	24	XXIV
3	III	25	XXV
4	IV	26	XXVI
5	V	27	XXVII
6	VI	28	XXVIII
7	VII	29	XXIX
8	VIII	30	XXX
9	IX	40	XL
10	X	50	L
20	XX	100	C
21	XXI	500	D
22	XXII	1000	M

Goodheart-Willcox Publisher

Figure 16.6 Arabic to Roman numeral conversions

Extend Your Knowledge ▶ Using Roman Numerals in Medicine

In the past, Roman numerals were used in conjunction with the *apothecary system* when writing prescriptions. The apothecary system was used for measuring and weighing drugs and solutions brought to the United States from England during the colonial period. Now, Roman numerals have been replaced mostly by the metric system. However, Roman numerals are still used in some pharmacies for prescription drug orders.

The Drug Enforcement Administration (federal agency that enforces federal drug laws) has created schedules for controlled substances. These schedules use Roman numerals to classify drugs. For example, a drug may be described as schedule I, II, III, IV, or V. The schedules represent the level of risk for potential abuse a drug may carry. Schedule I drugs have a high level of potential abuse. This includes drugs such as heroin, LSD, and ecstasy, which have no known medical use.

Apply It

1. Use the Internet to research examples of drugs that would be classified as schedule I, II, III, IV, and V.

2. How do criminal punishments differ among the different schedules of drugs? Will you be punished more for possessing a schedule IV drug than you would be for possessing a schedule II drug?

There are several things to remember about using Roman numerals:

- If a smaller numeral comes after a larger numeral, the smaller numeral is added to the larger one.

  XI = 10 + 1 = 11

- When the same numeral appears next to itself, the repeated numerals are added together.

  XXX = 10 + 10 + 10 = 30

- If two numerals that are the same appear together, with a smaller numeral in between, the result is as follows:

  XXIX = 10 + 10 + 9 = 29

- No numeral is repeated more than 3 times.

  XXX = 30
  XL = 40

Check Your Understanding ✓

Convert the following numbers to their Arabic or Roman equivalents.

1. XXXIV	4. 349	7. CL	10. CLVIII
2. D	5. XXIX	8. CLIV	
3. 501	6. 1,100	9. DC	

Data Analysis

The healthcare world produces a wealth of information each day. Hospitals need to keep track of inventory to maintain vital supplies, pharmacies need to be aware of the medications they have on hand, and health departments need to analyze rates of contagious disease outbreaks. Medical assistants, dental hygienists, and nursing assistants input information on spreadsheets and use charts and graphs to document height and weight, vital signs, and infant head circumference. These are just a few examples that demonstrate the importance of building a strong foundation in data analysis as part of your healthcare education.

Mean, Median, and Mode

The statistical tools of mean, median, and mode are three ways of analyzing data. Each of these tools will help you find a different type of statistic. To find the **mean**, total all numbers in your information and divide the result by the quantity of numbers you have been given.

mean
the mathematical average of data

> Example: Lori decides to calculate how much money she spent taking her beagle to the veterinarian in the past year. Her charges are listed in Figure 16.7.

After adding up the total of each bill, Lori determines she spent $795.00 on vet bills last year. Now she wants to know what the average amount was for each visit. To calculate the mean, or average, take the total Lori has paid ($795) and divide it by the number of visits (5).

$$\frac{\$795}{5} = \$159$$

On average, Lori spent $159 per vet visit.

The **median** is the number that falls exactly in the middle of a list of numbers organized in either ascending (*increasing*) or descending (*decreasing*) order.

median
the number exactly in the middle of a group of numbers listed in ascending or descending order

> Example: As Figure 16.7 shows, Lori's vet bills were $110, $110, $140, $165, and $270 (in ascending order). The median number is $140 because it is in the exact middle of the values (two above, two below).

Lori's Vet Expenses		
Month	**Services**	**Charges**
January	Checkup, shots	$140
March	Office visit, ear examination, ear medicine, nail trim	$165
May	Office visit, allergy testing, hypoallergenic food	$270
July	Office visit, allergy shots	$110
October	Office visit, allergy shots	$110

Goodheart-Willcox Publisher

Figure 16.7   Use the data in this table to calculate mean, median, and mode for Lori's vet bills.

In the example on the previous page, it was easy to identify the median because there were an odd number of bills. However, if you have an even-numbered list (let's say that Lori went to the vet six times), look for the *two* numbers that fall in the middle of the group. Add these two numbers together, and then divide the total by 2, because that's how many numbers were entered into the equation.

> Example: Imagine the numbers in your list are 1, 2, 3, 4, 5, and 6. The median numbers are 3 and 4.

Add 3 + 4 together and you get 7. Now divide by 2 because there were two median numbers.

> 7 ÷ 2 = 3.5, the median is 3.5

mode
the number that occurs most frequently in a set of numbers

The **mode** is the number that occurs most frequently in a set of numbers. Some lists of numbers do not have a mode, while others may have one or more. In the case of Lori's vet bills, the mode is $110 because it is the only number that appears twice in the list.

Spreadsheets and Databases

spreadsheet
a document containing rows and columns of data; useful for organizing numeric values and performing computer calculations

A **spreadsheet** is a document that displays information in rows and columns, and is usually created by a computer program. Each row and column contains cells that hold information in the form of words or numbers (Figure 16.8). Spreadsheet programs make it easy to perform mathematical operations on groups of numbers. You can easily add a column; calculate the mean, median, or mode of a column; or perform other mathematical operations on information organized in a column or a row. Inserting formulas into the spreadsheet will enable you to perform automatic calculations.

database
a collection of records such as addresses, phone numbers, and other patient information

A **database** is a detailed collection of related information organized for convenient access, generally using a digital device. An example of a database in a doctor's office is a specialized database with patient information such as name, address, telephone number, emergency contact number, Social Security number, health insurance information, and dates of office visits.

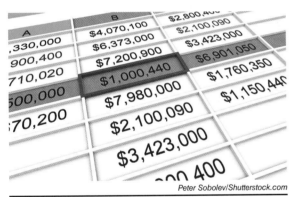

Peter Sobolev/Shutterstock.com

Figure 16.8 Spreadsheets are particularly useful for compiling and calculating numerical data.

Real Life Scenario   Using Mean, Median, and Mode in Healthcare

Five people who visited the Eastridge Hospital emergency room on Sunday were admitted with the following temperatures: 98.6°F, 101°F, 105°F, 98.6°F, and 98.6°F.

Over the course of the past week, the following number of meals was served each day in the Eastridge Hospital cafeteria:

Monday—145 meals
Tuesday—152 meals
Wednesday—192 meals

Thursday—230 meals
Friday—230 meals

Apply It

1. Calculate the mean, median, and mode of the patients' temperatures at Eastridge Hospital.

2. Calculate the mean, median, and mode for the number of meals served over the course of five days at Eastridge Hospital.

Charts and Graphs

Charts and graphs are used to display information clearly and quickly. Healthcare facilities use charts and graphs extensively. Temperature is often graphed on a patient's chart so the doctor can quickly view the fluctuations in a clear, easy-to-read manner.

Many graphs and charts are used throughout the healthcare world. The examples shown here depict the annual number of cases of influenza in one clinic. The same data is represented in four formats—a simple table, line graph, bar graph, and circle graph (or *pie chart*).

A simple table arranges dates and numbers of influenza cases in a clinic in rows and columns (Figure 16.9). A line graph shows the relationship of two or more numbers (Figure 16.10). This graph can also show trends across periods of time. A bar graph shows comparisons among categories; in this case, the months of the year (Figure 16.11 on the next page). For our purposes, the pie chart in Figure 16.12 on the next page presents the number of influenza cases by season.

Reading Graphs

When you read bar and line graphs, you will see a vertical axis called the *y axis* and a horizontal axis called the *x axis*. In Figure 16.10, the graph's *y* axis represents a clinic's total flu cases. The *x* axis represents the period of time in which the cases were recorded (January–December). Data was entered for each month, and the line connecting the data points illustrates trends in the number of flu cases. You can see that the flu cases were highest in the winter months, and that the number of cases declined in the summer months.

Month	Cases of influenza
Jan	55
Feb	50
Mar	45
Apr	35
May	26
Jun	14
Jul	7
Aug	6
Sep	7
Oct	25
Nov	31
Dec	40

Goodheart-Willcox Publisher

Figure 16. 9 A simple table

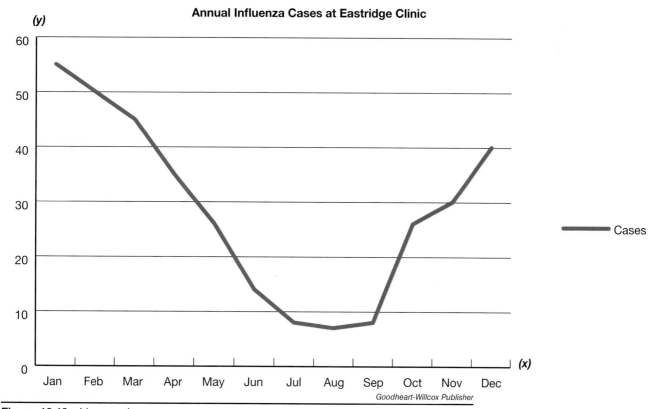

Goodheart-Willcox Publisher

Figure 16.10 Line graph

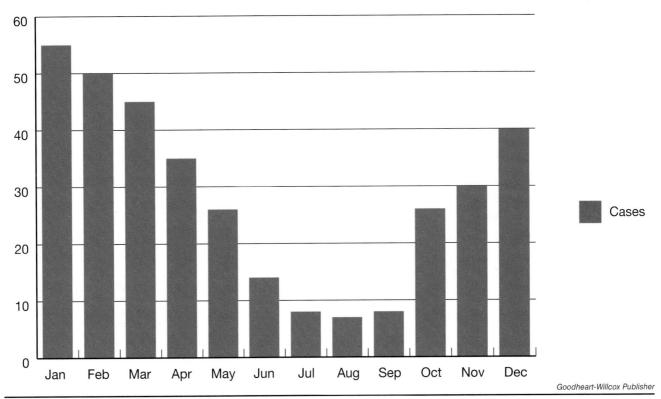

Figure 16.11   Bar graph

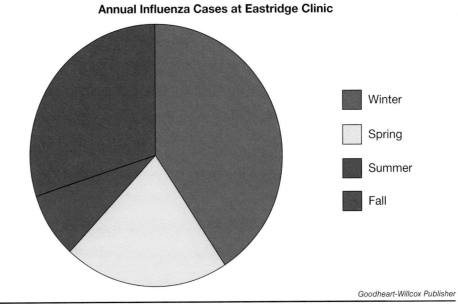

Figure 16.12   A circle graph is sometimes called a *pie chart*.

The bar graph in Figure 16.11 shows the same values represented on the *x* and *y* axes as Figure 16.10. In the case of a bar graph, the number of flu cases per month is easily read. Data trends are also easy to identify by comparing the height of each month's bar. Figure 16.12 is a circle graph (or *pie chart*), another way of showing relationships.

Check Your Understanding ✔

1. John works in sports medicine. Broken arms account for 1/4 of his patients' injuries, knee injuries make up another 1/4 of the cases, broken fingers account for 1/8 of his cases, 1/8 are elbow injuries, and 1/4 are shoulder injuries. Create a pie chart representing this data.

2. Emile works in the human resources department of Eastridge Hospital. His boss has asked him to make a bar graph showing how many total sick days hospital employees used during each month of the last year. Put the following data into a bar graph:

January: 190	April: 130	July: 110	October: 125
February: 195	May: 125	August: 100	November: 140
March: 165	June: 115	September: 110	December: 180

Measurement in Healthcare

When asked to measure something, most people in the United States use the **English system of measurement**. The United States is one of the few countries that have not converted to the metric system. The rest of the world has adopted the **metric system of measurement**.

The main differences between the metric and English systems of measurement can be found in the measurement units. All of the units in the metric system are organized by factors of ten, which provides a simple, consistent way of comparing the different units to each other. On the other hand, units of measurement in the English system are not logically related or consistent. In addition, while the English system uses many different units (ounces, pounds, quarts, gallons, feet, and inches, to name a few), the metric system has only three basic units: the gram, liter, and meter.

For most people, doing calculations using the metric system is much easier than doing calculations with the English system. The metric system is easier to work with because the English system does not have a logical relationship (such as the powers of 10) among the different units of measure. For example, legend has it that the length of a yard is based not on a logical connection but on the distance from King Henry I's nose to his thumb.

For these reasons, the metric system is universally used in science and medicine. Those who wish to have a career in healthcare must become comfortable using the metric system by understanding its terminology, including its basic units and its prefixes.

English system of measurement
a system of measurement commonly used in the United States; measurements are based on the inch, pound, gallon, and Fahrenheit degrees

metric system of measurement
a system of measurement using units related by factors of ten; measurements are based on the gram, liter, meter, and Celsius degrees

Did You Know?   The History of Measurement

The English system of measurement was originally based on the human body, nature, and everyday activities. For example, an acre originally was a measure of land based on the amount of land that could be plowed in a day. An inch was the width of a thumb. Such natural measures were fine for a simple, agricultural society. However, as trade and commerce grew, there was a need for more exact measures.

The metric system was developed by the French to create a system that uses units related by factors of ten and only three basic measurements for weight, volume, and length.

Basic Metric Measurements		
Metric System	**Measures**	**English System**
gram (g)	weight or mass	ounces and pounds
liter (l)	volume	cups, pints, quarts, and gallons
meter (m)	length	inches, feet, yards, miles

Goodheart-Willcox Publisher

Figure 16.13   Basic measurements as represented in the metric and English measurement systems

Metric Units

There are three basic units of measurement in the metric system—grams, liters, and meters (Figure 16.13). The gram (g) is the basic metric unit of measurement for weight. Weight is the physical measurement of an object subjected to the force of gravity. Scientists consider mass and weight the same within the gravitational field of Earth. In the English system, weight is measured in ounces and pounds.

The liter (l) is the basic metric measurement for the volume of liquid and gas. In the English system, volume is measured in cups, pints, quarts, and gallons.

The meter (m) is the metric unit for linear measurement (length). It is slightly longer than the English yard. Inches, feet, and miles are other English units of measurement for length.

Metric Prefixes

To properly use the metric system as a healthcare worker, you will need to recognize a variety of metric prefixes. These prefixes are added before the basic units (meters, grams, liters) to indicate the size of a particular metric unit. Figure 16.14 lists the metric prefixes, the related multiple of 10, and an example.

Converting Measurements

In addition to scientific use, the metric system is being used in industry, governmental agencies, education, and many other important areas in the

Metric Prefixes		
Prefix	**Multiple**	**Example**
nano-	1/1,000,000,000	1 nanometer=1/1,000,000,000 of a meter
micro-	1/1,000,000	1 microliter=1/1,000,000 of a liter
milli-	1/1,000	1 millimeter = 1/1,000 of a meter
centi-	1/100	1 centiliter = 1/100 of a liter
deci-	1/10	1 decimeter = 1/10 of a meter
deca-	10	1 decagram = 10 grams
hecto-	100	1 hectometer = 100 meters
kilo-	1,000	1 kilogram = 1,000 grams
mega-	1,000,000	1 megameter = 1,000,000 meters
giga-	1,000,000,000	1 gigameter = 1,000,000,000 meters

Goodheart-Willcox Publisher

Figure 16.14   Metric prefixes

Real Life Scenario — Converting Height and Weight to the Metric System

Angela is studying the metric system in a Nursing Science course. She is asked by her instructor to convert the following heights and weights of patients into meters and kilograms of the metric system. She can use a calculator. She knows that 1 pound = 0.45 kilograms and that 1 foot = 0.3048 meters.

Apply It

1. Ronald is 6 feet tall and weighs 200 pounds. His metric height and weight: _____

2. Isabel is 5 feet tall and weighs 150 pounds. Her metric height and weight: _____

3. Ashley is 5 feet 5 inches tall and weighs 130 pounds. Her metric height and weight: _____

4. Thomas is 5 feet 8 inches tall and weighs 145 pounds. His metric height and weight: _____

5. Ida is 4 feet 11 inches tall and weighs 115 pounds. Her metric height and weight: _____

United States. Being able to convert a measurement from the English system to the metric system, and vice versa, is a very useful skill to master. As a healthcare worker, you will likely find yourself converting English measurements to metric measurements more often than converting metric to English.

Consult the metric conversion chart in Figure 16.15 on the next page to convert values in the English system to the metric system. Find the English measurement that you wish to convert in the left-hand column. Then, multiply by the number in the middle column to convert to the related metric system value.

Example: 145 pounds = _____ kilograms
140 pounds × 0.45 = 65.25 kilograms

You can also convert from the metric system to the English system. To do so, divide the metric value by the number given in the middle column of the chart. Your answer is the related English system value.

Example: 100 grams = _____ ounces
100 grams ÷ 28.0 = 3.57, or rounded to 3.6 ounces

Check Your Understanding ✓

1. Calculate your weight, height, and body measurements (waist, hips, and chest), and then convert the English measurements to metric units.

2. Convert the mileage on your car to kilometers.

3. On a recent trip to Canada, you filled your gas tank with 40 liters of gasoline. How many gallons of gasoline did you put in your tank?

4. Convert 100 kilometers per hour into miles per hour.

5. Convert cups to liters: 10 cups, 4 cups, 20 cups, 14 cups

6. Convert quarts to liters: 2 quarts, 6 quarts, 10 quarts, 15 quarts

7. Convert pounds to kilograms: 100 pounds, 200 pounds, 150 pounds, 215 pounds

8. Convert feet to centimeters: 3 feet, 6 feet, 9 feet, 12 feet

9. Convert ounces to grams: 5 ounces, 7 ounces, 10 ounces, 14 ounces

10. Convert inches to millimeters: 5 inches, 2 inches, 10 inches, 12 inches

Conversion Table: English to Metric*		
When You Know ⬇	**Multiply By:** ⬇	**To Find** ⬇
Length		
inches	25.4	millimeters
inches	2.54	centimeters
feet	0.3048	meters
feet	30.48	centimeters
yards	0.9	meters
miles	1.6	kilometers
Weight		
ounces	28.0	grams
ounces	.028	kilograms
pounds	0.45	kilograms
short tons	0.9	tonnes
Volume		
teaspoons	5.0	milliliters
tablespoons	15.0	milliliters
fluid ounces	30.0	milliliters
cups	0.24	liters
pints	0.47	liters
quarts	0.95	liters
gallons	3.8	liters
cubic inches	0.02	liters
cubic feet	0.03	cubic meters
cubic yards	0.76	cubic meters
Area		
square inches	6.5	square centimeters
square feet	0.09	square meters
square yards	0.8	square meters
square miles	2.6	square kilometers
acres	0.4	hectares
Temperature		
Fahrenheit	$5/9 \times (F - 32)$	Celsius
Celsius	$(9/5 \times C) + 32$	Fahrenheit

Note: For all but temperature, when you know the metric measurement, divide by the same numbers given above to determine the English measurement.

BMI Calculation	US Customary	SI Metric
	$BMI = \dfrac{wt\ (lb)}{ht\ (in^2)} \times 703$	$BMI = \dfrac{wt\ (kg)}{ht\ (m^2)}$

Figure 16.15   English to Metric conversion table

Metric Temperature Measurement

Think It Through

Why do you think the United States has not converted from the English system of measurement to the metric system? Brainstorm a list of pros and cons to switching from the English system of measurement to the metric system.

The Celsius temperature scale (°C) is a metric scale used to measure temperature throughout the healthcare world. The Celsius scale is in general use wherever metric units are accepted, and it is used in scientific work everywhere. Many countries have adopted the Celsius scale, but the United States has not. Celsius is often reported with Fahrenheit in scientific journals and medical literature in the United States. The Fahrenheit temperature scale (°F) is the non-metric scale used in the United States to measure body temperature in healthcare facilities.

The freezing point of water on the Celsius scale is 0°, and the boiling point is 100°. The Fahrenheit scale is based on a system that is less logical and often more challenging to use. The freezing point of water on the Fahrenheit scale is 32°, and the boiling point is 212°.

Most healthcare facilities have conversion charts that can be used to convert temperatures on one scale to the other and vice versa. The conversions can also easily be made by using specific formulas.

Converting Temperatures from Fahrenheit to Celsius

The formula for converting Fahrenheit temperatures to Celsius is:

$$°C = \frac{5}{9} \times (°F - 32).$$

Example: °F = 98.6°

$$C = \frac{5}{9} \times (98.6 - 32)$$

$$C = \frac{5}{9} \times 66.6$$

$$C = \frac{5 \times 66.6}{9}$$

$$C = \frac{333}{9}$$

$$C = 37°$$

Converting Temperatures from Celsius to Fahrenheit

The formula for converting Celsius temperatures to Fahrenheit is:

$$°F = \frac{9}{5}(C) + 32.$$

Example: °C = 37°

$$F = \frac{9}{5} \times (37) + 32$$

$$F = \frac{9 \times 37}{5} + 32$$

$$F = \frac{333}{5} + 32$$

$$F = 66.6 + 32$$

$$F = 98.6°$$

Check Your Understanding ✓

Convert the following Fahrenheit temperatures to Celsius. Round to the nearest hundredth, if necessary.

1. 98.6°F

2. 100°F

3. 10°F

4. 37°F

5. 40°F

Convert the following Celsius temperatures to Fahrenheit.

6. 0°C

7. 5°C

8. 37°C

9. 100°C

10. 50°C

Answer the following questions.

11. While on vacation in Germany with your family, you become ill and need to visit a doctor. The doctor tells you that your temperature is 39°. Given your location, you assume, correctly, that he has given your temperature using the Celsius scale. Using the appropriate conversion formula, what is your Fahrenheit temperature?

12. You are a nurse at Eastridge Hospital and you have a patient from France. She asks you what her temperature is, and you tell her 103°F. She doesn't understand what this means. Convert her temperature into Celsius using the appropriate formula.

The 24-Hour Clock

24-hour clock
method of measuring time based on 24-hour-long segments; also called military time

12-hour clock
method of measuring time based on a 12-hour system in which a.m. and p.m. designations must be assigned to identify the proper time; used internationally

In the healthcare world, time is often expressed using the **24-hour clock**, which is commonly known as *military time*. A clear, concise way of accurately recording time is essential in a healthcare facility. Medical records are legal documents, so they must include accurate times. Time is critical when treatment, medication, and duration of procedures depend on accurate timekeeping.

The **12-hour clock** (which you typically use in your daily life) has the disadvantage of using just 12 numbers to designate 24 different hours. This means that each of those 12 numbers is used twice a day. Therefore, without the a.m. and p.m. designations, you cannot know for sure what time of day a particular number represents.

In contrast, the 24-hour clock designates every hour with a unique numerical time. When you say that it is 11:00 o'clock, do you mean 11:00 a.m. or 11:00 p.m.? If you are using military time, then those hours are written as 1100 and 2300, respectively. You don't need the a.m. or p.m. designation, and there is no chance for confusion.

Time on the 24-hour clock is always expressed in four digits. The first two digits represent the hours, and the second two digits represent the minutes. A 0 is placed in front of the hours 1 through 9 (01, 02, 03, and so on). Colons are not used to separate hours from minutes. Figure 16.16 shows how the 12-hour clock relates to the 24-hour clock.

Comparison of the 12-Hour Clock to the 24-Hour Clock			
12-hour clock	*24-hour clock*	*12-hour clock*	*24-hour clock*
1:00 a.m.	0100	1:00 p.m.	1300
2:00 a.m.	0200	2:00 p.m.	1400
3:00 a.m.	0300	3:00 p.m.	1500
4:00 a.m.	0400	4:00 p.m.	1600
5:00 a.m.	0500	5:00 p.m.	1700
6:00 a.m.	0600	6:00 p.m.	1800
7:00 a.m.	0700	7:00 p.m.	1900
8:00 a.m.	0800	8:00 p.m.	2000
9:00 a.m.	0900	9:00 p.m.	2100
10:00 a.m.	1000	10:00 p.m.	2200
11:00 a.m.	1100	11:00 p.m.	2300
12:00 p.m.	1200	12:00 a.m.	2400

Goodheart-Willcox Publisher

Figure 16.16   Conversion of the 12-hour clock to the 24-hour clock

Check Your Understanding ✓

Convert the following 12-hour clock times to military time.

1. 1:35 a.m.
2. 3:34 p.m.
3. 7:15 p.m.
4. 10:45 p.m.
5. 9:09 a.m.

Convert the following military times to the 12-hour clock.

6. 2345
7. 1450
8. 0256
9. 1145
10. 0637

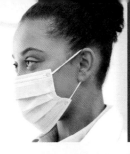

Summary

No matter what healthcare field you decide to enter, you will be required to perform some math calculations when doing your job. Decimals, percentages, basic algebra, ratios, and proportions are all important skills that will be used in your healthcare career.

Analyzing data is another skill for healthcare workers to learn and practice. You can use the mean, median, and mode, along with charts and graphs, to illustrate the relationships among numbers. Data analysis is a critical part of healthcare. Healthcare workers continuously compile statistics about the facility in which they work. Compiling this data may include gathering and updating patient information, keeping track of nosocomial infection rates, and tracking on-hand medical supplies.

Although the metric system of measurement is used in healthcare and science disciplines, the majority of the United States continues to use the English system. As you begin your healthcare career you must understand the metric system and its basic units—the gram, liter, and meter. Converting measurements of temperature from the metric, Celsius scale to commonly used Fahrenheit values is another important math skill for all healthcare students to master.

Because of its accuracy, the 24-hour clock (military time) is used in most healthcare settings. Healthcare workers must learn how to read and easily use military time. Maintaining accurate and proper records is dependent on the use of this timekeeping system.

Improving your math skills will not only benefit your career, but it can also make things easier in your daily life.

Review Questions

Answer the following questions using what you have learned in this chapter.

True or False

1. *True or False?* The English system is more logical than the metric system.

2. *True or False?* Algebra involves equations.

3. *True or False?* The 24-hour clock is the same as military time.

4. *True or False?* The term *percentage* means "per 100."

5. *True or False?* A yard is a metric measurement.

6. *True or False?* A spreadsheet displays information in rows and columns.

7. *True or False?* The mode is the number exactly in the middle of a group of numbers.

8. *True or False?* The statistical tool called the *mean* is a mathematical average of data.

9. *True or False?* 2200 is the same as 8:00 p.m.

10. *True or False?* The prefix *milli* is 1/1,000 of a meter.

Multiple Choice Assess

11. _____ is the branch of mathematics that substitutes letters for numbers.
    A. Algebra
    B. Arithmetic
    C. Geometry
    D. Statistics

12. Each of the following is a metric prefix *except* _____.
    A. nano-
    B. maxi-
    C. mega-
    D. giga-

13. The three basic statistical terms used to analyze information are _____.
    A. averages, median, sum
    B. median, mean, mode
    C. mean, estimate, prediction
    D. total, mode, sum

14. The mode of a set of numbers is _____.
    A. the average
    B. the sum of the numbers
    C. an estimation
    D. the number that occurs most frequently in a number set

15. Which of the following statements about decimal fractions is *true*?

    A. They are a special type of fraction that most people find easy to use.

    B. They are also called *decimals*.

    C. Decimal fractions represent parts of the whole.

    D. All of the above.

16. Which of the following is *not* a type of graph or chart?

    A. Roman graph

    B. bar graph

    C. pie chart

    D. line graph

17. Which of the following statements about the 12-hour clock is *true*?

    A. The 12-hour clock is used in all hospitals.

    B. The military uses the 12-hour clock exclusively.

    C. The 12-hour clock has unique numbers for each hour of the day.

    D. The 12-hour clock is commonly used in our everyday lives.

18. A gram measures _____.

    A. weight or mass

    B. volume

    C. length

    D. width

19. Which Arabic number is expressed as XXXIV in Roman numerals?

    A. 36

    B. 34

    C. 32

    D. 44

20. What is the answer when you convert the percentage 28.9% to a decimal fraction?

    A. 29

    B. .0289

    C. 0.289

    D. .00289

21. The doctor's order is 0.6 mg by mouth. The bottle of tablets is labeled 0.2 mg. How many tablets should the patient be given?

    A. 12

    B. 4

    C. 3

    D. 6

22. The bottle states 200 mg per 0.25 mL. The order calls for 400 mg. How many mL should be given?

    A. 0.5

    B. 5.0

    C. 1.25

    D. 0.125

Short Answer

23. What is the difference between the 12-hour clock and the 24-hour clock?

24. Explain how spreadsheets and databases might be used in a healthcare facility.

25. Which measuring system is used throughout most of the world? Why is this measuring system preferred?

26. What are the three basic units of measure in the metric system?

27. How are Roman numerals used in today's healthcare system?

Critical Thinking Exercises

28. What are the differences between the Fahrenheit and Celsius temperature scales? What might be the advantage of using the Celsius scale instead of the Fahrenheit scale?

29. Why is it important for members of a healthcare team to use the 24-hour clock?

30. Do you have a preferred type of graph or table to express data for analysis? pie chart? bar graph? line graph? simple table? Explain why you find one method better for expressing and analyzing data than the others.

31. Do you think that the United States should begin using the metric system and the 24-hour clock exclusively? Do you think this change will happen in the future? Why or why not?

32. Which type of calculation do you find the most confusing? decimal fractions? percentages? measurement conversions? algebra? basic arithmetic? Why? What can you do to feel more comfortable when performing the calculations that confuse you?

Additional Practice

Decimals

Answer the following questions without using a calculator.

1. 19.55 + 127 + 2,130.02 + 54.5 = _____

2. Round off each of the following numbers to the nearest tenth.
   A. 534.67
   B. 45.64
   C. 5.69

3. Round off each of the following numbers to the nearest one-hundredth.
   A. 3.456
   B. 43.333
   C. 57.892

4. A patient has a medical bill for $16,201.99. What is the balance remaining after her insurance company pays $12,961.59?

5. Convert the following fractions to decimal fractions.
   A. 5/16
   B. 43-2/5
   C. 4-4/7

Percentages

Answer the following questions without using a calculator. When necessary, round off to the nearest hundredth.

6. Convert 42% to a decimal fraction.

7. What is 20% of 150?

8. What is 6.5% of 645?

9. Convert 180% to a decimal fraction.

10. Convert 0.657 into a percentage.

11. One study has found that 25% of people who get the flu shot will still get the flu. If 15,230 people got the vaccine, how many people would still get the flu even with the vaccination?

12. In a health science class of 29 students, 12 students want to work in a hospital, 10 students want to work in a doctor's office, 3 students want to work in a clinic setting, and 4 are undecided. What percentage of students wants to work in a hospital?

13. Convert 85% to a decimal fraction.

14. Convert 5-3/4 into a percentage.

15. Convert 3.1416 into a percentage.

Ratios

Answer the following questions without using a calculator.

16. Convert 1:5 into a fraction.

17. In a chemistry laboratory, a student is asked to create a solution that contains 10 milliliters of a weak acid to 400 milliliters of distilled water. What is the ratio of the weak acid to the distilled water?

18. A student planning to be a dietician is surprised to learn that a gallon of ice cream contains 15 grams of fat, 12 grams of which are saturated fat. What is the ratio of saturated fat to the total fat in the gallon of ice cream?

19. Express the ratio 6:4 two different ways.

20. An instructor grades a health occupations class final. 24 students passed. 4 students failed the class. What is the ratio of students who passed to those who failed?

Algebra

Answer the following questions without using a calculator.

21. $x + 15 = 45$

22. $3x - 18 = 78$

23. $4x + 2 = 8$

24. $1/4\ x + 12 = 220$

25. $1/5\ x - 10 = 365$

26. Dr. Edward has x number of patients. Dr. Ryan has twice as many patients as Dr. Edward. Dr. Ryan has 42 patients. How many patients does Dr. Edward have? Show your work.

27. A doctor has ordered 80 mg of medication to be given to a patient by mouth. The medicine label indicates that one capsule contains 20 mg of medicine. How many capsules should be given to the patient to reach the required dosage?

28. The doctor has ordered that 120 mL of IV fluid be administered over 60 minutes with a tubing factor (how many drops per mL the tubing delivers) of 10 drops per milliliter. Determine the drops per minute using the following formula:

$$\frac{\text{number of milliliters to infuse}}{\text{number of minutes to infuse}} \times \text{tubing factor} = \frac{\text{drops per minute}}{\text{(gtt/minute)}}$$

Roman Numerals

Convert the following Arabic numbers to Roman numerals.

29. 1,002
30. 103
31. 545
32. 32
33. 145

Convert the following Roman numerals to Arabic numbers:

34. XI
35. LXIII
36. DXIV
37. CXXIV
38. CLVII

Data Analysis

Answer the following data analysis questions using what you have learned in this chapter.

39. Grace, a patient at Eastridge Hospital, has been running a fever for the past eight hours. Construct a line graph showing Grace's temperature at each hour. Then, look at the resulting graph and explain why this representation of the data might be helpful to a healthcare professional.

0600–102°F	1000–100.6°F
0700–102°F	1100–100°F
0800–101.6°F	1200–99.2°F
0900–101°F	1300–99°F

40. Construct a bar graph using the following patient data from Eastridge Hospital.

    2 patients have a temperature of 103°F

    5 patients have a temperature of 99.8°F

    7 patients have a temperature of 101.6°F

    12 patients have a temperature of 98.6°F

Measurement in Healthcare

Answer the following questions about metric units, metric prefixes, and measurements using the metric system.

41. A gram measures _____.
42. A liter measures _____.
43. A meter measures _____.
44. One kilogram is equal to _____ grams.
45. One milliliter is equal to _____ liters.
46. One hectometer is equal to _____ meters.
47. One decagram is equal to _____ grams.

48. One microliter is equal to _____ liters.
49. One inch is equal to _____ millimeters.
50. One gallon is equal to _____ liters.

Converting Measurements

Answer the following questions without using a calculator.

51. On Stan's hospital chart, the doctor notes that Stan must consume 2 liters of fluid per day. How many milliliters should Stan drink each day?

52. Convert the following measurements to liters.

    A. 769 kiloliters

    B. 77.2 deciliters

    C. 24 hectoliters

    D. 2,456 milliliters

53. The majority of adults have 5,000 to 6,000 mL of blood in their bodies. Convert this quantity to quarts.

54. Convert 68°F to Celsius.
55. Convert 100°C to Fahrenheit.
56. Convert 84°F to Celsius.
57. Convert 120 pounds to grams.
58. Convert 85 pounds to grams.
59. Convert the following weight to the metric system (meters and kilograms): 6 feet 2 inches, 185 pounds
60. Convert the following weight to the metric system: (meters and kilograms): 5 feet 4 inches, 135 pounds

The 24-Hour Clock

Convert the following 12-hour clock times to military time.

61. 2:30 p.m.
62. 11:30 p.m.
63. 4:15 p.m.
64. 3:30 p.m.
65. 10:00 a.m.
66. 1:45 a.m.

Convert the following military times to 12-hour clock time.

67. 0155
68. 1137
69. 0320
70. 1305
71. 1700
72. 2212
73. 2310
74. 0222
75. 1450

Chapter 17
Study Skills

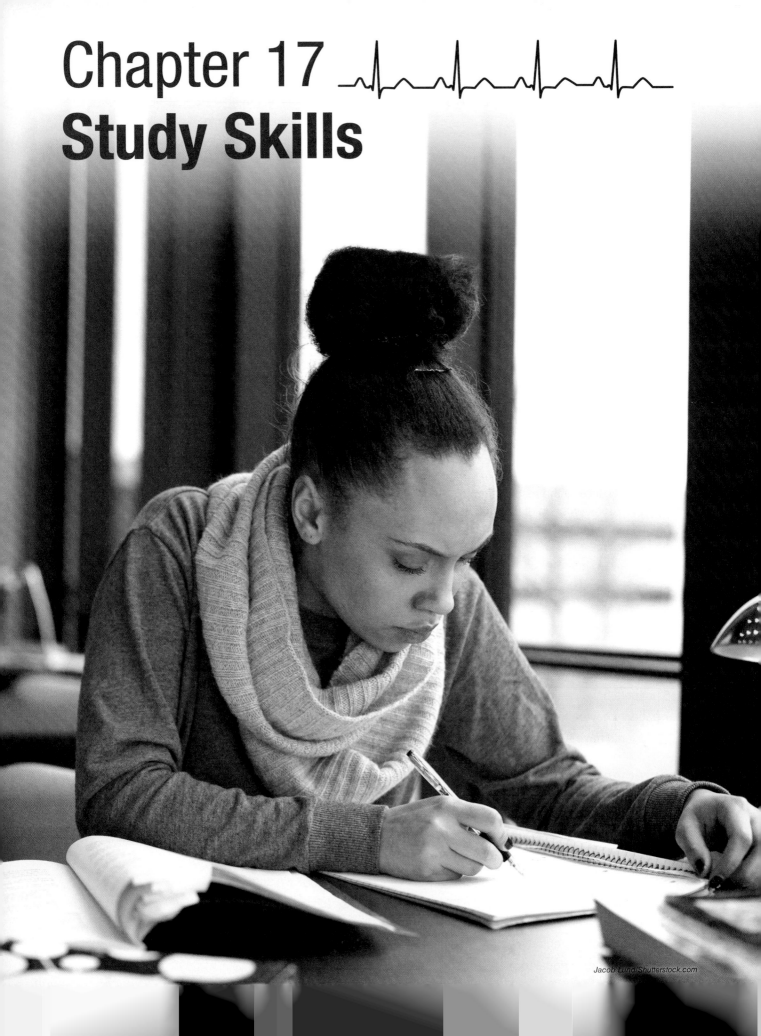

Jacob Lund/Shutterstock.com

Terms to Know

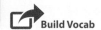

active reading

auditory learner

critical thinking

decoding

dyslexia

kinesthetic learner

learning styles

mnemonic devices

motivation

retention

thesaurus

time management

visual learner

vocabulary

Chapter Objectives

- Identify the importance of motivation, goals, confidence, and direction for achieving your career goals.
- Describe learning styles and their application for effective learning.
- List ways to effectively manage your time.
- Explain the concept of critical thinking and how this skill can be applied to your healthcare career.
- Discuss the benefits of daily reading.
- Identify techniques for improving your vocabulary.
- Explain the concept of active reading.
- Identify strategies to use when reading difficult and dense material.
- Explain what decoding is and how it relates to dyslexia.
- Discuss steps you can take to increase your reading speed.
- Explain ways to decrease eyestrain when reading or using a computer.
- Describe strategies for taking effective notes in class.
- Discuss ways of improving your memory.
- List effective ways to study for and take a test.
- Explain steps to take after finishing a test.

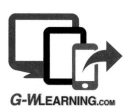

While studying, look for the activity icon to:

- **Build** vocabulary with e-flash cards and interactive games.
- **Assess** progress with chapter and unit review questions.
- **Expand** learning with animations and illustration labeling activities.
- **Simulate** EHR entry with healthcare documents.

G-WLEARNING.com

www.g-wlearning.com/healthsciences/

Learning is a lifelong adventure. People who enjoy success in life are often those who continue to study and learn throughout their lives. When pursuing a career in healthcare, you will be faced with many challenges in your field, including technological, societal, and economic changes. To succeed in the face of these challenges, you will need to be a lifelong learner and practice new skills in school, at work, and in your private life.

You may be undecided about what course of study you would like to pursue. Depending on your career goal, you could be looking at anywhere from six months of coursework to eight or more years of schooling. Regardless of your course of study, you will have opportunities to further your education even after you achieve your career goal.

This chapter will present a variety of approaches to mastering the skills every successful student needs. These skills include

- learning how to self-motivate;
- understanding your particular style of learning;
- managing your time well;
- understanding that effective studying relies on excellent reading skills;
- practicing critical thinking;
- listening carefully to instructors;
- taking effective notes;
- improving your memory; and
- preparing for, and taking, tests.

If you can build and improve your study skills, you will greatly increase your chances of achieving your career goals. Learning how to study effectively can bring you closer to a dream job. Good study skills may also help you advance up the career ladder.

Real Life Scenario   Understanding the Assignment

Madison is a first semester freshman at her local community college. She is taking her first science course, *Introduction to Anatomy and Physiology*. Madison has never been a top science student, and she is very nervous about taking this course. Her instructor speaks rapidly and has an accent she doesn't recognize. When Madison receives her first assignment, she does not understand what is required of her. The assignment is worth several points.

First, Madison consults a classmate, Ben. She explains to Ben what she *thinks* the instructor is asking for. Ben believes she is on the right track but has questions about the assignment himself.

Madison then asks her instructor for help, but she still does not grasp what the assignment is about.

Apply It

1. Have you ever been expected to comprehend an assignment and found that you did not? If so, what did you do? What would you suggest Madison do to ensure she understands her instructor's expectations?

2. Choose an activity you have encountered in this textbook and explain it to a classmate. What did you need to do to be sure your classmate understood the assignment?

Assessing Your Study Habits

Before you begin reading this section, take a moment to reflect on your study habits. Do you hit the books as soon as your teacher announces an upcoming test? Are you more successful when studying in a quiet environment, or do you prefer listening to music while studying? Some students have a hard time getting motivated to study before a test. Does that sound like you?

Analyzing your study habits now will allow you to better adopt and use the study skills presented in this chapter. Many factors influence your study habits. As you read this section, think about your level of motivation, whether or not you have trouble staying focused, and strategies for setting and meeting your goals.

Motivation

One important factor that shapes a person's study skills is the level of his or her motivation. **Motivation** is what causes us to act, whether that means baking cookies to satisfy a craving or researching new biomedical treatments to complete a homework assignment. When motivated, you are more likely to study for an important test, even though there are other things you might rather be doing. Motivation helps us reach our personal and career goals.

motivation
a process by which one initiates, guides, and maintains goal-oriented behavior

Staying motivated can be difficult. You might feel motivated at one moment, but you might lose that motivation when you experience a failure. Negative thoughts and concerns about the future can be distracting. At some point, everyone doubts their abilities. What separates the successful from the not-so-successful is whether one can stay motivated and keep moving forward despite those doubts.

Learning how to nurture motivating thoughts, ridding yourself of negative thinking, and focusing on the task you wish to complete can help you become motivated again. There are several strategies to help you stay motivated, including staying focused on your goal, being confident in your abilities, and establishing a direction as you pursue your goal.

Focusing on Your Goal

One way to stay motivated is to establish a goal and focus on ways to achieve that goal. Have you chosen a career goal? Let's say that you want to be a registered nurse. How can you achieve your goal? Talk to a career counselor at your school to find out about loans, grants, and scholarships for higher education. Your counselor may also know if work-study programs are available, and which nearby schools offer a nursing degree. Work with a counselor when applying for a medical course. Map out the courses you will be taking to help you move from being unfocused to focused. Keep your eye on the ball and do not let yourself be distracted from your goal (Figure 17.1). A lack of focus is the first barrier to motivation.

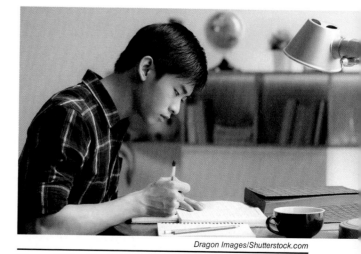

Dragon Images/Shutterstock.com

Figure 17.1 Staying focused on your goals is critical to academic and career success.

Think It Through

Do you have trouble listing your strengths or the positive aspects of your life? If so, do the negatives interfere with this exercise? What does that tell you?

Building Your Confidence

Lack of confidence can also affect your overall motivation. Past failures, bad luck, and personal inadequacies may cause you to lose confidence. You may use these problems as excuses for why you cannot succeed.

The way to get out of this negative mind-set is to focus on what's good in your life. Make a list of your strengths, your past successes, and the positive aspects of your life. It is human nature to take our positive achievements for granted and to focus on our failures. Tell yourself that you have the ability to be successful. Positive thoughts can motivate you to pick up your textbook and study for the test you are confident you will ace.

When you truly believe that you deserve success, you will find it easy to create ways to achieve your goal. Feeling confident in your abilities will enable you to be a successful student and healthcare worker.

Establishing a Direction

Once you have focused in on a goal, you need to establish a direction, or a specific strategy to achieve your career aspirations. If you do not have an established direction, you may lose motivation and begin to procrastinate. Procrastinating occurs when you put off an action until a later time. You may tell yourself that studying today is unnecessary because you will have time tomorrow or the next day, but this strategy often hampers your success.

If your motivation starts to disappear, establish your direction by creating a step-by-step plan that includes small tasks to accomplish as you work toward your ultimate goal. A first task might be studying to get a good grade on an upcoming biology quiz. Your next task can focus on a long-term goal such as planning your courses for the next year.

You will have periods of low energy, bad luck, and even failure. Do not let such periods block you from your career goal. Establish a goal, identify the direction you plan to take, and stay confident in your abilities to realize your career goal. These practices will help you stay motivated as you work toward academic and career success.

Learning Styles

Another way to improve your study habits is to determine how you learn best. Research shows that students can perform better on tests if they change their study habits to fit their learning styles.

Just as people have different personalities, they also possess a variety of **learning styles**. There are three basic learning styles—visual, auditory, and kinesthetic. We rely on our senses to process the information around us. As a result, some students best remember materials they have seen, others best remember materials that they have heard, and still others best remember materials they have experienced firsthand. Most people possess a combination of the three learning styles, but one style is often dominant.

learning styles
different ways that people learn; three basic types include visual, auditory, and kinesthetic; most people have a mixture of all three

Determining Your Learning Style

To determine your learning style, you may want to talk to your school's counselor. There are also learning style tests that can be found online. Just make sure the test comes from a credible source. Once you have determined your style, you must remember that there is significant variation in each style and each person. The following are descriptions of each style. See if you recognize your own traits in these descriptions. Remember that people can have more than one learning style.

The Visual Learner

Visual learners are those who learn by seeing things (Figure 17.2). You may be a visual learner if you are someone who

- may not enjoy or immediately understand a lecture;

- often enjoys colors and fashion;

- understands and appreciates charts and PowerPoint® presentations;

- may spell well but could forget your name; and

- needs quiet when you study.

visual learner
one who learns through seeing visual representations of ideas and concepts; charts, color-coded notes, and videos can be helpful tools for this learner

If you are a visual learner, the following suggestions may help you while studying:

- Create outlines to help learn the material.

- Copy what is on the board during a lecture.

- Take extensive notes, using color coding if possible.

- Make lists.

- Watch videos on the subject you are studying.

- Use flash cards.

- Use highlighters to circle key words and underline important phrases.

- If you study history, draw a timeline of events.

- Whenever possible, create an illustration to represent the topic being studied.

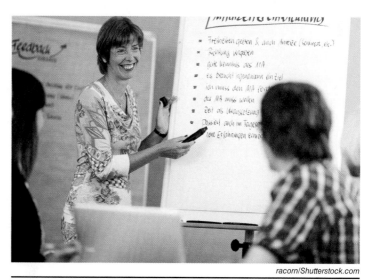
racorn/Shutterstock.com

Figure 17.2 Visual learners often appreciate instructors who use charts while teaching.

The visual learner usually does well on tests that require reading a map, writing an essay (if the student has studied using an outline), or showing a procedure. The more challenging tests for a visual learner are "listen and respond" tests, such as listening to a piece of music and answering questions about what you have just heard.

The Auditory Learner

auditory learner

one who learns best by listening; lectures, discussion, and talking about ideas and concepts are helpful tools for this learner

Auditory learners learn best by hearing things. You may be an auditory learner if you are someone who

- likes to read to yourself out loud;
- often enjoys giving speeches and presentations in class (Figure 17.3);
- does well in study groups;
- likes to teach others;
- is good at remembering names;
- enjoys music; and
- follows spoken directions well.

Auditory learners might use the following strategies when studying:

- record lectures (provided that you get permission from your instructor)
- repeat facts
- participate in group discussions
- use tapes when learning a language

Auditory learners may find timed tests challenging if the test requires reading passages and writing answers about the material. These learners are good at writing information in response to lectures they have attended. They can also excel at oral exams, such as those given in foreign language classes.

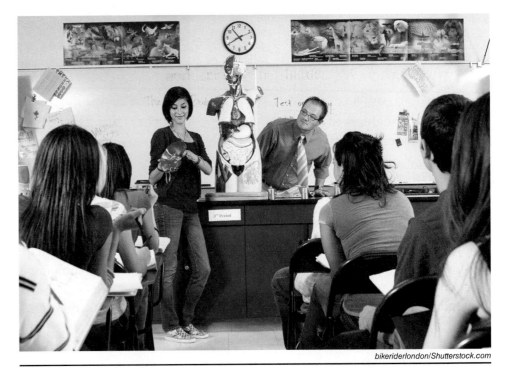

bikeriderlondon/Shutterstock.com

Figure 17.3 Auditory learners may enjoy giving presentations in class.

The Kinesthetic Learner

Kinesthetic learners are those who learn through hands-on experience. These learners are also called *tactile learners*. You may be a kinesthetic learner if you are someone who

- needs to move around in your seat after a short period of listening to an instructor;

- may have some trouble with spelling;

- may have less than perfect handwriting;

- loves active learning situations, such as conducting experiments in the lab (Figure 17.4);

- can study while listening to loud music;

- enjoys participating in sports;

- likes action movies; and

- needs to take breaks while studying.

kinesthetic learner
one who learns through experiencing and doing activities; labs and field trips can be helpful for this learner

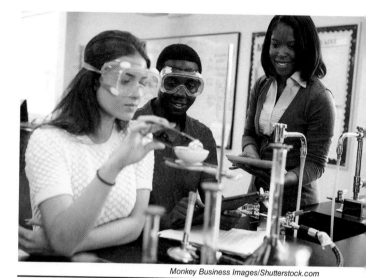
Monkey Business Images/Shutterstock.com

Figure 17.4   Lab activities are especially useful for kinesthetic learners.

Kinesthetic learners may do well studying with others. Memory games and flash cards may be helpful instructional tools for the kinesthetic learner. Some kinesthetic learners also appreciate when an instructor moves around while lecturing. In general, kinesthetic learners do better on tests with short definition, fill-in, and multiple choice questions; they may have a harder time with long, essay-heavy exams.

Sometimes an instructor's teaching style does not satisfactorily address a student's learning style. Understanding the differences among the learning styles will help you to deal with an instructor whose teaching methods favor a learning style that you do not possess. You might benefit from a conference with the instructor to explain how your style differs from his or her teaching methods. This will allow the two of you an opportunity to brainstorm ways you can succeed in the instructor's classroom.

Check Your Understanding ✓

1. Why is it important to be a lifelong learner?
2. Name three strategies for staying motivated.
3. What are three basic learning styles?
4. Which learning style might the following students favor?
   A. Jeff does not like to sit still.
   B. Maria finds charts to be helpful in class.
   C. Joanna is really good at remembering names.
   D. José enjoys loud music when studying.
   E. Rachel likes to color code her notes.

Time Management

time management
the process of planning and controlling the amount of time spent on specific activities to increase efficiency and productivity

Effective **time management** is an important skill for every student to learn, as it allows you to schedule time for studying. Successful, effective studying requires that you review material while you are alert and motivated. To study well, you must manage your time wisely. Most of us do not have the luxury of unlimited time, so we must make the most of the time we have for studying. Here are some tips for scheduling study time to effectively review your material:

- **Determine the best time of day to study**. Many people feel refreshed and clearheaded early in the morning. Others do their best studying after midnight.

- **Study the hardest or least interesting subject first**. Focusing on this information first will ensure that you have the energy to get through it. Save your favorite subjects for later. The fact that you enjoy those subjects should motivate you even if you have been studying for a while.

- **Get rid of distractions**. Try to eliminate or minimize distractions such as TV, music, the Internet, and your cell phone. Let others know that you need to study and will respond to them when you are done. If you have to leave your study area, write a note to yourself detailing what you were studying when you were interrupted.

- **Take advantage of downtime**. If you have to wait 20 minutes for a doctor's appointment or have an hour between classes, use this time to study. Always be prepared to sneak in short study periods that will allow you to accomplish small tasks. For example, write formulas or vocabulary terms that you have to memorize on an index card and carry them with you. iPads and other mobile devices are convenient study tools, and some educational programs offer student websites that you can visit using your smartphone.

- **Find the ideal study area**. Finding an area where you can study allows you to focus more quickly (Figure 17.5). You might do well studying in a well-lit, quiet library or even in a classroom environment. A desk with a comfortable, supportive chair can be helpful. Make sure you have all of the necessary supplies nearby, including a computer or tablet, pens, pencils, paper, and your textbook.

- **Join a study group**. Study groups may be unhelpful for students who are easily distracted by others. However, fellow students in a study group may be able to explain something that you do not understand. Such groups can be encouraging and give you energy that you did not have when studying alone (Figure 17.6).

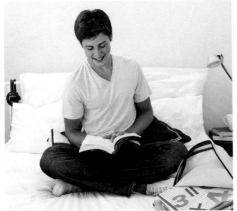

wavebreakmedia/Shutterstock.com

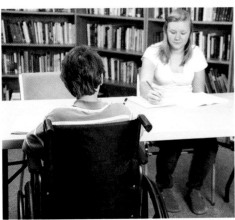

Lisa F. Young/Shutterstock.com

Figure 17.5 Some students prefer to study in their room, while others are more comfortable studying at a quiet table in the library.

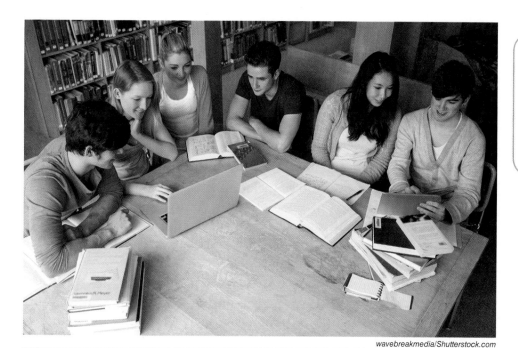

wavebreakmedia/Shutterstock.com

Figure 17.6 Studying in a group environment may be distracting for some students, but others find they study best with classmates.

Think It Through

Where do you study most effectively? What are the main distractions that you face while studying? How can you minimize these distractions?

It's important to occasionally evaluate your use of time to identify any potential time management issues. Take note of a study session in which you did not make any real progress. Ask yourself what you did that wasted time and blocked your progress. Being aware of the specific ways in which you managed your time poorly will help you improve in the future.

Extend Your Knowledge ▶ Cultural Attitudes toward Time

There are many different approaches to managing time, and these can vary among cultures. For example, in countries such as the United States, Great Britain, Norway, and Sweden, meetings usually start on time. However, in some South American countries, meetings may start at least half an hour late. In some cultures, arriving on time to an event may even be considered rude.

When studying with people of different cultural backgrounds, be aware of differences in their concept of time. Some students may not consider showing up late to a group study session to be rude or careless behavior. However, to maximize the time your study group has together, you should make sure all members know the planned start time for each study session.

Apply It

1. Use the Internet to research cultural differences related to time. Are schedules strictly enforced, or is there less pressure for events to happen at a particular time? For example, in some countries, buses leave when they are full, not according to a predetermined timetable.

2. Do you find that within your own group of friends, people have different concepts of time? For example, is someone always early, while another friend prefers to arrive "fashionably late"? How do these habits affect you?

Critical Thinking and Problem Solving

critical thinking
a process of actively and skillfully analyzing and evaluating information to draw a conclusion

Critical thinking and problem-solving skills often mark the difference between average and exceptional healthcare workers. Critical thinking is a process that involves examining and evaluating information. This process involves an attitude—a need to explore, question, and search for answers. Critical thinking helps a person analyze a situation, identify the important aspects of the situation, and reach intelligent conclusions.

Qualities of a critical thinker include the ability to ask relevant questions and to examine statements and arguments. Critical thinkers should not be judgmental or jump to conclusions, but should analyze the facts without emotion. To be a critical thinker, you must have an open mind and an interest in finding new solutions for problems.

Critical thinking can be used in every aspect of your life. For example, what evidence supports an article online that claims you can cure the common cold by eating 10 bananas a day? Where did the author of this article get his or her information? Which candidate will you support in the next presidential election? Will you simply follow your parents' political beliefs or are the candidates' opinions on a particular issue important to you?

If you are a critical thinker, you can see the whole picture and reach reasonable conclusions based on the facts. However, some common errors can derail effective critical thinking, such as making generalizations and false assumptions, rushing to judgment, and stereotyping.

- **Making generalizations**. A generalization occurs when a person concludes that something is true about another person or group without examining the facts. An example of this is *all children play video games and do not read*. Perhaps your neighbor's children constantly play video games rather than read, but that does not mean that *all* children behave in a similar manner.

Real Life Scenario Using Critical Thinking at Work

Two weeks ago, Mei's supervisor spoke to her about being late for work. Mei was on time last week, but this week she had many problems that prevented her from arriving at work on time. One morning, Mei's car wouldn't start, making her 15 minutes late. Another day this week Mei's babysitter ran late, preventing her from getting to work on time yet again. Today, she made it to work on time, but was 20 minutes late getting back to work after running errands at lunch. Mei's supervisor has requested a meeting with her to discuss this problem again.

Apply It
Think about this scenario from the perspectives of both Mei and her supervisor.

1. What might Mei's supervisor think about her continued tardiness? What would you do if you were Mei's supervisor?
2. What should Mei say to her supervisor during their meeting?
3. Brainstorm some ways this problem could be resolved.

- **Rushing to judgment**. Sometimes we make up our minds about something before we have all of the necessary information or facts. Perhaps you instantly dislike the new medical assistant, even though you don't really know him. Later on, you may realize that he reminded you of someone who once let you down, and that he is actually a skilled medical assistant and a great person. You rushed to judgment, and your initial impression was wrong.

- **Making false assumptions**. A false assumption is a belief or idea that you do not question. Imagine that a coworker tells you that the medical clerical supervisor in your new office is unfair and mean. When you first meet this supervisor, you assume she will be difficult to work with, and so you are very wary. Then you find out that she is quite warm and approachable. You based your assumption on another person's opinion, not your own experience.

- **Stereotyping**. A stereotype is a judgment held by a person or group about members of another group. An example of a stereotype is *all old people are cranky*. Learn to see individual differences within groups of people. Following stereotypes is lazy thinking.

You will need to think critically and problem solve throughout your life. As the world of healthcare—healthcare technology in particular—continues to evolve, you will have an ever-increasing need to obtain, analyze, understand, and share information. Becoming a skilled critical thinker will prepare you for success in your personal and professional life.

Check Your Understanding ✓

Each of the following quotes represents an error in critical thinking. Read each quote and then identify the mistake the speaker has made.

1. "Jeanine tells me that our new boss is unfriendly. I can't believe we are going to have another bad boss!"

2. "Our new boss is very young. She doesn't have the experience to do well in the job."

3. "All elderly patients have a tendency to be difficult. It is essential that you treat them with caution."

4. "Male nurses aren't as caring as female nurses."

5. "Oh, no. The new guy totally reminds me of my ex-boyfriend. I am going to stay clear of him!"

Reading to Learn

Reading is a critical element of perfecting your study skills. Being an effective reader will not only allow you to absorb the material in your textbook, it will also make you a better note-taker. In school, you will take notes from reading material as well as during lectures. Reading is the foundation of successful studying

Benefits of Reading

Experts recommend that people attempting to improve their reading skills should spend 20 minutes reading for pleasure each day (Figure 17.7). Why would experts recommend reading every day? The following are some benefits of reading:

- Keeping your brain active and stimulated through reading sharpens brain function.

- Knowledge is gained by reading. This new knowledge may help you handle challenges you face in school, at work, or in your personal life.

- Memory is enhanced by remembering concepts you have read.

- The growth of your vocabulary and exposure to different authors' writing styles through reading helps improve your writing skills.

- Enjoying a good book and getting lost in an interesting story can distract you from daily stresses, allowing you to relax.

- Reading promotes focus when you dedicate your attention to a story.

- Reading is free entertainment if you take advantage of local libraries.

Strong reading skills provide the basis for effective studying. By becoming a better reader, you will find it easier to take effective notes during lectures, and to outline and review your textbook and notes.

Vocabulary Building

vocabulary
a set of words known and used by a person

It can be an overwhelming challenge to read and understand a chapter in any book if you have a limited **vocabulary**. To read, write, and study well, you must have an adequate vocabulary.

When you embark on a career in healthcare, your vocabulary will expand as you learn medical terminology. A certain amount of memorization will take place when you are introduced to medical terms, but learning basic word elements will help you understand new medical terms. To progress in your healthcare education and career, it is critical that you become fluent in medical terminology.

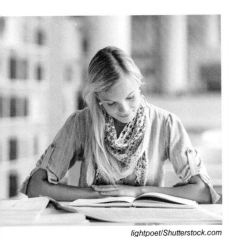
lightpoet/Shutterstock.com

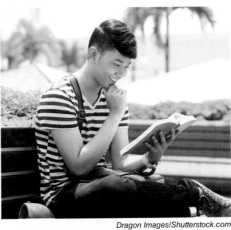
Dragon Images/Shutterstock.com

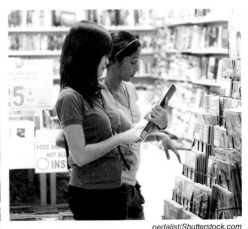
pedalist/Shutterstock.com

Figure 17.7   Make it a habit to read a variety of materials.

Do not be frustrated by a limited vocabulary—there are simple solutions to this problem. One solution is to always have access to a dictionary, medical dictionary, or **thesaurus** (Figure 17.8). There are many free dictionaries and thesauruses available on the Internet. Reliable dictionaries often have an app that can be downloaded on your smartphone or tablet to look up words when you are on the go. A traditional, printed dictionary or thesaurus is also a useful resource to add to your personal library.

thesaurus
a resource that identifies synonyms, or words with the same meanings

As you build your vocabulary, many instructors recommend you keep a list of new words you have learned. You can record new words, along with their definitions, in a notebook, on flash cards, or in an electronic list saved on your smartphone or computer. Keeping a word list is particularly important in vocabulary-heavy courses such as medical terminology. Review your word list each day and set a goal for how many new words you would like to learn every day or every week.

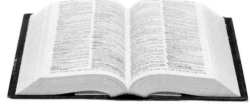

Mariusz Gwizdon/Shutterstock.com

In addition to building a word list and using references like dictionaries and thesauruses, there are many simple ways to improve your vocabulary:

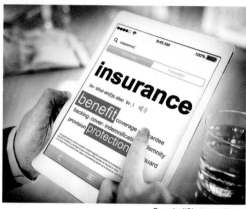

Rawpixel/Shutterstock.com

Figure 17.8 Having a print copy or digital dictionary at hand while reading makes it easy to quickly look up new vocabulary words.

- **Read every chance you get**. Frequent reading ensures that you are constantly coming in contact with new words. As you're reading, look up the definition of any word you do not understand, and then add the term to your word list.

- **Break down the word elements**. Medical terms are composed of basic word elements—prefixes, word roots, combining vowels, combining forms, and suffixes—that can be used to decipher terms' definitions.. Identifying these word elements can help you understand the term as a whole. You may want to recall what you learned about breaking down word elements in chapter 5.

- **Challenge yourself with word games**. Word games such as crossword puzzles, word jumbles, Boggle®, Scrabble®, or Bananagrams® are a fun way to learn and practice vocabulary (Many of these games are also available online.)

- **Listen to your friends, family, instructors, and coworkers for words you do not know**. Do not be afraid to ask others to define words you are unfamiliar with, or to look up the words later.

- **Highlight new words in lecture notes**. Later, you can write the definition above the highlighted word and add it to your word list.

- **Learn at least one word (or more) every day**. Buy a word-of-the-day desk calendar, and you will learn a new word every day for a year. Many online dictionaries offer you the option to subscribe to their word-of-the-day e-mails.

- **Use the new words you have learned**. Adding the new terms to your word list and using them in your daily vocabulary will help you remember these terms and expand your vocabulary.

Active Reading

active reading
reading with extreme concentration and focus; note taking and reading out loud are sometimes part of active reading

As you begin taking courses that are more demanding, you may wonder how you will find the time to read through the lengthy assignments given to you each week. Studies show that many students read without any strategy in mind. Adopting a reading strategy such as **active reading** will improve your level of **retention**.

Whether you are reading a novel on vacation, studying material for a test, or reading for a work assignment, you must become actively involved with the material you are reading. If you are not interested in the subject you are assigned to read, you will have a hard time retaining information you have read.

retention
the ability to remember information

Have you ever had the experience of finding yourself halfway through a chapter in a textbook but unable to remember what you have read? Your eyes moved across the page, but your brain did not process the information. Perhaps you were tired, distracted, or just bored by the topic. This is an example of passive reading—not being involved in processing the information. In contrast, active reading involves your level of concentration while reading.

Check Your Understanding ✔

1. Identify three benefits of reading.
2. List five strategies for improving your vocabulary.
3. Active reading will improve your level of _____.

Reading Difficult Material

Sometimes the strategies you use while reading easy and interesting material do not help when you are faced with a particularly challenging text. Perhaps the material is very dense and technical. Maybe the text itself is hard to read because the print is small, there are double columns on each page, the pages contain little white space, and no illustrations are included. What can you do in such situations to improve your reading experience and retain the material for a test?

When approaching difficult material, several techniques can be used to help you master the text:

1. Preview the reading assignment by scanning for key words, emphasized sections, headings, and end-of-chapter summaries. These will provide a foundation on which you can build an understanding as you read through the text.

2. After previewing the assignment, skim the chapter again, spending more time looking for key phrases and ideas.

3. After previewing and then skimming the chapter again, you are ready to read the assignment in more detail.

4. If you find you are still having a hard time understanding the chapter after completing steps 1–3, put the material down and take a break. Go for a walk, watch a television program, or tackle the material the next day when you are well rested after a good night's sleep.

5. Summarize each section that you read by writing down or explaining aloud what you think you have just read in your own words.

6. If you continue to have problems or questions, talk to your instructor. Take advantage of any study groups that exist for the course (Figure 17.9). Sometimes other people can explain a concept in a way that will help you understand.

7. When you are studying and come to something you do not understand, physically change positions. Walk around, stand while you read out loud, or find a different chair. Perhaps your body needs a stretch and a more comfortable position that will help your concentration.

8. Sometimes it is necessary to move ahead to the next section of the assignment. The next main point may help you better understand what you previously read.

9. Explore the library to find a similar textbook that may be written in a way that is easier for you to understand.

10. Explain the concept you are studying to another person to make sure that you are clear about what you have read.

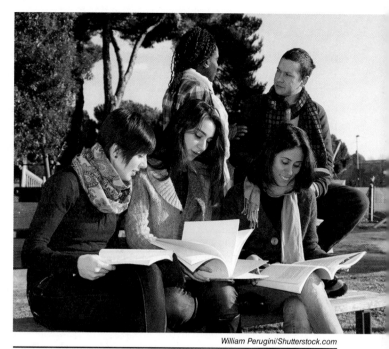

William Perugini/Shutterstock.com

Figure 17.9   Explaining concepts to the other members of your study group will help you make sure that you understand and retain the material you have been studying.

Think It Through

Have you ever been part of a study group? If so, was it a positive or negative experience? Can you think of any disadvantages of studying with others? How might such problems be resolved? If you have never worked with a study group, how could you join or create such a group?

Overcoming Reading Challenges

Some students may find reading to be a particularly challenging task. The good news is that you can improve your reading abilities by taking many of the steps included in this chapter. Some challenges to successful reading may be easy to overcome, like reducing eyestrain. Other challenges, such as the reading disability dyslexia or reading too slowly, may require dedication and time to overcome. Many resources are available to help you, including professionals at your school's learning center and other community resources. Above all, it is important that you have a positive attitude as you work to overcome any challenge you might face in school, work, or your personal life.

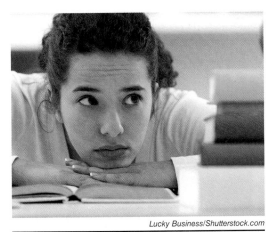

Figure 17.10 Reading problems can be frustrating, but it's important to overcome any feelings of frustration.

Maintaining a Positive Attitude

Sometimes improving your reading skills can feel like an impossible task—especially when it seems easier to watch the movie version of a novel, or listen to the news instead of reading about what's happening in the world. To maintain a positive attitude about reading, you have to get rid of any negative thoughts you associate with reading. Negative impressions such as, "I read too slowly to finish the long reading assignment for this course," will set you up for failure (Figure 17.10). It takes time and patience to become good at any task that is worthwhile. Did you learn to drive in a day?

Work on improving your attitude over time. The more you read, the more your reading skills will improve. Work to reverse any negative reading habits you have developed. This will allow your reading to improve, making reading a much more positive experience.

Decoding the Text

decoding
the process of breaking down words into recognizable parts

Decoding is the process that people use to break down words into units that are recognizable as parts of a word. The process of decoding can present a serious challenge to some readers, hurting their ability to comprehend, or understand the material. Signs of decoding problems include

- having trouble sounding out words;
- not recognizing words out of context;
- confusing the sounds that letters make;
- reading out loud at a slow pace;
- reading with little or no expression; and
- skipping over punctuation while reading.

Professional intervention is available for such problems, which are usually identified early in a student's life.

Extend Your Knowledge ▸ Reading Resources

Are you frustrated by your slow reading speed? Have you been told that your reading comprehension needs improvement? What kind of help is out there for you to improve your reading speed and comprehension?

Apply It

1. Speak to your school counselor about any help that might be available to you.

2. Research what help is available in your community. There could be courses or workshops on speed reading strategies that could be helpful.

3. Go online to see if there are strategies and techniques that might help you in your quest to become a stronger reader.

Dyslexia is a learning disorder that causes reading problems in the areas of decoding, comprehension, and retention of information. People with dyslexia may see words or letters in reverse order, have difficulty seeing similarities between words, or find it hard to remember sequences.

Dyslexia is a genetic (inherited) disorder that affects how the brain processes information. Although this disorder does not go away, people with dyslexia can learn strategies to become successful readers. Diagnosing dyslexia early in life may help a person develop the skills needed to read at the appropriate grade level. To learn more about strategies for treating dyslexia, talk to your school's counselor or an expert in the field.

Experts estimate that dyslexia affects as many as 15 percent of all Americans. Noteworthy individuals who have overcome dyslexia include Whoopi Goldberg, George Washington, Albert Einstein, and Thomas Edison (Figure 17.11).

Improving Your Reading Speed

Many students express a concern about their reading speed. Students can become overwhelmed by the volume of reading expected of them, and slow readers often fear that they cannot complete all the reading assignments on time.

Although this number varies greatly, the average adult reads about 250 to 300 words per minute. Many people believe that if you read rapidly, you will not comprehend as much as if you read at a slower pace; this is a myth. Research finds that there is little connection between rate of reading and comprehension of what you read. Identifying main ideas before you begin to read the chapter will increase your attention span and understanding of the material.

If you are serious about improving your reading rate, other strategies to increase your speed and understanding of what you read include:

- **Relaxing**. It is easier to read faster when you are relaxed. Feeling relaxed also helps you to concentrate on your subject. Stress interferes with your ability to focus and concentrate.

- **Sitting up at a desk or table**. Reclining on a couch or bed may prevent successful reading.

- **Overcoming bad habits**. There are many habits that you may have fallen into that can slow down your reading. Avoid reading every letter in a word; instead absorb whole words and phrases at a glance. Choose your reading environment carefully—is it too noisy, cold, or warm?

- **Skimming for main ideas**. If you are running out of time and are overwhelmed by the amount of reading you need to cover, skimming the text can be a good option. Read headings, subheadings, the first sentences of paragraphs, lists, graphs, and the summary at the end of the chapter. Notice italicized or bold words. Search for phrases such as "The four most important factors in…" and lists set off by numbers or bullets. Skimming can also be a good pre-reading tool to improve your comprehension when you have time to read the chapter in its entirety.

dyslexia
a learning disorder characterized by problems processing words; often causes difficulties when learning to read

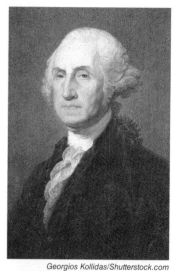

Georgios Kollidas/Shutterstock.com

Figure 17.11 Historians believe George Washington was dyslexic.

- **Timing yourself**. Assess your reading ability and determine reachable goals after timing yourself while reading. If you find you can easily read 35 pages in an hour, attempt to read the same amount in 50 minutes. Do you still understand the material when you read a bit faster? Push yourself to increase your reading speed while still retaining comprehension.

- **Being flexible**. Speed reading is not always useful. You may want to slow down when reading dense material and important subjects, such as your advanced calculus textbook. Vary your speed according to the type of material you are reading.

Avoiding Eyestrain

In today's digital world, eyestrain has become a major job-related complaint. Many students and healthcare workers spend a great deal of time in front of a computer screen while working on projects, researching online, and keeping up with social media. Stress and studying late into the night can also cause eyestrain. Some people also suffer from dry eyes, which can worsen eyestrain. Spending long periods of time reading your textbook can cause serious eyestrain as well.

If you find that your eyes tire easily, the following steps can help you to reduce eyestrain:

- **Make sure your eyes are healthy and properly corrected, if necessary**. Annual eye examinations are recommended to make sure you do not have any underlying eye problems (Figure 17.12). Eye examinations will ensure that you have proper vision and that your glasses or contact lens prescription is accurate and adequate for the work you are doing.

- **Reduce glare**. Glare can cause your eyes to tire quickly. If you are reading near a sun-filled window, close the blinds or curtains. Computer screens are a main source of glare (Figure 17.13). Installing an anti-glare screen on your monitor or adjusting the monitor's brightness can help reduce glare. Also, if you wear glasses, lenses can be treated with anti-reflective coating. This coating reduces the amount of light reflecting off your lenses.

- **Treat dry eyes**. Dry eyes can become a problem when reading for long periods of time. Remember to blink often or use artificial tears to moisten your eyes. Many work environments have especially dry air, which can increase dry eye problems. Staying hydrated at all times also helps. If your dry eyes persist, see your optometrist for further help.

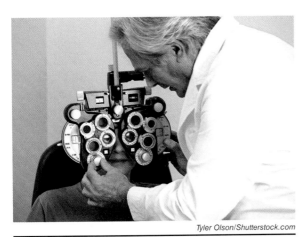

Tyler Olson/Shutterstock.com

Figure 17.12 Regular eye examinations will ensure your eyes are healthy.

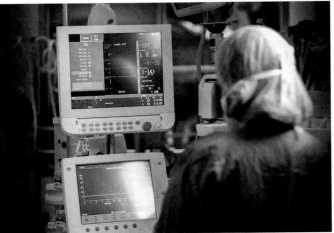

Oleg Ivanov IL/Shutterstock.com

Figure 17.13 The glare on a monitor, such as the bottom monitor in this operating room, can make the screen hard to read, often resulting in eyestrain.

- **Invest in computer glasses**. These glasses may or may not have a prescription lens, but do help your eyes focus on the computer screen rather than the glare. Computer glasses are designed to optimize your vision, reduce eyestrain, and prevent fatigued eyes and headaches.

- **Take time to exercise your eyes**. Focusing may become difficult after reading or looking at a computer screen for an extended period of time. Look away from your book or computer every 15 to 20 minutes and focus on a distant object for at least 30 seconds. Looking away relaxes your eye muscles and reduces eye fatigue. You can also shut your eyes and relax for a short time. Rolling your eyes and closing them tightly several times can also relax tired eyes.

- **Take frequent breaks during long reading sessions**. A break might include walking around your house for five minutes; getting something to drink; or stretching your arms, legs, back, neck, and shoulders. You might even want to develop a series of exercises to reduce tension and refresh your body before continuing to read.

Taking Notes

There are many reasons to take careful notes. Taking notes forces you to listen carefully and test your understanding of the material. When you are studying, your notes provide a list of important topics to remember for the test. Personal notes that you write down are usually easier to remember than what you read in a textbook. The action of writing down ideas helps reinforce the material (Figure 17.14).

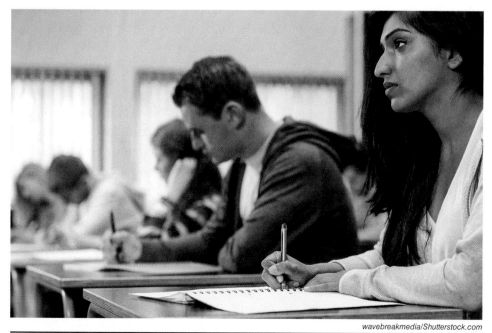

Figure 17.14 Well-written and organized notes can be one of your best study tools.

Instructors will typically give you clues as to what information is most important and might be on a quiz or test. Important material may be found in

- the information the instructor writes on the board;
- any material that is repeated and emphasized;
- word signals that indicate the number of important points in a chapter or covered by a subject;
- summaries given at the end of a lecture; or
- reviews that the instructor gives before quizzes and tests.

Once you are familiar with the instructor's lecturing methods and can identify the important topics of his or her lecture, you can perfect your note-taking skills. The following suggestions may be helpful for taking notes:

1. **Get organized**. It's important to have the materials you need for note taking on hand during class. This might include bringing a separate notebook to each class. If you use your tablet or laptop computer for note taking, create a separate document for each class's notes, and save these documents with an easily identifiable file name. You may want to create a folder for each semester or class.

2. **Be brief**. Use phrases and words instead of long sentences when taking notes. If you write down everything the instructor says, you will fall behind quickly and possibly miss important material.

3. **Write neatly**. Make sure that your handwriting is neat and legible. Unreadable handwriting will present a challenge when you are studying your notes. You may not remember what your notes mean when reviewing them for a test.

4. **Notes do not have to be exact**. Your job is not to write down exactly what the instructor is saying. However, formulas, definitions, and specific facts should be recorded exactly as they are presented. Review specific details in your textbook as well, if you have one for the class.

5. **Outline**. Outlines allow important points to stand out in your notes.

6. **Do not stop taking notes if you miss a point**. If you miss something, leave space on the page or in the document and come back to it later. Your instructor or classmates can help you fill in this information after the lecture.

7. **Color code your notes**. Using several different colored pens might help you better understand your notes when it comes time to study. One color could be used for points the instructor stresses, another for information that will be on the test, and a third color for points you do not understand. Highlighters can be very useful as well, especially for visual learners.

8. **Rewrite or type your notes after the lecture**. The repetition of rewriting or typing notes helps some students retain the material.

9. **Identify new vocabulary in your notes**. Consider using an equal sign (=) between a new term and its definition. For example, *procrastination = putting things off*. You may want to underline new words with two lines as well.

As you take notes, do not write down everything you hear. Be alert and attentive to the main points. It is important to stay focused and resist distractions. Notes should consist of key words or very short sentences. Keep notes in order and in one place, like a notebook with plenty of pages. After taking your notes, reread them and add extra points, spelling out unclear items. You may quickly forget the details of the lecture, so review the notes as soon as you can. Look over notes regularly before tests—these are an essential study tool.

Memorization

Before you study for your next test, you might want to learn a few strategies for boosting your ability to remember important information. There are a number of excellent techniques you can use to improve your memory. These strategies help you recall information and increase your retention of material presented in class, at work, or in your textbook.

Did You Know?   **Focusing on the Essence of a Chapter**

Studies have found that, when reading a textbook, people have an easier time learning material that comes at the beginning or end of the chapter. Recalling the information that comes in between can be difficult. Dedicate extra time to studying this information in the middle of the chapter. Remember that difficult material should be studied at the beginning of a study session, when you are most alert.

Mnemonic Devices

Mnemonic devices are techniques students often use to help memorize material. Using mnemonic devices helps translate information that may be hard to remember into a more memorable form, such as a song or funny saying. There are several types of mnemonics:

mnemonic devices
learning techniques such as rhymes, catchphrases, and acronyms used to help remember and retain information

- **Rhymes**. Turning a spelling rule or date in history into a rhyme will help you remember and use that rule. For example, "i before e, except after c" is a rhyme used to help spell words such as *receive*.

- **Spelling catchphrases**. To spell *potassium* correctly, you can remember that there is, "one tea, two sugars" in the word. This should help you recall the proper numbers of the letters *t* and *s* in the term.

- **Expression acronyms**. Many subjects will require you to memorize a specific order or number of things. For example, many biology students must memorize the classification of organisms. The phrase "Kids Prefer Cheese Over Fried Green Spinach" can be used to remember the order of Kingdom, Phylum, Class, Order, Family, Genus, Species.

You can invent your own mnemonic device to help you remember a specific piece of information. Get creative—sometimes the most amusing mnemonic devices are the easiest to remember!

Making Connections between Topics

Information is often organized into related groups in your memory. Grouping similar concepts and terms together may increase your chances of retaining this information. Make an outline of your notes and textbook readings to help you recognize related concepts. For example, when studying the history of healthcare, you might first study cultures that made significant impacts on ancient medicine and then study individuals who made exciting medical discoveries.

When you are learning unfamiliar material, take time to think about how this new material relates to things you already know. If you establish relationships between new ideas and existing knowledge, you can dramatically increase the likelihood of recalling the new information.

Visualizing Information

Many people, especially visual learners, benefit from visualizing the information they are studying. Focus on photographs, charts, and other graphics in your textbooks. If you do not have visual cues, create your own. Draw charts or figures in the margins of your notes, or use highlighters or pens in different colors to group related ideas in your study notes.

Did You Know?   **Cramming and Pulling All-Nighters**

Cramming and pulling all-nighters are not effective study methods. Reviewing materials over several study sessions gives you time to adequately absorb the information. Students who study regularly remember the material far better than those who did all of their studying in one last-minute session. Remember that being well rested makes learning much easier.

Alternating Your Study Routine

It may be helpful to occasionally change your study routine. If you often study in a specific location, try moving to a different spot during your next study session. If you study best in the evening, try spending a few minutes each morning reviewing material you looked at the previous evening. Occasionally changing your study routine will increase the effectiveness of your efforts and improve your long-term recall of the information.

How well you remember information depends on your attitude, interest level, awareness, mental alertness, distractibility, observation skills, memory devices, and willingness to practice remembering the material.

Test Taking

Have you ever said to yourself or heard someone say, "I'm just not a good test taker"? Everyone can improve their test-taking skills by thinking about taking a test in three parts:

1. test preparation
2. the test itself
3. after the test

Preparing to Take a Test

Preparing to take a test should start on the first day of class. The syllabus provided for the course will include the quizzes and tests you will be expected to complete. From the first day, you should be paying attention during class, taking good notes, and studying regularly.

Managing Your Schedule

Assess the amount of time you think a course will require. If possible, examine the syllabus and determine how much of your time will be required to complete the projects, papers, and test prep for this course. Is the final a take-home test or an in-class examination? Is this a subject that you love, or is it a required course that you are not excited to be taking? Take all these facts into consideration as you budget your time, and include other classes and your personal and professional responsibilities.

Attending Review Sessions

Review sessions present a wonderful opportunity to prepare for an upcoming test. Listen carefully to hints that the instructor may give about the test. This is the time to ask questions about any concepts you find confusing. You can also make an appointment with the instructor during his or her office hours to get extra help with material you do not understand. Ask the instructor about topics that will be emphasized on the test.

Real Life Scenario   **Last-Minute Cramming**

Ian always puts off studying until the night before a test. He has over 200 pages of reading to do for a test tomorrow in his Intro to Health Science class. Ian enjoys staying up late and feels that he does his best studying at night. Unfortunately, on the night before his test, Ian is especially tired and stressed after a busy day. He finds himself feeling sleepy after only an hour of reading.

Apply It

1. What reading strategies should Ian use to remain focused on the material?
2. What might he have done differently to prepare for the test?
3. Have you found yourself in a similar situation? If so, did it affect your test-taking performance?

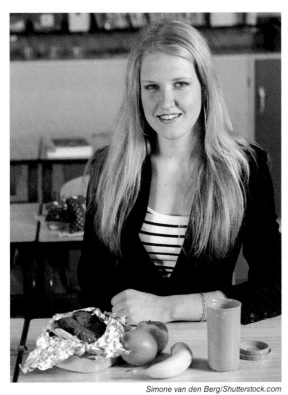

Simone van den Berg/Shutterstock.com

Figure 17.15 Eating a nutritious meal is especially important on the day of your test.

The Day of the Test

Review any material that will be on the test well before the examination, rather than the night before. Many students do not do well after staying up all night before the test to cram. You will most likely perform best when you are well rested. Go over practice tests, homework, sample problems, review material, the related textbook chapters, and class notes. Allow plenty of time to study all of these sources.

Eat before the test. Having nutritious food in your stomach gives you energy (Figure 17.15). Avoid heavy, sugary food that might make you groggy. Also be sure to visit the bathroom before going to your classroom. You do not want to be uncomfortable during the test.

On the day of the test, you should arrive at class early. Being late can cause you to feel stressed before the examination starts, instead of feeling relaxed and ready to go. Arriving a bit early may also give you a chance to look over your notes one more time. Be sure to set your alarm (and maybe a backup alarm as well) if your test is scheduled in the morning.

Taking the Test

Think It Through

Do you suffer from test anxiety? If so, has your stress affected how you have performed on a test? What other problems have you had with test taking? What strategies could you use to improve your test-taking ability?

There are many strategies you can use to more successfully take tests. A few of these strategies follow:

- First, make sure you put your name on the test.

- Be sure to bring proper writing instruments (pen or pencil—whichever your instructor tells you to use) with good erasers, if needed. If you are to use a calculator, be sure to bring it and any other approved resources (consider packing all of your test-taking resources the night before).

- If a clock is not available in the classroom, bring a watch so you can pace yourself.

- Try to stay relaxed. If you find yourself tensing up, take several deep breaths and then continue.

- Keep your eyes on your own test. Do not ask for trouble by appearing to cheat (Figure 17.16).

- When you receive the test, scan it to figure out how to budget your time.

- Pace yourself and do not rush. Read the entire question before you begin to answer it. Read everything carefully and pay attention to details.

- If you can, answer the questions that have been assigned the largest point value first.

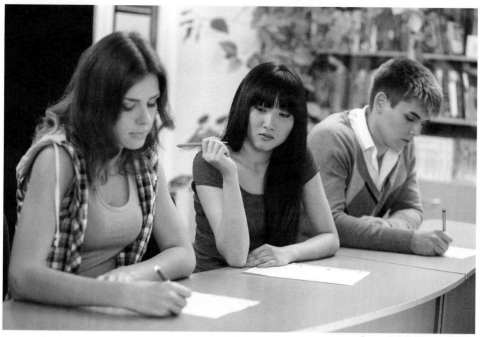

George Dolgikh/Shutterstock.com

Figure 17.16   Keep your eyes on your own test—even if you are not guilty of cheating, your teacher may interpret the situation as cheating.

- When you do not understand what a question is asking or what the instructions of the test say, ask your instructor for an explanation.

- Write legibly when answering all questions (especially essay questions). You do not want a question to be marked wrong because of poor handwriting.

- If you do not know an answer, skip the question and come back to it later. Other parts of the test may have information that will help you with the skipped question.

- Do not panic if everyone seems to be finished and you are not. Focus on your test and ignore everyone else.

After the Test

After your instructor passes back the test, you should look it over to make sure there are no grading mistakes. Make sure you understand why your answers were marked wrong. If the instructor does not go over the test, make time to ask him why a question may have been marked wrong.

If the instructor does go over the test in class, make notes on what he wanted to see in the answers for questions or problems that you got wrong. If you are not satisfied with your grade, ask if there are ways to improve your grade, such as retaking the test or obtaining extra credit. In college, extra credit may not be offered, so it is best to study harder and analyze how you might improve on the next test rather than rely on the possibility of extra credit.

If a test is returned to you, save it and use it as study material for future tests and quizzes in the class.

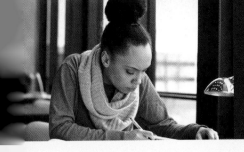

Chapter 17
Review and Assessment

Summary

In this chapter, you learned study skills every serious student needs to succeed. Maintaining your motivation and discovering your particular learning style are important factors when developing effective study habits.

Effective studying also depends on excellent reading skills. To read, write, and study well, you must first develop a strong vocabulary. Overcoming reading challenges can greatly improve study skills. Active reading can help improve your grades. Critical thinking is a skill that can be used in your personal life, at school, and at work. The critical thinking process involves analyzing and evaluating information to reach an intelligent conclusion. Critical thinking is especially helpful when taking tests and writing essays.

One way to ensure your studying is effective is to develop your memory. Using mnemonic devices, reading out loud, and making connections are all strategies for improving your recall. It is much easier to remember facts you have studied over time than what you reviewed when cramming the night before a test. Taking effective notes and actively listening in class will also improve your retention and recall of important information.

Mastering all of these study skills is important, but you must also know strategies for test taking to truly excel. Begin preparing for your tests as soon as possible. On the day of the test, arrive early and be prepared both mentally and physically for the exam period. When your graded test is returned, review the incorrect answers and make sure you understand why these answers are wrong.

Following the study tips, reading techniques, and test-taking strategies presented in this chapter will help prepare you for the rigorous demands of school and a career in healthcare.

Review Questions

Answer the following questions using what you have learned in this chapter.

True or False Assess

1. *True or False?* Kinesthetic learners typically have an easy time sitting still for long periods of time.

2. *True or False?* Critical thinking involves reaching reasonable conclusions based on important facts.

3. *True or False?* Using stereotypes is helpful when analyzing people.

4. *True or False?* Mnemonic devices are helpful when memorizing material.

5. *True or False?* Visual learners appreciate charts and PowerPoint® presentations.

6. *True or False?* Dyslexia is easily cured.

7. *True or False?* You can read rapidly and still understand what you are reading.

8. *True or False?* Active reading occurs when you have skimmed a passage but recall nothing of what you just read.

9. *True or False?* Retention means being able to remember information.

Multiple Choice Assess

10. A(n) _____ is a specific strategy implemented to help you achieve your goals.

    A. outline

    B. direction

    C. goal

    D. motivation

11. Which of the following should be done when preparing for a test?

    A. Pay attention during a lecture.

    B. Take clear notes.

    C. Budget your time to allow for ample studying.

    D. All of the above.

12. When taking a test you should _____.

    A. rush through the questions

    B. look around to see how your classmates are doing

    C. ignore the clock to avoid feeling rushed

    D. answer the questions with the highest point values first

13. Which of the following should *not* be done before taking a test?

    A. Eat a heavy, sugary meal before the test.

    B. Arrive to class at least five minutes early to take a test.

    C. Visit the bathroom before taking a test.

    D. Bring a watch so you can pace yourself.

14. All of the following concepts affect critical thinking negatively *except* _____.

    A. generalization

    B. rushing to judgment

    C. evaluating information

    D. stereotyping

15. After receiving your graded test, you should _____.

    A. immediately recycle the old test

    B. ask your classmates what grades they received

    C. check for grading errors

    D. look only at your score, disregarding the questions you answered incorrectly

16. Which of the following statements is *incorrect* when talking about the importance of motivation?

    A. Motivation is a process that guides a person toward a goal.

    B. Motivation is something that causes us to act.

    C. Motivation helps us reach our career goals.

    D. Motivation is always easy to maintain.

17. Which of the following statements about eyestrain is *false*?

    A. Eyestrain problems have increased as workers spend many hours in front of a computer screen.

    B. Eyestrain cannot be prevented.

    C. Eyestrain is particularly problematic when the air is dry.

    D. Eyestrain can be helped by using eye drops to add moisture to the eye.

18. When reading difficult material, it may be helpful to _____.

    A. summarize what you have read

    B. scan the document for key words and headings

    C. physically change positions

    D. All of the above.

19. _____ indicates a possible decoding problem.

    A. Reading with great expression

    B. Reading out loud at a slow pace

    C. An inability to recognize words out of context

    D. B and C only.

Short Answer

20. Explain motivation as it relates to studying.

21. List at least two strategies for improving one's self-confidence.

22. Describe the differences between visual, auditory, and kinesthetic learners.

23. What is a mnemonic device?

24. How might creating outlines contribute to effectively committing material to long-term memory?

25. What is time management and why is it important when studying?

26. Identify three benefits of reading.

27. What is active reading?

28. Describe dyslexia.

Critical Thinking Exercises

29. Most schools offer extensive resources to help students achieve their academic and professional goals. What resources are available to you at your school? Have you used any of these resources in the past? If not, do you plan on using these resources in the future?

30. Do you have any problems with motivation? If so, which motivation barriers do you experience? Will these motivation issues affect your ability to achieve your career goals?

31. Do you have short- and long-term goals for becoming a healthcare worker? List your goals and explain how you plan to accomplish them.

32. Make a list of all the things that keep you from listening well in each of your classes. How can you overcome these distractions?

33. In your experience, what is the best advice you can give someone who is about to take a very important test?

34. Think about a problem that could be solved through critical thinking and systematic problem solving. Apply this approach and analyze the steps used to solve the problem.

35. How much reading do you do every week? Track your reading time and create a chart listing how long you read, what material you read, and any challenges you experienced while reading.

36. Take a minute to think about your personal vocabulary. How would you rate your vocabulary? Does it need improvement? Does texting affect how you express yourself? Do you find yourself using excessive amounts of slang or swear words when trying to get your point across? Do you think people who use big words are snobby?

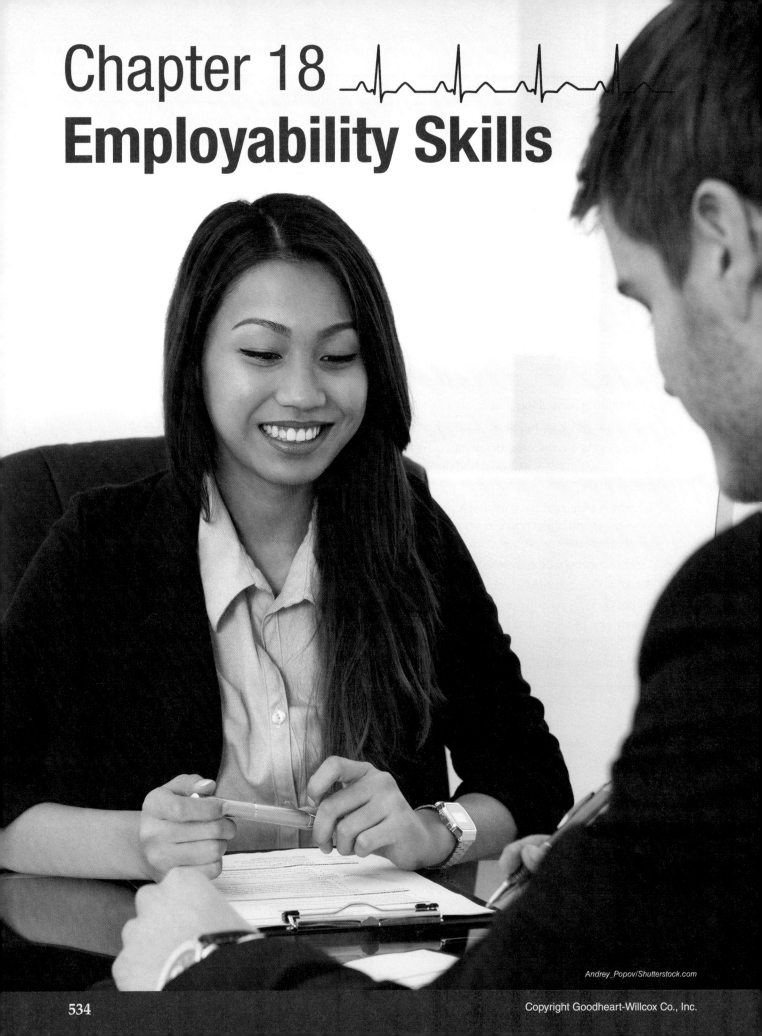

Chapter 18
Employability Skills

Andrey_Popov/Shutterstock.com

Terms to Know Build Vocab

career portfolio	empathy	patience
chain of command	enthusiasm	prioritizing
compassion	flexibility	professionalism
competence	integrity	punctuality
compromise	letter of introduction	résumé
conflict resolution	multitasking	soft skills
cover letter	networking	tact

Chapter Objectives

- Identify what professionalism means in the workplace.
- Describe the characteristics of a professional employee.
- Explain the benefits of demonstrating soft skills as a healthcare worker.
- Explain the importance of conflict resolution in the healthcare setting.
- Discuss why proper hygiene and appearance are necessary in the workplace.
- List the components of a healthy lifestyle.
- List ways you can prepare for employment.
- Identify a network to help you find employment.
- Create a career portfolio.
- Explain the importance of a properly completed job application.
- Discuss how to interview for a job.
- Identify ways to keep a job once you are hired.

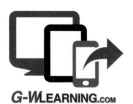

While studying, look for the activity icon to:

- **Build** vocabulary with e-flash cards and interactive games.
- **Assess** progress with chapter and unit review questions.
- **Expand** learning with animations and illustration labeling activities.
- **Simulate** EHR entry with healthcare documents.

Whether you are just beginning your health science education, or you are ready to apply for the job of your dreams, it is never too early or too late to develop career objectives. In this chapter, you will learn how to find the ideal job and put your skills to the test. First, in an effort to determine your career objectives, ask yourself the following questions:

- How should I be preparing today for my future career?

- What career do I hope to have in five years?

- Can I imagine myself in the same position in ten years, or will I want to advance up a career ladder?

- What skills do I need to develop to realize my career goals?

You may need to be employed while going to school to help finance your education. Choosing a job (or even a volunteer position) that can help you develop skills for your future career is a good idea. For instance, if you want to become a physical therapist, you might want to look into a job as a physical therapy assistant. If you are in high school or college and want to explore careers in healthcare, you might want to volunteer in a healthcare facility. If you are ready to begin your chosen career, you need to plan your employment search so that you have the best chance of obtaining a job in a competitive market.

Professionalism

professionalism
the conduct or attitude that is required to be the best employee that you can be; the act of contributing positively to an organization

What do you have to learn as a student to understand and practice **professionalism**? Professionalism is an attitude reflected by one's behavior. It includes the way you communicate, work, and view yourself and your coworkers. Although it may be early in your healthcare career or education, you still need to have pride in and a great attitude about your job—even if you are still working toward your preferred job.

Having a professional attitude will be a major key to your career success. Every healthcare organization looks for employees who possess skills that will make a difference in the lives of patients. Employees who will contribute positively to the organization are most desirable.

In this chapter, you will learn the skills that companies value and that make you employable. There is much competition for good jobs. Your professional attitude and excellent employability skills will greatly improve your chances of finding and keeping a fulfilling position.

Personal Characteristics

Successful healthcare workers not only have the skills and knowledge required for their job, but also possess particular personal characteristics that contribute to their success. Certain personal characteristics enable a healthcare worker to better execute responsibilities and improve interactions with everyone in the healthcare facility. Many of these personal characteristics concern interpersonal skills, or a person's ability to establish relationships with others.

Such characteristics are known as **soft skills**. Soft skills include social skills such as communication, friendliness, and having an optimistic personality. These skills enhance an individual's interactions with others.

It is also important for an employee to recognize social cues, including facial expressions, posture, and tone of voice, to name a few. Correctly reading social cues, which can sometimes be quite subtle, is important when working with patients who may say they are feeling fine when they are not.

As you begin your healthcare career, you will realize that no two patients are the same, and no two days will present the exact same challenges. **Patience** and **tact** are two skills that will help you navigate the many situations you will encounter throughout your career. These skills are especially important when addressing patients who may be angry, sick, or frightened.

Another helpful characteristic for healthcare workers to possess is **enthusiasm**. Have you ever worked with someone who was very negative and complained constantly? Imagine a person with such an attitude working closely with a sick patient. If you are enthusiastic about your work, your positive attitude will affect the people around you—including fellow workers, supervisors, and patients.

Flexibility is extremely important when working in healthcare. Changes are constant and may take place in procedures, instrumentation, staffing, or other aspects of the healthcare facility. Refusal to learn a new skill because you think the old way is better will not enhance your reputation as a valuable employee.

When you become a healthcare worker, you should embrace your role and do the absolute best you can. Errors in healthcare can be serious and should be avoided whenever possible. However, should an error occur, a supervisor should be notified immediately so that the error can be corrected, if possible, and patient harm can be prevented.

Courteous Behavior

You will work closely with a variety of people throughout your healthcare career. Being courteous to coworkers and patients will improve the quality of these relationships. Kind words, **compassion**, and **empathy** help to build the trust of others. Demonstrate a good attitude and offer patients, visitors, and coworkers a sincere smile whenever possible.

soft skills
personal characteristics that enable a person to have pleasant, effective interactions with others

patience
a skill that will help you interact calmly with coworkers and patients

tact
the ability to avoid giving offense through your words and actions

enthusiasm
an excited and positive attitude that you can bring to your work

flexibility
the ability to change or adjust your attitude and behavior to meet particular needs

compassion
deep awareness and concern for the suffering of others coupled with the desire to relieve this suffering

empathy
the act of identifying with and understanding another person's feelings or situation

---

Real Life Scenario   Developing Empathy

Ricky is a twenty-year-old student nurse. He recently began working in the geriatric department at Eastridge Hospital. Prior to this assignment, Ricky had little experience with the elderly. Ricky admits to his supervisor that he has trouble relating to his patients and finds some of them to be very difficult.

Apply It

1. How can Ricky change his behavior?

2. As a healthcare worker, you will likely provide care to people of all ages. Do you think you would have trouble relating to a particular age group? Why or why not?

Extend Your Knowledge ▶ Researching Great Leaders

Some people are natural leaders, while others shy away from leadership roles. Identify one great leader—either past or present—and research his or her contributions to the world. Write a brief, one-page report on the individual's life, paying particular attention to his or her leadership role. Then consider the following questions.

Apply It

1. What attributes do you think made this individual a strong leader?

2. How did the individual you researched treat the members of his or her team? Did she have a reputation for listening and taking the advice of others? Was he demanding of his team members or did his reputation for being a visionary draw others to his work?

One important aspect of a courteous attitude is respect, for both your coworkers and patients. Avoid using offensive language, gossiping, telling off-color or racist jokes, and other disrespectful behavior. A healthcare facility is no place for prejudice of any kind, and it is important that you respect those who are different from you (Figure 18.1). Show every patient, visitor, and coworker respect, regardless of his or her age, race, religion, or appearance.

Teamwork

Healthcare careers generally require employees to work cooperatively with others. When you are a team player, you need to put aside personal interests to achieve the common goal. If one of your coworkers asks you for help when you are tired, hungry, or about to go on a break, that is the time to put aside your own needs for a few minutes and be a team player. A big part of working in

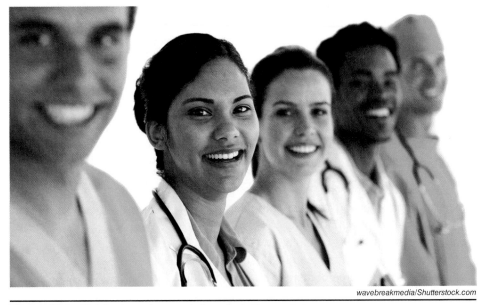

wavebreakmedia/Shutterstock.com

Figure 18.1   Celebrate and respect diversity in the workplace.

healthcare is putting the needs of others—specifically patients—before your own. This is why healthcare professions are often called the *helping professions*.

In healthcare, teams exist in many forms. Some examples include disaster response teams, emergency operations teams, hospital teams that care for the critically ill, teams for ambulatory patients, and teams in doctors' offices. Teams can be large or small, centralized or spread out, virtual or face-to-face. Regardless of the size of a team, some basic principles will be in place to help the team be effective.

Problem solving is often facilitated by working as a team. Team members offer unique perspectives, leading to better decisions when collaboration is embraced (Figure 18.2). Working together can lead to the development of bonds among team members. These bonds may enable the team to avoid unnecessary conflicts, since team members will have become better acquainted with each other.

Negotiation, assertive communication, gathering critical facts, expressing clear expectations, and utilizing mediation are effective techniques for managing team conflicts. Patients lose confidence in their caregivers when they can sense conflict among healthcare workers. Effective teamwork with little or no conflict is associated with increasing patient safety.

Effective leaders have specific attributes and attitudes. A leader must exhibit honest and ethical behavior. The leader must trust team members and delegate tasks readily. A leader must communicate well, both orally and in a written format. A misspoken word can potentially cause conflict and misunderstanding, and derail any progress the team has made. If the team leader is enthusiastic about team tasks, this enthusiasm may spread among the team members. A team leader should mentor members of the team and take every opportunity for teambuilding and communicating a vision of success and cooperation. A leader must also make sure that each team member is accountable for his or her part in the team.

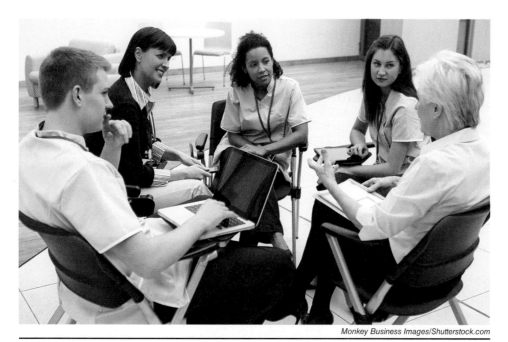

Figure 18.2   When members of a healthcare team work together, they not only strengthen their professional relationship, they are also more likely to provide patients with high quality care.

There are many types of leaders:

- autocratic (prefers to be the sole ruler)

- democratic (not afraid to share responsibility with other team members)

- laissez-faire (allows team members to operate on their own)

Studies find that democratic leaders with the attributes and attitudes previously listed will be the most effective leaders.

An effective team must contain active participants who have a commitment to the common goals of the team. Each member has to be sensitive to diversity in the team, whether it is racial, cultural, or otherwise. Team members should have positive attitudes, and each member's contribution should be valued. Trust must be present among the members, and can be earned when members show that they are reliable.

Team Dynamics

After a team is assembled, it still may take time for the team to become fully functioning and achieve its goal. Team members need to learn their roles, adjust to the way group members interact, and understand each other's behavior when working as a team. A team with a positive dynamic has members who trust one another. A team should work toward a collective decision, holding each member accountable for individual responsibilities that make the team operate successfully as a whole. Positive energy within the team also helps each member become more creative.

Poor team dynamics occur when

- leadership is weak, leading to a lack of direction and potential disagreements between team members;

- team members do not express their opinions, but simply agree with the leader to avoid possible conflict; and

- team members are uncooperative, refuse to participate, dominate the discussion, or use humor inappropriately.

Real Life Scenario — Strengthening Group Dynamics in the Workplace

Dr. Bishop is a dentist with a growing pediatric dental practice. Dr. Bishop recently sat down with his office manager, Ashley, to discuss her concerns about habitual tardiness among their employees. She stated that tardiness had begun to affect the smooth operation of the practice and the quality of care given to patients. Dr. Bishop asked Ashley to lead an employee meeting to discuss the problem of tardiness and brainstorm solutions.

Ten employees attended Ashley's meeting, and several had ideas about how to fix the problem of tardiness in the office. One dental assistant suggested that any employee arriving late should get a warning. After three warnings, the offender would be written up. One of the office hygienists felt that tardiness showed a lack of professionalism and proposed a time clock be installed. The office receptionist disagreed and felt that a time clock would be demeaning to employees and show a lack of trust. Voices were raised as everyone tried to talk at once.

Apply It

1. If you were Ashley, how would you proceed?

2. Would you characterize this as an example of a positive or negative team dynamic? Explain your answer.

3. How might Ashley, Dr. Bishop, and the other employees work to build a consensus and resolve this issue?

Consensus Building

A consensus is established when the majority of a team's members are in agreement. To reach a consensus, team members must participate and work together to achieve the team's goal. At times, team dynamics may become negative, preventing team members from agreeing on a path forward. In such cases, members must reach a consensus on which a majority agrees.

Methods for reaching a team consensus include the following:

- All team members should be given the chance to participate in the discussions.

- Team members should be allowed to give their input for all proposals.

- The team leader or leaders should make every attempt to reach a full agreement among all members of the team.

- Team members must be encouraged to keep the good of the whole team in mind.

- Individual preferences should not prevent the progress of the team.

Conflict Resolution

Good interpersonal skills and a respectful attitude do not ensure that you will get along with every person you encounter. Some interpersonal conflicts may be unavoidable in a stressful work environment. When people are rushed and under pressure, they don't always practice the best communication skills. Personalities may clash, and you may not always get along with your coworkers. To keep the work environment a pleasant and productive place, you should resolve any conflicts that arise on the job.

Conflict often occurs because personalities clash or because responsibilities and roles are misunderstood. Regardless of the reason, conflict can decrease the morale of a healthcare worker. Are you good at **conflict resolution**? It is important that you know how to handle conflict so it does not become a destructive force in your workplace.

conflict resolution
the process of alleviating or eliminating sources of discord or tension between individuals

A healthcare facility can be a fast-paced, stressful environment. A doctor may be impatient to get laboratory results back and yell at a laboratory assistant who has trouble finding the results in the computer. During stressful periods, it is important to remember that everyone is doing their best to get their jobs done. In such situations, a professional may not treat a worker in an assistant-level position with proper respect, which can cause conflict.

Real Life Scenario   Dealing with Conflict

Paula and Melissa are nursing assistants who often work together at Eastridge Hospital. Paula feels like she often does Melissa's duties for her. When there is an unpleasant mess to clean up, Melissa tends to disappear. Melissa takes long breaks, and Paula has trouble finding Melissa when she needs help. Melissa also avoids dealing with difficult patients.

Apply It

1. What should Paula do? Should Paula talk to Melissa? Should Paula approach her supervisor instead of speaking with Melissa?

2. Have you ever worked with someone like Melissa? If so, how did you resolve any conflict that arose between the two of you?

Think It Through

What do you think are some legitimate reasons for missing work? Can you think of some reasons that a supervisor would not accept? Have you ever had a job in which you had to work with a short staff because someone called in sick when he or she was not?

When conflict does arise in the workplace, there are a few options available for resolving the issue. Traditionally, the supervisor is responsible for managing conflict in the workplace. In healthcare facilities, employees often work as a team. Conflict within the team can destroy team efforts. Often, minor conflict can be resolved without the intervention of the supervisor if the individuals involved work through their issue together. The following list includes some potential methods for resolving conflict in the workplace:

1. Treat coworkers with respect—especially if you disagree with them on something. If a conflict does arise, meet with the person privately to honestly and calmly express your feelings about the situation. If your efforts are unsuccessful, talk to your supervisor about the problem. He or she may want the people involved in the conflict to have a discussion. Make sure all workplace conflicts remain professional instead of becoming personal.

2. Do not take sides when two coworkers have a conflict. Taking sides divides the team and may prevent you from doing your job well. It is also a mistake to confront a supervisor as a group with a complaint.

3. Remember that the goal of your healthcare career is to deliver outstanding care to patients. Any conflicts you might have should not get in the way of that mission.

4. Some facilities have procedures for handling conflict to reach a solution that everyone can accept. Often, **compromise** must be achieved for a conflict to be resolved. Holding on to rigid views without being open to hearing another person's solution is not professional behavior.

5. Listen to each other and agree to work toward a solution. It's important that you are open to compromise and attempt to find a solution. Do not bring other complaints into the conflict, but rather focus on one problem at a time.

You may experience conflict at some point in your healthcare career. Clear communication that focuses on active listening and dedication to resolving conflict in a positive manner will help your team grow stronger. Successful resolution of conflict will also allow you to provide professional patient care.

compromise
the settlement of differences in which each side makes concessions

multitasking
performing several jobs at once

prioritizing
the act of making decisions about the best order in which to perform multiple tasks so the most important tasks are completed first

integrity
the quality of being honest and having strong moral principles

competence
the ability to do your job well

Trustworthy Employees

Trustworthy employees are reliable, responsible, and competent. They are often good at **multitasking** and **prioritizing** their responsibilities to ensure all tasks are completed on time.

Integrity is a quality that inspires the trust of your employer. People with integrity are often honest and fair and follow their moral principles. Being able to say you are wrong and admit you have made a mistake shows integrity. Admitting to your supervisor that you are unsure of a procedure but are eager to learn is also a hallmark of an honest employee. Responding honestly when asked for your input can also show integrity.

To be a competent, trustworthy employee, you must possess the ability to do your job well. **Competence** is gained through training and experience.

If you prove that you are competent, or capable, you will gain the trust of your supervisor, coworkers, and patients.

Dependability is another quality of a trustworthy employee. You cannot be dependable without arriving on time for every scheduled shift. **Punctuality** is extremely important in the healthcare field (Figure 18.3). Arriving late could mean that a patient's procedure has to be delayed or rescheduled, paperwork is filed past its deadline, or another employee extends his or her shift to cover your absence. Poor attendance or frequent tardiness may affect your performance and lead to disciplinary actions or dismissal. Being both dependable and punctual will help you become a successful, trustworthy employee.

Loyalty to your employer and the facility for which you work is essential to being a trustworthy employee. If you talk behind your supervisor's back or continually criticize the way your facility functions, you are not proving yourself to be a loyal employee. If you feel that you cannot be an enthusiastic member of your team, you should seek other employment.

punctuality
the ability to be on time for work, appointments, and any other commitments

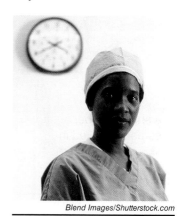
Blend Images/Shutterstock.com

Figure 18.3 Arrive at work at least five minutes early.

Attitude Is Everything

In the healthcare industry, a positive attitude can be the key to professional success. Employers often seek out self-motivated individuals who do not need to be directed to perform a task, but take the initiative to get things done without being asked. An energetic, ambitious employee with a good attitude is an asset to any organization (Figure 18.4).

Some situations may test your professionalism, such as being asked to learn new tasks or receiving criticism, but you should always maintain a good attitude. Employees who are open to learning new things are more employable than those who are resistant to learning new procedures, using updated computer software, or moving into new positions within the healthcare facility. Also, when received properly, criticism is often constructive—it can be used to improve your job performance. Try to have a good attitude about any criticism your supervisor may provide. Everyone makes mistakes, and it's important to recognize areas of your job performance that may need improvement.

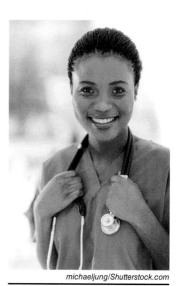
michaeljung/Shutterstock.com

Figure 18.4 Being enthusiastic about your work may make you more successful.

Chain of Command

In a healthcare facility, there is a clear **chain of command**, beginning with your immediate supervisor and continuing along the line until it reaches the director of the facility. If you work for a supervisor who is hard to talk to, you might be tempted to go to her supervisor. This may hurt your relationship with your supervisor, who may feel angry and embarrassed that you didn't come to her. Always make every attempt to speak with your supervisor about something that is bothering you. Your supervisor has been put in the position she is in because of her expertise, and you may find that you gain valuable information from her. Try your best to communicate any problems clearly and carefully.

chain of command
term that describes the levels of authority in an organization from the bottom to the top

Appearance and Hygiene

A well-groomed healthcare worker in appropriate dress can have a positive psychological effect on those he or she encounters while at work. People who are well-groomed pay attention to the details of their personal appearance. Before beginning your first day on the job, be sure to consult your facility's dress code. Different healthcare facilities may have variations in their dress codes. The following appearance and hygiene tips apply to most healthcare facilities:

- Take daily showers or baths, and wear deodorant. Be sure to wash your hair and style it appropriately for your job. Many positions require long hair to be pulled back or pinned up and off the collar for both safety and cleanliness (Figure 18.5).

- Brush your teeth at least twice a day, and be sure to floss (Figure 18.6). Good oral hygiene has been proven to prevent cardiovascular disease.

- Get plenty of sleep. Being well-rested will leave you feeling energized and may give you the appearance of someone who is excited to be at work.

- Depending on the facility's rules and the person's job, men may not be allowed to have facial hair. If facial hair is permitted, it should be washed regularly and neatly combed and shaped. Scraggly facial hair does not create a professional appearance.

- Avoid using perfume, aftershave, or cologne. Patients with breathing problems and those sensitive to strong odors may be adversely affected by the smell of these products.

- Makeup should be conservative and applied moderately.

- Limit any jewelry worn on the job to a watch, wedding band, and small stud or hoop earrings. Jewelry may cause injury to your patient or to yourself (an angry or struggling patient may grab your jewelry). Jewelry can also transmit bacteria. Healthcare workers required to wear gloves on the job may want to leave rings with stones at home because the stone may tear the glove.

- Fingernails should be kept clean and short to avoid scratching the patient. If nail polish is worn, it should be clear.

- Many healthcare jobs require employees to wear an identification name badge and a uniform or laboratory coat. These items must be worn as they identify the employee as a member of the healthcare team. Uniforms and lab coats must be kept clean and in good condition. If you have a healthcare job that does not require a uniform, you should dress according to the facility's dress code.

- Wear sensible, closed-toe shoes. If you are going to be on your feet all day, low heels and a comfortable shoe are a must.

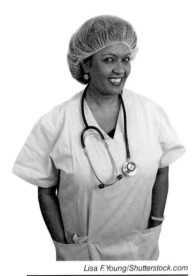

Lisa F. Young/Shutterstock.com

Figure 18.5 You may be required to wear a hairnet to ensure hygienic conditions in certain areas of the healthcare facility.

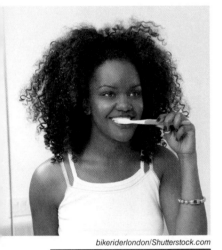

bikeriderlondon/Shutterstock.com

Figure 18.6 Maintaining good oral hygiene has many health benefits.

Check Your Understanding ✓

1. Why is it especially important for a healthcare worker to be punctual?
2. Name at least three techniques for consensus building.
3. What type of clothing and accessories are appropriate in a healthcare environment? What is inappropriate?

Preparing for Employment

There are many factors for an employer to consider in a potential hire. Each position is different and requires a specific set of skills. Just knowing how to do the job isn't always enough—your personality is important as well. What basic qualities are desirable in a new employee?

- The employer wants a skilled employee, capable of doing the job.

- The employer wants a dependable person who can prove that he or she has been a reliable team member in other jobs. This can be confirmed by checking the potential employee's past employer references.

- The employer wants someone who makes a good first impression, takes pride in his or her appearance, and is well spoken.

- The employer wants someone with a good attitude who conveys enthusiasm about the potential position. Asking informed questions about the position or the healthcare facility shows enthusiasm and interest in the job.

- The employer may want to see letters of recommendation from a person who has an academic or working relationship with the potential employee. Such letters provide a picture of personal characteristics, performance, experience, capabilities, and professional potential.

Building Your Career Portfolio

Your **career portfolio** contains the work you have done to prepare for a career or to get a specific job. Your portfolio can be used as you plan a high school course schedule, apply to college programs, or apply for a job. It is important to keep your portfolio up to date. Doing so will ensure that you have all the information you need for these tasks readily available.

A strong career portfolio should contain the following:

- an introductory letter
- a résumé and cover letter
- letters of recommendation
- records of paid and volunteer work experience
- samples of projects and presentations that illustrate your specific skills
- any certifications you have earned
- a list of school and community activities in which you have participated
- any scholastic and professional awards you have earned

Introductory Letter

A **letter of introduction** illustrates your personality, passions, and goals for your career. What experiences and interests have led you to this career? What goals have you set for yourself, and what can you contribute to this career?

career portfolio
an accumulation of documents and work related to a person's career planning and preparation

letter of introduction
a letter written by you to illustrate your personality, passions, and goals for your career

Include an example of one of your positive characteristics. Do *not* send this letter to potential employers. This letter is for your personal use, and it will help you consider your priorities as you begin your career journey. You can use the information in this letter as you fill out job applications and prepare for interviews.

The Resume

resume

a document that summarizes your education, work experiences, and other qualifications for employment; can be printed or submitted electronically

Your **resume** summarizes your educational background, work experiences, and other qualifications for employment. A resume can be sent to an employer along with a cover letter or given to an employer with a completed job application. The resume gives an employer a starting point for assessing your potential as an employee.

Preparing Your Resume

In some cases, you will be able to submit a hard copy of your resume rather than sending it to the employer electronically. When printing your resume, use standard 8 1/2- by 11-inch paper in white or off-white. Avoid using colored or patterned paper and colored typed font—this can detract from the information you are presenting.

Today, many employers ask you to submit your resume electronically. Known as an *e-resume*, this digital file is sent to potential employers via e-mail, or by uploading it onto the employer's website or a job search website. Detailed instructions for creating electronic formats of your resume can be found online. Employers may require you to submit the file in a specific format.

All information on your resume must be neatly organized with evenly spaced margins. Be sure to review your resume carefully for spelling, punctuation, and grammar errors. Include all of the important facts about your work history, schooling, and extracurricular activities. Ask your school counselor or a teacher to read your resume and use their constructive criticism to make revisions.

Did You Know?   Online Resources

Online resources are available to help you format and organize your resume. Your school likely has similar resources available to you. Consult your school's counselor if you have questions when preparing your resume.

What to Include on Your Resume

A resume alone will not get you a job, but a poorly written resume may rule you out for an interview. It is very important to make your resume concise. Most employers will not read through several pages of nonessential information. A well-prepared resume should not exceed one page of text.

Figure 18.7 is a sample resume you may use as a guide for creating your own resume. The format of your resume may vary, but this sample represents a very traditional approach in which the information is presented in a specific order.

Lauren E. Castle
22145 E. Rollins Avenue
Charlottesville, VA 22909
Home: 434-555-4356
Cell: 434-555-2681
E-mail: lcastle@e-mail.com

Objective
To obtain a position as a phlebotomist in a healthcare facility.

Education
Phlebotomy Technician Certification (CPT)
Atlantic Technical Institute for the Health Sciences, December 2017

Eastridge High School Diploma, June 2015

Experience
August, 2015–Present
Laboratory Aide, Jefferson Clinic, Charlottesville, VA
- Prepare specimens for testing at clinic laboratory
- Wash glassware used for laboratory testing
- Answer phones on weekends

October–December, 2015
60-Hour Externship, County Hospital, Charlottesville, VA
- Performed 100 phlebotomies under supervision
- Prepared specimens for testing in the main clinical laboratory
- Worked in satellite laboratories connected to hospital
- Gained exposure to on-the-job duties of a phlebotomist
- Learned to gain trust and confidence of patients

January–June, 2014
Junior Volunteer, County Hospital, Charlottesville, VA
- Worked in hospital gift shop
- Helped direct hospital visitors to patients
- Delivered flowers and reading materials to patients

Special Skills
Familiar with two hospital-based computer programs: FREEmed and Vitera. I also speak fluent Spanish, possess excellent people skills, am highly organized, and am able to prioritize multiple tasks.

Goodheart-Willcox Publisher

Figure 18.7   A sample résumé

Job Objective. The first section of a résumé is the job objective (or *career objective*). This allows the employer to immediately see which position you seek. There are probably many jobs available throughout the facility, and you may be rejected if your objective is poorly written or does not match the job opening.

Depending on the facility, job names or descriptions might be slightly different. You might have to change your job objective to match each position to which you are applying. Double-check your job objective before sending your résumé to each prospective employer.

Education. Your education is one of the most important features of your résumé, so this section should follow the job objective. The last school that you attended should appear first on the list. For each school, list the name, location, and dates attended. Also, state the diploma or degree you earned (or will earn, including your anticipated date of graduation) and what program you studied. If you did well, you might want to include your grade point average (GPA).

Work Experience. List your most recent job first. If you have a sparse work history, include internships, part-time jobs, summer jobs, or volunteer experience, even if such positions were not in a related field. Volunteer positions show an interest in your community. Including positions that may be unrelated lets the employer know that you are responsible and may have transferable skills.

Include the employer's name and location for each job listed. Also, include a brief description of your responsibilities, emphasizing any tasks or technical skills you gained that might relate to the job for which you are applying. Be sure to note any leadership experience gained with other employers. Use the past tense when describing a job that you no longer have. Use the present tense if the experience is current.

Honors and Activities. In this section, list the school and community organizations and activities in which you have participated. Offices held and honors received are also very important to list. Even if volunteer activities are not related to the position you are seeking, include them here. Community service activities may also impress a potential employer.

Special Skills and Related Courses. This section is an optional addition to your résumé. If you have a personal qualification that demonstrates a job-related skill or ability, you can list it here. These skills may include a language you speak fluently, computer skills that haven't been mentioned before, or courses related to the position for which you are applying.

The Cover Letter

cover letter
a letter that accompanies a résumé to provide additional information about the applicant's skills and experience; usually focuses on the applicant's qualifications for a particular job; also called cover message

You will also need a **cover letter** to accompany your résumé (Figure 18.8). Cover letters, which are sometimes called *cover messages* or *letters of application*, should be personalized for each position for which you apply.

The appearance of the letter is very important. Use the same paper that you used for the résumé, with a standard font size and style. Your letter should include a return address, date, inside address, salutation, body, and complimentary close. Again, make sure your letter is neat, clean, and free of spelling or grammatical errors. As with the résumé, a poorly constructed, misspelled cover letter may result in a potential employee never being called for an interview.

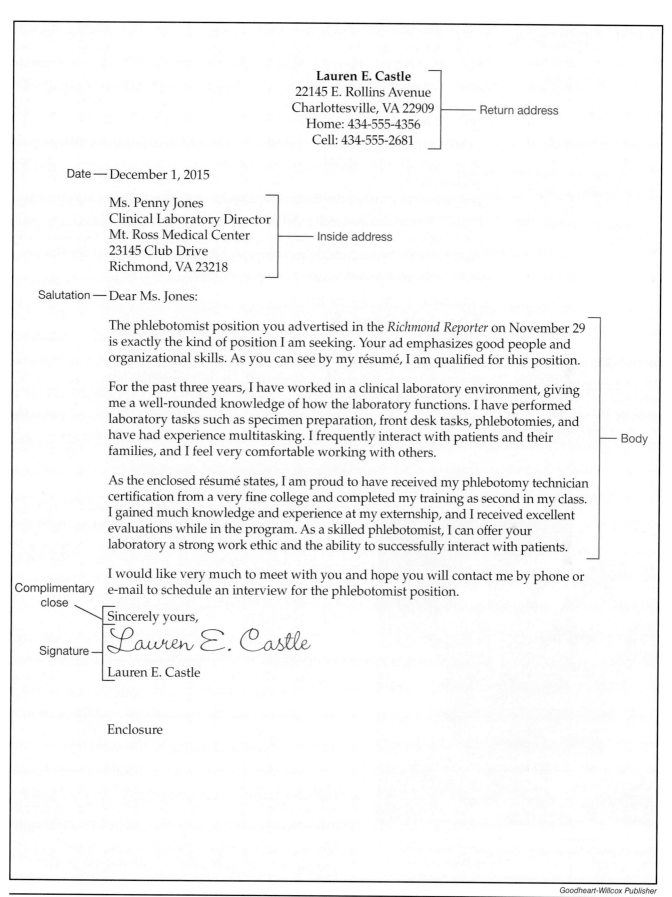

Return address — Lauren E. Castle
22145 E. Rollins Avenue
Charlottesville, VA 22909
Home: 434-555-4356
Cell: 434-555-2681

Date — December 1, 2015

Inside address — Ms. Penny Jones
Clinical Laboratory Director
Mt. Ross Medical Center
23145 Club Drive
Richmond, VA 23218

Salutation — Dear Ms. Jones:

Body — The phlebotomist position you advertised in the *Richmond Reporter* on November 29 is exactly the kind of position I am seeking. Your ad emphasizes good people and organizational skills. As you can see by my résumé, I am qualified for this position.

For the past three years, I have worked in a clinical laboratory environment, giving me a well-rounded knowledge of how the laboratory functions. I have performed laboratory tasks such as specimen preparation, front desk tasks, phlebotomies, and have had experience multitasking. I frequently interact with patients and their families, and I feel very comfortable working with others.

As the enclosed résumé states, I am proud to have received my phlebotomy technician certification from a very fine college and completed my training as second in my class. I gained much knowledge and experience at my externship, and I received excellent evaluations while in the program. As a skilled phlebotomist, I can offer your laboratory a strong work ethic and the ability to successfully interact with patients.

I would like very much to meet with you and hope you will contact me by phone or e-mail to schedule an interview for the phlebotomist position.

Complimentary close — Sincerely yours,

Signature — Lauren E. Castle
Lauren E. Castle

Enclosure

Figure 18.8   Make sure your cover letter includes all the important components shown here.

Think It Through

Networking may be extremely helpful in your job search. Building a network takes time, but it is well worth the effort. If you have not yet established a network, ask for advice about how to begin from your counselor, friends, and family.

When you are writing a cover letter, keep it short and focused. As with a résumé, you do not want to overload the potential employer with too many facts. Find out to whom you should direct the letter. This may be a human resources representative, hiring manager, or the supervisor for the posted position. This information may be found online, or you can call the company and ask for the name and title of the appropriate person.

When writing your letter, restrict its length to about three paragraphs. In the opening paragraph, identify the job or type of work you seek, and explain how you learned about the position. In the next paragraph, tell why you are right for the job. Briefly explain how your education and previous positions have prepared you for this work. Refer the potential employer to your enclosed résumé for more details. Finish your cover letter by asking for an interview and thanking the employer for considering you for the position. Make sure the employer knows where you can be reached.

The Job Search

networking

the process of developing contacts and relationships with people who are interested in your future employment

Job projections are favorable for those who wish to begin a career in healthcare, an industry that is one of the fastest growing in the United States. To obtain a job, you need to know how to begin the search and how to understand the job market. Job hunting takes work. How do you find potential employers? There are many sources to explore to find available jobs.

Networking

Networking involves making contact with people who are interested in your future employment and can help you search for jobs. These people should be familiar with your abilities and interests. After developing such a network, you may be in the position to help others looking for work (Figure 18.9). Networking works best when there is benefit to all involved.

There are many ways to build your network. Joining a professional or student organization may put you in touch with those who share your professional interests. You may meet local employers who participate as speakers in career and technical student organizations. Another option is volunteering in a workplace, such as a healthcare facility, where you can meet potential employers.

There are also exciting networking possibilities online. LinkedIn®, a social networking website for people seeking professional positions, will put you in contact with other people in your chosen field. Networking websites are expanding all the time, offering more options for employers to view your qualifications.

As you build your network, consider keeping a list of possible contacts in your career portfolio.

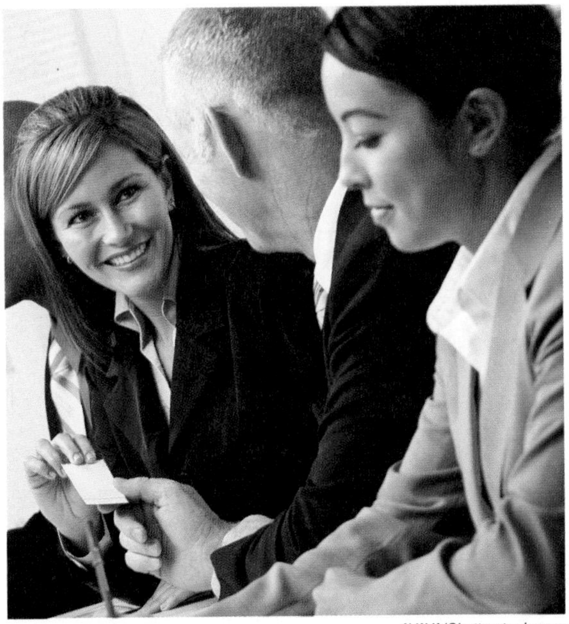

AVAVA/Shutterstock.com

Figure 18.9   Continue to build your network, even after accepting your first job. The connections you make throughout your healthcare career may lead to new opportunities or allow you to assist others in finding their dream job.

Resources at Your School

Many schools have a job placement office or a counselor who can help you find jobs in your community. Your school counselor may be able to review your résumé and offer feedback (Figure 18.10). Many schools also have a variety of online resources.

Your instructors can often guide you toward job opportunities. Instructors sometimes place students in internships that may lead to job offers. Employers may work directly with schools to fill open positions.

Your instructors know your skills and can attest to your excellent attitude in class, attendance record, and personal achievements. It is very important to make a good impression on your instructors; these individuals can be a valuable networking source as well.

Online Job Search

Many people have successfully found jobs on the Internet. There are thousands of employment options available online. If you do not have a computer at home, most public libraries and schools provide Internet access.

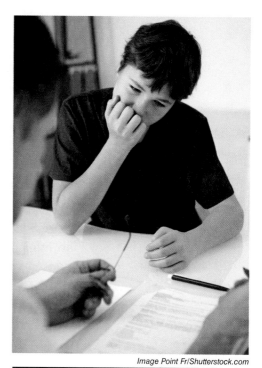

Image Point Fr/Shutterstock.com

Figure 18.10 Consider asking your school counselor to review your résumé before applying for a job.

Government websites sponsored by the United States Department of Labor, Employment, and Training Administration are good places to start your online job search. These sites display a great deal of information about the job market, listing job openings by type, title, and location. Another effective government source for researching careers is the *Occupational Outlook Handbook*.

There are also online job search engines that can be helpful. Some are specific to healthcare careers, while other, more general sites allow you to select healthcare as the career category you are seeking. If you have identified a facility where you might be interested in applying, visit the facility's website. Many companies post job listings on their websites.

Direct Employer Contact

Many people use direct contact with employers to find jobs. Make a list of possible employers by searching online, looking through the Yellow Pages, or contacting the Chamber of Commerce. You can also ask people in your network for employer contacts. Record the names, addresses, and phone numbers of employers who have job openings.

Next, contact the person who is responsible for hiring in each company. Such a person is often found in the human resources department of the facility. A human resources representative will know which jobs are available and how you can apply. It is common for facilities to post their job openings online. Some facilities may also have an automated job line that will list jobs available at the present time. You can access the job line information through a telephone extension for the facility.

Professional and Trade Journals

Many healthcare associations and organizations and related trades publish their own magazines and journals. Some of these journals may be found online, and many include advertisements for job openings. Some journals advertise both national and international job possibilities. Some national trade journals also list job opportunities by state. Journals and magazines published by state and local chapters of organizations can provide local job leads. These publications are also valuable resources because they contain up-to-date information about the latest developments in a given field.

Government and Private Employment Services

State employment offices are found in most large cities and towns. These offices can help job seekers find open positions within and outside the government. You can find the nearest state employment office by searching online.

At an employment office, you will be interviewed by an employment counselor to determine your skills and interests. Then you may be matched with positions that fit your profile. Once you have chosen a field, you will be directed to the employer(s) that may want to hire you. Only a small percentage of job seekers will find a job this way, so it is best to utilize many sources to find the job you want.

Private employment agencies are businesses that help match employers with job seekers. These agencies charge the job seeker or the employer for this service. For most entry-level jobs, the job seeker can expect to pay the employment agency. For most high-paying, professional jobs, the agency's fee is paid by the employer. Ask your school counselor to recommend a private employment agency. Some agencies specialize in certain jobs. As with the similar government agencies, only a small percentage of people find jobs this way.

Friends and Relatives

Friends and relatives can be effective sources for job leads. They may know of jobs that fit your skills. Make sure they are aware of your specific skills and background. Providing them with a résumé can also be helpful.

The Job Application

Some employers may only require you to submit your résumé when applying for a job, while others will ask that you also fill out an application. You may fill out several applications during your job search. It may be helpful to carry a personal fact sheet, especially when you are completing an application away from your records. A personal fact sheet includes all of the personal and professional information you will need to complete a job application (Figure 18.11). Carrying the fact sheet in your career portfolio will be especially helpful when applying for jobs. Like your letter of introduction, the fact sheet is for your own personal use during this process.

Personal Fact Sheet

Education	Name	Location	Date Attended	Date Graduated	GPA
Junior high school	_____	_____	_____	_____	_____
High school	_____	_____	_____	_____	_____
College	_____	_____	_____	_____	_____
Technical school	_____	_____	_____	_____	_____
Other	_____	_____	_____	_____	_____

Work Experience

Employer _____

Address _____
       (street address)   (city)   (state)   (zip)

Telephone _____ Employed from _____ to _____
                                        (mo./yr.)   (mo./yr.)

Job title _____ Supervisor _____

Starting salary _____ Final salary _____

Job duties _____

_____

Employer _____

Address _____
       (street address)   (city)   (state)   (zip)

Telephone _____ Employed from _____ to _____
                                        (mo./yr.)   (mo./yr.)

Job title _____ Supervisor _____

Starting salary _____ Final salary _____

Job duties _____

Skills _____

Honors and Activities _____

_____

Hobbies and Interests _____

_____

References

Name/Title _____

Address _____

Telephone (daytime) _____ E-mail _____

Name/Title _____

Address _____

Telephone (daytime) _____ E-mail _____

Name/Title _____

Address _____

Telephone (daytime) _____ E-mail _____

Figure 18.11   Your personal fact sheet is a helpful reference to take with you when applying or interviewing for jobs.

Do not submit an incorrect or sloppy application form. Read the entire application before beginning to fill it out. Carefully fill out the form using black or blue ink. Do not fill out the sections marked for employer use only. If the application asks you to print, do so. If the form is two-sided, be sure to answer the questions on both sides. Be aware that some applications are now online and require electronic completion.

If a question does not apply to you, write *does not apply* in the space provided. You may wish to omit your Social Security number. If so, write *will provide if hired* on the application.

If a question asks about wages or salaries, it may be best to write *open* or *negotiable* in that space. You do not want to limit your options. When filling out the employment history, remember to include part-time jobs. There may be questions asking you to describe the reason you left a job. Carefully draft your response to this question. Do not write negative comments about yourself or your former employer.

When handing in your application, you may want to include a résumé as well. The résumé may not be required, but it will provide additional details the human resources staff may find useful.

There are certain questions that cannot be asked on job applications or in a job interview (Figure 18.12). Knowing these questions can help you protect your rights. If you find a discriminatory question on an application, you can write *not clear* or *decline to answer*.

The Job Interview

Any job interview requires preparation and research. This could be one of the most important moments of your life—preparation is key! There are several things you can do before your interview to ensure you are properly prepared:

- Research the company or healthcare facility where you are interviewing—doing so shows that you are interested in what they do.

- Make a list of intelligent questions to ask your interviewer. These questions might be specific to the position or to the healthcare facility as a whole.

Illegal Questions for Job Applicants			
Subject	*Questions*	*Subject*	*Questions*
Race or national origin	What is the color of your skin, hair, or eyes? What is your race? What nationality are you? What is your ancestry? What language do you and your family speak at home? Is English your first language? What is your place of birth? Are you a naturalized citizen?	**Personal/ family**	What is your age? What is the date of your birth? Do you have a current photograph to attach to your application? Do you have any children, or are you planning to have children? What child care arrangements do you have?
Religion	What is your religion? What church do you attend? What religious holidays do you observe? Who is your religious leader?	**Sex and marital status**	Are you single, married, divorced, or widowed? Do you prefer to be addressed as Miss, Ms., or Mrs.?
Disabilities	Do you have any disabilities?	**Organizations**	To what organizations or clubs do you belong?

Goodheart-Willcox Publisher

Figure 18.12   Certain questions should not be asked during a job interview.

- Be sure to bring relevant materials with you—a pen, your résumé, the completed job application, and your list of questions. All of these items should be placed in your career portfolio.

- Decide what you are going to wear and lay it out the night before.

- Practice before the interview—think of how you might answer questions commonly asked during interviews (Figure 18.13).

- Make sure you know where to go for the interview and arrive at least 5 to 10 minutes early. Never arrive late for an interview.

- When you arrive for the interview, other employees may see you and judge your appearance and behavior. Act professionally at all times.

- Do not bring anyone with you to an interview, including children, parents, friends, spouses, or significant others.

Possible Interview Questions and Prompts

Tell me about yourself.

Why do you want to work for this facility or company?

What were your best subjects in school?

Why did you leave your last job?

Have you been fired from a job? If so, why?

What are your major strengths and weaknesses?

If you have ever had a conflict with a coworker, how did you resolve it?

How do you feel about working evenings, weekends, and holidays?

What are your salary requirements?

Where do you see yourself in five years? ten years?

Why should I hire you?

Goodheart-Willcox Publisher

Figure 18.13 Rehearsing answers to these prompts and questions will help prepare you for a job interview.

Check Your Understanding ✓

1. What tool should you use to collect and save your career planning and job search materials?

2. When should you arrive for a job interview?

3. What do you do if a question on a job application does not apply to you?

Dressing for the Job Interview

Think very carefully about what you want to wear to the interview. Your clothes and appearance will influence the employer's impression of you, just as your general appearance leaves an impression on patients and coworkers.

What to Wear

Try to dress one step above what will be worn on the job. If you are interviewing for a summer job with the recreation department, you might dress in a casual manner with clothes that are clean, neat, and ironed. Make sure your shoes are in good condition—polished, if necessary.

If you are interviewing for a position with a great deal of responsibility, you should take care to dress professionally (Figure 18.14). Men should wear a long-sleeved shirt with a tie. They may also want to wear a suit, sport coat, or blazer, if appropriate. Women in this position should wear a two-piece skirt or pant suit in a conservative color (navy, black, or brown). A blouse should be tailored with sleeves. Shoes should have a low heel and cover the toes. When in doubt, lean more toward professional than casual dress.

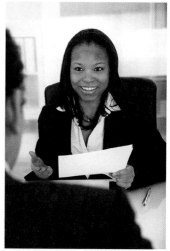

Andrey_Popov/Shutterstock.com

Figure 18.14 Dressing professionally and appropriately for a job interview may improve your chances of being hired.

What Not to Wear

When you are interviewing for a healthcare position, remember that the healthcare profession requires conservative dress. Because the healthcare employee is exposed to patients with a wide range of ages and points of view, piercings, tattoos, short skirts, cleavage, high heels, tight pants, and heavy makeup are not appropriate. Do not wear t-shirts with pictures or sayings on them, regardless of the job for which you are applying. No tattoos should be visible, and jewelry should be conservative. Do not wear athletic shoes, sandals, or boots. Cologne and perfume should not be worn.

Women should avoid wearing too much makeup—less is more. Short, tight clothing is not appropriate. Organize your purse or briefcase before the interview—you will look unprofessional and disorganized if you have to dig around in your purse or briefcase to find an item.

The Handshake

The first impression your potential employer will get from you is your overall appearance. The second impression may come when he or she shakes your hand. A firm handshake communicates confidence when coupled with direct eye contact (Figure 18.15). Do not get too close to the other person during a handshake. Present your hand, not your fingertips. Don't extend your hand first. Not everyone wants to shake hands.

Conducting Yourself during the Interview

Many employers use phone interviews to decide which applicants they would like to bring into the office for an in-person interview. In these cases, the phone interview is your first contact with an employer. These interviews are used to screen applicants before bringing them on-site, so you want to make a good impression. Take the call in a location where there is no outside noise (crying children, ringing phones, or background talking). Remember to speak slowly, clearly, and with confidence. Your attitude will come through on the phone as it does in person.

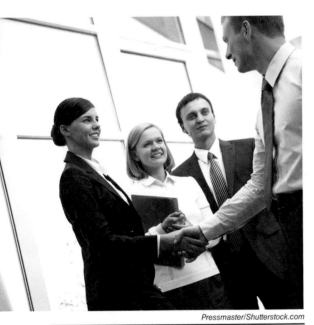

Pressmaster/Shutterstock.com

Figure 18.15 Direct eye contact and a firm handshake make a good impression on an employer.

For an in-person interview, there are more factors to consider. Do not sit until you are invited to do so by the interviewer. If you are already seated when an interviewer enters the room, stand to greet him or her. Introduce yourself if the interviewer has not stated your name. Smile and try to appear relaxed, even though you will probably be nervous.

When you are offered a seat, sit in a comfortable position, lean forward slightly, and do not slouch. Put your hands in your lap. If you cross your legs, cross them at your ankles rather than your knees. Avoid doing anything distracting, such as chewing gum, shifting nervously in your seat, playing with your hair, or avoiding direct eye contact. Keep the conversation positive throughout the interview. Do not mention reasons why it would be hard for you to take this job, such as child care problems or transportation challenges.

It may seem like the interviewer is asking you hard questions to get you to say the wrong thing. If you receive a question that you aren't prepared for, take a moment to think about your answer. Interviewers are interested in your ability to think on your feet. They are not interested in someone who gets flustered easily and is unable to come up with a reasonable answer.

When the interviewer has finished questioning you, you may be asked if you have any questions. Questions you might ask may include specific questions about the facility, or more general questions:

- What opportunities could this job present for me to learn and grow professionally?

- What is a typical workday like?

- What does the interviewer like about working for this particular facility?

- When does the interviewer think the decision will be made about the job?

Do not ask about salaries on a first interview. Be flexible regarding salary—it is best not to discuss compensation until you are offered the job. The employer will most likely promise to contact you in the future about the job. If you do not get the job, you may not get a call at all.

Real Life Scenario — Responding to Questionable Questions

Brianna has an interview with an employer for a part-time job in a long-term care facility over the summer. She is excited because if she gets this job, it will be a stepping stone for a career in this facility when she graduates.

Brianna's interviewer, Mr. Stone, asks her about her last name, which is Sanchez. He says he is curious about the origin of her name—specifically if it is Spanish, Mexican, or Filipino. Brianna recognizes that it is illegal for Mr. Stone to ask such a question.

Apply It

1. How should Brianna handle this situation?
2. Name three other examples of questions that are illegal for interviewers to ask.

After the Interview

Within two days of your interview, you should send a follow-up letter or e-mail. This brief note, written in a business-like manner, should thank the interviewer for his or her time. Draft another letter to thank anyone who referred you to the position. They may be pleased to get your feedback about how your interview went and to hear if you were offered a job.

If you go on many interviews, but are not offered any jobs, consider the following questions:

- Are you really qualified for this job? Maybe the jobs you're applying for require more experience and training than you currently have. You may have to start in an entry-level position that does not require experience.

- What is the job market like for the position you are seeking? Maybe you need to apply for jobs in neighboring towns or move to an area where there are more opportunities.

- Was your application filled out completely and properly? Did the application look neat? Did you cross out answers and attempt to write over the first answers? Did you read the application directions carefully?

- Did you present a résumé that was clear and appropriate for the jobs you wanted? Was the résumé neat and restricted to one page?

- Were you tired or excessively nervous during the interview? Did you project enthusiasm? Not asking questions about the job or seeming distracted during the interview could tell the interviewer that you are not really interested in the job.

- Did you lack confidence during the interview?

- Were you courteous with the interviewer? Did you get defensive when asked about your past employment?

- Were you late to the interview? Did you properly thank the interviewer?

Check Your Understanding ✔

1. Why should you avoid wearing perfume, cologne, or aftershave to a job interview?

2. Why would chewing gum during the interview be a bad idea?

3. How long after a job interview should you send a follow-up letter or e-mail?

The Job Offer

It is thrilling to be offered your first job in the healthcare world. Depending on where you live, jobs could be scarce, so you might feel very fortunate to receive a job offer. It is important to remember that your first job will likely be a stepping stone to a better-paying position with more responsibility.

When applying for an entry-level position in a healthcare facility, you may not know the salary for the position. You need to be realistic about the compensation and recognize that an entry-level job may lead to a better opportunity in the future.

Make sure you know what will be expected of you when you are offered a job. Ask specific questions about the job if information is not given to you by the employer. You may want to ask about work hours, salary, and other expectations not mentioned in the job description. Remember to be enthusiastic and optimistic about the job.

Rejecting the Job Offer

If after an interview you realize that the job is not a good fit for you, you will probably not accept an offer. Politely thank the interviewer and briefly explain why you feel you are not right for the job. Be direct, but polite. Although this specific position did not work out, you may want to apply for another job at the facility in the future.

The Art of Keeping a Job

Imagine you have studied your options for pursing a healthcare career and have completed the necessary coursework and training to begin your career. You carefully prepared a successful job search strategy, and you obtained your dream job. Now, how do you keep your new job? Here are a few suggestions that can help you be a valuable employee:

- **Show up on time.** Arriving early is even better than being on time. Always give yourself plenty of time to get to work in case of complications. Employers do not want to hear about your alarm clock not going off, your car battery dying, or the impossible traffic. Lack of punctuality may lead to disciplinary actions or dismissal.

- **Always look professional.** Wrinkled, dirty clothes and unwashed hair will not make a good impression on your employer. Pay attention to your grooming, hygiene, and appearance.

- **Present a positive attitude.** Complaining about your fellow employees, resisting any new tasks, and bringing your personal problems to the job are all signs of a bad attitude. Embrace any new task that you are asked to perform. Try as hard as you can to get along with other employees and keep personal drama out of the workplace.

- **Use appropriate language with patients and fellow employees.** Sarcasm shouldn't be used in the healthcare facility. People who do not use or understand sarcasm may be confused and even offended by it. Swearing is not tolerated in a healthcare facility, and using offensive language may be reason for termination.

- **Maintain appropriate relationships with coworkers.** You might think that flirting is harmless, but someone might feel your flirting is sexual harassment. You do not want to make fellow employees or patients feel uncomfortable. Overt sexual behavior can be punished through termination and even criminal charges.

- **Keep busy.** If your assigned task is finished, ask your supervisor for another. Help a coworker if you see that he or she is struggling to finish a task. Look around to see what needs to be done, and do it without direction or complaint.

- **Do not argue with a supervisor.** Some new employees feel like they know a better way to do a task than how it is being done in the workplace. You need to prove yourelf as an excellent employee before you can make suggestions. Do not correct your supervisor, especially in front of others.

- **Try to smile as much as possible.** Smiling more will show everyone that you are happy with your new job. You will also seem much more approachable and pleasant to be around (Figure 18.16).

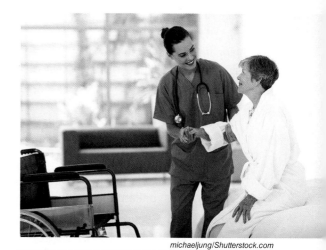

michaeljung/Shutterstock.com

Figure 18.16   A positive attitude and smile will improve your relationships with coworkers and patients.

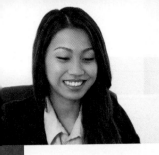
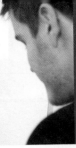

Chapter 18
Review and Assessment

Summary

If you have a professional attitude and appearance, you will be one step closer to becoming an excellent employee with a promising career future. Evaluating your personal characteristics may help you determine which area of healthcare is best for you. Practicing soft skills can improve your interactions with patients, visitors, and coworkers, and make you a better employee. Correctly recognizing social cues adds to your effectiveness when dealing with others.

Conflict resolution is very important in the healthcare setting. Excellent care for patients and a healthy work environment cannot be achieved if conflicts occur. Learning how to manage conflict is critical for the healthcare worker.

Preparing for the job search can be time-consuming. There are many sources for job leads including your personal network and the Internet. Your school may have invaluable resources to help you get leads for job openings.

Creating a well-written cover letter and résumé are necessary first steps to take when applying for jobs. As you fill out job applications, you must include accurate, complete information. Doing so improves your chances of getting an interview. Interviewing, whether in person or by phone, requires specific skills to present yourself in a positive light. Be confident in yourself and your ability to do the job.

Professional attitudes combined with employability skills will help you find a fulfilling job that fits your personal needs. These attitudes and skills will take a great deal of effort, but you will be rewarded for the time spent. Once you have your long-sought job, do everything in your power to keep it by being competent and having a great attitude in the workplace.

Review Questions

True or False Assess

1. *True or False?* Perfume should be worn while interacting with patients.

2. *True or False?* Conflict resolution is something *only* your supervisor needs to know.

3. *True or False?* Chewing gum during a job interview is unacceptable.

4. *True or False?* A firm handshake is important when interviewing for a job.

5. *True or False?* Only a small number of jobs are found through government and private employment agencies.

6. *True or False?* You should feel free to ask about a potential salary as soon as you are interviewed.

7. *True or False?* Soft skills include friendliness, optimism, and the ability to communicate well with others.

8. *True or False?* Making direct eye contact with a potential employer is a sign of dominance and should be avoided.

9. *True or False?* It is important to address your cover letter to a specific person instead of using *To Whom It May Concern*.

10. *True or False?* Employees in healthcare facilities never work as a team.

Multiple Choice Assess

11. Which of the following resources may be helpful when looking for a job?
    A. direct employer contact
    B. school resources
    C. friends and family connections
    D. All of the above.

12. Which of the following behaviors is considered unprofessional in the workplace?
    A. using coarse language
    B. gossiping
    C. wearing sloppy clothes
    D. All of the above.

13. When being criticized by an employer, you should do all the following *except* _____.
    A. resist being defensive
    B. listen carefully to what your employer is saying
    C. help determine a way to improve your performance
    D. question the validity of the criticism

14. _____ is the ability to avoid giving offense through your words and actions.

    A. Compassion

    B. Empathy

    C. Tact

    D. Competence

15. All of the following items should be included in a cover letter *except* _____.

    A. the correct name of the person who will read the cover letter

    B. a clearly written statement of the job you are seeking

    C. a short statement about your likes and dislikes

    D. a phone number where you can be reached

16. Which of the following would be inappropriate to include in the special skills section of your résumé?

    A. computer programs with which you are familiar

    B. languages you speak fluently

    C. gardening expertise

    D. ability to multitask

17. A well-written résumé should include each of the following *except* _____.

    A. a clear objective

    B. work experience

    C. education

    D. travel experiences

18. Which of the following statements is *not* true about a career portfolio?

    A. Your career portfolio should include letters of recommendation.

    B. Your portfolio should include a list of school and community activities in which you have participated.

    C. Your portfolio should include a list of contacts you have created by networking.

    D. Your portfolio should include flattering pictures of yourself.

Short Answer

19. Explain the ways in which healthy relationships can influence your career goals.

20. List five aspects of personal appearance necessary to look professional in the workplace.

21. Name three sources to explore to find available jobs.

22. Explain the importance of properly completing a job application.

23. What types of colors are appropriate for clothing you wear to a job interview?

24. Describe how to reject a job offer.

25. Identify three ways to keep a job once you are employed.

26. Explain what integrity is and why it is an important quality for healthcare workers to possess.

27. Why is respecting the chain of command particularly important in the workplace?

28. Explain why teamwork is important in the healthcare setting. How might consensus building contribute to better teamwork?

29. How might networking help you in your job search?

Critical Thinking Exercises

30. What aspects of practicing professionalism in attitude and appearance can be challenging for you, if any?

31. Have you ever interviewed for a job that you didn't get? What might have been the reasons for not getting the job?

32. What would you do if a potential employer acted unprofessionally during a job interview?

33. Do you have a job-seeking network? If not, how can you assemble one?

34. Do you have a potential employer that you would like to target when you finish preparing for your career? What are some ways you can begin to prepare for this future employment?

35. Prepare answers to each of the questions presented in Figure 18.13. Discuss your answers with a family member, friend, or teacher.

36. When working in a healthcare facility, you may be asked to take on a leadership role, whether it is heading a committee, becoming a supervisor, or just overseeing your coworkers in accomplishing a simple task. What specific leadership skills do you feel a healthcare professional should possess?

37. Take a moment to reflect on your own leadership abilities. Do you feel you have what it takes to be a successful leader in your future healthcare career? If so, list the qualities you feel will help you master a leadership role.

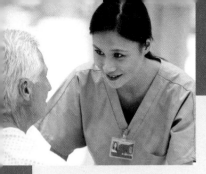

Review Questions

Answer the following questions using what you have learned in this unit.

True/False

1. *True or False?* The longest amount of time you should leave a person on hold after answering the telephone is two minutes.

2. *True or False?* Color coding your notes can be very helpful.

3. *True or False?* Using colored or patterned paper for your résumé is preferred.

4. *True or False?* The boiling point on the Celsius scale is 212°.

5. *True or False?* A liter is a basic metric measure of liquid volume.

6. *True or False?* In a hospital setting, there is no clear chain of command.

7. *True or False?* A circle graph may also be called a *pie chart*.

8. *True or False?* Auditory learners typically follow spoken directions well.

9. *True or False?* Most of the world uses the English system of measurement.

Multiple Choice

10. Which of the following describes how you might find the median of a group of numbers?
    A. total all numbers in a set and divide the result by the quantity of numbers
    B. find the number that falls exactly in the middle of a list of numbers
    C. look for the number(s) that occur most frequently in a set of numbers
    D. calculate all the odd numbers in a set

11. Which of the following statements about spreadsheets is *true*?
    A. They display information in rows and columns.
    B. They make it easy to perform mathematical operations.
    C. They allow you to insert formulas.
    D. All of the above.

12. Examples of mnemonic devices include all of the following *except* _____.
    A. rhymes
    B. sets of numbers
    C. acronyms
    D. spelling catchphrases

13. Which of the following items is acceptable for a woman to wear to a job interview?
    A. t-shirts with sayings and/or pictures
    B. tight pants
    C. a large amount of jewelry
    D. a woman's suit or pant suit in a conservative color

14. 1830 in military time is equivalent to _____ in 12-hour clock time.
    A. 5:30 p.m.
    B. 4:30 p.m.
    C. 6:30 p.m.
    D. 8:30 p.m.

Short Answer

15. What is the formula for converting a temperature from Fahrenheit to Celsius?

16. What is the difference between objective and subjective writing?

17. Name three cultural differences in nonverbal communication.

18. What are four benefits of reading every day?

19. Name five things you can do to keep a job once you are hired.

Critical Thinking Exercises

20. Discuss the first steps you would take to obtain a job.

21. Find a partner and take turns role playing as a job interviewer and job interviewee. The interview is for a position as a physical therapist.

22. When studying to become a healthcare worker, you may be required to read and understand complex technical material related to your field of study. What techniques might you employ to study and be able to understand such material?

23. In your chosen healthcare field, you will likely be required to clearly express ideas in writing, including documentation of patient status, incident reports, and more. What, if any, are your weaknesses when writing? spelling? punctuation? wordiness? sentence structure? How can you improve your writing skills?

24. In small groups, research and describe the roles of professional healthcare associations and regulatory agencies. As you work with classmates, focus on using your communication skills to build and maintain healthy relationships.

Career Exploration

Physician Assistant

Physician assistants, also known as PAs, are healthcare providers who are licensed to diagnose and treat illness and disease. Physician assistants can also prescribe medication for patients and provide many of the services that a doctor can provide. They can take medical histories, perform physical examinations, order and interpret laboratory tests, counsel patients, assist in surgery, and set fractures.

Physician assistants are usually supervised by doctors. PAs must be able to work as a team with doctors, surgeons, and other healthcare workers. Some PAs can also work in specialties other than primary care. Such specialties can include surgery, orthopedics, pediatrics, gerontology, and many others.

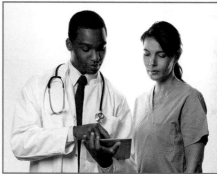
LarsZ/Shutterstock.com

Some people choose to become a PA because they cannot afford the necessary education to become a doctor, or they do not wish to dedicate at least six years to postgraduate education. The necessary education for this occupation typically includes a bachelor's degree and master's degree from an accredited program. To become a PA, you must be proficient in science and math, as well as having excellent written and spoken communication skills.

According to *Money Magazine*, physician assistant is one of the top ten best jobs in America. The starting salary for this job is $90,000.

Further Research

1. Research one of the related careers listed above using the *Occupational Outlook Handbook* and other reliable Internet resources. What is the outlook for this career? Are workers in demand, or are jobs dwindling?

2. Review the educational requirements for this career. What classes would you need to take to pursue a related degree?

3. What is the salary range for this job?

4. What do you think you would like about this career? Is there anything about it you might dislike? Compare the job you have chosen to research to the description of a physician assistant. Which job appeals to you more? Why?

Related Careers
Family and general physician
Nurse practitioner
Veterinarian
Paramedic
Back office medical assistant

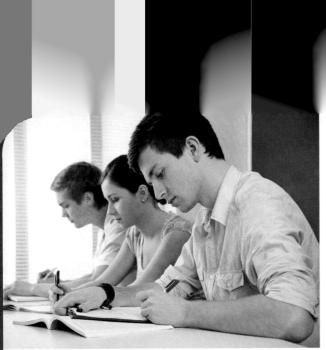

Alexander Raths/Shutterstock.com

Grammar Review

Terms to Know

 Build Vocab

adjective
adverb
capitalization
complex sentence
compound sentence
conjunction
consonants

contraction
grammar
interjection
noun
paragraph
parts of speech
preposition

pronoun
punctuation
simple sentence
verb
vowels

Lesson Objectives

- Explain the importance of mastering the elements of effective writing.
- Recognize the parts of speech.
- Understand why using proper grammar helps you communicate effectively.
- Explain why proper spelling is essential for healthcare workers.
- Describe why correct punctuation is an important part of clear writing.

As you learned in chapter 15, much of your daily life is spent communicating with others. Communication is always important, but it becomes especially critical when it takes place in a healthcare setting. To communicate effectively with coworkers, patients, and visitors in a healthcare facility, you must understand and observe the rules of correct grammar and spelling.

Grammar

When speaking or writing, using correct grammar helps you send a clear message that is easily understood. **Grammar** is the study of how words and their components combine to form sentences. Writing that contains grammatical errors makes the writer appear uneducated. As harsh as this seems, individuals are often judged simply based on poor writing skills and grammatical mistakes. Poor grammar can cause setbacks in certain situations, including your education and career.

It is important that you proofread, or review, your writing for grammatical errors. However, proofreading your own work is not effective if you do not know grammar rules or the correct spelling of words. You will present an unprofessional image to potential employers, patients, and coworkers if your writing has grammatical errors, misused words, and spelling mistakes. Instead of relying on a friend to review your work, use an online grammar check, read a grammar reference book, and edit your writing once more.

grammar
the study of how words and their components combine to form sentences

Real Life Scenario — Is Strong Grammar an Advantage?

Jenny and Drew are applying for the same job. They have each put together a résumé and filled out an application for the position. Drew took a considerable amount of time to craft his résumé and fill out the application, paying close attention to grammar and spelling. Jenny has a very busy schedule. She didn't take the time to carefully review her résumé and application for grammar and spelling mistakes, but she felt that her qualifications would be enough to get the job.

Apply It

1. Which applicant has the advantage if both candidates are equally qualified?
2. What impression might Jenny have given a potential employer by not proofreading her résumé and application?

Vowels and Consonants

When formulating words in the English language, the most basic building blocks are **vowels** and **consonants**. Written English has five vowel letters—a, e, i, o, and u (y may substitute for i). Consonants in the English language are the remaining letters of the alphabet—b, c, d, f, g, h, j, k, l, m, n, p, q, r, s, t, v, w, x, y, and z. Together, vowels and consonants form words. Each letter has a distinct sound, depending on where it appears in a word.

vowels
five letters in the English language: a, e, i, o, and u (sometimes y is substituted for i)

consonants
all letters of the English alphabet except a, e, i, o, and u

Parts of Speech

parts of speech
collective term for eight classifications of words that denote each word's function; in English these include noun, pronoun, verb, adjective, adverb, conjunction, preposition, and interjection

noun
a word that represents a person, place, or thing

Words in the English language are divided into eight different **parts of speech**. Parts of speech can be combined to form a complete thought, or *sentence*. A sentence can combine any or even all of the parts of speech listed in Figure BL1.1.

Nouns

A **noun** is a type of word that represents a person, place, or thing. Examples of nouns include *doctor*, *heart*, and *ambulance*. Nouns can be singular or plural (Figure BL1.2).

Proper Nouns. Nouns can be classified as *proper* or *common*. A proper noun begins with a capital letter no matter where it occurs in a sentence. Proper nouns name a specific item. A common noun is not capitalized and does not name a specific person, thing, or place.

> **Example** (common noun): writer
> **Example** (proper noun): Ernest Hemingway
> **Example** (common noun): city
> **Example** (proper noun): Chicago

Possessive Nouns. A possessive noun indicates ownership by the noun or a characteristic of the noun.

In most cases, plural nouns that end with an "s" are made possessive by adding an apostrophe after the "s".

> **Example**: The brothers' names all began with an M.

Plural nouns that do not end in "s" are usually made possessive by adding an apostrophe and an "s".

> **Examples**: *toys of children* would read: children's toys
> The nurse's smile made me feel welcome.

Parts of Speech		
Part	*Definition*	*Examples*
noun	a word naming a person, place, or thing	patient, clinic, medication
pronoun	a word taking the place of a noun	he, it, they
verb	a word showing action or state of being	help, run, is
adjective	a word describing a noun or pronoun	healthy, young, happy
adverb	a word describing a verb, adjective, or another adverb	rapidly, very, nearby
conjunction	a word connecting words, phrases, or sentences	and, or, but
preposition	a word relating nouns or pronouns to other words in a sentence	above, to, for
interjection	a word expressing strong emotion	STAT!

Goodheart-Willcox Publisher

Figure BL1.1   All English words can be categorized as one of the eight parts of speech.

Making Singular Nouns Plural		
Guidelines	**Singular**	**Plural**
For most nouns, add **s** to the singular form to create the plural form.	doctor	doctors
	X-ray	X-rays
	glove	gloves
For nouns that end in **sh**, **ch**, **s**, **x**, **z**, or similar sounds, add **es** to the singular form. In the case of z, the z is often doubled.	crutch	crutches
	box	boxes
	class	classes
	quiz	quizzes
For nouns that end in a consonant and a **y**, change the **y** to **i** and add **es**.	pharmacy	pharmacies
	nursery	nurseries
For nouns that end in **o** preceded by a vowel, add **s** to the singular form. For most nouns that end in **o** preceded by a consonant, add **s** to form the plural. For some exceptions, add **es**.	albino	albinos
	radio	radios
	memo	memos
	placebo	placeboes
For many nouns that end in **f** or **fe**, change the **f** sound to a **v** and add **s** or **es** to the singular form. For others, keep the **f** and add an **s**.	life	lives
	knife	knives
	strife	strives

Goodheart-Willcox Publisher

Figure BL1.2   Singular nouns can be made plural by following these guidelines.

Pronouns

A **pronoun** is a substitute for a noun. Common pronouns include *I, me, she, hers, he, him, it, you, they,* and *them*. Pronouns allow writing to flow smoothly without repeating nouns over and over.

pronoun
a word that can be substituted for a noun

Example: Jason didn't get the job, and *he* was very upset.

Verbs

A **verb** is a type of word that describes an action or a state of being, such as *waddle, walk, run, jump, have,* or *think*.

verb
any word that describes an action or a state of being

Example: Doctor Martin *diagnosed* his patient with strep throat.

Verbs such as *be, is, are, was, were,* and *am* can also show a state of being.

Example: I *am* hungry.

Helping Verbs. Certain verbs work with the main verb to show action. These are called *helping verbs*. These verbs have little meaning on their own, but they help make main verbs clearer. Helping verbs include *be, been, am, is, are, was, were, has, had, have, do, does, did, can, could, may, might, will, would, should, shall,* and *must*.

Examples: I *have* interviewed for that position.

I *should* study for the science examination.

Voice. Verbs also have different properties, including voice, mood, tense, person, and number. Voice can be either active or passive. Sentences using an active voice verb are considered more direct and easier to understand than those using passive voice. Passive voice is appropriate in some cases, such as in scientific papers to make conclusions sound more objective.

> **Example** (passive voice): The lecture *was given* by Dr. Brown.

> **Example** (active voice): Dr. Brown *gave* the lecture.

Extend Your Knowledge ▶ **Passive Versus Active Voice**

To become more aware of the use of passive voice, scan a newspaper article and underline every example you can find of passive voice verbs. Then, circle every example you can find of active voice verbs.

Apply It

1. Did you find more examples of passive or active voice verbs in the article? Why do you think the writer chose to use more of one verb type than the other?

2. Using a recent sample of your own writing, identify each time you used a passive verb. Then, substitute an active verb for each passive verb. How has changing the verbs altered your writing sample? Do you think it is stronger, weaker, or about the same as before?

Mood. The mood of a verb affects the way the writer wants the sentence to be understood. For example, mood can be used to express a fact or opinion.

> **Example**: The patient in pain *spoke* to the doctor.

Mood can also convey a command or request.

> **Example**: *Assist* the doctor with the procedure immediately.

Mood can also help to express doubt or uncertainty.

> **Example**: If I *were* you, I would pursue a career in healthcare.

Verb Tense. Verb tense will tell you if the action takes place in the present, past, or future.

> **Example**: Jerry *arrived* at the hospital last night. His doctors *are reviewing* his test results now, but he *will have* more lab work done tomorrow.

Verb Person. The person of a verb determines to whom the action or state of being refers. Verbs can refer to one of three persons: the person who is speaking (first person); the person being addressed (second person); or a person, or group of people, being discussed (third person).

A first-person verb is an action of the person who is speaking or writing.

> **Example**: I *am deciding* which career to pursue.

A second-person verb refers to an action of someone who is being addressed.

> **Example**: You *are going* to be a wonderful nurse.

A third-person verb refers to an action of someone being discussed.

Example: They *are going* to become physical therapists.

Verb Number. Verbs should agree in number with related nouns and pronouns. Verbs connected with "I" should always be singular.

Example: I *am* studying.

Verbs related to "you" are always plural.

Example: You *are* studying.

Verbs in the third person should agree in number with the nouns or pronouns.

Example: John and Laura *study* every day.

Adjectives

An **adjective** is a word that modifies or describes a noun or pronoun. Examples of adjectives include *big, cold, blue,* and *silly.* Adjectives provide details about the noun or pronoun that give you a better understanding of the person, place, or thing. Adjectives can come before or after the words they modify.

Examples: *Two* students failed the science test.
After studying all night, Denise is *tired*.

adjective
a word that modifies or describes a noun or pronoun

Adverbs

An **adverb** is a word that tells "how," "when," "where," or "how much." Some examples of adverbs include *easily, carefully, slowly, mainly, freely, often,* and *unfortunately.*

Examples: *Finally*, I finished my project.
Jennifer will have an interview *tomorrow*.
Sarah *quickly* finished the multiple choice section of her exam.

adverb
any word that tells how, when, where, or how much

Conjunctions

A **conjunction** is a word that joins other words, phrases (two or more words acting as a unit in a sentence), clauses (a group of words that contains a noun and a verb), or sentences. Examples of common conjunctions are *and, as, because, but, or, since, so, until,* and *while.*

Example: *While* I could become a nurse, I might also want to be a physical therapist *or* an occupational therapist.

conjunction
a word that joins other words, phrases, clauses, or sentences

Prepositions

A **preposition** is a word that connects or relates its object to the rest of the sentence. Examples include *to, at, by, of, under, beside, over,* and *during.*

Example: *During* an internship, you will be working *beside* an experienced medical professional.

preposition
a word that connects or relates its object to the rest of the sentence

Prepositional Phrases. A prepositional phrase consists of a preposition, its object, and related adjectives and adverbs.

Example: The patient is *in the examination room*.

Interjections

interjection
a word, phrase, or clause that expresses emotion

An **interjection** is a word, phrase, or clause that expresses emotion. An interjection often starts a sentence, but it can be contained within a sentence or stand alone. Examples of interjections include *oh, wow, ugh, hurray, eh,* and *ah.* Interjections should be used infrequently in workplace communications.

Interjections can appear at the beginning of a sentence that expresses strong emotion. Depending on how much emotion is expressed, a sentence containing an interjection can end with a period or an exclamation point. Interjections can also appear alone with an exclamation point.

Examples: *No,* don't let the patient walk without help!

Oh, you surprised me.

Ouch!

Did You Know? **Speaking and Verb Tense**

Many speakers are inconsistent when expressing verb tense. Some languages do not have verb tenses, so non-native English speakers sometimes find this very challenging. When in doubt, consult a grammar text.

Sentences

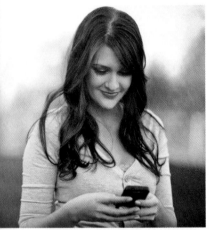

arek_malang/Shutterstock.com

Figure BL1.3 Slang used in text messages is not appropriate for workplace communication.

A sentence is a grammatical unit of one or more words that expresses an independent statement, question, request, command, or exclamation. A sentence typically has a noun (called the *subject*) as well as a verb (called the *predicate*). Sentences begin with a capital letter and end with the appropriate punctuation.

In this age of abbreviated messages in e-mails, text messages, and tweets, complete sentences are not often used to communicate (Figure BL1.3). In the workplace, however, complete sentences must be used to present professional communication skills and communicate a complete thought.

There are three types of sentences—simple, compound, and complex. The type of sentence you should use depends on how simple or complex an idea you wish to express.

Simple Sentences

simple sentence
a sentence that contains a subject and a verb, and which expresses a complete thought; independent clause

A **simple sentence**, also called an *independent clause,* contains a subject and a verb and expresses a complete thought. A noun or pronoun is always used as the subject of the sentence. In the following simple sentences, subjects are in green and verbs are in blue.

Examples: The nurse worked all weekend.

The patient began to cough loudly.

The phone rang at the nurse's desk.

Compound Sentences

compound sentence
a sentence that contains two independent clauses joined by a conjunction

A **compound sentence** contains two independent clauses joined by a conjunction. Except for very short sentences, conjunctions are always preceded by a comma. In the following compound sentences, subjects are in green, verbs are in blue, and the conjunctions and preceding commas are in red.

Examples: I tried to speak French, and my friend tried to speak English.

Darryl played basketball, so Maria went shopping.

James wants to be a physical therapist, but his mother wants him to be a doctor.

Complex Sentences

A **complex sentence** consists of an independent clause (a group of words that can stand alone) joined by one or more dependent clauses. In the examples shown here, the dependent clause is in blue.

complex sentence
a sentence that contains an independent clause and one or more dependent clauses

Examples: When he handed in his homework, the instructor smiled.

The instructor handed back the homework after she noticed an error.

The students are nervous because they have a test tomorrow.

Check Your Understanding ✓

Consider the examples listed here. Are these sentences? Or are they sentence fragments that do not constitute complete sentences?

1. Below the knee.
2. The calf is located below the knee.
3. The fact that Janice did not pass the anatomy test when she studied.
4. Janice studied a long time for the anatomy test and failed.
5. Because Larry is not comfortable with children, and he is assigned to work on the pediatric floor.
6. Larry worries that he will not be able to work on the pediatric floor because of his dislike for children.

The Paragraph

A **paragraph** is a part of a written composition, and consists of a collection of sentences all related to one topic. Paragraphs express one idea or present the words of a single individual. Each new paragraph should typically begin with an indented line.

paragraph
part of a written composition; consists of a collection of sentences related to one topic

An indent is signified by hitting the Tab key or inserting five spaces.

Example:

In our office, Tony is always the first one at work each morning. He was elected Employee of the Month three times because of how hard he works. Tony sets a good example for others.

I first met Tony when I was hired last year. He has always made me feel welcome in the office.

In a business letter, paragraphs are often not indented. Instead, the single-spaced paragraphs are separated by an extra line, or return, in between to clearly mark each paragraph.

Example:

Today there are many styles of writing paragraphs. Some styles include indenting paragraphs, and others do not.

Whichever style you choose, be consistent. Also, remember that a paragraph with more than six or seven sentences may be too long and will need to be broken up into two paragraphs. Chances are that there is more than one idea represented in that long paragraph.

Today, many instructors will tell you that they prefer you have at least two sentences in a paragraph. Be mindful of the length of your paragraphs. In general, paragraphs should be neither too short nor too long.

Punctuation

punctuation

the practice or system of using certain conventional marks or characters such as commas, question marks, and periods in writing

Punctuation is the practice or system of using certain conventional marks or characters in writing. Proper punctuation guides the readers and helps them understand the meaning of sentences.

End Punctuation

There are only three ways to end a sentence: a period (.), a question mark (?), and an exclamation point (!). The period is by far the most used mark of punctuation.

Periods. Paragraphs can contain several sentences, and the period is used to provide structure and separate thoughts by marking the end of each sentence. Periods are also used to divide parts of an abbreviation (p.m.) or signal the end of an abbreviation. An abbreviation is a shortened form of a word or letters used to represent a word or term. Figure BL1.4 provides a list of commonly used abbreviations in healthcare.

Today's accepted practices for many abbreviations that used to use periods have dropped the punctuation. Examples of this include academic degrees (BA, MA, AA) and two-letter state abbreviations (CA, TX, SC).

Question Marks. The question mark is used after a word or sentence that asks a question.

Example: What? Are you kidding?

Exclamation Points. Another form of end punctuation is the exclamation point. Exclamation points are used to express strong emotions.

Example: I passed my exam!

Internal Punctuation

Punctuation marks within a sentence are called *internal punctuation.* Internal punctuation marks include commas, dashes, parentheses, semicolons, colons, hyphens, apostrophes, and quotation marks.

Commas. Punctuation marks used to separate elements in a sentence are called *commas.* Commas provide breaks or pauses, helping readers to more easily understand a sentence. Commas are also used to separate items in a series.

Examples: Doctors, nurses, and physical therapists will be at the career fair.

Dorothy got the job by having an excellent résumé, an impressive application, and a great attitude.

Louis enjoyed his internship in Dr. Martin's office, but he was sorry he didn't choose an internship in a hospital setting.

Healthcare Abbreviations with Periods	
Term	**Abbreviations**
three times a day	t.i.d.
doctor	Dr.
company	co.
association	assoc.
orthopedics	ortho.

Goodheart-Willcox Publisher

Figure BL1.4 Some medical abbreviations are created using periods.

Some styles (preferred by newspapers and written communication in England) eliminate the last comma when separating items in a series. For example: *I prefer to wear a lab coat, a name badge and comfortable shoes.* Here, the comma that would typically appear after *name badge* is eliminated. However, the *Chicago Manual of Style* and most other style manuals dictate that a final comma appear before the conjunction, as shown in the previous examples.

Dashes. Also called *em dashes*, these punctuation marks separate elements in a sentence or signal an abrupt change of thought. The dash provides a stronger break than a comma.

> **Example**: I need my anatomy book—I lost it again—before the quiz.

There are also *en dashes*, which are shorter than em dashes, but longer than hyphens. The *en dash* is used to indicate a range of values, such as a span of time or a range of numbers.

> **Examples**: 8 a.m.–4 p.m.
> Monday–Friday
> 1993–2000

Parentheses. Parentheses are used to enclose words or phrases that clarify meaning or provide more information. When the entire sentence is enclosed by parentheses, the period should appear inside the closing parenthesis. If the parenthetical notation falls at the end of the sentence but only encloses a portion of it, the period should *follow* the closing parenthesis.

> **Examples**: I'll see you at the meeting at noon (3rd floor lounge).
> Please review the medical terminology abbreviations. (They are in Appendix A.)

Parentheses are also used to enclose numbers or letters in a list that is part of a sentence.

> **Example**: Your essay has errors in spelling (1), punctuation (2), and capitalization (3).

Semicolons. When a sentence requires a stronger break than a comma, a semicolon may be used. Semicolons are used to separate clauses or some items in a series. The separated clauses must be independent, meaning they are stand-alone clauses.

> **Example**: Our entire math class took the exam; everyone passed.

A semicolon can be used to separate items in a series when at least one item in the series already contains a comma.

> **Example**: I applied for an internship in Los Angeles, California; Seattle, Washington; and Las Vegas, Nevada.

Colons. When introducing elements in a sentence or paragraph, a colon may be used. The elements can be words, phrases, clauses, or sentences. The colon is a stronger break than a comma.

> **Example**: We need to study three things for the medical terminology quiz: abbreviations, prefixes, and suffixes.

Using Hyphens	
Rules for Use	**Examples**
Fractions shown in words	one-third, one-fourth
Numbers less than 100 with two words	thirty-one, fifty-three
Telephone numbers, Social Security numbers	1-888-2346, 558-34-1678
Between letters when a word is spelled out	Awkward is spelled a-w-k-w-a-r-d.

Goodheart-Willcox Publisher

Figure BL1.5 Follow these guidelines when using hyphens in written communication.

Hyphens. Hyphens are used to separate parts of a compound word. Hyphens are also used when spelling out numbers (Figure BL1.5).

Examples: My mother-in-law is a nurse.
twenty-four

Apostrophes. When forming possessive words and contractions, an apostrophe should be used. Possessive words show ownership. An apostrophe and a letter "s" are added to many nouns to create the possessive form. If the noun is plural, the apostrophe is placed after the letter "s."

Examples: Jennifer's test score was excellent.

The nurses' cars were parked in the hospital parking lot.

contraction
a shortened form of a word or term; one or more letters are omitted and replaced with an apostrophe to create one word

A **contraction** is a shortened form of a word or term. To form a contraction, omit one or more words and replace them with an apostrophe. This creates a single word.

Example: Rock 'n' roll became popular in the '50s.

Dr. Hartman didn't know the patient had high blood pressure until the patient's test results were returned.

Quotation Marks. Quotation marks enclose short, direct quotes and some titles (such as chapter titles or article titles). A direct quote is a restatement of someone's exact words. A quote does not have to be a complete sentence. Rather, it can be a word or phrase *within* a sentence that was said or written by another person. If a quote is long (several sentences in length or greater), it should be set apart from the paragraph. Long quotes that are set apart should not be enclosed in quotation marks.

Examples: "Why do you think you would be a good choice for this job?" asked the interviewer.

What did the administrator mean by "charitable giving?"

Capitalization Rules

capitalization
the use of an uppercase letter for the first letter of a word, and lowercase letters for the rest of the word; used for proper nouns

The following rules relate to **capitalization**. Capitalization is the use of an uppercase letter for the first letter of a word and lowercase for the remaining letters.

- A sentence always begins with a capital letter.
- Capital letters are used for headings in reports, articles, newsletters, and other documents. Capital letters are used for titles of books, magazines, and movies.

Examples: The Adventures of Huckleberry Finn, National Geographic

- Capitalize the first word and all other important words in a heading or title (conjunctions and prepositions are normally not capitalized).

Example: The Lion, the Witch, and the Wardrobe

- Proper nouns must always be capitalized.

Examples: Dr. Lang is my doctor.
I love Japanese food.

- Capitalize months, days, cities, states, and countries (Figure BL1.6).

Examples: January, Monday, New York, Great Britain

- Some abbreviations use capital letters.

Examples: HIPAA, UCLA, HTML, WI

- Capitalize titles that come before personal names.

Examples: Ms. Marquez, Dr. Fong, Officer Johnson

- Capitalize abbreviations for academic degrees and other professional designations that follow names.

Examples: Jacob White, LPN
Jessie Parks, RN, BSN, MSN

- Do not capitalize seasons.

Examples: fall, winter, spring, summer

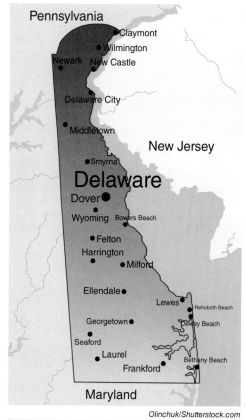

Olinchuk/Shutterstock.com

Figure BL1.6   The names of states and cities are proper nouns and must be capitalized.

Writing Numbers

As in all aspects of grammar, there are rules for expressing numbers as figures or words. Number guidelines are not as widely agreed upon as rules for punctuation and capitalization. The guidelines presented here should be used for general writing. If you are writing a research paper or an article for publication, find out if there are written number guidelines you must follow.

General guidelines for writing numbers include the following:

- Numbers one through nine should be spelled out as words. Numerals should be used for the number 10 and anything greater.

Examples: One supervisor and three workers were needed to solve the problem. The health unit coordinator ordered 25 black ink pens.

- Use words for numbers that are indefinite or approximate.

Examples: About twenty people applied for the job.
There were approximately ten thousand new cases of tuberculosis last year.

- When a number begins a sentence, it should be spelled out.

Example: Thirty copies of the report should be made.

- When two numbers come together in a sentence, use words for one of the numbers and numerals for the other.

Example: There are 11 twenty-year-old students in my class.

- Use words to express fractions. A hyphen comes between each word.

Example: The patient is to receive one-half of the dosage she previously had taken.

- When expressing time, use numerals followed by a.m. and p.m. designations. Always spell out the number that appears before the term *o'clock*. A colon is used between numerals expressing hours and minutes, but it is omitted when using military time (a 24-hour system).

Examples: 2:30 p.m.

eight o'clock

16:00 hrs.

1345

- Use numerals for days and years in dates. Do not write *th*, *nd*, *rd*, or *st* after a number.

Examples: I started my job on February 10, 2014.

I handed in my resignation at my last job on January 2, 2014.

Common Grammatical Mistakes

The purpose of using proper grammar is to ensure that what you write is easy to read and comprehend. Many employers immediately develop a negative impression when they receive a poorly written cover letter. Such cover letters will often cause the entire application to be tossed into the wastebasket without the employer even looking at the rest of the application.

Following grammar rules when you speak conveys to others that you are an intelligent and educated person, and that you are someone who recognizes that clear and concise language is easily understood.

The following list includes common grammar errors in the English language. Do you frequently make any of the errors listed here?

1. **don't versus doesn't**

   Incorrect: She *don't* answer questions in class.
   Rule: *Doesn't*, *does not*, or *does* are used for the third person singular (words like *he*, *she*, and *it* are third person singular words).
   Correct: She *doesn't* answer questions in class.

2. **double negatives**

   Incorrect: She *does not* dislike *no one* in her class.
   Rule: Double negatives can confuse the meaning of a sentence. Since *not* is negative, you cannot use *no one*, which is also negative, in this sentence.
   Correct: She *does not* dislike *anyone* in her class.

3. **gone versus went**

   Incorrect: I should have *went* to the lecture.
   Rule: *Gone* should be used with a helping verb.
   Correct: I should *have gone* to the lecture.

Incorrect: I *gone* to the game.

Rule: *Went* is used without a helping verb.

Correct: I *went* to the game.

4. **pronoun abuse**

Incorrect: *Me* and *my lab partner* did a great job on the assignment.

Correction: Rephrase the sentence without one of the subjects. Does it still make sense? Would you say "*Me* did a great job on the assignment"?

Correct: My lab partner and *I* did a great job on the assignment.

5. **its versus it's**

Incorrect: *Its* going to be hard to study with the beautiful weather today.

Rule: The contraction *it's* is used here because it stands for *it is*.

Correct: *It's* going to be hard to study with the beautiful weather today.

6. **good versus well**

Incorrect: You really spell *good*.

Rule: When an activity is being described, use *well*. When a condition or a state of being is described, use *good*.

Correct: You really spell *well*.

Another example: Lisa spelled *well* at the spelling bee; she looked *good* on stage wearing her new purple outfit.

7. **anxious versus eager**

Incorrect: Jenny was *anxious* to go to the graduation party in her honor.

Rule: In this case, Jenny was looking forward to her party but was not worried or uneasy, as the word *anxious* suggests.

Correct: Jenny was *eager* to go to the graduation party in her honor.

Another example: Jenny is *eager* to go to medical school after graduation, but her parents are *anxious* about the expense.

8. **affect versus effect**

Incorrect: Leonard's terrible cold *effected* his performance on the science test.

Rule: When you are referring to a thing (noun), you should use *effect* in almost all cases. When you are referring to an action (verb), you should use *affect*.

Correct: Leonard's terrible cold *affected* his performance on the science test.

Another example: The *effect* of Leonard's terrible cold was that his grade on the test was negatively *affected*.

9. **lay versus lie**

Incorrect: I asked the patient to lay down on the bed.

Rule: To *lay* is to place something (there always is a noun or a "something" that is being placed). To *lie* is to recline.

Correct: I asked the patient to *lie* down on the bed.

Another example: *Lay* your book on the table and *lie* down on the couch.

10. **lose versus loose**

Incorrect: I always *loose* my car keys.

Rule: *Loose* and *lose* are spelled similarly, but have very different definitions. *Loose* means something is not fastened, tied up, or confined, and that it is able to move freely. To *lose* something means you no longer have it or cannot find it.

Correct: I always *lose* my car keys.

Another example: I *lose* my lecture notes when they are *loose* in my binder.

11. **among versus between**

Incorrect: *Among* the two of us, I don't like to work with people.

Rule: *Among* refers to three or more individuals. *Between* refers to two individuals.

Correct: *Between* the two of us, I don't like to work with people.

Another example: *Among* the four of us, three want to be nurses.

12. **is versus are**

Incorrect: *Is* those two going to interview for the same job?

Rule: *Is* must be used with a singular noun. *Are* is used with a plural noun.

Correct: *Are* those two going to interview for the same job?

Another example: She *is* going to the interview, but Paul and Don *are* not going to interview for that job.

Spelling

In the classroom, as well as in the workplace, writing that contains spelling mistakes will detract from the message being delivered. If combined with a limited vocabulary and poor sentence structure, these mistakes will most likely earn you a poor grade, or you may be asked to redo your assignment.

Today, poor spellers may rely on the spell-check programs built into their word processors, but the automatic spell-check does not catch every misspelling. Your spell-check program may not recognize many medical terms that may have complicated spellings. Additionally, the program cannot help you if you substitute the wrong word, spelled correctly, for a word you intended to use.

The following are some basic English language spelling rules that should be followed closely:

- The letter *q* is followed by the letter *u*, with few exceptions.
- The letter *s* never follows the letter *x*.
- The letter *y*, not *i*, is used at the end of English words.

Examples: *my*, *by*, *why*, and *shy*

- When spelling a short vowel sound, only one letter is needed.

Examples: *bed*, *it*, *lot*, and *up*

- If a word ends with a silent *e*, drop the *e* when adding an ending that begins with a vowel.

Example: *rope* becomes *roping*; *come* becomes *coming*

- One of the most common spelling rules taught to elementary school children is: *i* before *e*, except after *c*, unless it says *a* (pronounced with a long *a*) as in *neighbor* and *weigh*.

Examples: *receipt*, *brief*, or *thief*

- When adding an ending to a word that ends with *y*, simply change the *y* to *i* if it is preceded by a consonant.

Example: *try* becomes *tries*; *fly* becomes *flies*

One of the most frustrating aspects of the English language is the number of exceptions to spelling rules. Memorization of spellings may be necessary, especially in the case of medical terminology, when you may have never encountered the terms before. Chapter 5 reviews many rules for learning to spell medical terms. Of course, when in doubt, look up the word in a standard or medical dictionary.

Figures BL1.7 and BL1.8 contain some of the most commonly misused and misspelled words in the English language. Do you have trouble spelling any of these words? Add your own problem words to this list.

Commonly Misused Words		
Word	**Definition**	**Example**
your	a possessive form	Your new scrubs are cute.
you're	a contraction form of *you are*	You're going to like the new doctor.
their	a possessive form	Their positive attitude made the patients more at ease.
they're	a contraction form of *they are*	They're going to take a small sample of blood.
there	a place or idea	I want to go there someday.
it's	a contraction form for *it is* or *it has*	It's almost time for Mr. Warner's medication.
its	indicates possession	The hospital room could not be used because its call button was broken.
then	expresses time	First we must distribute medication and then we will give the patient a bath.
than	used for comparison	Science is easier than English.
ensure	to make sure or certain	Safety education will help ensure safety in the workplace.
insure	refers to the provision of insurance; coverage against a specified loss	My new car is not yet insured.

Goodheart-Willcox Publisher

Figure BL1.7 Use this guide to ensure that you're using the correct words in your written communication.

Commonly Misspelled Words					
absence	cemetery	familiar	mysterious	precedence	ridiculous
accommodate	changeable	February	necessary	preference	sacrifice
accumulate	committee	fiery	ninety	preferred	schedule
achievement	conceivable	foreign	noticeable	prejudice	seize
acquaintance	conscience	forty	occasionally	prevalent	separate
acquire	criticize	fourth	occurred	principal	separation
advice	definitely	government	occurrence	principle	severely
advise	desperate	grammar	omitted	privilege	similar
amateur	dictionary	height	opportunity	probably	sophomore
analysis	disappearance	immediately	parallel	procedure	specifically
analyze	disappoint	independence	paralysis	proceed	specimen
apparatus	disastrous	inevitable	paralyze	profession	studying
apparent	discipline	intellectual	particular	professor	succeed
arctic	dissatisfied	intelligence	pastime	prominent	succession
arithmetic	effect	knowledge	performance	pronunciation	technique
ascend	eligible	laboratory	permissible	pursue	temperamental
athletic	encouragement	laid	personnel	quantity	tragedy
belief	environment	led	perspiration	quizzes	unanimous
believe	equipped	lightning	physical	recede	undoubtedly
boundaries	especially	loneliness	possession	receive	unnecessary
business	exaggerate	lose	possibility	recommend	villain
candidate	excellence	maintenance	practically	rhyme	weird
category	experience	mathematics	precede	rhythm	writing

Goodheart-Willcox Publisher

Figure BL1.8   This reference guide can be used to double-check spellings in your written communication.

Putting It All Together

Now that you understand how to use all the elements of grammar effectively, keep in mind these additional tips to ensure your written communications are as clear as possible.

1. **Use precise language.** Resist the urge to use vague words like *stuff* and *thing* in your writing. Do not use jargon or specialized language that your reader may not know.

2. **Keep your sentences short.** A very important rule to remember is that the longer the sentence, the more likely the reader will lose interest. Instead, use short, to-the-point sentences.

3. **Reread what you have written**. Spell-check is not perfect. It is helpful to read what you have written out loud to do your own spell-check. You may hear certain words repeated, or discover something that seemed fine when written but sounds unclear when read out loud.

4. **Seek feedback**. Your writing may not be as clear as you think. Ask someone to review your writing for clarity and grammatical errors (Figure BL1.9).

The ability to write clearly is becoming increasingly important. Excellent written communication skills will give you a significant advantage both when applying for a position and in your chosen profession.

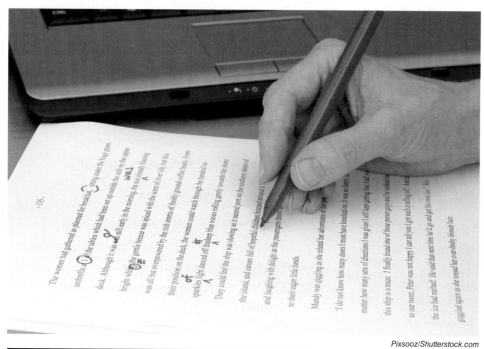

Pixsooz/Shutterstock.com

Figure BL1.9   A good proofreader will identify spelling mistakes, grammatical errors, and passages that need clarification.

Real Life Scenario

Testing Communication Skills in Interviews

Since obtaining his associate's degree six months ago, Jason has not been able to find a job related to his field of study. Jason is delighted when a friend tells him about a perfect position open in a well-paying company that offers benefits. After reading the job posting and description, Jason feels he is a great fit for this job.

Jason is surprised when he is scheduled for a lengthy interview. The process includes a writing exercise as well as a verbal interview. He feels confident after the verbal interview, and he sails through the writing portion. Jason is told he will hear about the job in two weeks.

Three weeks go by, and Jason has not heard anything. Jason decides to call the human resources representative at the company to ask if he got the job. Jason is told that his spelling and grammar are not up to the standard required for the position.

Apply It

1. How could Jason improve his writing skills?

2. Why do you think correct spelling and grammar usage are important to a healthcare worker?

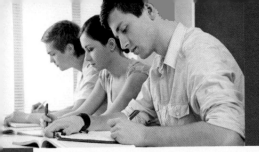

Summary

When you speak or write poorly, you may be judged as unprofessional or uneducated. Correct spelling, sentence structure, grammar, and punctuation are essential to your success as an employee. When working within the healthcare world, you must learn and use proper English.

Review Questions

Answer the following questions using what you have learned in this background lesson.

True or False Assess

1. *True or False?* The passive voice refers to noun usage.

2. *True or False?* Numbers one through nine should be spelled out in words.

3. *True or False?* The plural of *quiz* is *quizzes*.

4. *True or False?* An adjective is a word that describes a noun or pronoun.

5. *True or False? Among the two of us* is a correct usage of the word *among*.

6. *True or False? You spell good* is not correct grammar.

7. *True or False?* Words in the English language are divided into nine parts of speech.

8. *True or False?* Grammar is the study of how words and their components combine to form sentences.

9. *True or False? I always loose my house keys* is not a correct usage of the word *loose*.

10. *True or False?* A semicolon is used just like a colon.

Multiple Choice Assess

11. Which of the following statements about semicolons is *true*?
    A. They are the same as colons.
    B. They are used to separate clauses or some items in a series.
    C. Semicolons come before dashes.
    D. They are seldom used in formal writing.

12. Which of the following words is correctly capitalized?
    A. Summer
    B. wednesday
    C. october
    D. English language

13. All the following items are complete sentences *except* _____.
    A. Jimmy studies.
    B. Although Marie studied for the exam and hired a tutor.
    C. Jeffrey did not want to study but instead wanted to go surfing.
    D. Do not speak harshly to the patient.

14. What punctuation marks the end of a sentence?
    A. a period, comma, or dash
    B. a semicolon, colon, or question mark
    C. a period, question mark, or exclamation point
    D. a dash, period, or hyphen

15. Which of the following words is spelled correctly?
    A. beleive
    B. cemetary
    C. accomodate
    D. mathematics

16. Which of the following words can be used as an adjective?
    A. English
    B. tomorrow
    C. finally
    D. None of the above.

17. Which of the following words is *not* a conjunction?
    A. but
    B. until
    C. in
    D. since

18. Which of the following words is spelled incorrectly?
    A. prespiration
    B. accommodate
    C. arithmetic
    D. immediately
19. Which of the following words does *not* need to be capitalized?
    A. Tuesday
    B. Japanese
    C. Fall
    D. Jessie
20. Which of the following words is a pronoun?
    A. they
    B. them
    C. I
    D. All of the above.
21. Which of the following is *not* a part of speech?
    A. verb
    B. possessive
    C. adjective
    D. preposition
22. Which of the following words is *not* a proper noun?
    A. San Francisco
    B. Arnold
    C. January
    D. cat
23. Which of the following sentences is written in passive voice?
    A. I acted on my first instinct.
    B. Harry attended the party alone.
    C. She was given a grade of 100%.
    D. Joanne writes her notes in purple ink.

Grammar Review

Correct the grammar, punctuation, or spelling in the following sentences if necessary.

24. Its time for a coffee break.
25. Laura's supervisor asked her to separate the clean towels and washcloths from the dirty ones.
26. Your going to give an injection to the patient in Room 206B.
27. Do not loose your application.
28. They're coats are over their.
29. The pharmacist told me not to loose my reciept.
30. the luncheon is at noon first floor conference room.
31. I want to work in one of three cities, Atlanta, New York City, or Austin.
32. Dr. Evans said that I had three major problems in my essay spelling, punctuation, and passive verbs.
33. My sister in law is an occupational therapist.
34. Marie did well on her nursing exam.
35. These plays were written by shakespeare.
36. The class resumes in september.

Critical Thinking Exercises

37. If you are a poor speller, what can you do to ensure that your professional writing is free of spelling errors?
38. Over the next several weeks, take notes as you listen to the ways that people speak. List at least five grammar mistakes you hear from your friends and the media on a regular basis. Do you make any of these mistakes? What steps can you take to improve your grammar?

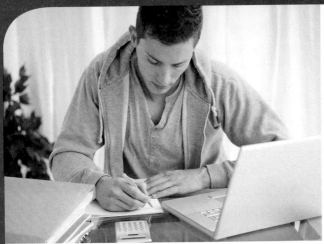

wavebreakmedia/Shutterstock.com

Math Review

Terms to Know

Build Vocab

addition
base ten system
common denominator
decimal numbers
division

fractions
mixed numbers
multiplication
nominal numbers
ordinal numbers

prime number
subtraction
whole numbers

Lesson Objectives

- Explain the different forms of numbers, including whole, mixed, decimals, and fractions.
- Perform basic mathematical computations such as addition, subtraction, multiplication, and division.
- Understand the use of fractions in the healthcare environment.
- Perform computations using fractions.
- Demonstrate how to use a calculator to perform functions of addition, subtraction, multiplication, and division.

No matter which healthcare field you choose, you will be required to perform some math calculations when doing your job. Of course, there are healthcare professions that will require more math skills than others, such as pharmacists, doctors, or registered nurses. At the minimum, you will be required to know how to add, subtract, multiply, and divide and to use the metric system. You will also be expected to understand and use decimals, fractions, and ratios. It is important that you are comfortable performing these basic math calculations.

This background lesson includes a review of these basic math skills. It will prepare you for some tasks that healthcare workers often encounter on a daily basis. There is a pretest online that covers this material. You may want to take the pretest before or after reviewing the lesson.

 Pretest

Numbers and the Base Ten System

The number system used for counting based on groups of ten is called the **base ten system**. Numbers that have more than one digit are defined by their place value. For example, the number 9,234,567 is read as nine million, two hundred thirty-four thousand, five hundred sixty-seven. If you understand the base ten system, you know that you can break that number down to 9 millions, 2 hundred thousands, 3 ten thousands, 4 thousands, 5 hundreds, 6 tens, and 7 ones. You could illustrate the number 9,234,567 as:

base ten system
numbering system used for counting that is based on multiples of ten

9,000,000 + 200,000 + 30,000 + 4,000 + 500 + 60 + 7

- the ones digit shows the number of ones (1)
- the tens digit shows the number of tens (10)
- the hundreds digit shows the number of hundreds (100)
- the thousands digit shows the number of thousands (1,000)
- the ten thousands digit shows the number of tens of thousands (10,000)
- the hundred thousands digit shows the number of hundreds of thousands (100,000)
- the millions digit shows the number of millions (1,000,000)

Check Your Understanding ✓

Read the following numbers out loud and identify the place value of each number. For example, how many ones, tens, hundreds, and thousands are in each number?

1. 540
2. 4,321
3. 98
4. 200,000
5. 4,444,444
6. 106
7. 2,435
8. 111,222
9. 12,432,000
10. 4

Types of Numbers

There are different types of numbers and each type is used for its own special purpose. The following descriptions of numbers will help you understand the differences between types.

Whole Numbers

whole numbers
numbers used for counting; do not contain decimal points or fractions; also known as integers

Whole numbers (also called *integers*) are the numbers you use to count, including zero. Whole numbers do not have decimal points and are not fractions or negative numbers. Examples of whole numbers include 1, 5, 10, 13, 20, and 0. Another name for whole numbers is *cardinal numbers*. A cardinal number (1, 2, 3, for example) is different from an ordinal number.

Ordinal Numbers

ordinal numbers
numbers that place objects in a series in order

When objects are placed in order, **ordinal numbers** are used to tell their position. If ten students were ranked according to their grades on the health occupations final, you would say that the student who got the top grade was in first place, the next student was in second place, and so on.

The first ten ordinal numbers are first, second, third, fourth, fifth, sixth, seventh, eighth, ninth, and tenth. They can also be written as 1st, 2nd, 3rd, 4th, 5th, 6th, 7th, 8th, 9th, and 10th.

Decimal Numbers

decimal numbers
numbers expressed with a decimal point; values left of the decimal are whole numbers and values to the right are fractions

Decimal numbers are expressed with a decimal point separating whole numbers and decimal fractions. Whole numbers appear to the left of the decimal point. Decimal fractions, or numbers with a value that is less than 1, appear to the right of the decimal point.

Examples: 10.5, 5.54, 3.1416, 152.71

Fractions

fractions
numbers that indicate part of a whole

Fractions are numbers defined as one or more parts of a whole number. Using fractions is an easy way to show portions less than one. Fractions are used to express parts of a whole, like the numbers that appear to the right of the decimal point in decimal numbers. Fractions are used in cooking, building, sewing, the stock market, and many other places.

Examples: 1/2, 3/4, 5/8

Mixed Numbers

mixed numbers
whole numbers followed by a remaining fraction

Mixed numbers are whole numbers with a fraction included.

Examples: 32-3/4, 1-1/2, 416-1/2

Negative Numbers

Negative numbers are less than zero. Negative numbers are also called *negative integers*.

Examples: −5, −100, −235

Percentages

The term *percent* means "per hundred." When you use a percentage, you divide a number into 100 parts. For example, a dollar can be divided into 100 pennies. One penny is 1/100th of a dollar. Sometimes, it is easier to express a percentage using the percent sign (%). For example, seven pennies can be expressed as 7% of a dollar.

Prime Numbers

A **prime number** is only divisible by itself and 1. If you try to divide a prime number by any other number, you will have a number and a fraction left over. A prime number must be a whole number greater than 1 (Figure BL2.1).

prime number
a number that is only divisible by itself and 1

Nominal Numbers

Nominal numbers name something—a telephone number, a house number, or a zip code. Nominal numbers do not show quantity or rank. They are used only to identify something.

nominal numbers
numbers that name or identify something

Examples: 417 Fern Avenue

The zip code for my hometown is 01796.

My office phone number is 708-555-5732.

Adding Whole Numbers

Addition is the process of combining two or more numbers. The numbers being added together are called *addends*. The addends of a written addition problem are separated by an addition sign (+). The answer to an addition problem is called the *sum*, and it comes after an equal sign (=).

addition
the process of combining two or more numbers to obtain their total value

Examples: 5 + 4 = 9

4 + 6 = 10

When you are adding numbers that contain two or more digits, it is best to write the numbers in a column, aligning the place value of the digits such as the ones, tens, or hundreds. Make sure the numbers in each column line up beneath one another. This alignment helps you add the correct numbers together. Always add the numbers in the right column first, before moving to the columns to the left.

2	3	5	7	11	13	17	19	23	29	31	37	41	43	47	53	59	61	67
71	73	79	83	89	97	101	103	107	109	113	127	131	137	139	149	151	157	163
167	173	179	181	191	193	197	199	211	223	227	229	233	239	241	251	257	263	269
271	277	281	283	293	307	311	313	317	331	337	347	349	353	359	367	373	379	383
389	397	401	409	419	421	431	433	439	443	449	457	461	463	467	479	487	491	499

Goodheart-Willcox Publisher

Figure BL2.1   Prime numbers

Example:

```
   21
+ 37
   58
```

This problem can be rewritten as:

```
  2 tens   and  1 ones
+ 3 tens   and  7 ones
  5 tens   and  8 ones  = 58
```

Sometimes, addition problems require you to carry over digits to the left.

Example:

```
   36
+ 45
```

First add the ones column (6 + 5 = 11) and carry the 1 (representing 10 ones) to the tens column. Then, add the tens column.

```
   1
   36
+ 45
   81
```

Example:

```
   788
+  57
```

Add the ones column and carry over the *1* to the tens column. Then, add the tens column, and carry the *1* to the hundreds column.

```
   11
   788
+   57
   845
```

Real Life Scenario   Supply Inventory

Carlos works in a doctor's office. One day, he is asked to take inventory of disposable surgery trays in the office. He finds 10 trays in exam room A's closet, 8 in exam room B's closet, and 24 in the supply cupboard.

Carlos is then asked to take inventory of boxes of alcohol swabs in the office. He counts 20 boxes in exam room A's closet, 18 in exam room B's closet, 12 in the reception room drawers, and 9 in the supply cupboard.

Finally, Carlos must total the number of patients that were seen by the doctor over the course of the

week (5 days). There were 20 patients seen on day 1, 35 on day 2, 40 on day 3, 34 on day 4, and 21 on day 5.

Apply It

1. How many trays are in the doctor's office?

2. How many boxes of alcohol swabs are in the office?

3. How many patients did the doctor see over the course of five days?

Subtracting Whole Numbers

Subtraction is the opposite of addition. When numbers are subtracted, one number is taken away from another. Simple subtraction is written as $6 - 2 = 4$, with the minus sign (–) indicating subtraction. The answer obtained in a subtraction problem is called the *difference*. Subtraction problems can be written in two ways:

subtraction
the process of removing one number from another number; the opposite of addition

$$\begin{array}{r} 54 \\ -\ 23 \\ \hline 31 \end{array} \quad \text{or } 54 - 23 = 31$$

You can check your answer by adding the difference to the number being subtracted. If your answer is correct, your total will equal the first number in the equation. To check this, $54 - 23 = 31$, you would add $31 + 23 = 54$.

Real Life Scenario   Subtraction in Everyday Life

As an emergency medical technician, Paul must keep track of various aspects of his job. For example, he has earned 14 vacation days this year and has already taken 8. If he wants to take some time off, he needs to know how many days he has left. As part of his job, Paul is required to complete 50 hours of continuing education every year. So far this year, he has completed 13 hours. Paul also puts in a lot of mileage while driving the ambulance. Last month, Paul recorded 675 miles traveled in his ambulance. This month, he has traveled 1,220 miles.

Apply It

1. How many vacation days does Paul have left?
2. How many hours of continuing education does Paul still need to complete to fulfill his requirement for the year?
3. How many more miles has Paul traveled this month than last month?

Subtracting by Borrowing Numbers

Some subtraction problems require that you "borrow" a number. When beginning a subtraction problem, align the numbers one on top of the other, as you do during an addition problem. Look at the rightmost column. If the number on top is smaller than the number on the bottom, you will have to "borrow" from the column on the left.

Consider the following subtraction problem:

$$\begin{array}{r} 34 \\ -\ 16 \\ \hline \end{array}$$

To subtract a larger number (6) from a smaller number (4), you must borrow 10 from the column to the left to complete the problem.

Example:

$$\begin{array}{r} 2\ ^{1}\!\!\!\!4 \\ \cancel{3}4 \\ -\ 16 \\ \hline 18 \end{array}$$

By borrowing the one 10 from the three 10s in the left column, 4 becomes 14. The 3 in the left column becomes a 2. When you subtract 6 from 14, you get 8, and 2 minus 1 equals 1, leaving you with an answer of 18.

Check Your Understanding ✓

1. $2,222 + 99 =$		5. $64 + 7 =$		9. $48 - 19 =$
2. $123,456 + 777 =$		6. $9,888 - 999 =$		10. $576 - 68 =$
3. $9,689 + 245 =$		7. $90,145 - 326 =$		
4. $68,834 + 8,834 =$		8. $11,103 - 871 =$		

Multiplication

multiplication

a mathematical operation that indicates how many times a number is added to itself; a shortcut for addition

Multiplication is a shortcut for addition. The standard symbol for multiplication is (×). Other ways of expressing multiplication include an asterisk (10 * 10 = 100) or parentheses (10)(10) = 100. The numbers to be multiplied are called the *multiplicand* (the first number) and the *multiplier* (the second number). The answer to a multiplication problem is called the *product*.

$$
\begin{array}{r}
87 \\
\times\ 15 \\
\hline
1305
\end{array}
$$

    87 ⟵ multiplicand
× 15 ⟵ multiplier
1305 ⟵ product

Throughout your healthcare career, you will encounter many situations that require the use of multiplication. The following is an example of one such situation.

	1	2	3	4	5	6	7	8	9	10	11	12
1	1	2	3	4	5	6	7	8	9	10	11	12
2	2	4	6	8	10	12	14	16	18	20	22	24
3	3	6	9	12	15	18	21	24	27	30	33	36
4	4	8	12	16	20	24	28	32	36	40	44	48
5	5	10	15	20	25	30	35	40	45	50	55	60
6	6	12	18	24	30	36	42	48	54	60	66	72
7	7	14	21	28	35	42	49	56	63	70	77	84
8	8	16	24	32	40	48	56	64	72	80	88	96
9	9	18	27	36	45	54	63	72	81	90	99	108
10	10	20	30	40	50	60	70	80	90	100	110	120
11	11	22	33	44	55	66	77	88	99	110	121	132
12	12	24	36	48	60	72	84	96	108	120	132	144

Goodheart-Willcox Publisher

Figure BL2.2   To use a multiplication table, choose one number from the top row and one number from the row on the left-hand side. Identify the cell where these two rows meet—this is the product of your multiplication problem.

Joy is working out the budget for the healthcare facility where she is employed. As part of her budgeting, Joy needs to know how much 12 boxes of latex gloves cost. Joy researches the price for one package and finds it costs $10.35. Joy could determine the cost of 12 boxes of gloves by adding $10.35 together twelve times, but that is time-consuming. Instead, Joy can find the answer using multiplication. The equation Joy must solve is: $\$10.35 \times 12 = ?$

To solve such a problem, you might want to memorize some basic multiplication problems. Using a multiplication table is the best way to practice this skill (Figure BL2.2). Knowing your multiplication tables allows you to calculate numbers quickly and without error.

To answer this problem using a multiplication table, you would multiply each digit separately to create partial answers. Then add the partial answers to find the final answer. Note that alignment of the numbers is very important!

```
    $10.35
  ×     12
```

First, multiply the ones digit of the multiplier (2) with each digit in the multiplicand. Because $2 \times 5 = 10$, you should place a 0 beneath the 5 and 2, and carry the 1 to the tens column, so it appears above the 3. Now, when you multiply 2×3, add 1 to the answer ($2 \times 3 = 6$; $6 + 1 = 7$). Place a 7 beneath the 3 and 1, and move on to the next digits. The first partial answer is 2,070.

```
         1
    $10.35
  ×     12
    ──────
      2070
```

Next, multiply the tens digits. Since you have already multiplied the ones column, place a *0* or *X* beneath the 0 in the ones column. Multiply 1 with each digit of the multiplicand ($1 \times 5 = 5$, $1 \times 3 = 3$, $1 \times 0 = 0$, and $1 \times 1 = 1$). The second partial answer is 10,350.

```
    $10.35
  ×     12
    ──────
      2070
     1035X
```

Now, add the two partial answers together to find the product. Because there is a decimal point in the number $10.35, the product also needs a decimal point. To determine the location of the decimal point, count the number of digits to the right of the decimal point in the multiplicand (two). Now, place the decimal point in the product so that there are two places to the right.

```
    $10.35
  ×     12
    ──────
      2070
  + 10350
    ──────
   $124.20
```

Real Life Scenario   Multiplying on the Job

For Elise, a respiratory therapist, multiplication is an important skill when working with her patients. But she can also use multiplication to determine information about her job, such as work hours and how many patients she has seen. Elise's supervisor has asked her to work 8-hour shifts for the next 3 weeks (Elise works 5 days a week). During each 8-hour shift, Elise sees 13 patients.

Apply It

1. How many total hours will Elise work during the next 3 weeks?

2. How many patients will she see in the next 3 weeks? Remember that Elise works 5 days a week.

Division

division

the process of determining how many times one number is present in another number

Division is a process that enables you to find how many times one number is present in another number. Division is the opposite of multiplication. Therefore, memorizing the multiplication table will help you solve division problems.

The most common symbol for division is ($\div$). The number that gets divided is called the *dividend*. The number that does the dividing is called the *divisor*. The answer to a division problem is called the *quotient*.

$$\begin{array}{r} 5 \leftarrow \text{quotient} \\ \text{divisor}\quad 3\,\overline{)\,15} \leftarrow \text{dividend} \end{array}$$

Division problems can be written several ways:

$$\frac{6}{3} \text{ or } 3\,\overline{)\,6}$$

Many situations will arise during your career requiring the use of division. The following is an example of how you might use division in a healthcare setting.

> Hazel is the front office medical assistant in charge of buying new chairs for the medical office's reception room. She is given a budget of $745 to purchase five new chairs. What is the most that Hazel can pay for each chair while staying in budget? The equation Hazel must solve is 745 ÷ 5 = ?

To begin, divide 5 into the first digit of the dividend (7). Because 5 goes into 7 only one time, write a 1 above the 7. Next, multiply the 5 and 1, and write the product (5) below the 7. Then, subtract the 5 from the 7, which gives you the remainder of 2.

$$\begin{array}{r} 1 \\ 5\,\overline{)\,745} \\ \underline{5} \\ 2 \end{array}$$

Real Life Scenario — Calculating Volunteer Hours and Student Loans

Even before you enter the healthcare field, math skills can help you understand important information you need for school. As you improve your math skills, try applying them in situations such as the ones described here.

Madison is a high school senior who wants to be an LPN (licensed practical nurse). Madison's school counselor recommends volunteering at a hospital to observe the daily responsibilities of an LPN. The volunteer program at the local hospital requires a commitment of 100 volunteer hours to complete the program.

Steven decides he wants to become an EMT. He will need a student loan to pay for the required classes. The cost of an EMT program is $1,195 with additional fees for textbook rentals of $240. After training, he will have to pay back the loan at $100 a month.

Apply It

1. If Madison volunteers for 5 hours a week, how many weeks will it take her to complete her volunteer commitment?

2. Assuming there is no interest on the loan, how many months will it take Steven to pay back his student loan?

Now, bring the 4 from the 745 down next to the 2. Divide 5 into 24. Because 5 goes into 24 four times, write a 4 next to the 1 in the quotient. Multiply the 4 and the 5 and put the result (20) below the 24. Subtract the 20 from the 24 and write the difference (4) beneath the 20.

```
      14
 5 ) 745
      5
     ───
     24
     20
     ───
      4
```

Next, bring the third digit (5) down so that it is next to the 4. Divide 5 into 45. Write the answer (9) next to the 4 in the quotient. Because $9 \times 5 = 45$, the difference is 0 and there is no remainder. Hazel has $149 to spend on each chair for the reception room.

```
      149
 5 ) 745
      5
     ───
     24
     20
     ───
     45
     45
     ───
      0
```

Remainders

Some numbers do not divide perfectly into others. In such division problems, there is a *remainder*, or number left over after dividing all of the numbers in the dividend by the divisor. A remainder can be expressed by using a lowercase *r*, or as a fraction. For example, a problem with a quotient of 7 and a remainder of 2 would be written as: 7 r.2 or 7-2/7.

Example:

```
      5
 5 ) 26
     25
     ───
      1
```

Because 2 is less than 5, you should instead determine how many times 5 goes into 26. Because $5 \times 5 = 25$, and $26 - 25 = 1$, this quotient is 5 with a remainder of 1. This quotient can be expressed in the following ways:

- 5 r.1
- 5-1/5
- 5.2

Check Your Understanding ✓

1. $100 \times 10 =$	5. $15.20 \times 9 =$	9. $10,439 \times 426 =$
2. $325 \times 35 =$	6. $457 \div 3 =$	10. $40,200 \div 9 =$
3. $220 \div 20 =$	7. $547.89 \times 40 =$	
4. $1,425 \div 5 =$	8. $546.20 \div 4 =$	

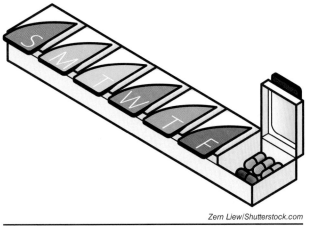

Zern Liew/Shutterstock.com

Figure BL2.3   A seven-day pill box can represent a fraction. In this image, 1/7 of the pill box is open and 6/7 are closed.

Fractions

Fractions, decimals, and percentages are mathematical concepts that express numbers that are part of a whole (Figure BL2.3). These three concepts will be especially important for anyone entering the healthcare field to understand. Fractions are one or more parts of a whole number. Fractions are written in the following way:

1/2 or $\dfrac{1}{2}$ 13/15 or $\dfrac{13}{15}$ 5/7 or $\dfrac{5}{7}$

The number written above or before the line is called the *numerator*. The number written below or after the line in a fraction is called the *denominator*. The denominator is the number of parts into which the fraction is divided. When reading fractions, you always read the top number first, followed by the bottom number.

$$\frac{\text{Numerator}}{\text{Denominator}}$$

Fractions with the Same Denominator

common denominator
the number that can be divided evenly by all of the denominators in a group of fractions

When adding or subtracting fractions that have a **common denominator**, you only add or subtract the numerator.

Example: $\dfrac{9}{8} + \dfrac{6}{8} + \dfrac{4}{8} = \dfrac{9+6+4}{8} = \dfrac{19}{8}$

If adding the fraction leaves you with a numerator that is divisible by the denominator, the fraction must be reduced. This can be done by dividing the numerator by the denominator.

The answer $\dfrac{19}{8}$ must be reduced by dividing $19 \div 8 = 2\dfrac{3}{8}$

Because 8 goes into 19 twice, the answer includes a 2 next to the remaining fraction, which is 3/8. This creates the mixed number of 2-3/8.

Subtraction of fractions with common denominators is similar to addition.

Example: $\dfrac{10}{9} - \dfrac{5}{9} - \dfrac{4}{9} = \dfrac{10-5-4}{9} = \dfrac{1}{9}$

Fractions with Different Denominators

To add or subtract two or more fractions that have different denominators, you must find a lowest common denominator.

Example: $\dfrac{1}{2} + \dfrac{2}{5} + \dfrac{4}{10} = ?$

To find the lowest common denominator for 2, 5, and 10, consider the multiples of each number.

Multiples of 2: 2, 4, 6, 8, **10**…

Multiples of 5: 5, **10**, 15, 20…

Multiples of 10: **10**, 20…

The lowest common denominator is 10.

For the first two fractions that do not already have a denominator of 10 (1/2 and 2/5), you need to multiply both the numerator and denominator by the number that will produce a denominator of 10. So the fraction 1/2 will have its numerator and denominator multiplied by 5 to equal 5/10. The fraction 2/5 will have its numerator and denominator multiplied by 2 to become 4/10. The fraction 4/10 already has a common denominator of 10. So the problem becomes:

$$\frac{5}{10} + \frac{4}{10} + \frac{4}{10} = \frac{13}{10} = 1\frac{3}{10}$$

Subtracting fractions is done through the same process used to add fractions. First, find a common denominator, then subtract the numerators, and write the answer using the common denominator.

Multiplying Fractions

When multiplying fractions, you don't need to find a common denominator. Instead, simply multiply across the fraction (numerator × numerator, and denominator × denominator).

Example: $\frac{3}{4} \times \frac{2}{3} = \frac{6}{12}$

(3 × 2 = 6 and 4 × 3 = 12) = 6/12

The fraction 6/12 needs to be reduced (or *simplified*). You are trying to get the smallest possible number for both the numerator and denominator. To reduce this fraction, you would divide 6 into the top number and 6 into the bottom number (6 goes into 6 once, 6 goes into 12 twice).

The fraction 6/12 becomes 1/2.

Real Life Scenario   Using Fractions in Healthcare

Fractions express parts of a whole. In healthcare, this can mean a portion of a prescription, the remainder of syringes left in a supply closet, or the number of patients being treated.

Dennis has been told that his blood pressure is bordering on high. Dennis' doctor has given him a prescription to reduce his blood pressure. The prescription calls for Dennis to take half of a pill daily for 45 days, and then have his blood pressure checked to see if there is improvement.

Leeann is a nurse's aide on the surgical floor of a busy hospital. On this floor, 1/4 of the patients will have surgery on Monday and will go home on Wednesday. Another 1/4 of the remaining patients will go home on Thursday.

Apply It

1. How many pills will Dennis need so he can take half a pill every day for 45 days?

2. If no new patients arrive on the surgical floor where Leeann works, what fraction of the patients will be left on Friday?

Dividing Fractions

The process of dividing fractions is very unique and requires the use of the reciprocal fraction. To identify a fraction's reciprocal, turn the second fraction in the problem upside down to switch the numerator and denominator. For example, the fraction 5/8 would become 8/5. Then, multiply the first fraction and the inverted second fraction. There is no need for a common denominator.

$$\text{Example: } \frac{3}{4} \div \frac{5}{8} = \frac{3}{4} \times \frac{8}{5} = \frac{24}{20} = \frac{6}{5} = 1\frac{1}{5}$$

Note that the answer was reduced from 24/20 to 6/5 by dividing the numerator and denominator each by 4. The fraction 6/5 was then converted to a mixed number. When dividing mixed numbers, you will need to convert them to fractions first.

Converting Mixed Numbers to Fractions. A mixed number (5-1/2) is composed of a whole number (5) and a fraction (1/2). If you want to convert 5-1/2 into a fraction, you must first multiply the whole number (5) by the denominator of the fraction (2). Now you have determined how many one-halves there are in 5 (10). Next, add the numerator (1) to give you 11/2. 11/2 is another way of expressing 5-1/2.

Check Your Understanding ✔

Convert the following mixed numbers to fractions.
   1. 6-1/2   2. 7-1/4   3. 1-1/8

Reduce the following fractions to their simplest form.
   4. 6/18   5. 10/80   6. 14/17

Complete the following calculations.
   7. 1/8 + 4/8 + 3/8 =   11. 7/16 − 1/8 =   15. 5/8 × 3/4 =
   8. 1/2 + 1/4 + 3/8 =   12. 1/2 − 1/4 =   16. 4/8 ÷ 1/8 =
   9. 1/2 + 3/5 + 2/10 =   13. 1/4 × 2/3 =   17. 3/4 ÷ 1/8 =
  10. 7/8 − 5/8 =   14. 1/8 × 5/8 =   18. 9/10 ÷ 1/4 =

Using a Calculator

Healthcare workers are required to perform math calculations when doing various tasks, such as determining medication dosages, working in a healthcare facility's accounting department, or determining the salt content of a low-sodium diet. Even though calculators are on hand in most cases, you should understand the fundamentals of mathematics. You never know when you may have to solve a problem by knowing how to manipulate the numbers rather than using a calculator.

You are likely familiar with the calculator's functions, but a brief review of how to add, subtract, multiply, and divide using a calculator follows. Many calculators perform much more complex functions, such as graphing, calculus, and trigonometric operations.

When used correctly, a calculator saves valuable time and ensures accuracy, especially in the case of complex problems (Figure BL2.4). Double-check your answers by performing the calculation at least twice—wrong entries will result in wrong answers.

Entries are made by pressing certain numbers and symbols on the keyboard of the calculator (Figure BL2.5). The information entered appears in the display area above the keyboard. It is always helpful to check the display area after entering a number to make sure you've entered it correctly.

- **Addition.** Enter the first addend of your problem and then press the (+) key. Enter the second addend. Press the (=) key and the sum will appear on the display.

- **Subtraction.** Enter a number and press the (−) key. Next, enter the number to be subtracted from the first number. Then press the (=) key to find the difference.

- **Multiplication.** Enter the multiplicand and press the (×) key. Next, enter the multiplier and press the (=) key. The product will appear on the display.

- **Division.** Enter the dividend, press the (÷) key, and enter the divisor. After pressing the (=) key, the quotient will appear on the display.

- **Calculating a percentage.** Say you need to identify 20% of 50. Enter 50, press the (×) key, enter 20, and then press the (%) key. The answer (10) will appear on the display. If your calculator does not have a (%) key, you can calculate this percentage by multiplying 50 by 0.2.

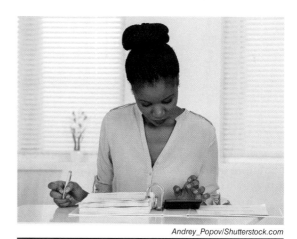

Andrey_Popov/Shutterstock.com

Figure BL2.4   Using a calculator will make it easier to complete math problems while on the job.

Common Symbols on a Calculator	
Key	**Function**
C	clears all entries
CE	clears last entry
.	enters a decimal point
+	adds
−	subtracts
×	multiplies
÷	divides
%	calculates percentage
=	calculates the final answer

Goodheart-Willcox Publisher

Figure BL2.5   Common symbols on a calculator

Real Life Scenario   Calculator Uses in Healthcare

Although math skills are essential for healthcare workers to learn, there will be situations in which you'll be able to use a calculator. In those situations, you should take care to use the calculator correctly. This will ensure that you get an accurate answer to your question. Use a calculator to solve problems in the situations described here.

Karen works in the accounting department of Eastridge Hospital. Her boss has asked her to calculate how many employees make over $50,000 each year. Karen finds that the hospital employs 450 people. Of those employees, 75 make over $50,000.

Gail is studying to become a cardiac care nurse. She learns that the heart pumps about 65 milliliters of blood every time it beats. Gail measures her own pulse and finds that her heart beats 75 times per minute.

Apply It

1. What is the percentage of employees at Eastridge Hospital who make over $50,000?

2. How many milliliters of blood does Gail's heart pump per minute? per hour?

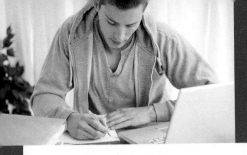
Summary

Basic math skills such as recognizing types of numbers; understanding fractions; and practicing addition, subtraction, multiplication, and division are important for anyone planning to enter the healthcare field.

Many healthcare workers use calculators to help solve math problems. During your health science education, some instructors will allow you to use calculators, but others may not. Calculators can stop working during exams or at work. You may be required to take professional exams for getting licenses or certification, which will probably not allow using calculators. It is best to know how to solve basic math problems without the calculator.

Review Questions

Answer the following questions using what you have learned in this background lesson.

True or False Assess

1. *True or False?* Whole numbers have decimal points.
2. *True or False?* Fractions are numbers defined as one or more parts of the whole.
3. *True or False?* A prime number is only divisible by itself and 1.
4. *True or False?* Multiplication is *not* a shortcut for addition.
5. *True or False?* The fraction 8/12 needs to be reduced.
6. *True or False?* If you have a calculator, there is no need to improve your math skills.
7. *True or False?* Addition is the opposite of multiplication.
8. *True or False?* 5th is an ordinal number.
9. *True or False?* Your telephone number is known as a *nominal number*.
10. *True or False?* 100 – 21 = 79

Multiple Choice Assess

11. The top number of a fraction is called the _____.
    A. denominator
    B. numerator
    C. reciprocal
    D. remainder

12. Which of the following statements about division is *true*?
    A. Division problems can be written several ways.
    B. The most common symbol for division is (÷).
    C. The number that gets divided is called the *dividend*.
    D. All of the above.

13. Which of the following statements about multiplication is *false*?
    A. Multiplication is a shortcut for subtraction.
    B. The standard symbol for multiplication is (×).
    C. Other symbols for multiplication are parentheses (1)(8) or an asterisk (*).
    D. The numbers to be multiplied are called the *multiplicands*.

14. Which of the options shown here is the correct answer to the following multiplication problem?

    [1-3/4 × 2-2/3 =]

    A. 4-2/3
    B. 3-2/3
    C. 4-1/3
    D. None of the above.

15. Which of the options shown here is the correct answer to the following division problem?

    [812 ÷ 4 =]

    A. 200
    B. 198
    C. 103
    D. 203

16. Which of the options shown here is the correct answer to the following fraction division problem?

    [3/4 ÷ 3/8 =]

    A. 1-1/2

    B. 2-3/4

    C. 2-1/2

    D. 2

17. Which of the following statements about fractions is *not* true?

    A. Fractions express numbers that are part of a whole.

    B. The number above the line in a fraction is called the numerator.

    C. When adding or subtracting fractions with common denominators, you only add the numerators.

    D. In healthcare, you will be working only with fractions.

18. Reduce the following fraction to its simplest form:

    [14/17]

    A. 14/17

    B. 7/17

    C. 2/7

    D. None of the above.

19. Which of the options shown here is the correct answer to the following fraction multiplication problem?

    [2-1/2 × 1-1/4 =]

    A. 3-1/2

    B. 4-1/2

    C. 3-1/8

    D. 4

20. Which of the following is *not* a mixed number?

    A. 416-1/2

    B. 4,567-1/2

    C. 43.200

    D. 62-1/4

Short Answer

21. Explain the concept of a common denominator.

22. What is the base ten system in math?

23. What are the differences between ordinal and nominal numbers?

24. Explain the concept of "borrowing numbers" in subtraction.

25. What are *remainders* in division?

Critical Thinking Exercises

26. Some students argue that learning basic math skills such as the multiplication tables is not important because the calculator can do all math calculations for them. Why is it important to learn basic math skills? How will basic math skills be used during your healthcare career?

27. Why do you think so many people are frightened by math? Are you one of those people? If so, what could you do to increase confidence in your math skills?

28. How often do you use a computer or a calculator to work with numbers? Can you do calculations in your head without pencil, paper, or electronics?

29. Interview someone you know who works in heathcare. Ask how often he or she uses math on the job.

30. Which math courses are you taking now in preparation for a healthcare career? Do you work with a counselor to make sure the math you are planning to take will be sufficient for job options you are exploring?

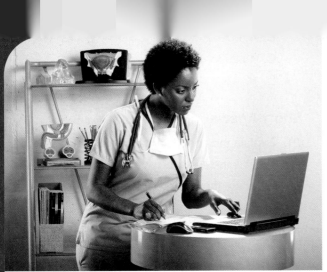

REDAV/Shutterstock.com

Computer Technology Review

Terms to Know

 Build Vocab

cloud technology
computer hardware
computer virus
download
firewall
hackers

Internet
malware
podcasts
software
upload
virtual learning environment (VLE)

Wi-Fi
word processing
World Wide Web

Lesson Objectives

- Discuss hardware components of a computer.
- Explain the most common types of software for computers.
- Explain simple ways to troubleshoot problems with your computer.
- Understand how the Internet functions and its uses related to medical issues.
- Identify what is meant by *cloud technology* and *Wi-Fi*.
- Explain the functions and uses of a Virtual Learning Environment.
- Discuss threats that can derail computer systems.
- Discuss how to keep your computer as safe as possible from disruptions.

As technology continues to evolve, healthcare workers must adjust rapidly to expanding responsibilities related to the use of technology (Figure BL3.1). It is important for healthcare workers to embrace technology rather than be frightened by it. As you learned in chapter 10, healthcare technology will offer endless opportunities to learn new skills and be a part of exciting new paths to improve healthcare for everyone. In any discussion of computers, it is helpful to start with the basics, such as computer hardware, software, and peripheral devices.

Hardware

Computer hardware consists of physical devices that make up the computer system (Figure BL3.2). Examples of computer hardware include a monitor, keyboard, and mouse.

- **Monitor.** The monitor lets you see what the computer is processing by displaying the information on a screen. Today, there are many technologies used to give the monitor display a high resolution, including liquid crystal diodes (LCD) and organic light-emitting diodes (OLED).

- **Central processing unit (CPU).** The central processing unit serves as the "brain" of a computer. All functions of the computer are processed by the CPU. The CPU can be contained in the "tower" of a desktop computer, the base of a laptop computer, or the base of a monitor. The CPU provides the machine's computing power and is the most important element of a computer system.

- **Mouse.** A mouse controls the cursor on the computer screen and allows the user to control the computer's functions by clicking. Some mice have two buttons, each of which has a special purpose, while others have only one. Advancing technologies have offered alternatives to traditional mice, such as external touchpads. These function much like the touchpad on a laptop—the user can "click" by tapping, or double-tapping the touchpad with a fingertip.

- **Keyboard.** A keyboard is a device used to enter text commands into the computer. Keyboards can be plugged into a USB port on the computer or connect wirelessly. Some computers do not use keyboards, but function with touch screens instead.

- **Printer.** This device prints processed information on paper, creating a hard copy.

- **CDs and DVDs.** CDs and DVDs are physical items that store information to be opened on the computer. These are inserted into computer disk drives located on the CPU.

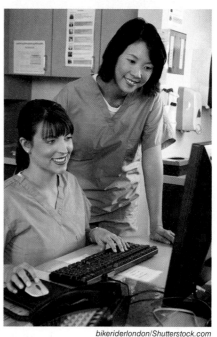

bikeriderlondon/Shutterstock.com

Figure BL3.1 Healthcare workers rely on various computer technologies to do their jobs.

computer hardware
physical components of a computer system; includes the computer, keyboard, monitor, and mouse

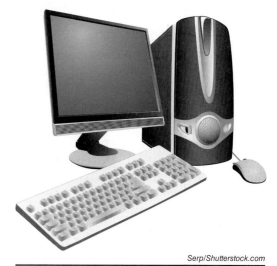

Serp/Shutterstock.com

Figure BL3.2 Basic computer hardware includes a monitor, mouse, keyboard, and a tower that houses the central processing unit (CPU).

- **Modem.** This device transmits data to and from a computer by way of a telephone or other communication line.

- **Router.** This device, which is attached to a modem, allows multiple users and computers to share Internet access, files, and data. Some routers are wired and some are wireless.

- **Scanner.** A scanner is connected to a computer and is used to copy documents and photographs. This device converts scanned items into digital files. Scanners are often combined with printers in one machine.

- **Digital Cameras.** Digital cameras have almost entirely replaced film cameras. In these cameras, photos are captured on memory cards rather than film. Digital cameras can be plugged into a computer's USB port, and pictures are transferred onto the computer's hard drive. Webcams are video cameras that are plugged into, or built into, computers and are used for videoconferences or video chatting.

Within the computer, there are several critical devices that allow it to process information. The CPU serves as the computer's brain and is responsible for running the computer's software. Other devices work with the CPU to process data. Some of these devices include the following:

- **Motherboard.** All hardware in the system is connected to the motherboard. The motherboard is the primary printed circuit board in the computer.

- **Hard Drive.** The hard drive serves as permanent storage for files and programs.

- **Random Access Memory (RAM).** RAM is memory that plugs into the motherboard.

- **Power Supply.** The power supply sends power to the other hardware systems so they can operate.

- **Disk Drives.** These drives are used to insert CDs, DVDs, or other file storage devices into the computer. A USB flash drive is also used to store data for periods of time (Figure BL3.3). A flash drive is sometimes called a *thumb drive*, *keychain drive*, or *jump drive*. This small unit can be plugged into a computer's USB port. Flash drives can transfer data into or out of the computer.

- **Video Card.** This part of the computer system converts code from the CPU so that it can be viewed on the monitor.

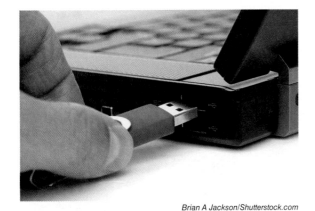

Figure BL3.3 A USB flash drive is a great tool for saving and transferring small amounts of data.

Software

software
programs that allow a user to interact with a computer; computer programs; in contrast to hardware

Software refers to programs and data that are stored digitally within the computer. In contrast, hardware consists of storage, processing, and display devices. Software allows a user to interact with the computer.

Two types of software are *operating system software* and *application program software*. Operating system software directs the computer's hardware. Application program software directs the computer to perform specific tasks. Three commonly used types of software include databases, spreadsheets, and word processing programs.

Databases and spreadsheets are important tools for storing, organizing, and using information (see chapter 16). Databases are computer files that contain a collection of related information entered and sorted by category. Patient names and all related medical information can be put into a database, with information such as the patient's medication record being able to be pulled out separately. Spreadsheets are documents that may include a combination of text and numbers, and which are often used for financial accounting. Microsoft Access is an example of database software, while Microsoft Excel is spreadsheet software.

Word processing programs are some of the most commonly used software. These programs allow the user to enter, edit, save, and print words on a computer. Most word processing programs are able to check and correct the grammar and spelling of the entered text. Microsoft Word is a commonly used word processing program.

word processing
software that allows the user to enter, edit, save, and print text through a computer

File organization is an important component of effectively using your computer. Computer files are the modern equivalent of paper documents. Files on a computer can be organized similarly to files in a filing cabinet. All the files can be put into a large folder using the file explorer tab or its equivalent. This folder can be called *documents*. Then, the large folder can be divided into separate folders for each category of documents, such as *personal, work, pictures*, and so on.

Did You Know?   **Software Usage**

Some of the most popular software includes tax preparation software, accounting software, anti-virus software, and word processing software. What software do you use most often? Your software may vary slightly based on the type of computer you use. Are you an Apple user or a Windows user?

Basic Computer Troubleshooting

There are many different things that could cause a problem with a computer. In some cases, you may need to use several different approaches before you find a solution. Many problems are easy to fix. Sometimes, you may involve a professional to help you find the solution. The following tips may be helpful:

- **Pay attention to error messages.** If something goes wrong with the computer, it may send you an error message. Reading these carefully can help you solve the computer's problem or relay information to a professional.

- **Always check the cables.** If you're having trouble with a specific piece of computer hardware, such as your monitor or keyboard, an easy first step is to check all related cables to make sure they're properly connected. If your power supply is not properly plugged in, you will get no response from the computer.

Internet
an electronic communications network that connects computer networks and computer facilities around the world

World Wide Web (WWW)
a means of accessing the Internet by using an HTTP web address

Wi-Fi
technology that enables electronic devices to exchange data wirelessly over a computer network; *also known as* wireless fidelity

- **Check the power cord.** If your computer does not start, begin by checking the power cord to confirm that it is plugged securely into the back of the computer case and the power outlet. If the cord is plugged into an outlet, make sure it is a working outlet. To check your outlet, you can plug in another electrical device, such as a lamp or cellphone, and see if it receives power. If the computer is plugged into a surge protector, make sure it's turned on. You may have to reset the surge protector by turning it off and then back on. You can also plug a lamp or other device into the surge protector to verify that it is on.

- **Monitor the settings.** Did you change any settings? If you did, you might want to change them back to the way they were. The simple change you made could be causing a problem that you're experiencing.

- **Restart the computer.** When all else fails, one of the best things to try is restarting the computer. This can solve several basic issues you may experience with your computer.

The Internet

The **Internet** is composed of a multitude of computer networks around the world joined together (Figure BL3.4). The **World Wide Web** (WWW) allows people to access the information available on the Internet (Figure BL3.5). Both the Internet and World Wide Web allow healthcare workers to exchange information and access resources at impossibly fast speeds.

When a person accesses the Internet, he or she is *online*. A user has to have the appropriate software and a modem to get online. A connection to the Internet can be provided by a phone line, a cable line, or a digital subscriber line (DSL). You may use a search engine, such as Google, Yahoo, or Bing, to find information online.

Wi-Fi is a popular technology that enables electronic devices to exchange data wirelessly over a computer network. Many people use Wi-Fi to get online using their smartphones. Wi-Fi is often found in many homes, businesses, and cafés, allowing people to access the Internet wirelessly using a laptop, tablet, or e-reader.

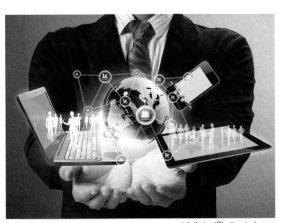
violetkaipa/Shutterstock.com

Figure BL3.4 The Internet is formed by multiple computer networks that are connected to each other.

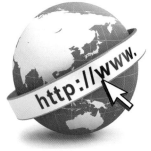
smatch/Shutterstock.com

Figure BL3.5 Accessing information on the Internet is easy when browsing on the World Wide Web.

Going Online at Work

One thing to remember about going on the Internet when at work is that you are responsible for limiting your use to work-related activities. Your employer will have Internet usage guidelines and can monitor your time spent online. Do not expect privacy while using the Internet at work. Do not send inappropriate e-mails or visit inappropriate websites. You could lose your job if you do not limit your use of the computer to work-related tasks.

Many people, including adults and teens, send text messages several times a day. Personal texting during work time is not allowed in most work environments. You should also put your smartphone away when at work.

Extend Your Knowledge ▶ **Podcasts**

Podcasts are audio or video files downloaded and played on a computer, tablet, smartphone, or similar device. Podcasts appear as episodes updated daily or weekly. Podcasts can be entertaining and/or informative. Teachers can use podcasts in instructional settings. There are interesting podcasts that discuss recent medical information.

Apply It

1. Have you ever seen or listened to a podcast?
2. Has an instructor ever used podcasts in any of your classes?

podcasts
multimedia files that are downloaded and played on a computer, tablet, or smartphone

Cloud Technology

Cloud technology is Internet-based computing in which programs and data are stored at remote locations rather than on your computer. These remote locations have a high capacity for data, allowing them to store more information than the typical onsite data storage facility. Items stored in the "cloud" can be accessed quickly using a variety of devices such as laptops, tablets, or smartphones.

cloud technology
Internet-based technology that stores programs and data at remote locations instead of on your computer

Cloud technology presents exciting possibilities for the healthcare community. The transition to electronic medical records has increased the data storage requirements of many healthcare facilities. Facilities must be able to store a large amount of information and access it quickly. Healthcare facilities using cloud technology to store data must be certain their cloud storage provider has tough security measures in place. Medical records are sensitive materials, and patient confidentiality must be maintained.

One specific benefit and application of cloud technology in the healthcare world is a doctor being able to treat a patient who is on vacation. Any doctor should be able to access the patient's medical records from his or her primary doctor via the "cloud." The records could then be updated to include any procedures performed and medication prescribed by the off-site doctor.

Virtual Learning Environments

A **virtual learning environment (VLE)**—which may also be called a *course management system* (CMS) or *learning management system* (LMS)—brings learning materials to students using the World Wide Web. VLEs support student learning outside the classroom at any hour of the day, seven days a week. VLEs allow institutions of learning to educate not only traditional full-time students, but also those who cannot be on campus due to health, geographic, or time restrictions. These systems track student progress, allow students to collaborate with one another, offer assessment programs, and include various communication tools. Blackboard Learning System is a popular VLE.

virtual learning environment (VLE)
an online learning system that brings classroom materials to students via the Internet

Internet Research

As an Internet user, you have access to an overwhelming amount of information. Many reliable healthcare websites exist to provide accurate information, but it is always best to consult your doctor before following an online diagnosis or treatment plan. Websites sponsored by US government organizations such as the National Institutes of Health or the Department of Health and Human Services provide valuable healthcare resources. The Centers for Disease Control and Prevention (CDC) is another good government source of information. Websites of various health organizations, such as the Mayo Clinic, may also be worth visiting.

The Internet makes it possible to gather up-to-date data on exciting new research. Are you curious about new advances in treating breast cancer? Do you want your résumé to have a new, modern format? This information is out there for you to discover. The Internet opens up many prospects for learning, and also makes practical information for everyday living available and easily accessible.

While the Internet can be an excellent source of information, it is also filled with quite a bit of misinformation. Some misinformation can be completely inaccurate, misleading, or even dangerous to patients seeking help for a health problem. If you are looking for answers on the Internet, you may want to use the following questions to evaluate the information you are receiving:

1. What is the purpose of the website? Who sponsors and authors the website?

2. Does the website list other sources you can use to learn about this information?

3. How often is the website updated?

4. Where else on the Internet can you find details and verification about the information you are reading?

5. Which people in your life with expertise in the area can you ask about what you are reading on the website?

One of the dangers of misinformation is that someone will self-treat a health problem after reading an inaccurate or misleading article online. Some healthcare professionals have become concerned about the information available to their patients online. Health information websites and pharmaceutical companies may have a financial agreement in which a pharmaceutical company sponsors the website. This may lead the hosts of the website to recommend a drug that is not the best treatment option for a particular illness but is produced by their sponsor.

On the other hand, health information websites can help a person answer questions concerning symptoms of an illness—encouraging that person to consult a doctor. The lesson to learn here is that you must be an intelligent consumer and consult a reputable doctor who will make a diagnosis and develop a treatment plan.

Check Your Understanding ✓

1. List one example of hardware and one example of software.
2. What does *WWW* stand for?
3. What is cloud technology?
4. What is the purpose of a virtual learning environment?
5. What is one question you can ask to determine the validity of a website?

Computer Disruptions

Malware is malicious or destructive software. Malware is used by attackers to disrupt computer operation, gather sensitive information, or gain access to private computer systems. Commonly used types of malware include worms, Trojan horses, and spyware. Some **computer viruses** are also classified as malware (Figure BL3.6). Cookies (small pieces of data left on your computer by the websites you visit) may share your personal information.

> ## Did You Know?   Transferring Files
>
> **Upload** and **download** are terms that refer to types of electronic data transfers. The difference between them is the direction in which the files are being transferred. Files are uploaded when they are transferred from a computer or other electronic device to a central server. When files are downloaded, they are transferred from a server to a smaller peripheral unit, such as a computer, smartphone, or other device.

Spyware

Spyware is any software that covertly (without your knowledge) gathers user information through the computer's Internet connection, often for advertising purposes. Spyware can often be a hidden component of software that is free for download on the Internet. Once installed, the spyware can watch user activity on the Internet and send the information to someone else. Spyware can also obtain e-mail addresses, passwords, and credit card numbers.

malware
destructive software used to disrupt computer operation, gather sensitive information, or gain access to a private computer

computer viruses
malware designed to copy itself into other programs; may cause the affected computer to operate incorrectly or corrupt the computer memory

upload
transmission of a file from a computer or other electronic device to a central server

download
transmission of a file from one computer system to another; usually transmitting from a larger computer system to a smaller one

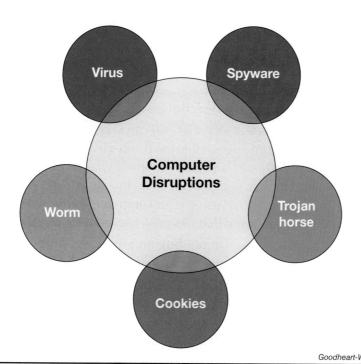

Goodheart-Willcox Publisher

Figure BL3.6   Computer disruptions come in many forms and from various sources.

Worms and Trojan Horses

A computer worm is a type of malware designed to install itself on a computer. Once installed, the worm sends personal data to another party without the user knowing.

Another serious form of malware, a Trojan horse, initially seems to be useful software. However, this malware does extensive damage once it is installed or run on a computer. A user can be tricked into opening a Trojan horse because it appears to be legitimate software or files.

Trojan horses vary in their destruction. Some are designed to be annoying rather than destructive and might, for example, continuously change your desktop icons. Others cause serious damage by deleting files and destroying system information.

Computer Viruses

Computer viruses are software programs designed to destroy computer information. Viruses replicate (duplicate) themselves, spreading from computer to computer through Internet downloads, e-mails, and other sources. These viruses can destroy files and damage hardware.

Most healthcare facilities store information on large computers and must protect data from viruses through vigilant monitoring. Personal computers and laptops are more difficult to monitor. Comprehensive, reliable anti-virus software is a necessity for all computers. This software must be updated frequently as new viruses are developed every day.

Do not download attachments from any suspicious e-mails sent by an unknown person or company. Doing so may infect your computer with a virus that is capable of destroying programs, data, and possibly the computer hardware. Viruses can also spread themselves by attaching to your e-mails.

Avoiding Malware

hackers

people who break into computer systems to access data, steal personal information, and sometimes cause harm to a computer system

Unfortunately, these examples of malware are just a few of many computer disruptions that are active today. Computer **hackers** continue to think up new and evolving malware to victimize computer users.

The single most important step that you can take to protect your computer from malware is to install and use well-known anti-virus software. The software will update itself regularly and constantly monitor your computer for malware. Most anti-malware scanners will provide tools to automate these tasks so that they take place when you are not using your computer. Anti-virus software will protect you when you visit a site that has been hacked and infected.

Avoid fake anti-malware. Do not buy anti-malware software advertised in pop-up ads. Legitimate software isn't sold this way, and these programs can actually load malware onto your machine rather than protect you from it.

Delete e-mails with suspicious attachments and do not open the attachments. E-mail attachments are one of the most popular ways to spread malware. If you don't know what an e-mail is or whom it is from, delete the e-mail immediately rather than opening it.

Malware often comes from unconventional websites. Download and install software only from websites you know and trust. The following are symptoms that suggest a virus or spyware is present in a computer:

- The computer slows down.
- The anti-virus program is turned off.
- The system freezes or crashes.
- The hard drive light is on because the hard drive is constantly working.
- The user receives alerts from a firewall that an unknown program is trying to access the Internet.
- New browser icons appear in the menu.

Computer Protections

Because new methods of computer disruption are developed daily, your computer needs constant protection from intrusion. While anti-virus software will protect you from some threats, sometimes a higher level of security is required. This is especially true in a healthcare facility that must protect its patients' personal information.

Firewall

A **firewall** is a software program or a piece of hardware developed to prevent a hacker from accessing personal information on your computer. A firewall filters incoming and outgoing information for potential threats while also preventing security breaches from remote log-ins. Windows operating systems include a built-in firewall that can be kept on at all times. A firewall is also included in some routers and modems.

firewall
software program or piece of hardware designed to prevent unauthorized access to a computer system

Password Protection

Using passwords to control access to the files on your computer helps protect those files and any personal information they may contain. Design strong passwords that cannot be easily guessed by another person. Use at least eight or more characters for the passwords, combining letters and numbers. Including both uppercase and lowercase letters in your password is also helpful. Do not use the same password for multiple accounts, and be sure to change your password frequently. When you are assigned a password in a healthcare facility, you must not share it with anyone.

Check Your Understanding ✓

1. What is the difference between a worm and Trojan horse?
2. List three symptoms found in a computer that has been affected by malware.
3. What is the purpose of a firewall?
4. How is the term *cookie* used when discussing computer disruptions?
5. List the guidelines for creating a strong password.

Think It Through

Have you ever experienced malware on your computer? Are you currently running anti-malware software? Reliable, free software programs are available to protect your computer from malware. Be sure to renew your software when you get a notice that it is expiring. If you are not protected, you are extremely vulnerable to malware.

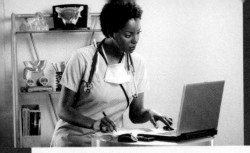
Summary

Regardless of which healthcare career you choose to pursue, you will be using computers and other complex technology to perform your job duties. Successful healthcare workers are confident in their computer skills and willing to learn the latest advances.

Understanding basic computer technology is helpful when working with computers. Basic knowledge includes various software programs, simple troubleshooting, cloud technology, virtual learning environments, and podcasts. Using the Internet effectively to exchange information and access reliable resources will be invaluable skills for an employee. However, it's important to evaluate information found online for accuracy and to practice safe browsing. Avoid opening e-mails or downloading software from unknown sources, as these may contain malware.

It is especially important to protect your computer from viruses and other malware when working in a healthcare facility. Sensitive, confidential patient information must be protected from computer disruptions such as viruses, spyware, and computer hackers.

Review Questions

Answer the following questions using what you have learned in this background lesson.

True/False

1. *True or False?* Employers in many workplaces can monitor your activity on the Internet while you are at work.

2. *True or False? CPU* stands for central progression unit.

3. *True or False?* Medical information found on the Internet is always accurate.

4. *True or False?* Scanners are categorized as software.

5. *True or False?* Podcasts can be used for classroom instruction.

6. *True or False?* Uploading a file means transferring a file from your computer to an outside location.

7. *True or False?* You only need one password for all computer applications.

8. *True or False?* You should always pay attention to error messages on your computer.

9. *True or False?* Cloud technology stores your information at a remote location.

10. *True or False?* If your computer is running slowly, the computer could be infected with malware.

Multiple Choice Assess

11. _____ is *not* a type of computer disruption.
    A. A cookie
    B. A virus
    C. Spyware
    D. Destructo-ware

12. The term _____ describes devices that are connected to the computer.
    A. databases
    B. malware
    C. software
    D. hardware

13. Programs and data are stored at remote locations and accessed online when _____ is used.
    A. a USB flash drive
    B. cloud technology
    C. remote saving
    D. a jump drive

14. _____ enable online learning and include student tracking, assessment, and communication tools.
    A. Cookies
    B. Firewalls
    C. Virtual learning environments
    D. Podcasts

15. A computer virus is capable of _____.

    A. destroying hardware

    B. duplicating itself

    C. spreading through e-mails

    D. All of the above.

16. A computer scanner is _____.

    A. used to listen to police calls

    B. considered software

    C. never combined with any other device

    D. used for converting scanned items into digital files

17. Troubleshooting methods include all of the following *except* _____.

    A. turning the computer off and back on

    B. checking all the cables

    C. hitting the tower twice

    D. checking the power cord

18. Which of the following definitions describes a firewall?

    A. can be a software program or piece of hardware

    B. prevents hackers from accessing your computer information

    C. filters incoming and outgoing information from malware threats

    D. All of the above.

19. Which of the following is *not* an indication that your computer might have malware?

    A. the system freezes or crashes

    B. the system slows down

    C. the anti-virus protection is turned off

    D. the computer boots up successfully

20. Which of the following items is *not* software?

    A. podcasts

    B. word processor

    C. spreadsheets

    D. databases

Short Answer

21. Give three examples of computer hardware. Explain the function of each item.

22. Give three examples of computer software. Explain the function of each item.

23. What is the difference between the Internet and the World Wide Web?

24. What is malware?

25. Why is it important for healthcare facilities to maintain powerful firewalls that protect their computer system?

Critical Thinking Exercises

26. What steps have you taken to protect the data on your computer? Have you ever experienced an intrusion into your computer? If so, what could you have done to prevent this computer disruption?

27. Are your computer skills up to par? Do you feel confident in your abilities to use complex computer systems like the ones found in most healthcare facilities? If not, what can you do to improve your computer skills?

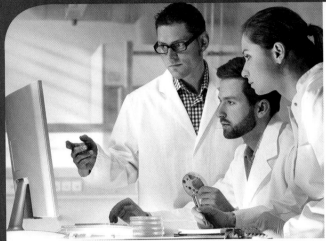

Alexander Raths/Shutterstock.com

Science Review

Terms to Know

 Build Vocab

empirical
hypothesis

induction
science

scientific method

Lesson Objectives

- Define *science*.
- Identify the six steps of the scientific method and understand how the process can be used to solve a problem.
- Discuss the importance of the scientific method pioneers who helped develop scientific thinking.
- Identify categories of science that are relevant to healthcare.
- Describe a science career related to healthcare.

What is **science**? How does it apply to healthcare careers? Science is a system of acquiring knowledge through observation and experimentation to describe the natural world.

Modern medicine is based on well-established laws, principles, and practical findings in many scientific areas of study, including chemistry, physics, biology, anatomy, and physiology. Pursuing a career in the healthcare field means that, in most cases, you have been exposed to many science courses throughout your education.

Depending on the career that you choose, you may study disciplines that fall into the category of the natural sciences. The natural sciences comprise disciplines that study the physical world, including biology, physics, chemistry, and geology. This does not include the social sciences and the abstract sciences such as mathematics.

science
a system of acquiring knowledge through observation and experimentation to describe the natural world

The Scientific Method

To derive conclusions about the world around them, scientists use the **scientific method** to logically formulate, test, and evaluate a problem or hypothesis. A **hypothesis** is a supposition or proposed explanation made based on limited evidence as a starting point for further investigation.

The application of the scientific method has resulted in many medical discoveries. These discoveries relate to the functions of the human body, the diagnosis and treatment of disease, and the development of new drugs and machines used in patient care. Doctors use the scientific method to arrive at diagnoses and determine the appropriate treatment to use.

Medical advances such as new surgical procedures and vaccines have been made by applying the scientific method. The scientific method can be used for problem solving in school or at work. The scientific method may also be helpful when evaluating information found on the Internet, in newspapers, or given to you by friends or coworkers.

scientific method
a method designed to logically formulate, test, and evaluate a problem or hypothesis

hypothesis
an idea or suggestion often developed to explain something, the cause of which is unknown

The History of the Scientific Method

No one person can be said to have invented the scientific method. Elements of this method can be traced back to ancient people who found it to be a natural way of obtaining reliable knowledge. The accomplishments of the individuals listed here contributed to the development of the scientific method:

- Aristotle (384–322 BCE), a Greek philosopher who is one of history's great thinkers, worked to find reliable knowledge by studying phenomena, or observable facts and events (Figure BL4.1).

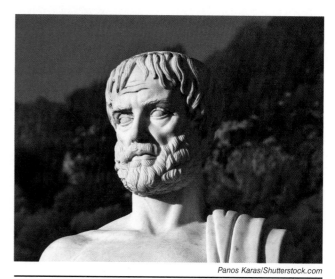

Panos Karas/Shutterstock.com

Figure BL4.1 Aristotle

empirical

term that means based on, concerned with, or verifiable by observation or experience rather than theory or pure logic

induction

term that describes reasoning that moves from specific observations to broader generalizations

- Roger Bacon (1214–1294) was an English philosopher and Franciscan friar (Figure BL4.2). Bacon was influenced by writings of Muslim scientists. He described a cycle of observation, hypothesis, experimentation, and verification that led to many important discoveries. Bacon was considered to be a modern experimental scientist because he placed emphasis on **empirical** and scientific study.

- Galileo Galilei (1564–1642) was an Italian physicist, mathematician, astronomer, and philosopher (Figure BL4.3). He is often described as the *father of the scientific method* because he put together pieces of the method that were developed by others. Galileo developed a system that combined observation, hypothesis, mathematical deduction (starting from a broad idea and narrowing the idea down to a hypothesis), and confirmation.

- Francis Bacon (1561–1626), an English philosopher, statesman, scientist, and author, played a very important role in the advancement of scientific thought (Figure BL4.4). Bacon proposed a research method called **induction**—reasoning that moves from specific observations to broader generalizations. Bacon also urged scientists to keep records of experiments and exchange data to share newly discovered knowledge.

- René Descartes (1596–1650) was a French philosopher, mathematician, and physicist (Figure BL4.5). Descartes developed the use of mathematical methods in scientific inquiry. His goal was to add elements of precision and certainty to many fields of study.

Thanks to these great thinkers, and many who followed, the world has a framework for developing and executing scientific investigation that produces accurate and reliable findings. The medical field, in particular, has benefitted greatly from the development of the scientific method.

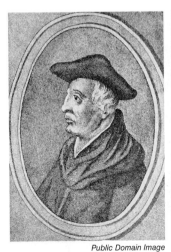

Public Domain Image

Figure BL4.2   Roger Bacon

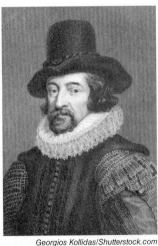

Georgios Kollidas/Shutterstock.com

Figure BL4.3   Galileo Galilei

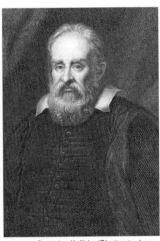

Georgios Kollidas/Shutterstock.com

Figure BL4.4   Francis Bacon

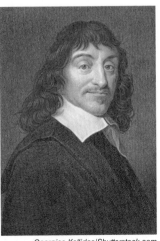

Georgios Kollidas/Shutterstock.com

Figure BL4.5   René Descartes

Other intellectuals who helped to refine the scientific method include Sir Isaac Newton, Charles Darwin, Albert Einstein, and Benjamin Franklin.

Using the Scientific Method

Scientific method steps and procedures vary from one scientific field to another, but the general principles are the same. Following is a six-step method, along with an example that highlights how the scientific method can be applied in an everyday situation.

1. **The question**: The goal of research using the scientific method is to find an answer to an important question. The question should be worthwhile and able to be answered through the collection and analysis of data.

   During a fishing trip, Brandon slips while climbing down to the river and twists his ankle. The experience is painful, causing Brandon to ask, "What have I done to my ankle?"

2. **Hypothesis**: A hypothesis is an educated guess as to what your research will reveal about the question you have asked. By the end of the process, a hypothesis will either be confirmed or rejected.

   Brandon suspects that he has sprained his ankle.

3. **Research and collecting data**: Research involves recording observations and collecting data to determine whether your hypothesis is accurate.

   Because Brandon is out of town and cannot consult his family doctor, he decides to treat the sprain by icing his ankle. The ice seems to help, and Brandon wraps his ankle securely with a bandage to prevent the ankle from moving. At this point, Brandon's assumption that his ankle is sprained seems to be reasonable.

4. **Interpreting the data**: Examine the collected data and establish whether it is sufficient to begin determining the result of your study. If not, further research may be required to come to an accurate result and conclusion.

   Two weeks have passed since the accident and Brandon continues to have ankle pain. The swelling in his ankle has increased, and Brandon finds it difficult to walk. Brandon decides to visit a local clinic to have the ankle evaluated.

5. **Results**: After collecting and interpreting the data, it is possible to determine the results of a study. Was the hypothesis confirmed? Did the interpretation of the data collected reveal that it was incorrect?

   An X-ray shows that Brandon has a cracked bone in his ankle. His original ankle sprain hypothesis was proven false and rejected.

6. **Conclusion**: The conclusion of a study consists of a concise statement expressing the key findings of the study.

   Surgery is immediately performed on Brandon's ankle to repair the broken bone. A plate is attached to the bone to prevent it from shifting its position.

Scientists working to solve healthcare problems often use the scientific method. These scientists are asking questions related to the diagnosis and treatment of disease, as well as developing safe drug therapies and diagnostic machines for their patients. After drawing conclusions and either rejecting or confirming their hypothesis based on their use of the scientific method, scientists often share their results with others. Such communication can inspire additional experiments and often results in exciting discoveries in healthcare.

Check Your Understanding ✔

Think of a problem that could be solved by using the scientific method. Divide a piece of paper into two columns. In the left column, list the six steps of the scientific method. In the right column, follow the example of Brandon's sprained ankle and use the steps to solve your problem.

Healthcare-Related Science Disciplines

There are numerous disciplines, or specialized areas, that fall under the broad category of science. Many science courses are relevant when studying for a career in healthcare. Whether you are hoping to go into the research field in an effort to discover new medical uses for lasers, or you want to work in the financial office of a hospital, you will encounter science disciplines. Depending on the type of degree you wish to pursue, you will be required to take at least two or three science courses (Figure BL4.6). These courses may include anatomy and physiology, biology, chemistry, botany, bioengineering, health sciences, physics, or computer science.

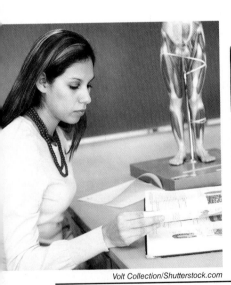
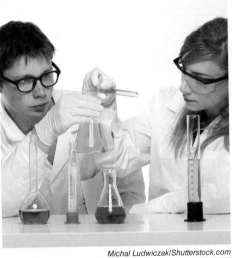
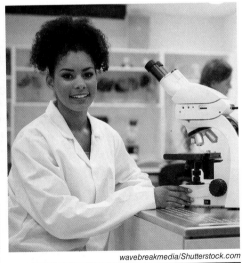

Volt Collection/Shutterstock.com   Michal Ludwiczak/Shutterstock.com   wavebreakmedia/Shutterstock.com

Figure BL4.6   Developing a strong science background will be beneficial to your future healthcare career.

Education for most healthcare careers focuses on how the human body works (or animal bodies, in the case of veterinary medicine). Studying the inner workings of the human body will help you provide patients with the proper care—analyzing medical records, treating wounds, or administering medication. Knowing how your body works will improve your ability to maintain good health. This knowledge will also help you be an educated partner to your doctor when solving potential health problems in the future.

Healthcare Science

Healthcare scientists, often known as *clinical scientists*, work on the cutting edge of medicine, researching and developing new treatments and equipment (Figure BL4.7). This profession does not often include any patient interaction, with most work being done in a laboratory. Healthcare science covers a range of categories, which are generally subdivided into the following three main categories:

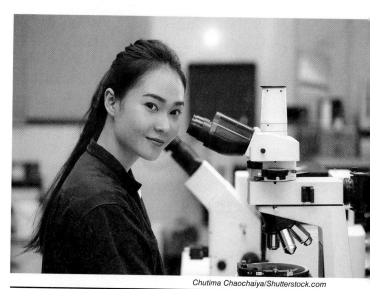

Chutima Chaochaiya/Shutterstock.com

Figure BL4.7   Healthcare scientists can focus on life sciences, physiological sciences, or clinical engineering and physical sciences.

- **Life sciences** involve the study of illness and disease (pathology), pharmacy, genetics, and embryology, which is used in fertility treatments.

- **Physiological sciences** include the study of the body and organs. This covers categories such as audiology and neurology.

- **Clinical engineering and physical sciences** focus on developing techniques and technology such as radiography, ultrasound, and nuclear medicine for diagnosis and monitoring of patients.

Preparing for a career in healthcare science requires an undergraduate degree in healthcare science and often a master's degree as well. A strong science background is mandatory. Many colleges now offer this major.

Check Your Understanding ✓

1. Define *science*.
2. How did Francis Bacon contribute to the scientific method?
3. Name one step in the scientific method.
4. What is one science course that is related to healthcare?
5. What do the physiological sciences include?

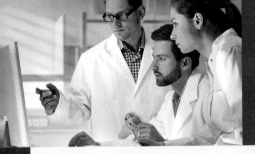

Summary

Science is a system of acquiring knowledge through observation and experimentation to describe the natural world. The scientific method is used to obtain reliable knowledge. Several famous pioneers of science helped develop the scientific method. These famous scientists include Aristotle, Roger Bacon, Galileo Galilei, René Descartes, and Francis Bacon. The method consists of a question, a hypothesis, research and data collection, interpretation of the data, analysis of results, and a conclusion. It can be used throughout the medical field to diagnose illness, invent new therapies, design and develop new technologies, and discover new drug treatments.

Modern medicine is based on many scientific disciplines, and the student who wants a career in healthcare must take several science courses, such as anatomy and physiology, physics, biology, human growth and development, and chemistry. Healthcare scientists focus on the cutting edge of medicine, including life sciences, physiological sciences, clinical engineering, and physical sciences.

Review Questions

Answer the following questions using what you have learned in this background lesson.

True or False Assess

1. *True or False?* "Study" is a step in the scientific method.
2. *True or False?* The scientific method was invented in the 1930s.
3. *True of False?* Today, the scientific method is not used often.
4. *True or False?* A healthcare scientist works primarily in a laboratory.
5. *True or False?* Plato invented the scientific method.

Multiple Choice Assess

6. Which of the following individuals was *not* credited for contributing to the development of the scientific method?
   A. Francis Bacon
   B. Bill Gates
   C. René Descartes
   D. Galileo Galilei

7. Which of the following individuals is often called the *father of the scientific method*?
   A. René Descartes
   B. Galileo Galilei
   C. Roger Bacon
   D. Benjamin Franklin

8. Which of the following terms describes reasoning that moves from specific observations to broader generalizations?
   A. hypothesizing
   B. empiricism
   C. induction
   D. criticism

9. Which of the following terms means based on, concerned with, or verifiable by observation or experience?
   A. inductive
   B. empirical
   C. deductive
   D. critical

10. Which of the following is *not* a step in the scientific method?
    A. hypothesis
    B. researching and interpreting data
    C. conclusion
    D. criticizing data

11. Which of the following subjects is *not* considered a natural science?

A. mathematics

B. physics

C. biology

D. geology

12. Education for most healthcare careers focuses on _____.

A. physics

B. reproduction

C. microbiology

D. how the body works

13. A doctor or scientist would use the scientific method for which of the following?

A. diagnosis of a disease

B. determining a course of treatment for a patient

C. developing a new drug

D. All of the above.

Short Answer

14. Name three people whose accomplishments and discoveries contributed to the development of the scientific method.

15. List the six steps in the scientific method.

16. Name four categories of science that are relevant to healthcare.

17. List three categories of study that are considered life sciences.

18. Describe *induction*.

Critical Thinking Exercises

19. Give an example of how you might use the scientific method to solve the following problem. A 14-year-old named Jennifer Castle has a rash all over her face. Her mother says that it looks like acne. Jennifer's mom buys several kinds of over-the-counter acne medicine for her and tells her not to eat chocolate. Jennifer's rash doesn't go away. Finally, Mrs. Castle takes her daughter to the dermatologist. "It isn't acne," says the doctor. "Did you change face soap?"

20. Develop two problem scenarios that you can solve with the scientific method. Describe how the scientific method can be applied to each scenario.

21. Which science courses have you taken? Which science courses interest you the most? Which courses do you plan to take and why? How do you think these courses will contribute to a future career in healthcare?

22. Look up the definition of a scientific theory. How does it differ from a hypothesis? What do you think must happen to a hypothesis for it to become a theory?

23. Research someone who contributed to the scientific method but was not discussed in this chapter. Examples include Sir Isaac Newton, Charles Darwin, Albert Einstein, or Benjamin Franklin. Write a one-page report about this person's contributions to the scientific method's development.

24. Research a healthcare-related science discipline that interests you. What types of courses would you have to take to focus on this discipline? Write a short plan that you could follow if you wanted to eventually work in that discipline.

Glossary

12-hour clock: Method of measuring time based on a 12-hour system in which a.m. and p.m. designations must be assigned to identify the proper time; used internationally. (16)

24-hour clock: Method of measuring time based on 24-hour-long segments; also called military time. (16)

A

abdominal quadrants: The four divisions of the large abdominal area. (5)

acronyms: Words formed from the first letters or parts of other words. (5)

active listening: The act of listening intently to not only hear the words being spoken, but to understand the complete message being sent. (15)

active reading: Reading with extreme concentration and focus; note taking and reading out loud are sometimes part of active reading. (17)

activity of daily living (ADL): Any basic self-care task, including grooming, bathing, and eating. (13)

addiction: A physical or psychological need for a habit-forming substance, such as drugs or alcohol, or an activity, such as shopping. (8)

addition: The process of combining two or more numbers to obtain their total value. (BL2)

adjective: A word that modifies or describes a noun or pronoun. (BL1)

administration unit: The unit of measurement used when giving a patient a drug. (16)

adolescence: The stage of life following the onset of puberty during which a young person develops from a child into an adult. (9)

advance directive (AD): A legal document in which a patient gives written instructions about healthcare issues in the event the patient becomes unable to make such decisions in the future. (3)

adverb: Any word that tells how, when, where, or how much. (BL1)

aerobe: An organism that requires oxygen to live. (4)

aerobic exercise: Exercise that requires the heart to deliver oxygenated blood to working muscles. (8)

Affordable Care Act (ACA): Passed into law in 2010 for a major regulatory overhaul of US healthcare; also called *Obamacare*. (1)

algebra: The branch of mathematics that substitutes letters for numbers; involves solving for the unknown. (16)

allergen: Any substance that causes an allergy. (12)

ambulation: The ability to walk from one place to another. (13)

anaerobe: An organism that requires little or no oxygen to live. (4)

anaphylaxis: A severe allergic reaction that can affect the whole body. (12)

anatomical position: A standing position in which the feet are parallel and the arms and hands are at the sides, palms facing out. (5)

anatomy: The study of the structure of the body. (6)

anesthesia: Loss of feeling with or without the loss of consciousness. (1)

ankylosis: The stiffening or immobility of a joint resulting from disease, trauma, surgery, or bone fusion. (13)

anorexia nervosa: An eating disorder characterized by low weight, fear of gaining weight, and food restriction. (8)

antibiotics: Drugs that slow the growth of, or destroy bacteria; used to treat infections. (1)

antibody: A protein produced by the immune system; circulates in the plasma in response to the presence of foreign antigens. (6)

antigen: Any foreign substance, either outside or inside the body, that causes the immune system to produce antibodies. (6)

antihistamine: A drug that slows down or stops the actions of histamine, the substance that causes an allergic reaction. (12)

antisepsis: The process of using an antiseptic to prevent or inhibit the growth of pathogenic organisms. (4)

anus: The opening at the end of the gastrointestinal (GI) tract, where solid waste leaves the body. (11)

Apgar scale: A measure used to determine the health of a newborn based on heart and respiratory rates, muscle tone, responsiveness, and body color. (9)

aphasia: A collection of language disorders caused by brain damage. (15)

apical pulse: The pulse located at the bottom left portion of the heart. (11)

apnea: Lack of breathing. (11)

arbitration: A cost-effective alternative to litigation. (3)

asepsis: Term that describes the absence of bacteria, viruses, and other microorganisms. (4)

asphyxia: A lack of oxygen that causes breathing to stop; may be caused by an obstruction or swelling of the trachea. (12)

assault: Any words or actions that lead an individual to fear that he or she will be harmed by another person. (3)

associate's degree: A two-year college degree, often offered through a community college and awarded after completing 60 credit hours or more in a semester system. (2)

atherosclerosis: Buildup of plaque on the inner lining of an arterial wall over time that causes the arteries to harden and may lead to a myocardial infarction. (7)

atony: Lack of sufficient muscular tone. (13)

atrophy: A decrease in size or *wasting* away of a body part or tissue. (13)

auditory learner: One who learns best by listening; lectures, discussion, and talking about ideas and concepts are helpful tools for this learner. (17)

aural: Of or relating to the ear or the sense of hearing. (11)

autism: Mental condition present from early childhood, most often characterized by difficulty communicating, forming relationships, using language, and understanding abstract concepts. (7)

autoclave: A machine used frequently in healthcare facilities to kill all microorganisms and their spores on a surface. (4)

automated external defibrillator (AED): A medical device that delivers an electric shock through the chest to the heart to stop an irregular heart rhythm and allow a normal heart rhythm to resume. (12)

axillary temperature: Temperature taken in the axilla, or armpit. (11)

B

bachelor's degree: A four-year college degree awarded after 120 credit hours or more in a semester system. (2)

bacteria: Small, one-celled microorganisms that cannot be seen by the naked eye; can be pathogenic (cause disease). (4)

base ten system: Numbering system used for counting that is based on multiples of ten. (BL2)

battery: Touching a person without consent. (3)

biohazard sharps container: A puncture-resistant container used for disposing of waste-contaminated sharps, including needles, scalpels, glass slides, and broken glassware. (4)

biopharmaceuticals: Prescription drugs that are produced as a result of biotechnology. (10)

biopsy: A piece of tissue removed from the body for examination; the process of removing tissue for examination. (4)

biotechnology: Technology that uses biological processes, organisms, or systems to develop products intended to improve the quality of human life. (10)

biotechnology research and development: Highly science-oriented career pathway that uses living systems and organisms to create and develop products used in healthcare. (2)

bipolar disorder: Mental disorder characterized by alternating periods of euphoria, or an elevated mood, and depression. (8)

bloodborne pathogens: Infectious microorganisms in human blood that can cause disease. (4)

body alignment: The optimal placement of body parts so that bones are used efficiently and muscles have to do less work to get the same effect. (13)

body cavities: Spaces in the body that contain organs; the human body is divided into the dorsal and ventral cavities. (5)

body image: A person's thoughts and feelings about how he or she looks. (8)

body mass index (BMI): A method that uses height and weight to determine whether a person is at a healthy weight, overweight, or underweight. (7)

body mechanics: The proper use of body movements to prevent injury during the performance of physical tasks, such as lifting and sitting. (4)

body planes: Imaginary planes, or flat surfaces, that divide the body into sections; include sagittal, coronal, and transverse planes. (5)

bonding: The act of developing an emotional connection between a parent or caregiver and a baby. (9)

bone marrow: Soft, spongy, blood-forming tissue found inside bones. (6)

bradycardia: A slow pulse of less than 60 beats per minute. (11)

bradypnea: An unusually slow rate of breathing, typically under 12 breaths per minute. (11)

Brazelton Neonatal Behavioral Assessment Scale: A test given to a newborn that measures reflexes and responses to sounds, touch, and light. (9)

bulimia nervosa: An eating disorder characterized by bingeing and purging. (8)

C

caduceus: An emblem of medicine in the United States. (1)

cancer: Uncontrolled cell growth. (7)

capitalization: The use of an uppercase letter for the first letter of a word, and lowercase letters for the rest of the word; used for proper nouns. (BL1)

carcinoma: Cancerous tumor derived from epithelial cells. (7)

cardiopulmonary resuscitation (CPR): An emergency lifesaving procedure in which a series of chest compressions and rescue breaths are given to a person whose breathing or heartbeat has stopped; supports blood circulation and breathing. (12)

career ladder: Term for the progression from an entry-level position to higher levels of pay, skill, and responsibility. (2)

career portfolio: An accumulation of documents and work related to a person's career planning and preparation. (18)

carotid pulse: A pulse taken at either of the two main arteries located on each side of the neck. (11)

carpal tunnel syndrome: A painful, progressive hand and arm condition caused by compression of a key nerve in the wrist; can be caused when wrists are not supported during keyboard use. (4)

cell membrane: The outer layer of a cell that holds the cell together. (6)

Celsius (°C): The metric measurement used for temperature; the freezing point of water is 0° and the boiling point is 100°. (11)

Centers for Disease Control and Prevention (CDC): A division of the United States Department of Health and Human Services that focuses on disease outbreaks and prevention in the United States. (1)

central nervous system (CNS): Part of the nervous system that includes the brain and the spinal cord. (6)

certification: Recognition given for completing a course of study and/or passing a certification exam. (2)

chain of command: Term that describes the levels of authority in an organization from the bottom to the top. (18)

chain of infection: The sequence of events that allows infection to move from one source or host to another. (4)

chemotherapy: Treatment of a disease with chemical agents. (7)

chromosome: Threadlike structure found in the nucleus of most living cells; carries genetic information. (6)

chronic disease: A disease of long duration. (7)

civil law: Directives that pertain to disputes between individuals, organizations, or a combination of the two in which monetary compensation is awarded; also known as *tort law*. (3)

cloning: The creation of an organism that is an exact genetic copy of another; a clone has identical DNA to its parent. (10)

cloud technology: Internet-based technology that stores programs and data at remote locations instead of on your computer. (BL3)

combining form: Term that describes a word root and a combining vowel together; used to form medical terms. (5)

combining vowel: Letter used to combine two word roots, or a word root and a suffix; usually an *o*. (5)

common denominator: The number that can be divided evenly by all of the denominators in a group of fractions. (BL2)

communicable disease: A disease that is caused by pathogens and can be transferred from one living thing to another. (7)

compassion: Deep awareness and concern for the suffering of others coupled with the desire to relieve this suffering. (18)

competence: The ability to do your job well. (18)

complementary and alternative medicine (CAM): Health practices used in place of or in conjunction with traditional Western medicine; also known as *integrative health*. (8)

complex sentence: A sentence that contains an independent clause and one or more dependent clauses. (BL1)

compound sentence: A sentence that contains two independent clauses joined by a conjunction. (BL1)

compromise: The settlement of differences in which each side makes concessions. (18)

computer hardware: Physical components of a computer system; includes the computer, keyboard, monitor, and mouse. (BL3)

computer on wheels (COW): A mobile computer used to access and enter patient information while moving around the healthcare facility; often rolled into a patient's hospital room. (10)

computer virus: Malware designed to copy itself into other programs; may cause the affected computer to operate incorrectly or corrupt the computer memory. (BL3)

concentration: The dosage strength of a drug; describes the amount of medication per administration unit. (16)

confidentiality: The practice of allowing only certain individuals the right to access information; ensures that others do not obtain the personal information of patients. (3)

conflict resolution: The process of alleviating or eliminating sources of discord or tension between individuals. (18)

conjunction: A word that joins other words, phrases, clauses, or sentences. (BL1)

consonants: All letters of the English alphabet except *a*, *e*, *i*, *o*, and *u*. (BL1)

contraction: A shortened form of a word or term; one or more letters are omitted and replaced with an apostrophe to create one word. (BL1)

contracture: A condition characterized by the tightening or shortening of a body part, such as muscle, tendon, or skin, due to lack of movement. (13)

contraindicated: Term that describes any situation or condition that causes a particular type of treatment to be improper or undesirable. (13)

copayment: A fixed amount (for example, $15) paid for a covered healthcare service, usually when service is provided; amount varies depending on type of health insurance a person has. (1)

cover letter: A letter that accompanies a résumé to provide additional information about the applicant's skills and experience; usually focuses on the applicant's qualifications for a particular job; also called *cover message.* (18)

criminal law: Directives that pertain to a crime in which the guilty party is punished by incarceration and possible fines. (3)

critical thinking: A process of actively and skillfully analyzing and evaluating information to draw a conclusion. (17)

cyanotic: Blue discoloration of the skin. (12)

cytoplasm: Transparent, gel-like substance inside of every cell; cellular activities occur here. (6)

D

database: A collection of records such as addresses, phone numbers, and other patient information. (16)

decimal numbers: Numbers expressed with a decimal point; values left of the decimal are whole numbers and values to the right are fractions. (BL2)

decimals: Fractions that are expressed in the base 10 system; also known as decimal fractions. (16)

decoding: The process of breaking down words into recognizable parts. (17)

decubitus ulcer: A skin sore that is a result of lying in one position too long; caused by pressure that interferes with blood circulation to the skin. (13)

deductible: The amount you owe for covered healthcare services before your health insurance plan begins to pay. (1)

defamation: Damaging someone's good name or reputation. (3)

delegate: To assign the accountability and responsibility of one's task to another worker. (14)

dementia: Condition characterized by a decrease in mental ability, including loss of memory, impaired judgment, and disorientation. (7)

deoxyribonucleic acid (DNA): Genetic material shaped like a double helix; part of all living cells. (6)

depression: Mood disorder causing a persistent feeling of sadness and loss of interest. (8)

diabetes mellitus: A disease caused by insufficient utilization of insulin resulting in an increased amount of glucose in the blood and urine. (7)

diagnostic-related groups (DRGs): A system that categorizes patients according to their diagnoses. (2)

diagnostic services: A healthcare pathway offering careers in implementing procedures to determine causes of diseases or disorders. (2)

diastolic pressure: Part of a blood pressure reading that is taken when the heart muscle relaxes. (11)

differentiation: Process through which cells of the body vary according to their specific function. (6)

digital: An electronic readout of numbers. (11)

direct contact: A type of infection transmission in which the pathogen travels directly from one host to another, such as in person-to-person transmission. (4)

discharge plan: A set of instructions regarding the patient's treatment and medications for use after leaving a healthcare facility. (14)

discrimination: The act of unfairly treating a person or a group of people differently from others. (3)

disease: Any condition that interferes with the normal function of the body. (7)

disinfection: The use of antimicrobial agents on nonliving objects or surfaces to destroy or deactivate microorganisms. (4)

disorder: An abnormality of function; a pathological condition. (7)

division: The process of determining how many times one number is present in another number. (BL2)

do not resuscitate (DNR) document: A legal document made by a patient, which states that CPR or other advanced cardiac life support should not be performed if a patient stops breathing or a patient's heart stops. (3)

doctorate: A degree awarded after two to six years of education beyond the bachelor's degree; available in many disciplines. (2)

dorsal recumbent position: A position in which a patient lies on her back with the knees flexed and separated. (5)

dosage unit: The unit of measurement that indicates a drug's weight or action. (16)

download: Transmission of a file from one computer system to another; usually transmitting from a larger computer system to a smaller one. (BL3)

drug-resistant bacteria: Strains of a bacterium that have adapted and are no longer controlled or killed by normal antibiotic treatment. (7)

durable power of attorney: A legal document that grants another person the authority to make legal decisions for you. (3)

duty of care: A legal obligation for healthcare personnel to take reasonable care to avoid causing harm to a patient. (3)

dyslexia: A learning disorder characterized by problems processing words; often causes difficulties when learning to read. (17)

dyspnea: Difficult breathing usually observed as shortness of breath. (11)

E

edema: Excess build-up or retention of fluid in the bodily tissues that causes swelling, usually in the legs and feet. (11)

electronic health record (EHR): A digital record that contains information about a patient and spans his or her entire medical history and experiences. (2)

electronic medical record (EMR): A digital record that contains information from a single medical practice or even a single stay in one healthcare facility. (10)

emancipated minor: A person under 18 years of age who has legally established that he or she does not live with parents. (3)

embolus: A mass, most commonly a blood clot, that becomes lodged in a blood vessel and obstructs the flow of blood. (13)

emotional intelligence (EI): The measure of one's ability to be aware of, control, and express one's emotions and to maintain successful interpersonal relations. (8)

empathy: The act of identifying with and understanding another person's feelings or situation. (18)

empirical: Term that means based on, concerned with, or verifiable by observation or experience rather than theory or pure logic. (BL4)

endocrine glands: Glands that secrete chemical substances called hormones, which regulate body functions; part of the endocrine system. (6)

endorphins: Hormones secreted within the brain during exercise that reduce the sensation of pain or stress. (8)

English system of measurement: A system of measurement commonly used in the United States; measurements are based on the inch, pound, gallon, and Fahrenheit degrees. (16)

enthusiasm: An excited and positive attitude that you can bring to your work. (18)

epidemic: An outbreak of a disease that affects many people and spreads rapidly. (1)

equations: Mathematical statements containing expressions composed of numbers and/or letters; two sides of an equation are separated by an equal sign and must be equal to one another. (16)

ergonomics: The practice or science of maximizing efficiency and preventing discomfort or injury during the time a person is performing work tasks. (4)

ethics committee: A committee made up of individuals who consider ethical problems in the healthcare facility and recommend solutions for resolving the issues. (3)

euphoria: Emotional and mental condition in which a person experiences intense feelings of well-being, happiness, and excitement. (8)

exhalation: Breathing out; also called *expiration*. (11)

exocrine glands: Glands that contain a duct, allowing them to secrete their enzymes directly at the site of action; part of the endocrine system. (6)

expiration date: The date on which a medication is no longer fit for use. (16)

F

Fahrenheit (°F): The English system of measurement used for temperature; the freezing point of water is 32°F and the boiling point is 212°F. (11)

fetal alcohol syndrome (FAS): Term that describes conditions such as cognitive disabilities resulting from prenatal exposure to alcohol. (9)

fibrillation: An irregular heart rhythm. (12)

fire triangle: Term for the three elements—fuel, heat, and oxygen—needed to start and maintain a fire. (4)

firewall: Software program or piece of hardware designed to prevent unauthorized access to a computer system. (BL3)

flexibility: The ability to change or adjust your attitude and behavior to meet particular needs. (18)

Food and Drug Administration (FDA): A government agency that regulates products in the food and drug industries and develops nutrition facts labels to help consumers make informed food choices. (1)

foot drop: A condition characterized by the inability to lift the front part of one or both feet due to weakness or paralysis of the muscles in the foot; causes the toes to drag on the ground while walking. (13)

formed elements: The solid components of blood, including red blood cells, white blood cells, and platelets. (6)

Fowler's position: A position in which a patient lies in bed with the head of the bed elevated 45°. (5)

fractions: Numbers that indicate part of a whole. (BL2)

fungi: Parasitic organisms that live in the soil or on plants; include disease-causing microorganisms such as yeasts and molds. (4)

G

gait belt: A device made of canvas, nylon, or leather that is used by healthcare workers to safely move (transfer) patients to a standing position or to assist them during walking. (13)

generic name: The official name assigned to a drug in the United States. (16)

genetic engineering: The manipulation of genetic materials to eliminate undesirable traits or to ensure desirable traits. (10)

genomic medicine: A branch of medicine that studies a person's DNA sequences, which carry genetic information. (1)

geriatrics: The care of aging people. (9)

gerontology: The study of the aging process. (9)

gestation: The period between fertilization and birth; also known as *pregnancy*. (9)

Good Samaritan laws: Laws that protect people from legal action after voluntarily giving emergency medical aid while using reasonable care. (3)

grammar: The study of how words and their components combine to form sentences. (BL1)

grand mal seizure: A generalized seizure in which a person may experience a loss of consciousness and violent muscle contractions. (12)

guardian: A court-appointed person who may make decisions for a patient who is mentally or physically incapable of making such decisions. (3)

H

hackers: People who break into computer systems to access data, steal personal information, and sometimes cause harm to a computer system. (BL3)

hand hygiene: Hand washing with a detergent or antimicrobial soap and water, or by applying an alcohol-based hand rub; considered the single most important way to prevent the spread of infection. (4)

handoff reports: Reports used during a shift change or change in the level of patient care to explain a patient's current situation. (10)

hands-only CPR: Uninterrupted chest compressions given to restore heartbeat and promote blood circulation; an alternative procedure for those not trained in conventional CPR. (12)

health informatics services: Career field considered to be a bridge between medicine and technology, and which provides critical support to all other medical services; includes positions such as medical clerical worker, human resource workers, and medical records workers. (2)

Health Information Technology for Economic and Clinical Health (HITECH) Act: Legislation passed to improve healthcare through increased use of health information technology (HIT). (10)

Health Insurance Portability and Accountability Act (HIPAA): An act approved by the US Congress in 1996 and fully enforced in 2006; includes a privacy provision for patient health records. (3)

health literacy: An individual's ability to obtain, communicate, and understand basic health information and services, allowing him or her to make appropriate health decisions. (8)

health maintenance organizations (HMO): Managed care organizations that provide prepaid, comprehensive healthcare at a flat rate and for a fixed period of time through a network of participating healthcare professionals and hospitals; policyholders select a primary care physician (PCP) and referrals from the PCP must be obtained to see a specialist. (1)

healthcare simulation: The use of learning tools to show what a medical emergency looks like or how a healthcare procedure is performed. (10)

Heimlich maneuver: A series of abdominal thrusts performed to remove an object that is lodged in a person's airway, preventing the person from breathing. (12)

hemorrhage: Excessive blood loss over a short period of time due to an internal or external injury. (12)

hepatitis: Inflammation of the liver. (7)

Hippocratic Oath: A promise of professional behavior made by doctors beginning their careers; promises ethical and honest practice of the medical profession. (1)

holistic health: A wellness approach that advocates for treating the patient as a whole, rather than just the symptoms of disease, because the body works as a combination of physical, emotional, mental, and spiritual health. (8)

homeostasis: State of internal balance achieved by adjusting the physiological systems of the body. (6)

hormones: Chemicals secreted by endocrine glands to regulate body functions. (6)

hospice: A type of care designed to relieve pain and reduce suffering in terminally ill patients. (1)

hospital emergency codes: Signals used in hospitals to alert staff to various emergencies; examples include Code Red (fire) and Code Blue (cardiac arrest). (4)

human reproduction: Process that occurs when the male sex cell and female sex cell unite to create a new human being. (6)

hypertension: A condition in which blood pressure is too high. (11)

hyperventilation: Breathing too quickly. (11)

hypotension: A condition in which blood pressure is too low. (11)

hypothermia: A body temperature below 95°F. (11)

hypothesis: An idea or suggestion often developed to explain something, the cause of which is unknown. (BL4)

hypoventilation: Breathing too slowly. (11)

hypoxia: A lack of adequate oxygen. (11)

I

ideal body weight (IBW): The healthiest weight for an individual; determined primarily by height, but also takes gender, age, build, and muscular development into account, using adjusted statistical tables. (11)

immobility: A condition characterized by a limited, or complete lack of, ability to move. (13)

immunity: Ability to resist pathogens. (6)

incident reports: Forms used in a healthcare facility to document both safety- and non-safety-related events that are not part of a routine operation in the facility. (4)

incurable disease: A disease that cannot be cured or adequately treated. (7)

indirect contact: A type of infection transmission in which the pathogen takes an indirect path—such as through food, air, or clothing—to its next host. (4)

induction: Term that describes reasoning that moves from specific observations to broader generalizations. (BL4)

infant: Term that describes a child from thirty days after birth until the first birthday. (9)

infection control: Term for all efforts made to prevent the spread of infection. (4)

inflammation: A localized reaction in which part of the body becomes reddened, swollen, hot, and often painful, especially as a reaction to injury or infection. (7)

informed consent: A form, given to a patient by a doctor, explaining the benefit and risks of a procedure; the patient accepts the risk by signing the informed consent form. (3)

inhalation: Breathing in; also called *inspiration*. (11)

integrity: The quality of being honest and having strong moral principles. (18)

interjection: A word, phrase, or clause that expresses emotion. (BL1)

Internet: An electronic communications network that connects computer networks and computer facilities around the world. (BL3)

intravenous (IV): Existing or taking place within, or administered into, a vein or veins. (11)

invasion of privacy: Intrusion on another's personal life; applies to personal information as well as a person's body. (3)

isolation rooms: Rooms in a healthcare facility used to prevent the spread of infections, either by containing patients who have contagious diseases or by protecting immune-compromised patients from infectious diseases. (4)

J

job shadowing: A job exploration tool that involves following an employee while he or she completes the tasks of a job you find interesting. (2)

joint: Physical point of connection between two bones; also known as an *articulation*. (6)

K

kinesthetic learner: One who learns through experiencing and doing activities; labs and field trips can be helpful for this learner. (17)

knee-chest position: A position in which a patient rests his or her body weight on the knees and chest. (5)

L

laryngeal mirror: A device used to examine the mouth, tongue, and teeth. (14)

lateral position: A position in which a patient lies on his or her side. (5)

learning styles: Different ways that people learn; three basic types include visual, auditory, and kinesthetic; most people have a mixture of all three. (17)

letter of introduction: A letter written by you to illustrate your personality, passions, and goals for your career. (18)

libel: Damaging someone's good name or reputation in writing. (3)

licensure: Recognition given by a state agency when a person meets the qualifications for a particular occupation; given after the person passes a licensure examination; required to practice. (2)

ligaments: Tough bands of fibrous tissue that connect bone to bone. (6)

lithotomy position: A position in which a patient lies on her back with the feet in stirrups and knees flexed and separated. (5)

lymph: Colorless fluid from the body's tissues that carries white blood cells; collects and transports bacteria to the lymph nodes for destruction; carries fats from the digestive system. (6)

lymphocyte: White blood cell that destroys pathogenic microorganisms. (6)

M

malignant: Term that describes a life-threatening tumor; also known as *cancerous*. (7)

malpractice: Any misconduct or lack of skill that results in patient injury; also known as *professional liability*. (3)

malware: Destructive software used to disrupt computer operation, gather sensitive information, or gain access to a private computer. (BL3)

managed care: A general term for any healthcare plan that emphasizes wellness and provides healthcare through a network of doctors, hospitals, and other healthcare providers. (1)

Maslow's hierarchy of needs: A theory of human needs developed by American psychologist Abraham Maslow. (9)

master's degree: Academic degree awarded by a college or university to those who complete from one to two years (depending on the degree) of prescribed study beyond the bachelor's degree. (2)

material safety data sheet (MSDS): A document containing comprehensive information about a particular chemical used in a healthcare facility; each chemical used has a corresponding MSDS. (4)

mean: The mathematical average of data. (16)

median: The number exactly in the middle of a group of numbers listed in ascending or descending order. (16)

Medicaid: A program jointly funded by state and federal taxes that provides medical aid for low-income individuals of all ages; managed by the states. (1)

medical ethics: Standards concerned with whether a healthcare worker's actions are right or wrong. (3)

medical law: Standards concerned with whether a healthcare worker's actions are legal or illegal. (3)

medical specialties: Specific areas of medicine that are often named according to a body system. (7)

Medicare: A federal health insurance program for persons 65 or older and disabled individuals. (1)

menstrual cycle: The monthly process in which the uterus grows a new lining and then sheds that lining during the menstrual period if a pregnancy does not occur. (6)

metabolism: Term for the chemical processes, occurring within a living organism, that maintain life. (6)

metastasis: The spread of cancerous cells from their place of origin to other parts of the body via the bloodstream. (7)

Methicillin-resistant *Staphylococcus aureus* **(MRSA):** An antibiotic-resistant bacterium responsible for a difficult-to-treat infection; sometimes prevalent in hospitals, prisons, schools, and nursing homes. (4)

metric system of measurement: A system of measurement using units related by factors of ten; measurements are based on the gram, liter, meter, and Celsius degrees. (16)

microscope: An instrument that uses a lens to magnify objects too small to be seen with the naked eye. (1)

mixed numbers: Whole numbers followed by a remaining fraction. (BL2)

mnemonic devices: Learning techniques such as rhymes, catchphrases, and acronyms used to help remember and retain information. (17)

mode: The number that occurs most frequently in a set of numbers. (16)

monogenic disease: A disease that is caused by a flaw in one gene. (7)

morphology: The science or study of the form and structure of organisms. (4)

motivation: A process by which one initiates, guides, and maintains goal-oriented behavior. (17)

multiplication: A mathematical operation that indicates how many times a number is added to itself; a shortcut for addition. (BL2)

multitasking: Performing several jobs at once. (18)

myocardial infarction: Heart attack. (7)

N

National Institutes of Health (NIH): A division of the Department of Health and Human Services that conducts research and provides information to promote and improve public health through 27 different agencies. (1)

necrotic: Term that describes dead cells or tissues. (13)

Needlestick Safety and Prevention Act: A law enacted in 2000 requiring employers to identify, evaluate, and introduce safer medical devices to avoid needlesticks. (4)

needlesticks: Any accidental punctures of the skin by needles; can be dangerous in a healthcare setting because the puncture can cause a potentially serious infection. (4)

negligence: Performing an act that a reasonable person would not have done, or not doing something that a reasonable person would have done in the same or a similar circumstance, resulting in harm to a patient. (3)

neonate: Term that describes a baby from birth to one month. (9)

neoplasm: Tumor; can be either malignant or benign. (7)

networking: The process of developing contacts and relationships with people who are interested in your future employment. (18)

nominal numbers: Numbers that name or identify something. (BL2)

noncommunicable disease: A disease that cannot be passed from one living thing to another, and which is caused by genes, diet, behavior, and other factors. (7)

nonverbal communication: Any form of communication that does not involve speech, including gestures, the way one sits, eye contact (or lack of), and facial expressions; also known as *body language*. (15)

nosocomial infections: Infections acquired in hospitals and other healthcare facilities; also known as *healthcare-acquired infections*. (4)

noun: A word that represents a person, place, or thing. (BL1)

nucleus: The "brain" of a cell; directs all activities and contains genetic information. (6)

O

objective writing: Writing based on evidence you can see and evaluate. (15)

Occupational Safety and Health Administration (OSHA): A government agency that creates regulations to prevent work-related injuries, illnesses, and deaths. (1)

ombudsman: A member of the healthcare team who ensures that patients are not abused and that their legal rights are protected; investigates complaints and advocates for patient rights. (3)

on-hand dose: The amount of medication per capsule or other delivery method. (16)

ophthalmoscope: A lighted medical device used to examine the interior of the eyes. (14)

oral prophylaxis: Term for actions taken to maintain oral health and prevent the spread of disease. (14)

ordinal numbers: Numbers that place objects in a series in order. (BL2)

organs: Two or more groups of tissues working together to perform specific functions. (6)

OSHA Bloodborne Pathogens Standard: Guidelines developed by the Occupational Safety and Health Administration (OSHA) that list potentially infectious materials and mandate all healthcare workers to proceed at all times as if the materials are infectious. (4)

OSHA Hazard Communication Standard: Rules established by the Occupational Safety and Health Administration (OSHA) that require employers to educate employees about chemical hazards in the workplace. (4)

otoscope: A lighted medical device used to examine the ear and eardrum. (14)

P

palliative care: Term for measures taken to treat symptoms and pain even though the treatment will not cure a disease; use of comfort measures. (9)

paragraph: Part of a written composition; consists of a collection of sentences related to one topic. (BL1)

parasites: Organisms that live in or on another organism. (4)

parts of speech: Collective term for eight classifications of words that denote each word's function; in English these include noun, pronoun, verb, adjective, adverb, conjunction, preposition, and interjection. (BL1)

pathogens: Disease-producing microorganisms. (1)

patience: A skill that will help you interact calmly with coworkers and patients. (18)

Patient Self-Determination Act: A law passed by the US Congress in 1990 that requires most healthcare institutions to inform a patient about his or her rights at the time of admission. (3)

Patients' Bill of Rights: Summary of a patient's rights regarding fair treatment and appropriate information. (3)

percentage: An amount per one hundred. (16)

peripheral nervous system (PNS): Collective term for nerves that lie outside the central nervous system; transmits information from the CNS to all parts of the body. (6)

personal protective equipment (PPE): Equipment worn by workers to protect them from serious workplace injuries or illnesses. (4)

petit mal seizure: A generalized seizure in which the person has impaired awareness and responsiveness, and may lose consciousness. (12)

pH scale: System for measuring a substance's acidity or alkalinity; ranges from 0 to 14. (6)

phagocytosis: Process in which white blood cells surround, ingest, and destroy a foreign invader. (6)

physiology: The study of the function of the body. (6)

plaque: A sticky substance found on teeth. (14)

plasma: The liquid component of blood. (6)

platelets: Part of the formed elements; play an important role in blood clotting; also called *thrombocytes*. (6)

podcasts: Multimedia files that are downloaded and played on a computer, tablet, or smartphone. (BL3)

post-traumatic stress disorder (PTSD): An anxiety disorder that may develop after exposure to a terrifying event or ordeal in which severe physical harm occurred or was threatened. (7)

posture: Position of the body when sitting or standing. (13)

potentially infectious materials (PIM): Substances designated by OSHA that require healthcare workers to proceed as if they are infectious. (4)

preferred provider organizations (PPO): Health insurance organizations that contract with a network of preferred providers from which the policyholder can choose; often involves an annual deductible payment for service, but patients do not have a designated primary care physician and may self-refer to specialists. (1)

prefix: The part of a word that comes before the word root; changes the meaning of the word root. (5)

premium: The amount an insured person pays to his or her insurance company to maintain coverage. (1)

prenatal: The life stage before birth; during or relating to pregnancy. (9)

preposition: A word that connects or relates its object to the rest of the sentence. (BL1)

preschoolers: Term that describes children between the ages of three and five. (9)

preteens: Term that describes children between the ages of 10 and 12. (9)

prime number: A number that is only divisible by itself and 1. (BL2)

prioritizing: The act of making decisions about the best order in which to perform multiple tasks so the most important tasks are completed first. (18)

probe: A long, thin medical instrument with a blunt end used for exploration into body cavities. (11)

professionalism: The conduct or attitude that is required to be the best employee that you can be; the act of contributing positively to an organization. (18)

prone position: A position in which a patient lies facedown. (5)

pronoun: A word that can be substituted for a noun. (BL1)

proportion: A statement of the equality of two ratios. (16)

prosthesis: An artificial device that replaces a missing part of the body such as a limb. (10)

proteomics: Field of biotechnology concerned with analyzing the structure, function, and interactions of the proteins produced by the genes of a particular cell, tissue, or organism. (7)

protozoa: Microorganisms that depend on a host cell to survive and replicate; can cause serious illness. (4)

proxemics: The study of humans' use of space; includes physical territory and personal territory. (15)

psychoanalysis: A method of analyzing and treating mental and emotional disorders through sessions in which the patient is encouraged to talk about personal experience and dreams. (1)

puberty: A stage of life beginning between the ages of 8 and 14; indicates sexual reproduction is possible. (6)

pulse oximeter: A medical device usually applied to the fingertip to indirectly measure the amount of oxygen saturation in the blood. (11)

punctuality: The ability to be on time for work, appointments, and any other commitments. (18)

punctuation: The practice or system of using certain conventional marks or characters such as commas, question marks, and periods in writing. (BL1)

Q

quality improvement (QI): Term for policies that motivate or require healthcare facilities to monitor and evaluate their services based on predetermined criteria for the purpose of improving those services. (4)

quarantine: The process of isolating people who have been exposed to infectious or contagious disease. (1)

R

radial pulse: The pulse located on the thumb side of the wrist. (11)

ratio: A mathematical expression that compares one quantity with another, similar quantity. (16)

reasonable care: Legal protection for the healthcare worker if proven that the worker acted reasonably as compared to other members of the profession in the same or a similar situation. (3)

red blood cells: Part of the formed elements; contain hemoglobin, which carries oxygen and carbon dioxide to and from the body's cells; also called *erythrocytes*. (6)

respiration: The act of supplying oxygen to the cells and removing carbon dioxide; also called *breathing*. (6)

résumé: A document that summarizes your education, work experiences, and other qualifications for employment; can be printed or submitted electronically. (18)

retention: The ability to remember information. (17)

rickettsiae: Parasites that normally choose fleas, lice, ticks, or mites as their host organisms; can cause severe infections. (4)

Roman numerals: Letters used by the ancient Romans to represent numbers. (16)

rooting reflex: The natural inclination of newborns to turn their head toward a food source when the side of their mouth is stroked. (9)

rule of nines: A method of calculating the surface area of the body that has been affected by burns. (12)

S

sanitization: The use of antimicrobial agents on objects, surfaces, or living tissue to reduce the number of disease-causing microorganisms. (4)

science: A system of acquiring knowledge through observation and experimentation to describe the natural world. (BL4)

scientific method: A method designed to logically formulate, test, and evaluate a problem or hypothesis. (BL4)

scope of practice: Tasks that an employee is legally allowed to perform based on his or her training and certification. (3)

self-advocacy: Refers to an individual's ability to effectively communicate, convey, negotiate, or assert his or her own interests, desires, needs, and rights. (1)

self-esteem: The personal level of satisfaction about oneself and one's abilities. (8)

semi-Fowler's position: A position in which the a patient lies in bed with the head of the bed elevated at 30°. (5)

sender-receiver communication model: A model designed to describe communication between two people. (15)

sexual harassment: Unwanted sexual advances and other forms of offensive sexual behavior; both men and women can be sexually harassed. (3)

sexually transmitted infection (STI): An infection transferred from one person to another through sexual contact. (6)

sharps: Needles or any other objects that could puncture or cut the skin. (4)

shock: A condition in which the body experiences a lack of sufficient oxygen available to the organs and tissues. (12)

simple sentence: A sentence that contains a subject and a verb, and which expresses a complete thought; independent clause. (BL1)

Sims' position: A position in which a patient lies on his or her left side, with the right leg drawn up high and forward, the left arm along the back, and the chest forward resting on the bed. (5)

slander: Saying something that damages someone's good name or reputation. (3)

soft skills: Personal characteristics that enable a person to have pleasant, effective interactions with others. (18)

software: Programs that allow a user to interact with a computer; computer programs; in contrast to hardware. (BL3)

speculum: A medical device designed to enter a body opening such as the vagina, rectum, or nose, making those areas visible for an examination. (14)

sphygmomanometer: A specialized manual or digital medical device used to measure blood pressure; also called a *vital sign machine*. (11)

spreadsheet: A document containing rows and columns of data; useful for organizing numeric values and performing computer calculations. (16)

standard of care: Reasonable and prudent care that a practitioner of similar qualifications would have performed in the same or similar situation. (3)

standard precautions: A set of basic practices intended to prevent transmission of infectious diseases from one person to another. (4)

startle reflex: The natural inclination of a baby's limb and neck muscles to contract in response to a loud noise or jolt. (9)

statute of limitations: The amount of time during which any legal action may be taken; after such time a lawsuit may not be filed (3)

stem cells: Cells in the body that evolve into specific cells in a particular organ system. (6)

stereotype: An impression that is formed from a small amount of information or one example, assuming that the information or example represents a whole person, group of people, or situation. (15)

sterilization: The act of killing all microorganisms and their spores on a surface; methods of sterilization in a healthcare facility may include hot pressurized steam, dry heat, and gas. (4)

stertorous breathing: Breathing that sounds like snoring. (11)

stethoscope: A medical device used to listen to body sounds such as breathing, heartbeats, and lung and bowel sounds; composed of two earpieces connected by flexible tubing with a diaphragm at its end. (11)

stress: The body's physical, mental, and emotional response to change, trauma, or challenging situations. (8)

stroke: A medical emergency in which blood flow to a part of the brain is cut off. (7)

subjective writing: Writing based on evidence you cannot evaluate. (15)

substance abuse: The use of drugs or alcohol, or a misuse of prescription medication. (8)

subtraction: The process of removing one number from another number; the opposite of addition. (BL2)

sudden infant death syndrome (SIDS): Unexpected death that occurs for unknown reasons during the first few months of a baby's life. (9)

suffix: The part of a word that is added after the word root to change its meaning. (5)

suicide: Intentionally ending one's life. (8)

suicide cluster: Multiple suicides that occur within a community during a relatively short period of time. (8)

suicide contagion: Term for the copying of suicide attempts after hearing about another person's suicide. (8)

supine position: A position in which a patient lies faceup. (5)

support services: A sector of a healthcare facility that plays a critical role in providing a clean, safe environment for all who enter a healthcare facility. (2)

syncope: Fainting. (12)

syndrome: A group of symptoms that together indicate a disease. (7)

systolic pressure: Part of a blood pressure reading that is taken when the heart muscle contracts and pushes blood through the artery. (11)

T

tachycardia: A fast pulse of over 100 beats per minute. (11)

tachypnea: Rapid, shallow breathing due to the lungs only partially filling. (11)

tact: The ability to avoid giving offense through your words and actions. (18)

telemedicine: A field of medicine in which communication and information technologies are used to provide patients with medical care at remote locations. (10)

temporal artery temperature: Temperature taken on either side of the head, where the temporal arteries are located. (11)

tendons: Fibrous tissues that connect muscles to bone. (6)

terminal disease: A disease that eventually ends in death. (7)

therapeutic services: Career path that offers hands-on experience with patients and focuses on changing the health status of a patient over time. (2)

thesaurus: A resource that identifies synonyms, or words with the same meanings. (17)

thrombus: A blood clot that forms in a blood vessel and remains at the site of formation. (13)

time management: The process of planning and controlling the amount of time spent on specific activities to increase efficiency and productivity. (17)

tissues: Groups of cells that work together to accomplish a task. (6)

toddlers: Term that describes children between the ages of one and three. (9)

traction: The use of a pulling force to treat muscle and skeletal disorders. (13)

trade name: The name assigned to a drug by its manufacturer. (16)

Trendelenburg position: A position in which a patient lies flat on his or her back with the head of the table lowered at a 45° angle. (5)

trochanter roll: A rolled towel or blanket placed along the hip that prevents the hips from rotating externally. (13)

tympanic temperature: Temperature taken in the ear. (11)

U

United States Public Health Service: Federal agency that dates back to the late 1700s whose mission is to promote public health. (1)

upload: Transmission of a file from a computer or other electronic device to a central server. (BL3)

V

vaccination: The use of medicines that contain weakened or dead bacteria or viruses to build immunity and prevent disease. (1)

values: The concepts, ideas, and beliefs that are important and meaningful to a person. (3)

vectors: Carriers—such as insects, rodents, or other small animals—that spread pathogens from host to host. (4)

verb: Any word that describes an action or a state of being. (BL1)

verbal communication: Expressing your thoughts out loud; also known as *speaking*. (15)

virtual learning environment (VLE): An online learning system that brings classroom materials to students via the Internet. (BL3)

viruses: Pathogenic microorganisms, much smaller than bacteria, that depend on a living cell to survive; cause many serious diseases and illnesses. (4)

visual learner: One who learns through seeing visual representations of ideas and concepts; charts, color-coded notes, and videos can be helpful tools for this learner. (17)

vocabulary: A set of words known and used by a person. (17)

vowels: Five letters in the English language: *a, e, i, o,* and *u* (sometimes *y* is substituted for *i*). (BL1)

W

white blood cells: Part of the formed elements; fight infection in the body; also called *leukocytes*. (6)

whole numbers: Numbers used for counting; do not contain decimal points or fractions; also known as *integers*. (BL2)

Wi-Fi: Technology that enables electronic devices to exchange data wirelessly over a computer network; also known as *wireless fidelity*. (BL3)

word elements: Parts that are used to form medical terms; include the word root, prefix, suffix, combining vowel, and combining form (word root plus combining vowel). (5)

word processing: Software that allows the user to enter, edit, save, and print text through a computer. (BL3)

word root: The body or the main element of a word. (5)

worker's compensation: A form of government insurance that provides wage replacement and medical benefits for employees injured at work. (1)

World Health Organization (WHO): An agency of the United Nations that is concerned with international public health. (1)

World Wide Web: A means of accessing the Internet by using an HTTP web address. (BL3)

Index

D

E

F